HEAD AND NECK PATHOLOGY

Other books in this series:

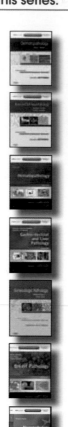

Busam: *Dermatopathology*,
978-0-443-06654-2

Folpe & Inwards: *Bone and Soft Tissue Pathology*,
978-0-443-06688-7

Hsi: *Hematopathology*, 2e
978-1-4377-2606-0

Iacobuzio-Donahue & Montgomery: *Gastrointestinal and Liver Pathology*, 2e,
978-1-4377-0925-4

Nucci & Oliva: *Gynecologic Pathology*,
978-0-443-06920-8

O'Malley & Pinder: *Breast Pathology*, 2e,
978-1-4377-1750-0

Prayson: *Neuropathology*, 2e,
978-1-4377-0949-0

Sidawy & Ali: *Fine Needle Aspiration Cytology*,
978-0-443-06731-0

Tubbs & Stoler: *Cell and Tissue Based Molecular Pathology*,
978-1-4377-1948-2

Zander & Farver: *Pulmonary Pathology*,
978-0-443-06741-9

Zhou & Magi-Galluzzi: *Genitourinary Pathology*,
978-0-443-06677-1

122.00

122.00

HEAD AND NECK PATHOLOGY

A Volume in the Series
FOUNDATIONS IN DIAGNOSTIC PATHOLOGY
SECOND EDITION

EDITED BY
Lester D. R. Thompson, MD
Consultant Pathologist
Department of Pathology
Southern California Permanente Medical Group
Woodland Hills Medical Center
Woodland Hills, California

SERIES EDITOR
John R. Goldblum, MD, FCAP, FASCP, FACG
Chairman, Department of Anatomic Pathology
The Cleveland Clinic Foundation
Cleveland Clinic Lerner College of Medicine
Case Western Reserve University
Cleveland, Ohio

ELSEVIER
SAUNDERS

ELSEVIER
SAUNDERS

1600 John F. Kennedy Blvd.
Ste 1800
Philadelphia, PA 19103-2899

HEAD AND NECK PATHOLOGY, SECOND EDITION   ISBN: 978-1-4377-2607-7
(A VOLUME IN THE FOUNDATIONS IN DIAGNOSTIC PATHOLOGY SERIES)

Notices

Knowledge and best practice in this field are constantly changing. As new research and experience broaden our understanding, changes in research methods, professional practices, or medical treatment may become necessary.

Practitioners and researchers must always rely on their own experience and knowledge in evaluating and using any information, methods, compounds, or experiments described herein. In using such information or methods they should be mindful of their own safety and the safety of others, including parties for whom they have a professional responsibility.

With respect to any drug or pharmaceutical products identified, readers are advised to check the most current information provided (i) on procedures featured or (ii) by the manufacturer of each product to be administered, to verify the recommended dose or formula, the method and duration of administration, and contraindications. It is the responsibility of practitioners, relying on their own experience and knowledge of their patients, to make diagnoses, to determine dosages and the best treatment for each individual patient, and to take all appropriate safety precautions.

To the fullest extent of the law, neither the Publisher nor the authors, contributors, or editors assume any liability for any injury and/or damage to persons or property as a matter of products liability, negligence or otherwise, or from any use or operation of any methods, products, instructions, or ideas contained in the material herein.

Library of Congress Cataloging-in-Publication Data
Head and neck pathology / edited by Lester D.R. Thompson.—2nd ed.
    p. ; cm. — (Foundations in diagnostic pathology)
  Includes bibliographical references and index.
  ISBN 978-1-4377-2607-7 (hardcover : alk. paper)
  I. Thompson, Lester D. R. II. Series: Foundations in diagnostic pathology.
  [DNLM: 1. Head and Neck Neoplasms. 2. Head—pathology. 3. Neck—pathology. WE 707]
  616.99'491—dc23
                                                  2012008543

Executive Content Strategist: William Schmitt
Senior Content Development Specialist: Kathryn DeFrancesco
Publishing Services Manager: Patricia Tannian
Senior Project Manager: Kristine Fecherty
Design Direction: Lou Forgione

Printed in China

Last digit is the print number: 9 8 7 6 5 4 3 2 1

To Friends who make me laugh and cry,
to Family who make me what I am,
and to Pam, whose love is unconditional

Contributors

Carol F. Adair, MD
Staff Pathologist
Department of Anatomic Pathology
Baylor University Medical Center
Dallas, Texas

Walter C. Bell, MD
Associate Professor
Department of Pathology
University of Alabama at Birmingham
Birmingham, Alabama

Margaret Brandwein-Gensler, MD
Professor
Head, Surgical Pathology Section
Division of Anatomic Pathology
Department of Pathology
University of Alabama at Birmingham
Birmingham, Alabama

John W. Eveson, PhD, FRCPath
Emeritus Professor
Department of Head and Neck Pathology
School of Oral and Dental Science
University of Bristol
Bristol, United Kingdom

Uta Flucke, MD
Pathologist
Department of Pathology
Radboud University Nijmegen Medical Centre
Nijmegen, The Netherlands

Nina Gale, MD
Professor
Institute of Pathology
Faculty of Medicine
University of Ljubljana
Ljubljana, Slovenia

Francis H. Gannon, MD
Professor
Departments of Pathology and Immunology
    and Orthopedic Surgery;
Director
Residency and Fellowship Programs
Department of Pathology and Immunology
Baylor College of Medicine
Houston, Texas

Jennifer L. Hunt, MD, MEd
Aubrey J. Hough, Jr., MD Endowed Professor and Chair
Department of Pathology and Laboratory Medicine
University of Arkansas for Medical Sciences
Little Rock, Arkansas

James S. Lewis, Jr., MD
Associate Professor
Department of Pathology and Immunology
Department of Otolaryngology Head and Neck Surgery
Washington University in St. Louis
St. Louis, Missouri

Susan Müller, DMD, MS
Professor
Department of Pathology and Laboratory Medicine
Department of Otolaryngology Head and Neck Surgery
Winship Cancer Institute
Emory University School of Medicine
Atlanta, Georgia

Brenda L. Nelson, DDS, MS
Head
Department of Anatomic Pathology
Naval Medical Center San Diego
San Diego, California

Mary S. Richardson, DDS, MD
Professor
Director of Surgical Pathology
Department of Pathology and Laboratory Medicine
Medical University of South Carolina
Charleston, South Carolina

Pieter J. Slootweg, DMD, MD, PhD
Professor
Department of Pathology
Radboud University Nijmegen Medical Centre
Nijmegen, The Netherlands

Lester D. R. Thompson, MD
Consultant Pathologist
Department of Pathology
Southern California Permanente Medical Group
Woodland Hills Medical Center
Woodland Hills, California

Kevin R. Torske, DDS, MS
Chairman and Program Director
Department of Oral and Maxillofacial Pathology
Naval Postgraduate Dental School
Bethesda, Maryland

Foreword

The study and practice of anatomic pathology are both exciting and overwhelming. Surgical pathology, with all of the subspecialties it encompasses, and cytopathology have become increasingly complex and sophisticated, and it is not possible for any individual to master the skills and knowledge required to perform all of these tasks at the highest level. Simply being able to make a correct diagnosis is challenging enough, but the standard of care has far surpassed merely providing a diagnosis. Pathologists are now asked to provide large amounts of ancillary information, both diagnostic and prognostic, often on small amounts of tissue, a task that can be daunting even to the most experienced pathologist.

Although large general surgical pathology textbooks are useful resources, they by necessity could not possibly cover many of the aspects that pathologists need to know and include in their reports. As such, the concept behind Foundations in Diagnostic Pathology was born. This series is designed to cover the major areas of surgical and cytopathology, and each edition is focused on one major topic. The goal of every book in this series is to provide the essential information that any pathologist, whether general or subspecialized, in training or in practice, would find useful in the evaluation of virtually any type of specimen encountered.

Dr. Lester Thompson, a renowned and prolific head and neck and endocrine pathologist, formerly of the Armed Forces Institute of Pathology and currently with the Southern California Permanente Medical Group, Woodland Hills, California, has edited an outstanding, state-of-the-art book on the essentials of head and neck and endocrine pathology. In the first editions of this series, these topics were separated into two separate editions. However, given the significant overlap in content, the decision was made to combine these topics into one comprehensive edition. This area is one of those topics in surgical pathology that virtually every surgical pathologist encounters with great frequency, but in fact, few actually have formal training in this area. As such, a comprehensive reference such as this has great practical value in the day-to-day practice of any surgical pathologist. The list of contributors includes some of the most renowned pathologists in this field, all of whom have significant expertise as practicing pathologists, researchers, and renowned educators. Each chapter is organized in an easy-to-follow manner, the writing is concise, tables are practical and easy to reference, and the photomicrographs are of incredibly high quality. There are thorough discussions pertaining to the handling of biopsy and resection specimens, as well as frozen sections, which can be notoriously challenging in this area.

The book is organized into 28 chapters, including separate chapters that provide thorough overviews of non-neoplastic, benign, and malignant neoplasms of the larynx, hypopharynx, trachea, nasal cavity, nasopharynx, paranasal sinuses, oral cavity, oropharynx, salivary glands, ear, temporal bone, gnathic bones, and the neck. Similarly, chapters describing the non-neoplastic benign and malignant neoplasms of the thyroid gland, parathyroid gland, and paraganglia system are included.

I am truly grateful to Dr. Thompson and all of the contributors who put forth a tremendous effort to allow this book to come to fruition. It is an outstanding addition to the Foundations in Diagnostic Pathology series, and I sincerely hope you enjoy this comprehensive volume and find it to be useful in your everyday practice.

John R. Goldblum, MD

Preface

It is staggering and startling to contemplate the extreme increase in knowledge over the past few years. Amazing discoveries about disease etiology, diagnosis, and treatment have become available. Anybody can access these findings easily by starting a computer and putting in a few simple words into a search engine. This exponential expansion in knowledge must, however, be tempered with wisdom. Wisdom encompasses perspicacity, with the necessary sophistication to separate the wheat from the chaff, distilling the information evaluated into a balanced and useful piece of information. This ability is central to being an effective and exceptional pathologist.

This edition of the book presents information in a highly templated format, which will allow the discerning pathologist the ability to reach the correct diagnosis in selected disorders of the larynx, sinonasal tract, ear and temporal bone, salivary gland, oral, gnathic, and neck regions. With the constraints of page number and the limits of book bindings, it is impossible to present all of the current concepts of disorders of the Head and Neck and Endocrine organs. However, it is hoped that the major disorders herein presented will provide sufficient information for busy surgical pathologists to make appropriate diagnoses in their daily work. It is my goal for the pathologist to distill pertinent clinical, imaging, laboratory, macroscopic, microscopic, histochemical, immunohistochemical, ultrastructural, and molecular results into a comprehensive diagnosis, which will result in superior patient management.

Lester D. R. Thompson, MD

Acknowledgments

Every Wednesday morning for the past 15 years, I have prayed with Dr. Francis H. Gannon, even though we may be anywhere in the world. This time is devoted to praying for those with whom we work, for family and friends, and for patients. It is a time for gaining perspective, developing understanding, seeing things from a different viewpoint, and always providing a sense of balance, calmness, and peace. It is a great way to start the day, knowing that no matter what may happen, things will turn out for the best in the long run. As I think of all of the people over the years for whom we have prayed, many in that list are to be thanked for how they have influenced and helped me in my undertakings. Although I cannot possibly ever give credit to all as I should, I have instead focused on just a few who have been the most influential:

Drs. Elisabeth and Douglas Wear, for their commitment to me in college, financial support in medical school, and influence to become a pathologist.

Drs. Reesa and Donald Chase, who provided a fun way to learn pathology during medical school at Loma Linda.

Dr. Yao-Shi Fu, for his early and persistent attempts to get me into head and neck pathology while a resident at University of California, Los Angeles.

Dr. Dorothy Rosenthal, for her unique way of blending so many parts of pathology into a meaningful whole.

Dr. Sunita Bhuta, for her steadfast support and commitment to seeing me become an excellent diagnostician, while also writing concise reports that people understood.

Dr. Clara Heffess, who taught me everything I know about endocrine pathology, while still remaining a friend and surrogate mother.

Dr. Dennis Heffner, whose ability to expound on the esoterica of pathology while still understanding its practical points, allowed me to blossom at the Armed Forces Institute of Pathology.

Dr. Bruce Wenig, for always encouraging another publication, another project, and another lecture.

My parents, Dr. and Mrs. Ronald Thompson, who instilled in me a work ethic bar none, a curiosity that will never kill a cat, and a kindness that puts all into perspective.

My brother, Dr. Glynn M. Thompson, who has always been the "wind beneath my wings," allowing me to enjoy the spotlight when he should have.

And for my wife, Pamela A. Thompson-Thompson. The enormous sacrifices she has endured to see me achieve professional success cannot be overemphasized. There are so many countless days, nights, weekends, and holidays that have been spent with me "worshipping" the computer, while she has waited patiently for me to finish just "one more project." This type of Agape love is unique and so treasured. She makes life worth living.

So many gave professional assistance at Elsevier, but I would like to specifically thank Kathryn DeFrancesco and Kristine Feeherty for their constant editorial assistance and guidance, and William R. Schmitt for his immediate replies to whatever the query!

Although axiomatic, the responsibility for any errors, omissions, or deviation from current orthodoxy is mine alone!

Lester D. R. Thompson, MD

Contents

HEAD AND NECK PATHOLOGY

Non-Neoplastic Lesions of the Nasal Cavity, Paranasal Sinuses, and Nasopharynx

■ **Margaret Brandwein-Gensler** ■ **Walter C. Bell**

■ RHINOSINUSITIS

CLINICAL FEATURES

RHINOSINUSITIS—DISEASE FACT SHEET

Definition
- Sinonasal inflammation secondary to multiple possible etiologic factors

Incidence and Location
- Common
- Involves the mucosa of the nasal passages and paranasal sinuses

Morbidity and Mortality
- May result in secondary polyps, sinus obstruction, mucocele formation, and extension of infection into orbital soft tissues or meninges

Gender and Age Distribution
- Equal gender distribution
- Age dependent on underlying etiology

Clinical Features
- Nasal congestion and drainage
- May be associated with sneezing and itching
- Headache, tenderness over sinuses
- Fever with bacterial etiology
- Otitis media

Radiographic Findings
- Mucosal thickening
- Air-fluid levels with acute bacterial sinusitis

Prognosis and Treatment
- Excellent prognosis with appropriate antimicrobial therapy for bacterial sinusitis and endoscopic sinus surgery to correct structural impairment

---

Rhinosinusitis is a common inflammatory disorder involving the nasal cavity and paranasal sinuses. Symptoms vary according to the underlying etiology, but in all forms, there is mucin hypersecretion leading to nasal stuffiness and discharge.

Acute rhinosinusitis is typically caused by viral and bacterial infections. A number of different upper respiratory viral infections can lead to "the common cold," most often rhinoviruses, parainfluenza viruses, influenza viruses, adenoviruses, and respiratory syncytial viruses. Bacterial sinusitis often occurs as a superimposed infection secondary to severe viral upper respiratory infections. It may also develop secondary to an anatomic structural abnormality preventing appropriate aeration. Bacterial sinusitis causes mucopurulent discharge, headache, fever, and pain over the involved sinuses.

Imaging studies show sinus opacification or air-fluid levels. In nonimmunocompromised individuals, acute bacterial sinusitis is usually caused by *Streptococcus pneumoniae* or *Haemophilus influenzae,* transmitted via ororespiratory droplets. However, with the introduction of the seven-valent pneumococcal vaccine in children, there has been a shift in the causative agents for acute sinusitis for both children and adults. Brooks and colleagues demonstrated decreasing incidence of *S. pneumoniae* and increasing incidence of *H. influenzae.* Bacterial sinusitis in patients with AIDS is usually caused by *Pseudomonas aeruginosa* or *Staphylococcus aureus.* If not appropriately treated, bacterial sinusitis may progress to involve surrounding tissues with serious consequences, such as orbital cellulitis, meningitis, intracranial abscess formation, or cavernous sinus thrombosis.

Chronic sinusitis is defined as a symptomatic sinusitis lasting longer than 12 weeks. It is most often caused by allergies or may be caused by structural alterations leading to impaired sinus aeration or drainage. An association with environmental irritants, such as second-hand smoke, has also been demonstrated. Allergic rhinosinusitis is common, affecting 10% to 30% of adults worldwide. It is a type I hypersensitivity, immunoglobulin E (IgE) mediated response, most commonly to pollens, animal dander, dust mites, or molds. Exposure to these agents causes nasal congestion, rhinorrhea, sneezing, and itching. When an allergic etiology is suspected, skin testing may be appropriate to confirm the diagnosis and to identify the offending allergen.

Acute exacerbation of chronic sinusitis is often associated with anaerobic bacterial infections such as

Peptostreptococcus sp., *Fusobacterium* sp., and *Propionibacterium acnes*. Chronic sinusitis may be complicated by the development of sinonasal polyps (discussed later in this chapter), which can lead to further impairment of sinus aeration and drainage. Mucosal edema may lead to obstruction of the sinus osteum and development of an obstructive mucocele. Collected secretions cause expansion of the sinus resulting in sinus pain, and may even cause bone remodeling and skull deformity. Secondary bacterial infections in this setting result in development of a mucopyocele.

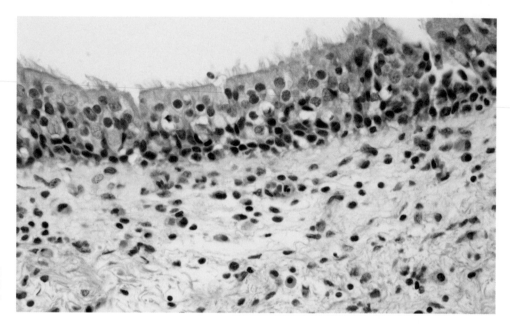

FIGURE 1-1

Sinusitis. Respiratory mucosa with a mixed chronic inflammatory infiltrate composed predominantly of lymphocytes and plasma cells.

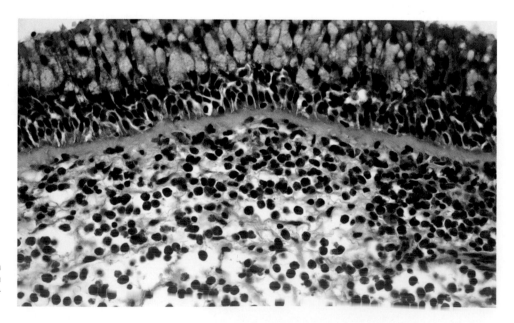

FIGURE 1-2

Allergic sinusitis. Respiratory mucosa with a prominent eosinophilic infiltrate and a thickened basement membrane, suggestive of an allergic etiology.

PATHOLOGIC FEATURES

GROSS FINDINGS

Gross specimens from endoscopic sinus surgery typically consist of fragments of bone and sinus mucosa. Gross changes are typically minimal with thickening of the mucosa due to edema. A purulent exudate may be seen in cases of bacterial infection. Polyps may be present, which appear glistening and transparent.

MICROSCOPIC FINDINGS

In general, specimens from patients with chronic sinusitis show mucosal edema with a mixed inflammatory infiltrate, typically consisting of mature lymphocytes admixed with plasma cells, eosinophils, neutrophils, and macrophages (Figure 1-1). The surface epithelium often exhibits squamous metaplasia. Thickening of the basement membrane is common in chronic sinusitis and is seen even after resolution of the process. In allergic rhinosinusitis, the inflammatory infiltrate is dominated by eosinophils (Figure 1-2). Acute bacterial sinusitis will demonstrate increased numbers of neutrophils.

DIFFERENTIAL DIAGNOSIS

The clinical differential diagnosis of chronic sinusitis includes systemic diseases such as Wegener granulomatosis and Churg-Strauss syndrome (both discussed later). Briefly, Wegener is characterized by the classic triad of vasculitis, granulomatous inflammation, and aseptic necrosis. Similarly, Churg-Strauss shows vasculitis and granulomatous inflammation but is notable for

its marked eosinophilia. Although necrosis may be seen in acute rhinosinusitis, it is typically associated with abundant neutrophils and does not have the typical geographic, granular character of the necrosis in Wegener. Moreover, granulomas and vasculitis are not expected as a usual feature in rhinosinusitis, although granulomas could be present in association with sarcoidosis or with mycobacterial infections. Nonetheless, if the diagnosis of Wegener or Churg-Strauss is under consideration, then cytoplasmic antineutrophil cytoplasmic antibody (c-ANCA) studies may be helpful (although not to differentiate between the two). In younger patients with recurrent sinusitis, the diagnoses of immotile cilia syndrome and Kartagener syndrome (immotile cilia, bronchiectasis, and situs inversus) require consideration. Ultrastructural examination of shed respiratory cells is useful in confirming abnormal cilia morphology. Brush biopsy samples submitted in gluteraldehyde can be used for visualizing the ultrastructure of ciliated cells.

PROGNOSIS AND THERAPY

The treatment of acute sinusitis should involve eradication of the causative bacteria and improvement of sinus drainage and aeration. Sinus puncture and irrigation allow for specimen collection for bacterial culture, and thus the initiation of directed antimicrobial therapy. It also relieves symptoms due to sinus pressure. Endoscopic sinus surgery can address anatomic causes of impaired drainage. Topical sprays and oral vasoconstrictors can be used to reduce edema and further aid sinus drainage. Amoxicillin, clarithromycin, and azithromycin are the recommended first-line antimicrobials to cover *S. pneumoniae, H. influenzae, Moraxella catarrhalis*, and anaerobic bacteria.

Chronic sinusitis requires at least 3 to 4 weeks of antimicrobial therapy, ideally guided by culture results. Amoxicillin-clavulanate, second-generation cephalosporins, and erythromycin-sulfisoxazole are recommended first-line antibiotics. Other individualized supportive therapies include steroids, decongestants, nasal irrigations, mucolytic agents, antihistamines, and antiallergic immune therapies. Patients should be supported with smoking cessation programs. Patients who are refractory to medical therapy or have evidence of anatomic obstruction may undergo (endoscopic) sinus surgery.

RHINOSINUSITIS—PATHOLOGIC FEATURES

Gross Findings

- Fragments of bone and sinus mucosa, possibly with edema
- Polyps may be present, glistening and transparent

Microscopic Findings

- Mucosal edema with mixed inflammatory infiltrate
- Eosinophils may be prominent
- Squamous metaplasia of the surface epithelium
- Thickened basement membrane

Pathologic Differential Diagnosis

- Wegener granulomatosis, Churg-Strauss syndrome, immotile cilia syndrome (in young patients)

■ SINONASAL POLYPS

Sinonasal polyps have a multitude of etiologies: allergy, vasomotor rhinitis, infectious rhinosinusitis, diabetes mellitus, cystic fibrosis, aspirin intolerance, and nickel exposure. However, they are most frequently caused by repeated bouts of sinusitis. Sinonasal polyps are the result of an influx of fluids into the lamina propria of the Schneiderian mucosa. Occasionally, antral (maxillary) polyps may expand and prolapse through sinus ostia, presenting as intranasal or nasopharyngeal masses. These are referred to as antrochoanal polyps and represent 4% to 6% of all sinonasal polyps. Angiomatous polyps are traumatized, vascularized nasal choanal polyps often associated with fibrosis.

CLINICAL FEATURES

About 20% of patients with nasal polyps have asthma, and conversely about 30% of asthmatic patients have polyps. These patients will often present with rhinorrhea, stuffiness, nasal discharge, headaches, sinusitis, and other nonspecific sinonasal symptoms. Nasal polyps may be also associated with aspirin intolerance and bronchial asthma (Samter triad). Between 10% and 20% of children with cystic fibrosis have nasal polyps. Generally, nasal polyps in children are uncommon, and 29% of such polyps in children are associated with cystic fibrosis.

RADIOLOGIC FINDINGS

Sinonasal polyps may appear as single or multiple expansile masses within the nasal cavity and/or paranasal sinuses (Figure 1-3). One can also see mucus retention and/or thickened mucosa within the affected sinus. If the ethmoid complex is involved, it appears widened; however, the delicate ethmoid septae remain intact. In contrast, a solid tumor—either benign or malignant—will destroy the ethmoid septae. Angiomatous polyps usually are present in the nasal cavity. On angiography, these polyps have only a few demonstrable feeding vessels compared with the rich vascular supply of a nasopharyngeal angiofibroma.

PATHOLOGIC FINDINGS

GROSS FINDINGS

Sinonasal polyps are usually smooth, glistening and translucent, and gray/pink in color (Figure 1-4). Antrochoanal polyps are firmer and not translucent. Angiomatous polyps have a similar appearance but may appear erythematous due to increased vascularization.

MICROSCOPIC FINDINGS

Typical sinonasal polyps contain a moderate degree of chronic inflammation within an expanded lamina propria (Figure 1-5). The mucoserous glands are present and may demonstrate goblet cell hyperplasia (Figure 1-6). If the polyps are allergic in nature,

SINONASAL POLYPS—DISEASE FACT SHEET

Definition
- Multifactorial etiologies, resulting in expansion of the lamina propria by fluids, protein, and fibrosis

Incidence and Location
- Common
- Nasal cavity, paranasal sinuses (maxilla and ethmoids)

Morbidity and Mortality
- Bone remodeling may lead to facial asymmetry

Gender and Age Distribution
- Equal gender distribution
- Wide age distribution, but uncommon in children (raises the possibility of cystic fibrosis if in a child)

Clinical Features
- Rhinorrhea, nasal stuffiness, obstruction, and, rarely, anosmia
- Chronic headache
- Etiologies are legion but include allergy, infection, diabetes, aspirin sensitivity, asthma, cystic fibrosis, nickel exposure

Prognosis and Treatment
- Prognosis is excellent, although management of underlying etiology is considered best treatment
- Conservative endoscopic removal and improved sinus ventilation

SINONASAL POLYPS—PATHOLOGIC FEATURES

Gross Findings
- Smooth, glistening, gelatinous, translucent
- Antrochoanal polyp has a narrow stalk, firm, nontranslucent

Microscopic Findings
- Mucosa may be metaplastic but is usually intact
- Edematous lamina propria with lymphoplasmacytic infiltrate, with occasional eosinophils (depends on etiology)
- Mucoserous glands may have goblet cell metaplasia
- May have "stromal atypia" with myofibroblastic cells
- Antrochoanal polyps are fibrotic with reduced or absent glands
- Pseudoangiomatous change, infarction, organization, and secondary infections may result

Pathologic Differential Diagnosis
- Chronic sinusitis, Schneiderian papilloma, inverted type rhabdomyosarcoma, nasopharyngeal angiofibroma, allergic fungal sinusitis, lymphoma

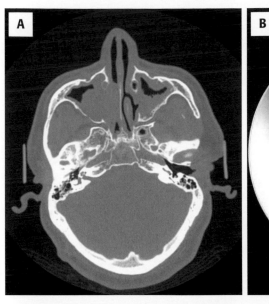

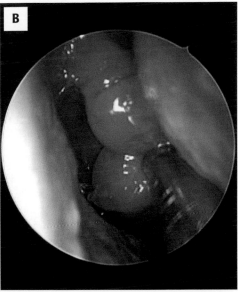

FIGURE 1-3

A, Multiple polyps are identified in the nasal cavity and in both maxillary sinuses. There is also extensive mucosal thickening of chronic sinusitis. **B**, Endoscopic view of multiple, shiny, translucent polyps within the nasal cavity. *(Courtesy of Dr. G.G. Calzada.)*

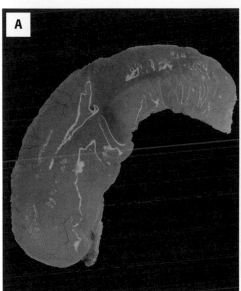

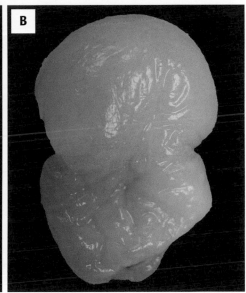

FIGURE 1-4

A and **B**, Two different sinonasal tract polyps, both showing a glistening, wrinkled surface, with a translucent appearance.

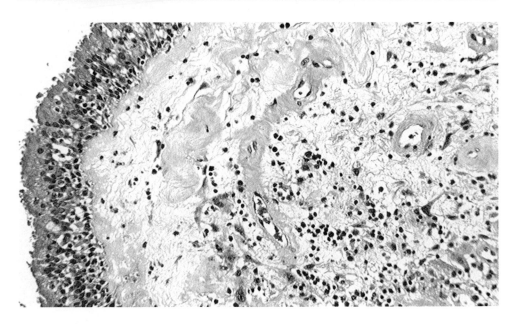

FIGURE 1-5

Sinonasal polyp. This polyp has an inflammatory infiltrate and a loose connective tissue stroma.

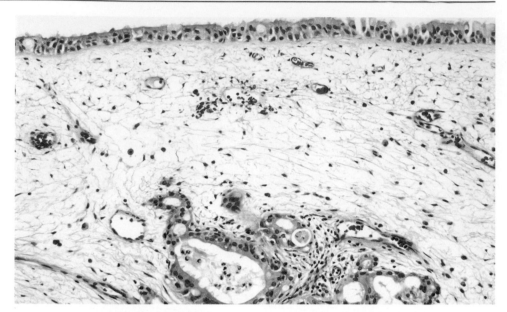

FIGURE 1-6

Sinonasal polyp. Seromucous glands are noted with chronic inflammation and an edematous stroma.

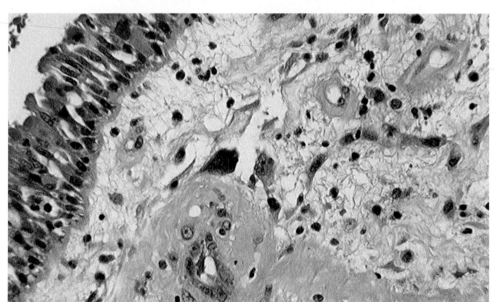

FIGURE 1-7

Atypical, single, myofibroblastic cells can be seen in sinonasal tract polyps.

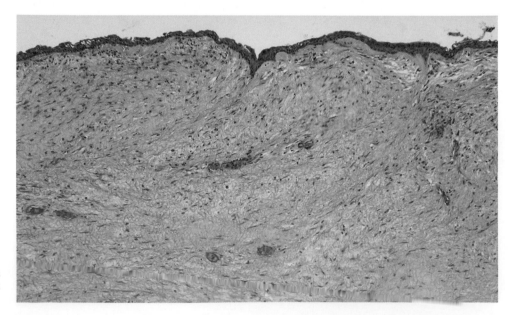

FIGURE 1-8

An antrochoanal polyp has dense fibrosis and decreased to absent mucoserous glands.

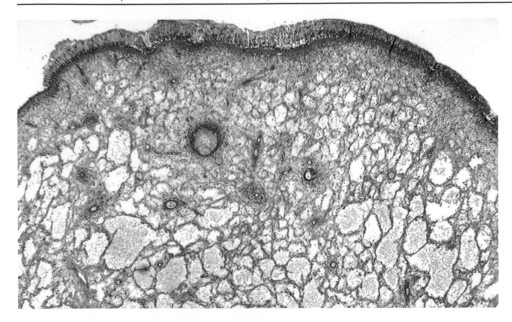

FIGURE 1-9
Angiomatous polyp. A pseudoangiomatous appearance is seen in this polyp with multiple, dilated vascular channels.

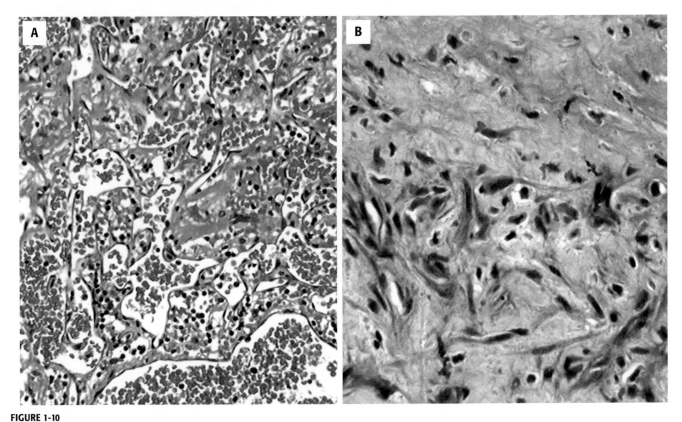

FIGURE 1-10
A, An infarcted polyp undergoing organization with a rich vascular ingrowth. **B**, Fibrosis with reactive and atypical stromal myofibroblasts seen in a postinfarct polyp.

then a prominent eosinophilic infiltrate is seen. Stalk torsion can result in dispersed, single, bizarre reactive fibroblasts within the lamina propria, so-called "stromal atypia" (Figure 1-7). Antrochoanal polyps are fibrotic, and the underlying mucoserous glands are diminished or absent (Figure 1-8). Angiomatous or pseudoangiomatous (lymphangiomatous) polyps contain proliferating thin-walled vessels in a loose, edematous to myxoid matrix (Figure 1-9). Polyps of all types may undergo infarction, organization, or secondary infection, sometimes giving rise to difficulties in diagnosis (Figure 1-10). Also, polyps may coexist with other sinonasal tract disorders, which should be carefully excluded.

DIFFERENTIAL DIAGNOSIS

Chronic sinusitis may cause slight stromal edema but usually does not result in polypoid tissue fragments. Schneiderian papillomas may be polypoid but are characterized by the proliferation of a transitional/respiratory epithelium and an inverted growth pattern. Rhabdomyosarcoma tends to be more cellular, with a layering or aggregation of atypical spindle cells. Muscle markers (myogenin, MYOD1, myoglobin, desmin) will also distinguish these two entities. Nasopharyngeal angiofibromas, seen exclusively in males, arise from the posterior nasal choanae and fill the nasopharynx. They are characterized by variably sized vessels (both with and without smooth muscle) embedded in collagenized stroma with plump spindled to stellate cells.

Polyps may become secondarily infected, so infectious agents must be excluded if there is a heavy acute inflammatory infiltrate or allergic mucin, a thick, pasty (inspissated) light green to brown collection of mucus with inflammatory debris. Lymphomas within the sinonasal tract contain an atypical population of lymphoid cells and will show immunophenotypic restriction.

PROGNOSIS AND THERAPY

The prognosis is excellent, as these are benign reactive lesions. However, removal of the underlying etiologic agent, if known, results in significantly reduced morbidity. Polyps are usually amenable to conservative endoscopic removal and improved sinus ventilation.

■ NASAL GLIAL HETEROTOPIA

Nasal glial heterotopia (NGH) is a congenital malformation of displaced, mature glial tissue (choristomas) in which continuity with the intracranial meningeal component has become obliterated. (The term NGH is preferred to "glioma," which implies a tumor.) By contrast, an encephalocele represents herniation of brain tissue and leptomeninges through a bony defect of the skull; continuity with the cranial cavity is maintained.

CLINICAL FEATURES

NGH most frequently presents during infancy but occasionally may be identified in older children and adults. Most cases present as small, firm subcutaneous nodules at or near the bridge of the nose in children or infants. These are classified as extranasal NGH and constitute

the majority (60%) of cases. Approximately 10% of NGHs are characterized as mixed, with both subcutaneous and intranasal components. Last, approximately 30% of NGHs are characterized as intranasal and manifest as polypoid lesions within the superior nasal cavity (Figure 1-11). Patients present with nasal obstruction, along with nasal polyps, chronic sinusitis, nasal drainage, and chronic otitis media. It is important to obtain imaging studies before biopsy, to ascertain the lack of continuity with the central nervous system and avoid postbiopsy complications. Meningitis and/or cerebrospinal fluid (CSF) rhinorrhea either before or after surgical manipulation suggests the possibility of an encephalocele.

RADIOLOGIC FEATURES

NGH forms a sharply demarcated, expansile mass, either extranasally or in the superior nasal cavity (Figure 1-12). Intracerebral extension needs to be excluded; this

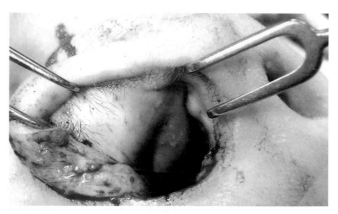

FIGURE 1-11
Nasal glial heterotopia can present as a purely intranasal polyp.

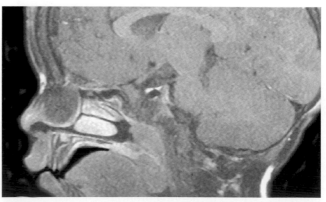

FIGURE 1-12
Nasal glial heterotopia. Sagittal T1-weighted, fat-suppressed magnetic resonance image of an anterior nasal fossa nasal glial heterotopia that comes up to the anterior skull base but has no intracranial component. There is no caudal distortion of the undersurface of the frontal lobe.

NASAL GLIAL HETEROTOPIA—DISEASE FACT SHEET

Definition
- Congenital malformation of displaced, mature glial tissue without an intracranial connection

Incidence and Location
- Uncommon
- Location: extranasal (60%), intranasal (30%), mixed (10%)

Morbidity and Mortality
- If an encephalocele (intracranial connection), then meningitis or cerebrospinal fluid leak may develop

Gender and Age Distribution
- Equal gender distribution
- Most frequent during infancy, rare in adults

Clinical Features
- Mass, often over the glabella/nasal bridge
- Nasal obstruction
- Chronic sinusitis and nasal drainage
- Otitis media

Radiographic Findings
- Sharply demarcated mass without any identifiable intracranial connection

Prognosis and Treatment
- Excellent prognosis, although up to 30% may "recur" if incompletely excised

NASAL GLIAL HETEROTOPIA—PATHOLOGIC FEATURES

Gross Findings
- Smooth, homogeneous, glistening cut surface
- Can be firm if there is extensive fibrosis
- Polyp if within the nasal cavity

Microscopic Findings
- Nasal glial heterotopia resembles gliosis
- Glial tissue blended with fibrosis below intact surface
- Astrocytic cells may show gemistocytic change
- Encephaloceles appear identical to normal brain tissue, but degeneration may result in loss of neurons

Ancillary Studies
- Trichrome highlights glial tissue (red) in contrast to fibrosis (blue)
- S100 protein and glial fibrillary acidic protein react with glial tissue

Pathologic Differential Diagnosis
- Encephalocele and fibrosed nasal polyp

would appear as a tract or a cribriform plate defect. If an intracerebral communication is found, particularly one including communication of CSF, then the lesion is better classified as an encephalocele. Even with high-resolution CT scans and MRI, the connection may be small and inapparent.

PATHOLOGIC FEATURES

GROSS FINDINGS

These tumors have a smooth, homogeneous, glistening cut surface, similar to brain tissue. They may be firm, due to a fibrous tissue component.

MICROSCOPIC FINDINGS

NGH resembles gliosis. The glial tissue is blended with fibrosis, often below an intact skin or surface mucosa (Figure 1-13). It is composed of nests and masses of fibrillar neuroglial tissue with a prominent network of glial fibers. Astrocytic cells may show gem-

istocytic changes (Figure 1-14). Neuronal cells are rarely (10%) identified. Choroid plexus, ependymal cells, and pigmented cells with retinal differentiation have rarely been reported. It is imperative to stress that fibrosis may obscure the glial tissue (Figure 1-15), often requiring histochemistry and immunohistochemistry for their recognition. Encephaloceles appear identical to normal brain tissue, but degeneration may result in loss of neurons. In such cases, distinction from NGH requires radiographic and clinical correlation.

ANCILLARY STUDIES

Trichrome will separate fibrous connective tissue (stains blue) from the glial tissue (stains bright red). The glial tissues will react strongly and diffusely with glial fibrillary acidic protein (GFAP) (Figure 1-15) and S100 protein.

DIFFERENTIAL DIAGNOSIS

The most common entity to be distinguished from NGH is a fibrotic nasal polyp. Large astrocytic cells may be misidentified as histiocytes, but immunohistochemical expression of GFAP is diagnostic for glial cells. The diagnosis of a fibrotic polyp requires the exclusion of neural tissue.

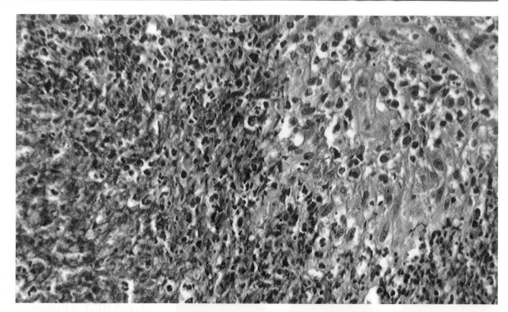

FIGURE 1-32

The blue, granular bionecrotic material associated with a small vessel being destroyed (*top right*).

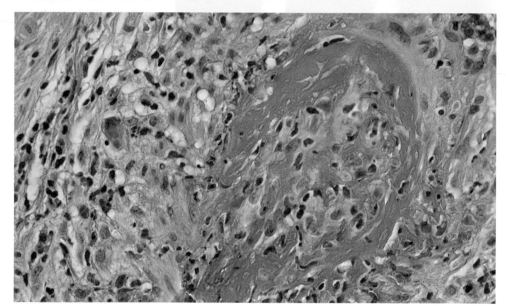

FIGURE 1-33

The vessel wall is destroyed, showing epithelioid histiocytes, isolated giant cells, and a fibrinous degeneration of the wall in this example of vasculitis in Wegener granulomatosis.

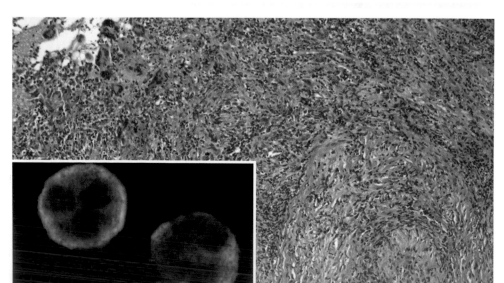

FIGURE 1-34

Rarely, giant cells may be present (*top left*), but well-formed granulomas are absent. Note the vessel wall in *bottom left*, with destruction by the inflammatory process in an example of vasculitis. *Inset*, Cytoplasmic antineutrophil cytoplasmic antibody shows a granular cytoplasmic pattern in a case of Wegener granulomatosis.

sinusitis, microscopic polyangiitis (MPA), Churg-Strauss syndrome, extranodal NK/T-cell lymphoma, nasal type, and cocaine abuse. Infectious granulomatous sinusitis can be seen with chronic invasive fungal sinusitis. It may also develop as extension of chronic granulomatous meningoencephalitis secondary to acanthamoeba in the setting of immunosuppression. MPA is a related small vessel vasculitis that affects the lungs, kidneys, and skin. It is associated with ANCA against myeloperoxidase (MPO-ANCA). Churg-Strauss syndrome usually affects the lungs and is associated with asthma, peripheral eosinophilia, pulmonary infiltrates, and polyneuropathy, as well as sinusitis. NK/T-cell lymphoma is characterized by cytologically atypical cells and vascular destruction and demonstrates specific immunohistochemical findings. Cocaine abuse may sometimes mimic the findings of WG due to the vasoconstrictive effects of amphetamines and the granulomatous response elicited by various substances used to "cut" cocaine. Using polarization may identify the talc, for example, often used to cut cocaine, although talc is not always associated with cocaine use.

PROGNOSIS AND THERAPY

Outcome depends on the extent of disease, as well as the type of therapy, which is directed by disease severity. Symptomatic relapses are common. Immunosuppression is the therapeutic mainstay; cyclophosphamide and glucocorticoids are most often used in combination. Side effects of therapy need to be monitored.

■ RESPIRATORY EPITHELIAL ADENOMATOID HAMARTOMA

Respiratory epithelial adenomatoid hamartomas (REAHs) represent benign proliferations of sinonasal minor mucoserous glands. These uncommon hamartomas are composed of small glandular epithelial islands in a mesenchymal background but lack any components from other germ cell layers.

CLINICAL FEATURES

REAHs are more common in men than in women, with a peak incidence in the 6th decade. Patients complain of unilateral nasal obstruction, epistaxis, and recurrent sinusitis, symptoms identical to chronic rhinosinusitis or polyps.

RESPIRATORY EPITHELIAL ADENOMATOID HAMARTOMA (REAH)—DISEASE FACT SHEET

Definition
- A benign proliferation of mature sinonasal tissue presenting as a polyp

Incidence and Location
- Rare
- REAH usually in the nasal cavity

Gender and Age Distribution
- Male > female
- Peak in 6th decade

Clinical Features
- Unilateral nasal obstruction
- Epistaxis
- Recurrent sinusitis

Prognosis and Treatment
- Cured with conservative but complete excision

RADIOLOGIC FEATURES

A unilateral nasal mass arising from the posterior nasal septum or the lateral nasal wall is seen in approximately 80% of cases. In the remaining cases, the mass may be in the nasopharynx or the paranasal sinuses.

PATHOLOGIC FEATURES

GROSS FINDINGS

REAHs are exophytic, polypoid, rubbery to firm, tan-white to red-brown lesions, measuring up to 6 cm in largest dimension.

RESPIRATORY EPITHELIAL ADENOMATOID HAMARTOMA— PATHOLOGIC FEATURES

Gross Findings
- Exophytic, polypoid, up to 6 cm masses
- Firm, tan-white to red-brown

Microscopic Findings
- Proliferation of mature respiratory glandular tissue with invagination from the surface epithelium
- Glands surrounded by thick basement membrane material
- Multilayered, columnar, respiratory epithelium with cilia

Pathologic Differential Diagnosis
- Schneiderian papilloma, inverted type; intestinal-type adenocarcinoma; inflammatory polyps

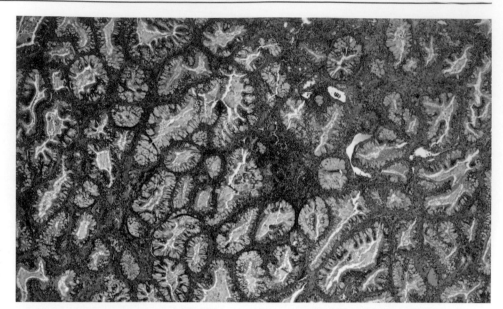

FIGURE 1-35

Respiratory epithelial adenomatoid hamartoma. Multiple small glandular proliferations are noted in the stroma. There is no
"stromal" reaction, although there is a
prominent basement membrane.

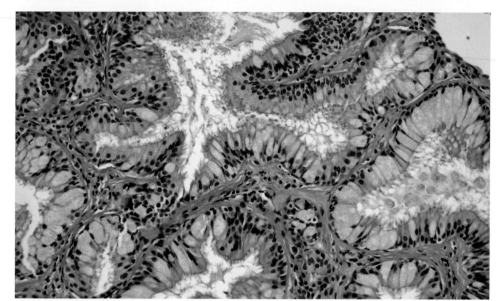

FIGURE 1-36

Respiratory epithelial adenomatoid hamartoma. Well-circumscribed glandular profiles
are surrounded by basement membrane
material. There is a pseudostratified columnar epithelium.

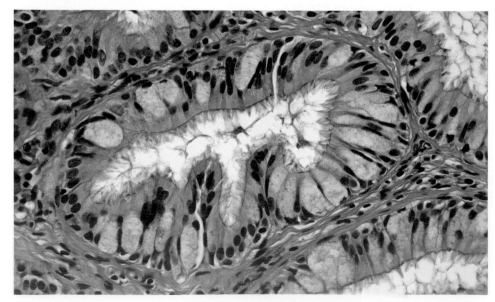

FIGURE 1-37

Respiratory epithelial adenomatoid hamartoma. The epithelium is histologically
benign with abundant cilia noted on the
surface. There is nuclear stratification
as would be expected in a respiratory
epithelial adenomatoid hamartoma.

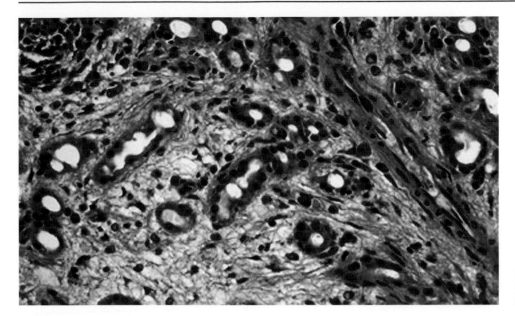

FIGURE 1-38
Multiple small ductoglandular units are present in this example of serous hamartoma.

MICROSCOPIC FINDINGS

These polyps are composed of prominent glandular proliferations lined with ciliated respiratory mucosa (Figure 1-35). The glands are often in continuity with the surface but are usually surrounded by a thickened, dense, pink basement membrane material that separates these invaginations from the fibrotic, edematous, and focally inflamed stroma (Figure 1-36). The epithelium has multilayered, columnar, respiratory-type epithelium, with prominent cilia noted (Figure 1-37). The epithelium is reactive for cytokeratin 7; the basal cells are reactive for p63 and 34βE12. Occasionally, cartilage or bone is also present, and some authors have termed these lesions chondro-osseous respiratory epithelial adenomatoid hamartomas (COREAHs).

Sinonasal serous hamartoma appears to be a related entity existing on a spectrum with REAH. Serous hamartomas are rare lesions characterized by a proliferation of *small ductoglandular elements,* which, similarly to REAHs, are in continuity with the surface epithelium (Figure 1-38). Hybrid lesions have been described with budding of the serous glands from the respiratory epithelium-lined glands of REAHs. The serous glands often lack myoepithelial cells on immunohistochemical staining.

DIFFERENTIAL DIAGNOSIS

The differential diagnosis includes Schneiderian papilloma, inverted-type (inverted papilloma [IP]), intestinal-type adenocarcinoma (ITAC), and inflammatory polyps.

The inverted islands of IP may retain luminal respiratory epithelium, but in general there is a hyperplastic squamous epithelium. Small mucous cysts filled with debris are present, but goblet cells or mucoserous glands are rare. Moreover, the epithelial groups are not usually surrounded by a thickened basement membrane. Well-differentiated ITAC is composed of back-to-back glands without a basal reserve layer or basement membrane material and does not have ciliated respiratory epithelium. A lobular architecture is maintained. Inflammatory polyps, with fewer glands, lack the "adenomatoid" appearance of epithelium within the stroma.

PROGNOSIS AND THERAPY

Conservative but complete excision is curative, with little chance of recurrence, if any.

■ MYOSPHERULOSIS

CLINICAL FEATURES

Myospherulosis is an iatrogenic foreign body reaction resulting from the interaction of erythrocytes with petroleum, lanolin, or traumatized fat tissue. Patients will usually have a history of previous sinus surgery that used petroleum-impregnated packing. The clinical presentation includes persistent sinusitis, facial pain, and swelling. These patients tend to have a significantly higher chance of developing adhesions and are likely to require additional therapy.

PATHOLOGIC FEATURES

Numerous variably sized (up to 100 μm) pseudocysts are seen yielding a "Swiss cheese" appearance on low-power magnification. Heavy fibrosis often surrounds these cysts (Figure 1-39). Within these cystic spaces are sac-like structures ("parent bodies") with a nonrefractile thin membrane containing brown, discolored, misshapen erythrocytes (Figure 1-40). Unlike microorganisms, the erythrocytes will not react with silver impregnation stains. In contrast, a hemoglobin stain will confirm their origin.

DIFFERENTIAL DIAGNOSIS

The differential diagnosis includes coccidiodomycosis and *Rhinosporidium*. The "capsule" of myospherulosis is only approximately 1 μm thick, so it is not as thick, and neither double walled nor birefringent, compared with

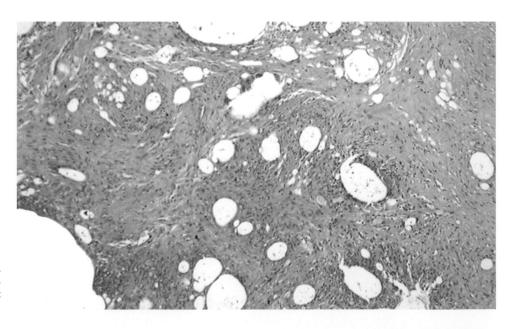

FIGURE 1-39

Myospherulosis. Heavy fibrosis and multiple vacuoles are noted with inflammation. Small aggregates of "eosinophilic globules" are seen in the spaces.

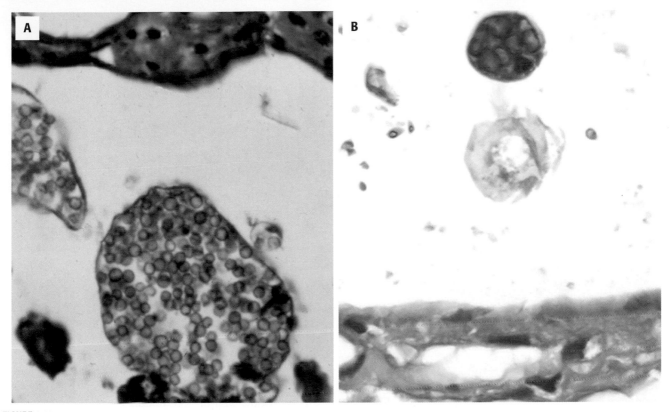

FIGURE 1-40
Myospherulosis. **A**, The encysted erythrocytes in myospherulosis mimic fungal spores. **B**, Small degenerated erythrocyte nuclei are housed in a ball within the lumen of this cyst.

the capsules of *Coccidioidomyces* and *Rhinosporidium*, respectively.

PROGNOSIS AND THERAPY

Myospherulosis is amenable to conservative treatment, although patients who have this response to surgery are more likely to require revision surgery. Therefore, nasal packing with lipid-based ointments should be avoided in patients who have previously been diagnosed with myospherulosis.

SUGGESTED READINGS

The complete suggested readings list is available online at
   www.expertconsult.com.

2

Benign Neoplasms of the Nasal Cavity, Paranasal Sinuses, and Nasopharynx

■ Lester D. R. Thompson

■ SCHNEIDERIAN PAPILLOMAS

The mucosae of the nasal vestibule and the superior wall of the nasal cavity are lined by squamous and olfactory mucosa, respectively. The remaining nasal mucosa consists of ciliated columnar epithelium of ectodermal origin known as the Schneiderian membrane. Three benign neoplastic papillomatous proliferations arise from the Schneiderian membrane: exophytic, fungiform or everted papillomas (EPs); inverted or endophytic papillomas (IPs); and columnar, cylindrical cell, or oncocytic papillomas (OPs). They are defined as a group of benign epithelial neoplasms arising from sinonasal (Schneiderian) mucosa. Although these entities share a number of features and are classified as "Schneiderian papillomas," there are sufficient clinical and microscopic differences to regard them as three distinctive clinicopathologic entities. The overall lack of mixed papillomas and their relation to human papilloma virus (HPV) are sufficiently different to lend further credence to this separation.

CLINICAL FEATURES

Sinonasal Schneiderian papillomas (SSPs) are a rare disease with an estimated annual incidence of 0.6 per 100,000 population, representing <5% of all sinonasal tract tumors. Males are affected much more commonly than females (4:1), with most patients presenting in the latter years of life (mean, 5th to 8th decades). Children are rarely affected. Clinical symptoms are nonspecific and include unilateral nasal obstruction, followed by epistaxis, rhinorrhea, facial pressure, and headaches. Often, patients report previous intranasal surgery before a diagnosis of SSP is firmly established. Physical examination usually demonstrates a unilateral polypoid mass in the nasal cavity.

SSPs show a remarkable anatomic distribution according to histologic type: EPs arise almost exclusively on the nasal septum (up to 8% may be lateral); IPs and OPs affect the lateral nasal wall, middle meatus, and less often the paranasal sinuses (maxillary, ethmoid, sphenoid, frontal sinuses). Rarely, exceptions are noted. Less than 3% of cases are bilateral and usually reflect extension of the disease from one side to the other. Rarely, cases are seen as primary lesions in nasopharyngeal or middle ear mucosa.

RADIOLOGIC FEATURES

Plain x-rays, computed tomography (CT), and magnetic resonance imaging (MRI) routinely show a unilateral polypoid mass filling the nasal cavity, although variable based on the extent of disease. Displacement of the nasal septum and opacification of sinuses are also frequently seen. Pressure erosion of the bone is present in approximately 45% of cases. Intratumoral calcification is extremely rare.

PATHOLOGIC FEATURES

GROSS FINDINGS

EPs have been described as gray-tan cauliflower-like, papillary or mulberry-like verrucous papillary proliferations attached to underlying mucosa by a narrow stalk. IPs usually are large, multinodular, firm, bulky, polypoid lesions with deep clefts and intact mucosa (Figure 2-1). Often, resections for IPs include fragments of bone. Grossly, OPs are usually small and fragmented and consist of soft pink, tan to brown papillary fragments of tissue.

SCHNEIDERIAN PAPILLOMA—DISEASE FACT SHEET

	Exophytic Type (32%)	Endophytic Type (62%)	Oncocytic Cell Type (6%)
Definition	A papilloma derived from the Schneiderian membrane composed of exophytic, papillary fronds with fibrovascular cores lined by multiple layers of well-differentiated stratified epithelial cells	A papilloma derived from the Schneiderian membrane with proliferation and invagination into the underlying stroma	A papilloma derived from the Schneiderian membrane displaying exophytic fronds and endophytic invaginations lined by multilayered columnar oncocytic cells
Incidence and Location	Uncommon (~6/1,000,000-population) Nasal septum	Uncommon (~6/1,000,000-population) Lateral nasal wall, middle meatus, and less often the paranasal sinuses (nasopharynx and middle ear are rare)	Rare Lateral wall of nasal cavity
Morbidity and Mortality	Morbidity associated with nasal obstruction and epistaxis No mortality	Intracranial invasion Malignant transformation in up to 27% of cases	Nasal obstruction, bleeding Rare cases of malignant transformation
Gender, Race, and Age Distribution	Male > female (4:1) Adults (mean, 6th decade)	Male > female (4:1) Adults (mean, 6th decade) uncommon in children	Equal gender distribution 6th decade
Clinical Features	Unilateral nasal obstruction Epistaxis Rhinorrhea Headaches	Nasal obstruction Epistaxis Rhinorrhea Facial pressure Headaches	Nasal obstruction Epistaxis
Prognosis and Treatment	Excellent long-term prognosis, although recurrences develop (up to 50%) Meticulous and complete surgical resection	Excellent long-term prognosis (excluding cases with malignant transformation) Recurrences up to 60%, depending on type of surgery Malignant transformation in up to 27% of cases Meticulous, complete surgical resection	Excellent prognosis Very rare examples of malignant transformation Meticulous and complete surgical resection

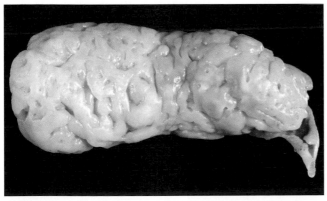

FIGURE 2-1

Surgical specimen of an inverted Schneiderian papilloma with a polypoid appearance. The cerebriform surface shows numerous clefts due to exuberant endophytic epithelial proliferation.

MICROSCOPIC FINDINGS

Exophytic

EPs consist of branching, exophytic proliferations composed of fibrovascular cores lined by well-differentiated stratified squamous epithelium (Figure 2-2). The epithelium ranges from basal and parabasal cells (Figure 2-3) to well-differentiated keratinized cells with a granular cell layer and surface keratin with hyperkeratosis (Figures 2-4 and 2-5). However, surface keratinization is uncommon. There may be intraepithelial or luminal ciliated or goblet cells. The stroma usually contains variable numbers of seromucus glands. Mitotic figures and atypical cells are distinctly uncommon in EP. Malignant transformation is vanishingly rare.

Endophytic

IP consists of a markedly thick, inverted, or endophytic growth of nonkeratinizing transitional cells (Figure 2-6). The inverted areas are surrounded by a well-formed basement membrane and do not show "invasive" growth (Figure 2-7). The epithelium in IP undergoes squamous maturation with superficial cells adopting a flattened orientation (Figure 2-8). Surface keratinization and a granular cell layer are uncommon (seen in approximately 10%). Distinct cell borders and cleared cytoplasm (due to glycogen) are frequent

SCHNEIDERIAN PAPILLOMA—PATHOLOGIC FEATURES

	Exophytic Type	Endophytic Type	Oncocytic Cell Type
Gross Findings	Gray-tan, cauliflower-like or verrucous papillary proliferation attached to mucosa by narrow stalk	Large, multinodular, firm polypoid lesions. Deep clefts of inverted but intact mucosa. Fragments of bone in surgical specimen	Small fragments of soft, fleshy, pink, tan, papillary tissue
Microscopic Findings	Branching, exophytic proliferations with fibrovascular cores lined by well-differentiated stratified squamous epithelium. Basal and parabasal cells, well-differentiated keratinized cells, granular cell layer, surface keratin. Intraepithelial or luminal ciliated or goblet cells. Stroma with seromucus glands	Markedly thick, inverted neoplastic proliferation replacing mucoserous glands and ducts (noninvasive). Transitional/squamoid epithelium with numerous intraepithelial microcysts containing macrophages, mucin, and cellular debris. Distinct cell borders with glycogenation. May have ciliated columnar cells or surface keratinization. Foci of cytologic atypia. Stroma ranging from edematous, myxomatous, to fibrous with an inflammatory infiltrate. No seromucus glands in stroma. Transformation to carcinoma (in situ or invasion) may occur (usually squamous cell carcinoma)	Both exophytic and endophytic patterns. Multiple layers of columnar oncocytic epithelium. Tumor cells have well defined borders with eosinophilic or granular oncocytic cytoplasm. Round nuclei with small nucleoli. Cilia may be present focally on the surface. Intraepithelial cysts. Rare malignant transformation
Immunohisto-chemistry Features		Co-expression of columnar and squamous epithelial keratins by the same cells	Mitochondrial histochemical stains (PTAH)–positive. Cytochrome c oxidase positive
Pathologic Differential Diagnosis	Cutaneous squamous papilloma, inflammatory nasal polyp, papillary squamous cell carcinoma	Sinonasal polyp, respiratory epithelial adenomatoid hamartoma, carcinoma	Rhinosporidiosis and low-grade papillary sinonasal adenocarcinoma

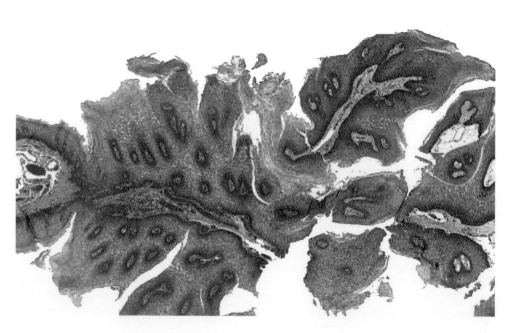

FIGURE 2-2

Exophytic Schneiderian papilloma of nasal septum lined by markedly thickened well-differentiated squamous epithelium

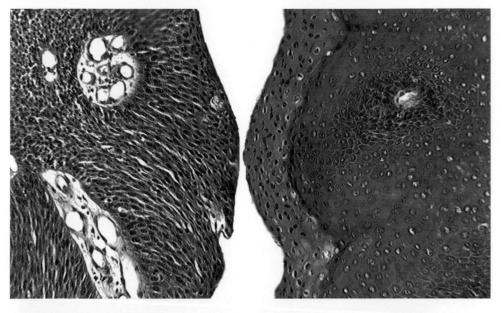

FIGURE 2-3

A basal-parabasal appearance to this exophytic Schneiderian papilloma is noted on the left, while a more well-differentiated keratinized epithelium with parakeratosis is noted on the right.

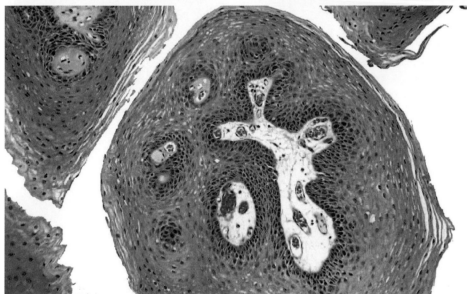

FIGURE 2-4

Exophytic Schneiderian papilloma with papillary "finger-like" projections with a fibrovascular core lined by squamous cells.

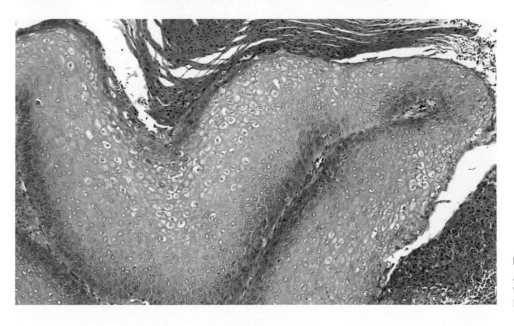

FIGURE 2-5

An exophytic Schneiderian papilloma with koilocytic atypia, hyperkeratosis, and parakeratosis.

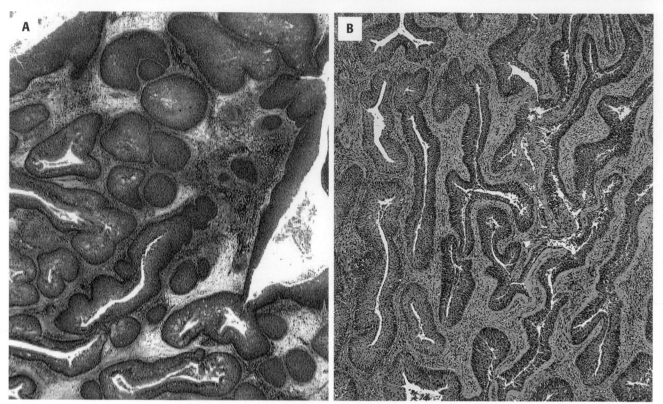

FIGURE 2-6

A and **B**, Inverted Schneiderian papillomas with nests of cells deep in the stroma. Note the "squamous" versus transitional type epithelium within the different tumors.

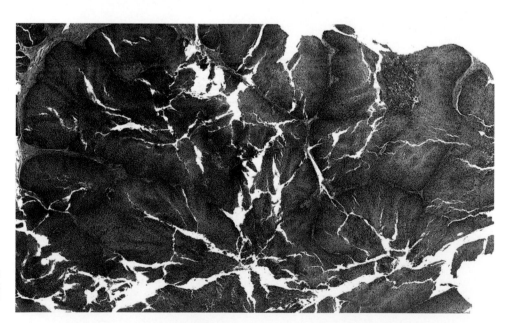

FIGURE 2-7

A large inverted Schneiderian papilloma showing a well-developed endophytic growth, but still arranged as a polypoid structure overall.

findings. Cellular pleomorphism may be present, but is focal and not associated with dyskeratosis or increased mitotic activity. A characteristic feature is the presence of numerous intraepithelial microcysts containing macrophages, mucin, and cell debris (Figure 2-8). These microcysts are more numerous close to the luminal surface. Mucous cells may be interspersed. Mitotic activity is variable, but usually limited to basal and

parabasal cells. Occasionally, the luminal surface may be lined by ciliated columnar cells. The stroma ranges from edematous, myxomatous, to fibrous, usually showing a conspicuous absence of seromucous glands. An inflammatory infiltrate composed of a variable mixture of neutrophils, eosinophils, small lymphocytes, and plasma cells with occasional germinal centers is a consistent finding (Figure 2-9). Concurrent nasal

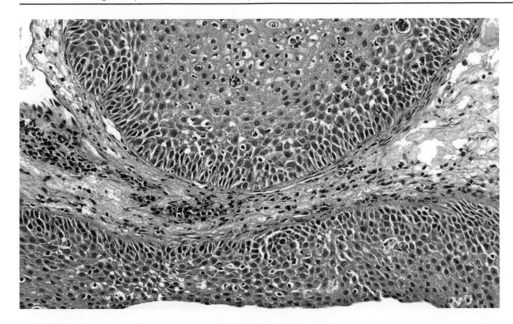

FIGURE 2-8

Typical nonkeratinizing squamous epithelium found in an inverted papilloma. Intraepithelial cysts with occasional macrophages are present.

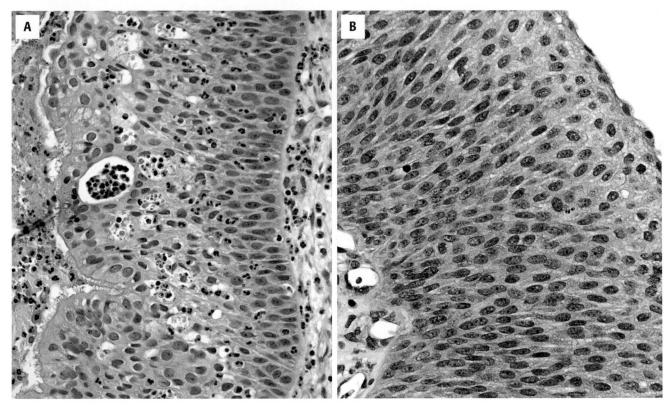

FIGURE 2-9

A, A large number of inflammatory cells and small micro-abscesses are noted in this inverted Schneiderian papilloma. **B**, There is a lack of inflammatory elements within this area of Schneiderian papilloma. However, the transitional-type epithelium is easily identified.

inflammatory polyps may be present. Surface keratinization is uncommon. Malignant transformation can be seen, identified as conventional in situ and invasive squamous cell carcinomas (Figure 2-10). When carcinoma is present, it is synchronous in 60% and metachronous in 40%.

Oncocytic Cell Papilloma

OPs are characterized by a proliferating multilayered columnar or oncocytic epithelium (Figure 2-11). Most OPs have an exophytic branching papillary appearance with long delicate fibrous cores. The individual tumor cells show well-defined cell borders with eosinophilic or

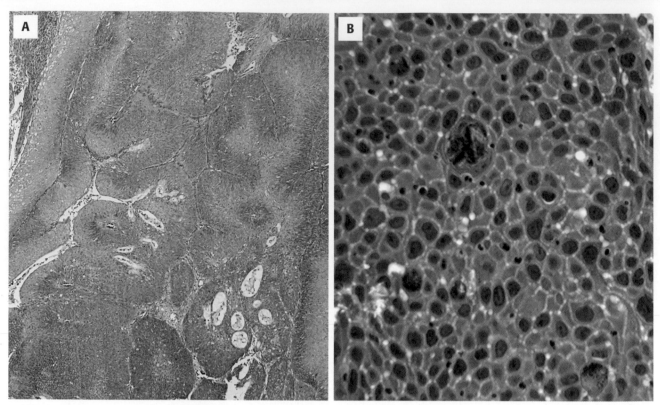

FIGURE 2-10

Malignant transformation of an inverted Schneiderian papilloma demonstrates an increased cellularity and lack of maturation (**A**), while nuclear pleomorphism and atypical mitotic figures are seen on high power (**B**).

granular oncocytic cytoplasm. The nuclei are round, centrally located, and uniform. Small to medium nucleoli are readily seen. Occasional surface cells show well-defined cilia (Figure 2-12). Numerous small intraepithelial mucous cysts are also typically seen in these tumors. Mitotic figures are uncommon in OP. Unlike IP, seromucus glands are present in the submucosa of OP. Malignant transformation of OP is uncommon, but can be seen.

ANCILLARY STUDIES

ULTRASTRUCTURAL FEATURES

While unnecessary for diagnosis, electron microscopy shows that IPs consist of stratified transitional-like cells, with areas of basal and squamous differentiation, characterized by cytoplasmic bundles of tonofilaments. Occasional goblet cells with mucin granules can also be identified. The tumor cells show long microvilli-like processes joined by well-developed desmosomes. Cytoplasmic glycogen and lysosomes are prominent. The basement membrane is thin and discontinuous in many areas.

IMMUNOHISTOCHEMICAL FEATURES

Immunohistochemical studies are not necessary for the diagnosis or classification of SSP. Interestingly, the co-expression of keratins typical of columnar and squamous differentiation by the same cells appears to be characteristic of Schneiderian papillomas and is not seen in non-neoplastic mucosa. The cells of OP are immunoreactive with cytochrome c oxidase as would be expected in an oncocytic cell.

MOLECULAR TECHNIQUES

In situ hybridization and polymerase chain reaction have convincingly demonstrated an etiologic role for human papillomavirus (HPV) in SSP, although variation in technique and serotypes of HPV sought yield variable results. The low-risk HPV types 6 and 11 are by far the most commonly identified. The presence of HPV does not seem to increase the risk of malignant transformation. Inverted papillomas do not harbor key genetic alterations associated with malignant transformation, such as p53, which is only seen in cases with malignant transformation.

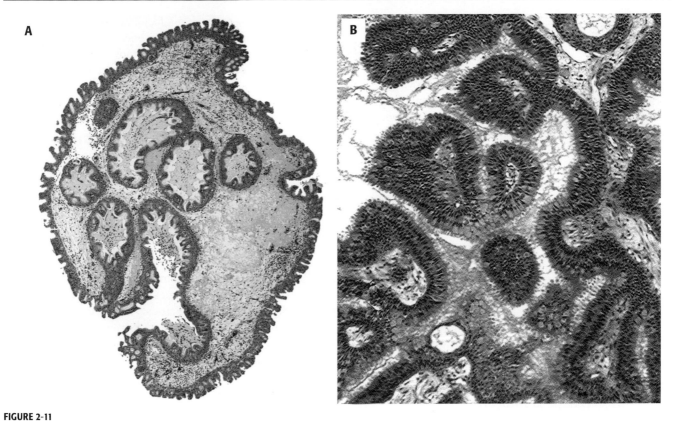

FIGURE 2-11

A and **B**, Multilayered oncocytic epithelium arranged in a focal "tram-track" architecture. Cilia are abundant at the surface of this complex papillary growth, showing an "endophytic" growth.

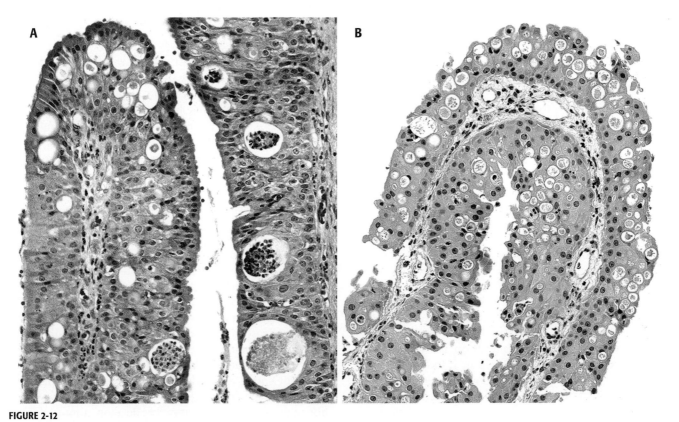

FIGURE 2-12

A and **B**, Oncocytic cell Schneiderian papilloma with stratified columnar respiratory epithelium with oncocytic cells and small neutrophilic abscesses. These structures are within the epithelium.

DIFFERENTIAL DIAGNOSIS

The differential diagnosis depends on the histologic type of papilloma, and includes sinonasal polyps, cutaneous squamous papilloma, verruca vulgaris, papillary squamous cell carcinoma, respiratory epithelial adenomatoid hamartoma (REAH), low-grade papillary adenocarcinoma, and rhinosporidiosis. *Sinonasal polyps* have marked stromal edema and inflammation with a nonproliferative epithelium, lacking intraepithelial microcysts. *Verruca vulgaris* has prominent keratinization with verrucoid or papillomatous growth, keratohyaline granules, and koilocytes, while lacking intraepithelial mucocytes. *Papillary squamous cell carcinomas* are characterized by papillae with fibrovascular cores lined by clearly malignant squamous epithelium. It is important to bear in mind the possibility of a carcinoma arising in a Schneiderian papilloma. *REAH* is a rare hamartoma with epithelium arranged in a glandular distribution. *Low-grade papillary sinonasal adenocarcinoma* has an infiltrative growth, with acinar, cystic, or trabecular growth. *Rhinosporidiosis* has characteristic sporangia and endospores within the stroma, below the epithelium rather than the microcysts within the epithelium of IP and OP.

PROGNOSIS AND THERAPY

The long-term prognosis of SSP without in situ or invasive carcinoma is excellent. However, there is a considerable recurrence rate, often dependent on the extent of the tumor and initial surgical approach used. If inadequately removed, recurrences or persistence develops in up to 60 % (more common for inverted than the other types), usually developing within 5 years of initial presentation. Multiple recurrences are not uncommon. Given the anatomic confines, if neglected, significant morbidity may be experienced. There is no correlation between the number of recurrences and the development of carcinoma, if it occurs. Carcinoma develops in up to 27 % of all cases, usually the inverted (up to 27 %), followed by oncocytic (up to 17 %), and rarely in the exophytic type. Most carcinomas are keratinizing squamous cell carcinoma, although verrucous squamous cell carcinoma, mucoepidermoid carcinoma, small cell carcinoma, adenocarcinoma, and sinonasal undifferentiated carcinoma are reported. The carcinoma may be seen synchronously or metachronously with the papilloma. Papilloma may still be present, limited, or absent, depending on the development of the tumor. If carcinoma develops, it may invade and destroy vital structures of the region. Prognosis for carcinoma is similar to primary squamous cell carcinoma.

The treatment of choice is surgery, whether endoscopic, snare avulsion, or by a more radical excision (lateral rhinotomy and medial maxillectomy, Caldwell-Luc procedure, craniofacial resection or midfacial degloving). Meticulous removal is imperative if recurrences are to be averted. Chemotherapy and radiation therapy are not of benefit, although radiation may be used in rare cases to treat unresectable cases.

■ LOBULAR CAPILLARY HEMANGIOMA (PYOGENIC GRANULOMA)

Lobular capillary hemangiomas (LCHs) are a relatively common, benign vascular neoplasm of capillary loops, representing about 25 % of all nonepithelial sinonasal tract neoplasms and about 10 % of all head and neck hemangiomas. Although the term "pyogenic granuloma" preceded "lobular capillary hemangioma" as the diagnostic term for these lesions, it is a misnomer. LCHs are not "purulent," "infectious," or "granulomatous." While the pathogenesis is unknown, local trauma and hormonal factors (pregnancy or oral contraceptive use) are suggested etiologic agents (hence, *epulis gravidarum* as another name). Nose picking, nasal packing, cauterization, shaving/hair removal, and nonspecific microtrauma are all associated etiologic findings. There are isolated cases which are part of Sturge-Weber or von Hippel-Lindau syndrome.

CLINICAL FEATURES

About one-third of mucosal LCHs arise in the nasal cavity (about 60 % present in the oral cavity). When in the oral cavity, the gingiva is most frequently affected, while in the nasal cavity, the anterior nasal septum (Little area or Kiesselbach triangle) accounts for about 60 % of cases; 20 % involve the nasal vestibule and 20 % affect the turbinates. These lesions usually affect boys under the age of 15, females in their reproductive years and, less commonly, older adults of either gender. Patients with an inherited syndrome tend to be younger at initial presentation. Overall, females are affected more frequently than males (2:1), but in the pediatric group (up to 18 years), males are much more frequently affected than females.

Patients typically present with intermittent, painless episodes of unilateral epistaxis (in about 95 % of cases). The lesions tend to bleed easily, often with only slight trauma. Large lesions may cause nasal obstruction (in up to 35 % of cases). Tumors may present as a rapidly growing, painless, hemorrhagic mass, with patients experiencing symptoms for a relatively short duration. Rhinoscopy generally shows a well-defined, sessile or polypoid, red to purplish mass. Often, there is mucosal ulceration with a fibrinous exudate. Patients who develop tumors during pregnancy may show spontaneous involution postpartum, as hormone levels return to normal.

**LOBULAR CAPILLARY HEMANGIOMA
(PYOGENIC GRANULOMA)—DISEASE FACT SHEET**

Definition

- Benign vascular tumor with lobular architecture composed of variable size vessels with proliferating endothelial cells

Incidence and Location

- Common
- Anterior nasal septum (60%), nasal vestibule (20%), turbinates (20%)

Gender and Age Distribution

- Boys <15 years
- Females in reproductive years
- Older adults no gender differences

Clinical Features

- Intermittent, painless epistaxis
- Nasal obstruction

Prognosis and Treatment

- Excellent prognosis with no significant recurrences
- Complete endoscopic resection with bleeding control

**LOBULAR CAPILLARY HEMANGIOMA
(PYOGENIC GRANULOMA)—PATHOLOGIC FEATURES**

Gross Findings

- Sessile, polypoid, or nodular red to purplish mass
- Ulceration is common

Microscopic Findings

- Lobular architecture with mixture of thin and thick blood vessels
- Central vessel surrounded by cellular lobule of closely packed capillaries
- Plump endothelial cells with bland nuclear features and scanty to moderate eosinophilic cytoplasm
- Frequent mitotic figures
- Edematous to fibrotic stroma with mixed inflammatory infiltrate
- Ulcerated surface with fibrinous exudate simulating granulation tissue

Immunohistochemical Features

- Endothelial cells positive for CD31, CD34, factor VIII–RAg
- Actins positive in pericytes and smooth muscle cells

Pathologic Differential Diagnosis

- Nasopharyngeal angiofibroma, glomangiopericytoma (sinonasal-type hemangiopericytoma), angiosarcoma

Radiographic studies, such as ultrasound and angiography, show the anatomic site, extent, and vascular nature of the lesion, and identify feeder vessels and allow for presurgical embolization. Other studies can help to confirm the diagnosis, if required.

PATHOLOGIC FEATURES

GROSS FINDINGS

LCHs are polypoid (Figure 2-13), nodular, or sessile masses with pink or gray-tan color. They are often soft and compressible submucosal masses. Frequently, the surgical specimen is ulcerated (about 40% of cases) and partially covered with a yellow to white fibrinous exudate.

There is a wide range in size (1 to 8 cm), with a mean of about 1.5 cm.

MICROSCOPIC FINDINGS

The term "lobular capillary hemangioma" properly describes the microscopic appearance of this benign vascular tumor. At low power, the polypoid LCH exhibits a distinct lobular architecture with a mixture of thin and thick blood vessels comprising the center of the lesion (Figure 2-14). Surface ulceration with fibrinoid material can be seen (Figure 2-15), sometimes with a collarette of epithelium on either side of the ulcerated area. The lobules are quite cellular and composed of small, closely packed capillaries with slit-like or indistinct lumina

(Figure 2-16). The endothelial cells are plump with bland nuclear features and scant to moderate eosinophilic cytoplasm (Figure 2-17). Mitotic activity within the lobules is readily identified. The center and superficial portions of LCH show well-formed capillaries or large angulated vessels with branching lumina. These vessels may have thick walls resembling small arteries or venules. There is usually an intimate association of spindled pericytes within the perivascular spaces. The stroma ranges from edematous to fibrotic, the latter well developed in older lesions. A variable inflammatory infiltrate composed of small lymphocytes, plasma cells, mast cells, and neutrophils is also present. The inflammatory infiltrate is most prominent in the surface of ulcerated tumors. Ulcerated tumors also exhibit a fibrinous exudate and areas indistinguishable from conventional granulation tissue (Figure 2-15).

ANCILLARY STUDIES

While unnecessary in the vast majority of cases, the endothelial cells are positive for vascular markers such as CD31, CD34, and factor VIII–RAg, as well as variable staining with estrogen and progesterone receptors. Actin stains highlight pericytes and smooth muscle cells. Reticulin will highlight the endothelial cells, while elastic stains highlight fibers in the vessel walls. Although not used in diagnosis, a clonal deletion (21) (q21.2q22.12) has been identified.

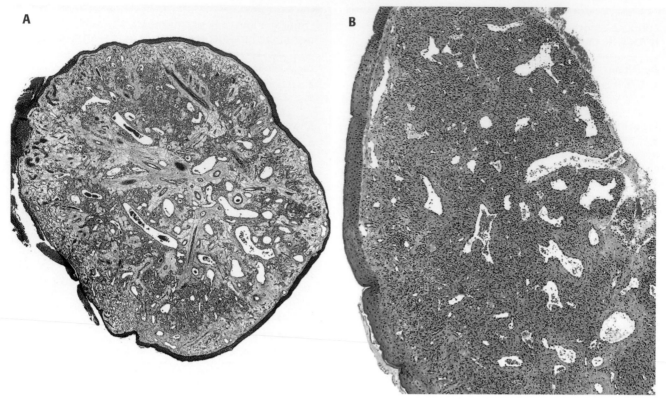

FIGURE 2-13

A, A lobular arrangement around large patulous vessels is seen in this lobular capillary hemangioma (LCH) at low power. **B**, LCH with lobular architecture demonstrating cellular lobules interspersed with larger dilated blood vessels.

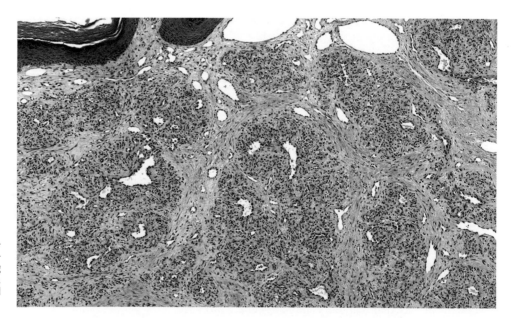

FIGURE 2-14

The surface keratinized squamous epithelium (*top left*) is overlying a well-developed lobular pattern of proliferating vessels. There is a "tight" architecture, with a central patulous vessel surrounded by slit-like vascular channels.

DIFFERENTIAL DIAGNOSIS

This benign tumor must be separated from nasopharyngeal angiofibroma (NPA), glomangiopericytoma (sinonasal-type hemangiopericytoma), and angiosarcoma. The lobular architecture is not seen in other vascular tumors. The vascular component of *NPA*, which develops exclusively in males, is separated by thin to thick collagen fibers and spindle or stellate stromal cells. *Glomangiopericytoma* is a cellular tumor composed of fascicles of oval to spindle cells with a characteristic perivascular hyalinization and interspersed mast cells and eosinophils. *Angiosarcoma* is

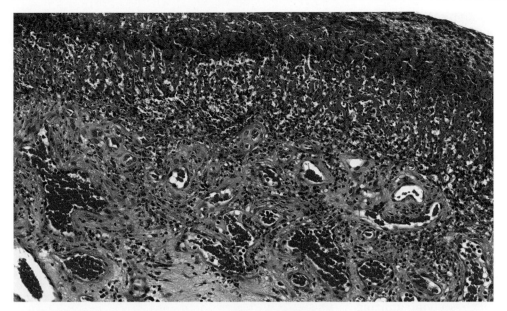

FIGURE 2-15

This lobular capillary hemangioma shows surface ulceration and a "granulation tissue–like" reaction. The characteristic lobular pattern was noted more deeply in this tumor.

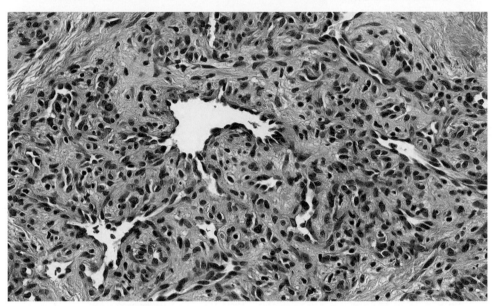

FIGURE 2-16

Central vessel surrounded by lobules of endothelial-lined capillaries. There is no significant pleomorphism and no significant inflammatory infiltrate in this image.

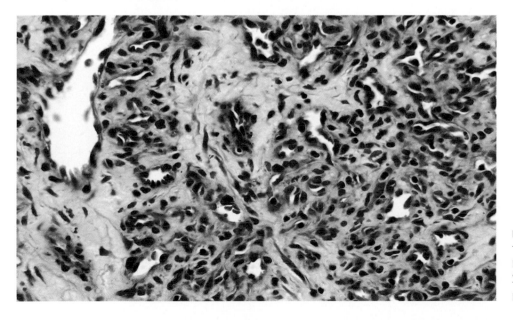

FIGURE 2-17

The lobule is quite cellular and is composed of prominent endothelial cells admixed with inconspicuous pericytes. The lobule contains and is surrounded by variably sized blood vessels.

widely infiltrative, composed of atypical endothelial cells lining freely anastomosing vascular channels, while showing increased mitoses. *Sinonasal polyps* have more of a haphazard vascular proliferation, but are surrounded by an edematous to fibrotic stroma with mucoserous glands and eosinophils.

PROGNOSIS AND THERAPY

LCHs are benign tumors which do not recur after complete resection. When recurrences are seen, they tend to develop more often in children. Axiomatic, biopsy should be avoided due to profound epistaxis, which may develop. Planning of the resection should include imaging studies to investigate the extent of the tumor and allow for possible presurgical embolization. Excision is best accomplished by wide endoscopic resection, utilizing YAG laser to control potential bleeding. The resection should include a rim of normal mucosa/submucosa. Aplasia of the nasal cartilages could result in potential disfigurement in young patients, so caution should be used in choosing between various surgical options.

■ GLOMANGIOPERICYTOMA (SINONASAL-TYPE HEMANGIOPERICYTOMA)

This tumor has been referred to by a number of names, including *hemangiopericytoma-like tumor*, *sinonasal-type hemangiopericytoma*, and *glomangiopericytoma*. This is an uncommon sinonasal tract neoplasm demonstrating perivascular myoid phenotype, showing hybrid differentiation between glomus (myoid) and hemangiopericytoma (pericytic), hence the preferred term *glomangiopericytoma (GPC)*. This lesion is distinctly different from soft tissue–type hemangiopericytoma.

CLINICAL FEATURES

GPC is a rare neoplasm (<0.5% of all sinonasal neoplasms), observed slightly more frequently in females than males (1.2:1). The age at presentation is variable and ranges from in utero to 90 years, with a mean in the 7th decade. Most patients complain of nasal obstruction, epistaxis, and less commonly, nasal discharge, pain, sinusitis, difficulty breathing, and headaches. Symptoms are usually present for less than one year. Physical examination usually reveals a unilateral, polypoid mass in the nasal cavity, with rare bilateral involvement (<5%). The paranasal sinuses are uncommonly affected. There are rare patients who have an association with osteomalacia.

GLOMANGIOPERICYTOMA—DISEASE FACT SHEET

Definition
- A sinonasal tumor demonstrating perivascular myoid phenotype

Incidence and Location
- Rare neoplasm (<0.5% of all sinonasal tract neoplasms)
- Lateral nasal cavity
- Paranasal sinuses uncommonly affected

Morbidity and Mortality
- Rare malignant tumors

Gender, Race, and Age Distribution
- Slight female predominance (1.2:1)
- Mean, 7th decade (range, in utero to 90 years)

Clinical Features
- Nasal obstruction
- Epistaxis
- Nasal discharge, pain, and headaches

Prognosis and Treatment
- Indolent neoplasm with excellent prognosis (>90% 5-yr survival)
- Recurrences in up to 30%
- Rare malignant neoplasms (2%)
- Complete surgical resection

RADIOLOGIC FEATURES

Radiologic studies are not distinctive. Plain x-rays and CT scans typically show sinus and nasal opacification by a polypoid nasal mass (Figure 2-18). Bone erosion and sclerosis are seen in a significant number of cases. There may be nonspecific sinusitis concurrently. Cribriform plate involvement is not seen.

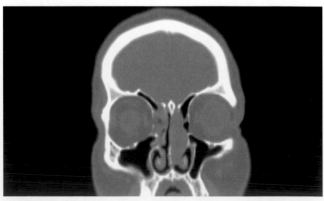

FIGURE 2-18
A computed tomography scan showing a polypoid mass filling the nasal cavity. Note there is no true bone destruction and the sinuses are unremarkable.

PATHOLOGIC FEATURES

GLOMANGIOPERICYTOMA (SINONASAL-TYPE HEMANGIOPERICYTOMA)—PATHOLOGIC FEATURES

Gross Findings

- Polypoid masses
- Mean, 3 cm
- Solid, beefy, fleshy masses with areas of hemorrhage

Microscopic Findings

- Subepithelial unencapsulated cellular tumor
- Closely packed cells, short fascicles, and storiform-whorled pattern
- Vascular channels (staghorn) demonstrating prominent peritheliomatous hyalinization
- Uniform, syncytial arrangement of oval to elongated cells
- Round to spindled nuclei
- Mast cells and eosinophils
- Moderate to severe nuclear atypia and a mitotic rate of >4 per 10 high-power fields associated with an increased risk of developing recurrent disease or dying with disease

Immunohistochemical Features

- Positive for vimentin, smooth muscle actin, muscle-specific actin, factor XIIIa
- Negative bcl-2, keratins, CD31, factor VIII–RAg, desmin, CD117

Pathologic Differential Diagnosis

- Hemangioma, solitary fibrous tumor, glomus tumor, leiomyoma, monophasic synovial sarcoma, fibrosarcoma, and malignant peripheral nerve sheath tumor

GROSS FINDINGS

The generally polypoid tumors range up to 8 cm (mean, approximately 3 cm). Tumors in female patients tend to be larger than male patients. The tumors are beefy-red to grayish-pink, soft, edematous, fleshy to friable masses, often demonstrating hemorrhage.

MICROSCOPIC FINDINGS

GPC is a subepithelial well-delineated but unencapsulated cellular tumor, effacing or surrounding the normal structures (Figure 2-19). There is usually a well-developed zone of separation between the surface epithelium and the tumor. Bone remodeling can be seen, but not true invasion. The tumor is composed of closely packed cells, forming short fascicles and sometimes exhibiting a storiform, whorled, or palisaded pattern, interspersed with many vascular channels (Figure 2-20). The latter are in the form of capillary-sized to large patulous spaces that may have a "staghorn" or "antler-like" configuration. A prominent peritheliomatous hyalinization is characteristic (Figure 2-21). The neoplastic cells are uniform, elongated to oval, and possess vesicular to hyperchromatic, round to oval to spindle-shaped nuclei, and lightly eosinophilic cytoplasm (Figure 2-22). The cells are often syncytial in appearance. Mild nuclear pleomorphism and occasional mitotic figures may be present, but necrosis is not found. Extravasated erythrocytes, mast cells, and eosinophils are nearly ubiquitously present (Figure 2-23). Occasionally, tumor giant cells (Figure 2-23), fibrosis, or myxoid degeneration may be seen. Rarely, lipomatous change and hematopoiesis

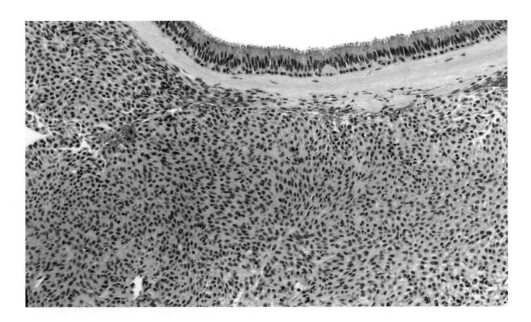

FIGURE 2-19

Characteristic diffuse growth within the submucosa with effacement of the normal components of the submucosa. The overlying respiratory epithelium remains intact, separated by dense collagenized stroma.

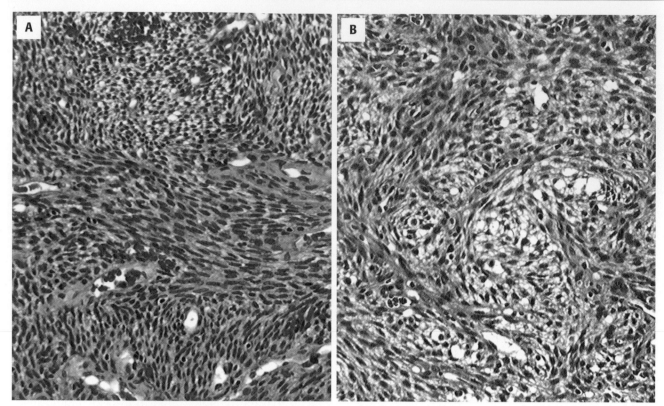

FIGURE 2-20
Closely packed cells in short fascicles (**A**) or a vague storiform pattern (**B**). Many vessels are present.

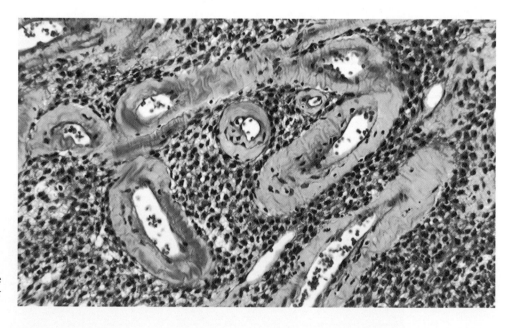

FIGURE 2-21
A characteristic histomorphologic feature is the presence of prominent perivascular hyalinization.

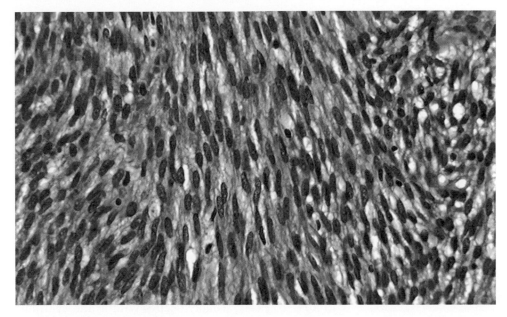

FIGURE 2-22

A syncytial arrangement of streaming, short spindled cells. The nuclei are oval. Mast cells are seen. Vascular spaces are not prominent in this field.

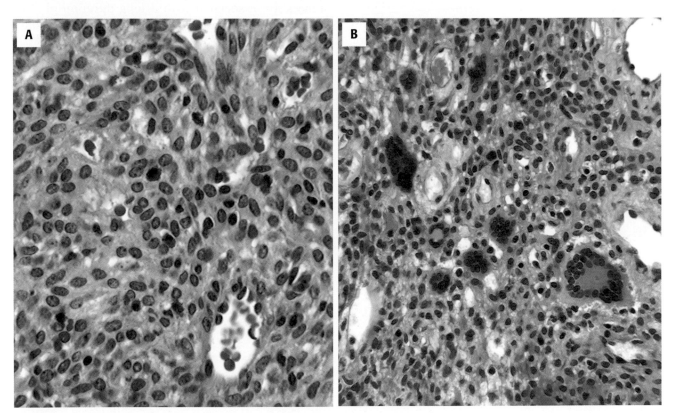

FIGURE 2-23

A, Eosinophils and mast cells are common in glomangiopericytoma, along with extravasated erythrocytes. **B**, Occasionally, tumor giant cells can be seen.

can be seen. Concurrently, other tumors may also be present, including solitary fibrous tumor, fibrosarcoma, respiratory epithelial adenomatoid hamartoma, and sinonasal polyps. Moderate to severe nuclear atypia and a mitotic rate of >4/10 high-power fields (HPFs) have been associated with an increased risk of developing recurrent disease or dying with disease.

ANCILLARY STUDIES

ULTRASTRUCTURAL FEATURES

Electron microscopy studies have shown that GPCs are composed of spindle and stellate cells surrounding non-neoplastic vessels and endothelial cells. The tumor cells contain bundles of microfilaments with dense bodies and subplasmalemmal plaques consistent with true pericytic differentiation. Micropinocytotic vesicles are demonstrable in some tumors.

IMMUNOHISTOCHEMICAL FEATURES

The tumor cells are diffusely positive for vimentin, smooth muscle actin, muscle-specific actin, FXIIIa and β-catenin (Figure 2-24). Occasional focal staining for CD34 is noted in the lesional cells, but it is not as strong as in the endothelial cells. The neoplastic cells are negative with bcl-2, keratins, CD31, factor VIII–RAg, desmin, CD99, and CD117 in the vast majority of cases.

DIFFERENTIAL DIAGNOSIS

The differential diagnosis of GPC includes a variety of benign and malignant spindle cell tumors, but usually can be limited to hemangioma, solitary fibrous tumor, glomus tumor, leiomyoma, meningioma, monophasic synovial sarcoma, fibrosarcoma, and malignant peripheral nerve sheath tumor. *Hemangiomas* are lobular, frequently exhibit surface ulceration, and do not grow in a fascicular architecture. *Solitary fibrous tumor (SFT)* is often hypocellular; has thick, ropey, stromal collagen; lacks inflammatory cells; and is diffusely positive for CD34 and bcl-2 (Figure 2-25). *Glomus tumors* are composed of round, epithelioid cells forming cellular nests with organoid appearance and are exceptionally rare in the sinonasal tract. *Leiomyomas* of the sinonasal tract show a perivascular distribution with larger spindle cells. They are desmin positive in addition to the actins. All the *sarcomas* usually have significant pleomorphism, mitotic activity, and necrosis.

PROGNOSIS AND THERAPY

GPCs are indolent, with an overall excellent survival rate (>90% 5-yr survival) achieved with complete surgical excision. Recurrence, which develops in up to 30% of cases, usually occurs within one year, but may occur many years after the initial surgery. Recurrences are associated with a long duration of symptoms, bone invasion, and severe nuclear pleomorphism. Aggressive-behaving GPC (malignant GPC) is uncommon (2%), and usually exhibits the following features: large size (>5 cm), bone invasion, severe nuclear pleomorphism, increased mitotic activity (>4/10 HPFs), atypical mitotic figures, necrosis, and proliferation index >10%.

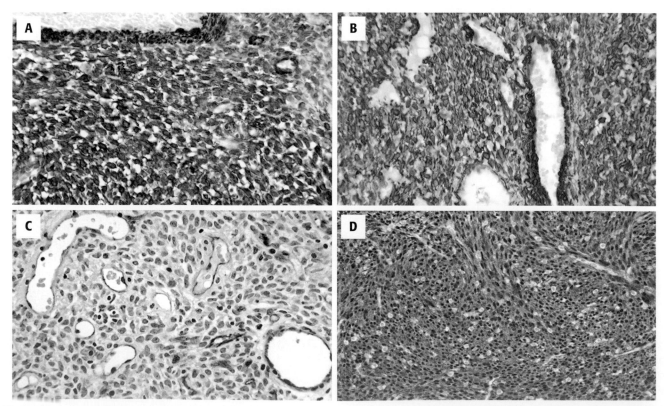

FIGURE 2-24

A variety of different immunohistochemistry studies can be seen. **A**, Muscle specific actin **B**, Smooth muscle actin. **C**, No reaction in the neoplastic cells with CD31. **D**, The nuclei and cytoplasm show a strong β-catenin reaction.

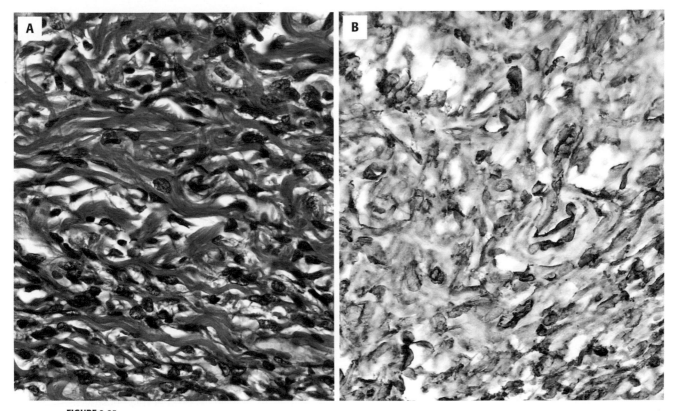

FIGURE 2-25
A, A solitary fibrous tumor has a haphazard cellular arrangement with heavy fibrosis. **B**, CD34 strongly highlights the lesional cells.

■ NASOPHARYNGEAL ANGIOFIBROMA

The term "juvenile" angiofibroma is a misnomer since angiofibromas do not arise exclusively in the young. Nasopharyngeal angiofibromas (NPAs) are benign, highly cellular and richly vascularized mesenchymal neoplasms that arise in the roof of the nose and nasopharynx in males. It is a rare tumor, accounting for <1% of all nasopharyngeal tumors, arising in the fibrovascular stroma of the posterolateral wall of the roof of the nose. Localization studies have determined that the point of origin for most NPAs is the region where the sphenoidal process of the palatine bone meets the horizontal ala of the vomer and pterygoid process. This junction forms the superior margin of the sphenopalatine foramen and the posterior margin of the middle turbinate. The tumor is thought to be testosterone dependent, with a puberty-induced growth that can be blocked with estrogen or progesterone therapy. There is a reported association with familial adenomatous polyposis.

CLINICAL FEATURES

NPA affects almost exclusively boys and adolescent to young men, with a mean age of 15 years. NPAs are uncommon tumors with an estimated incidence of 1 in 150,000 males, with fair-skinned and red-haired males more commonly affected in Caucasian patients (these features are not seen in Central and South Americans, Africans, or Asians). If a female is affected, testicular feminization has to be excluded by chromosome analysis. The most common symptoms of NPA are nasal obstruction, spontaneous epistaxis, and nasal drainage, present for 12-24 months in most patients. Other patients may present with facial deformities, proptosis, rhinolalia, deafness, sinusitis, otitis, and a bulging palate resulting from extension of the tumor into soft tissues of the face and orbit. Endoscopic examination usually shows a mass involving the posterior nasal wall. Various staging systems have been proposed, with size and location determining the outcome (Table 2-1).

RADIOLOGIC FEATURES

On plain x-rays, NPAs are characterized by a soft tissue mass causing bowing of the posterior wall of the maxillary sinus and distortion and posterior displacement of the pterygoid plates (Holman-Miller sign). Bony margins may be eroded, but are obvious. CT and MRI show the extent of the tumor as well as possible surgical approach (Figure 2-26). Angiography identifies the feeder vessel(s)

TABLE 2-1

System for Staging Juvenile Nasopharyngeal Angiofibroma

Stage	Description
Stage I	Tumor limited to the nasopharynx with no bone destruction
Stage II	Tumor invading the nasal cavity, maxillary, ethmoid, and sphenoid sinuses with no bone destruction
Stage III	Tumor invading the pterygo-palatine fossa, infratemporal fossa, orbit and parasellar region
Stage IV	Tumor with massive invasion of the cranial cavity, cavernous sinus, optic chiasm, or pituitary fossa

NASOPHARYNGEAL ANGIOFIBROMA—DISEASE FACT SHEET

Definition

- A benign, highly cellular, and richly vascularized mesenchymal neoplasm that arises in the nasopharynx in males

Incidence and Location

- Uncommon, incidence of 1/150,000 males
- <1% of nasopharyngeal tumors
- Posterior nasal wall, roof of nose and nasopharynx

Morbidity and Mortality

- Intracranial extension in some patients
- Mortality up to 9% related to hemorrhage and intracranial extension

Gender and Age Distribution

- Males (exclusively)
- Peak age, 15 years (range, 6 to 29 years)

Clinical Features

- Nasal obstruction, spontaneous epistaxis, nasal drainage
- Facial deformities, proptosis, and a bulging palate
- Sinusitis, rhinolalia, otitis, tinnitus, deafness

Radiographic Features

- Soft tissue density with bowing of the posterior maxillary sinus
- Bony margins may be eroded
- Angiography identifies feeder vessels and permits presurgical embolization

Prognosis and Treatment

- Benign but locally aggressive neoplasm
- Recurrences in about 20%, most commonly intracranial, and usually within first 2 years
- Complete surgical resection with preoperative embolization or hormonal therapy
- Radiotherapy for unresectable intracranial tumors

and allows for presurgical embolization The dense tumor blush is characteristic (Figure 2-26). Due precautions are suggested before taking biopsies from these tumors because of the risk of life-threatening bleeding.

PATHOLOGIC FEATURES

GROSS FINDINGS

Most NPAs are round or nodular, nonencapsulated masses with a sessile or pedunculated base. The tumors may be large (up to 22 cm), although the mean size is 4 cm. The surface of the tumors is largely covered by intact mucosa with focal areas of ulceration and superficial hemorrhage. The cut surface is variable and shows dilated vascular channels, which give the tumors a spongy appearance. In less vascular areas, the tumors appear solid and fibrotic (Figure 2-27).

MICROSCOPIC FINDINGS

The microscopic appearance of NPA resides in the dynamic combination of three elements: an abnormal vascular network, a connective tissue stroma, and

NASOPHARYNGEAL ANGIOFIBROMA—PATHOLOGIC FEATURES

Gross Findings

- Round or nodular, nonencapsulated masses with sessile or pedunculated base
- Intact mucosa with focal areas of ulceration and superficial hemorrhage
- Cut surface showing dilated vascular channels which give the tumors a spongy appearance or solid, fibrotic tumors
- Mean size, 4 cm

Microscopic Findings

- Combination of abnormal vascular network, a connective tissue stroma, and stromal cells
- Vascular network with variable sized vessels, from thin-walled, slit-like to large irregular vessels
- Muscle layer is absent, focal, pad-like, or circumferential
- Endothelium is attenuated, but can be plump
- Spindle, stellate, angular stromal cells in collagenized background
- Inflammatory cells usually absent
- Increased fibrosis with treatment; embolic material may be seen

Immunohistochemical Features

- Vessel walls positive with vimentin
- Endothelial cells positive for CD34, CD31, androgen, estrogen and progesterone receptors, factor VIII–RAg
- Stromal cells positive for vimentin, β-catenin, androgen receptors

Pathologic Differential Diagnosis

- Lobular capillary hemangioma, sinonasal polyps, peripheral nerve sheath tumor, solitary fibrous tumor, desmoid tumor (desmoid-type fibromatosis)

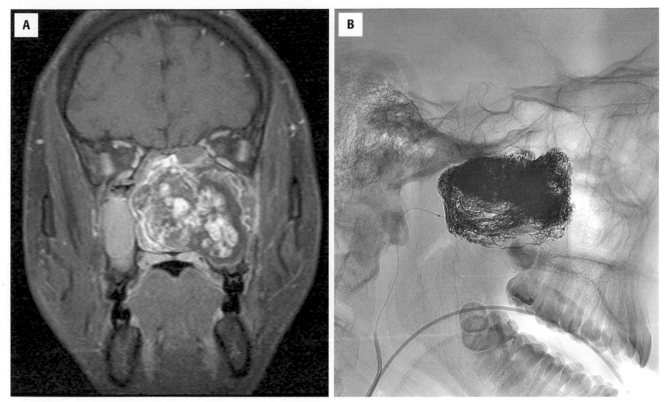

FIGURE 2-26

A, A magnetic resonance image shows a large mass within the nasopharynx, nasal cavity, and maxillary sinus. Note the bright signal within the tumor. **B**, A dense blush showing the rich vascularity of the angiofibroma.

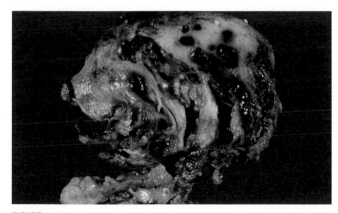

FIGURE 2-27

Nasopharyngeal angiofibroma with smooth surface. The cut surface shows a solid mass with large hemorrhagic areas corresponding to feeding vessels. Note how it is molded to the shape of the turbinate tissue as it has filled into the nasal cavity.

stromal cells (Figure 2-28). The vascular network consists of mostly thin-walled, slit-like ("staghorn") or dilated vessels, with calibers ranging from capillary to large, patulous vessels (Figure 2-29). The muscular layer can be absent, focal and pad-like, or circumferential (Figure 2-30). Elastic fibers are typically absent, one of the reasons for the profuse bleeding (vessels cannot contract down). The vascular spaces and lining endothelium appear to be resting directly on the connective tissue stroma (Figure 2-31). The endothelial cells may be plump but are usually attenuated. The fibrous connective tissue stroma consists of plump spindle, angular, or stellate-shaped cells, and a varying amount of fine and coarse collagen fibers (Figure 2-32). Focally, the stroma may be acellular with a hyalinized appearance, or show myxoid changes (especially in embolized specimens). The nuclei of the stromal cells are generally cytologically bland (Figure 2-31), but they may be multinucleated or show some degree of pleomorphism in the more cellular areas. The chromatin is finely and evenly dispersed. Large stromal cells with abundant cytoplasm resembling ganglion cells can be identified. Mitotic activity and nuclear atypia are not features of typical NPA. Mast cells may be seen, but other inflammatory elements are usually absent (except if there is surface ulceration). Long-standing lesions show increased fibrosis and diminished vasculature. Treatment with hormones results in increased collagenization of the stroma with fewer, but thicker walled vessels. In specimens excised after embolization treatment, the tumor often shows areas of infarction, and emboli can be seen in some blood vessels (Figure 2-33). Sarcomatous transformation is an exceedingly uncommon event, usually following massive doses of radiation.

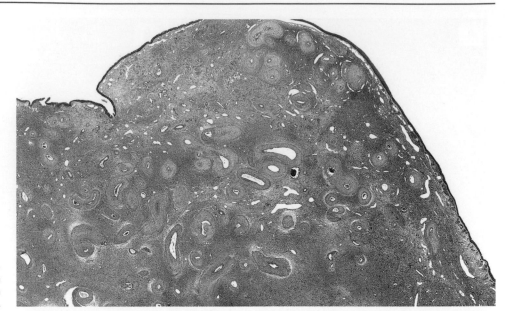

FIGURE 2-28

The intact respiratory epithelium (*top*) overlies a richly vascular neoplasm with variably sized vessels surrounded by a cellular fibroblastic stroma with collagen.

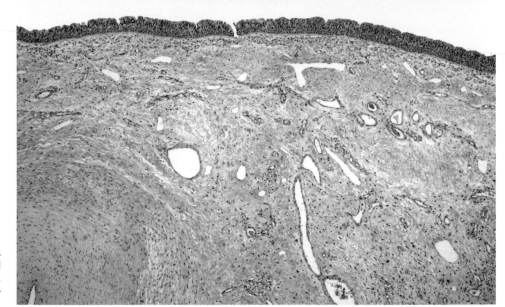

FIGURE 2-29

Smooth muscle–walled vessels, patulous vessels, and capillaries are all surrounded by the characteristic collagenized stroma. The respiratory epithelium (at the top) is uninvolved.

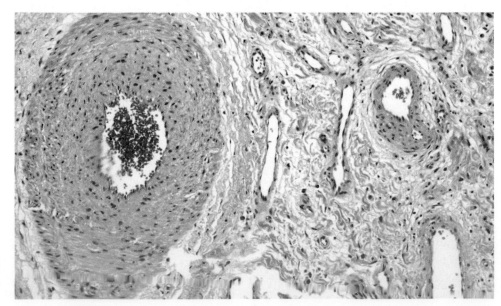

FIGURE 2-30

Note the remarkable variability in the nature of the vessels. Muscle-walled vessels, pad-like muscle, and no muscle are all seen in the vessels of this field.

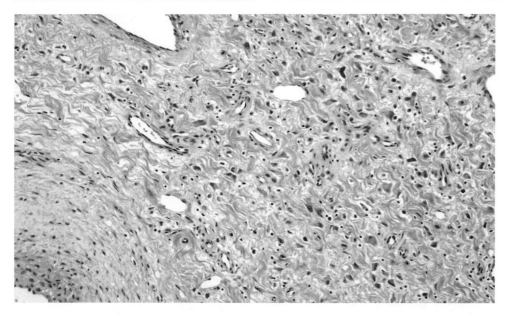

FIGURE 2-31

Thin-walled and thick-walled vessels surrounded by dense, "keloid-like" collagen. Stellate fibroblasts are noted, giving a slightly "atypical" appearance.

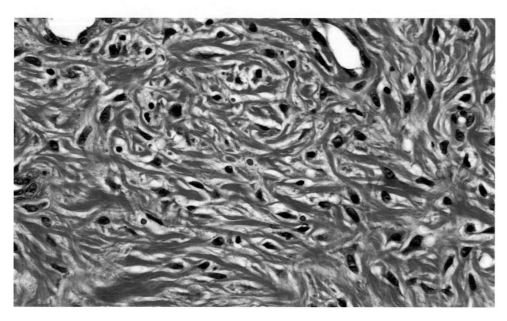

FIGURE 2-32

Heavily collagenized stroma demonstrates only a few stellate fibroblastic cells within heavily collagenized stroma, with a vessel at the top.

ANCILLARY STUDIES

ULTRASTRUCTURAL FEATURES

Ultrastructurally, the stromal cells contain lobulated nuclei, intranuclear inclusions, variable amounts of rough endoplasmic reticulum and thin filaments, hemidesmosomes, focal basal lamina, and prominent pinocytotic vesicles, suggesting a hybrid mesenchymal cell (myofibroblast). The presence of intranuclear dense bodies in stromal fibroblasts is an uncommon but characteristic feature. These nuclear bodies resemble large perichromatin granules. The stromal fibroblasts are surrounded by abundant mature collagen fibers.

IMMUNOHISTOCHEMICAL FEATURES

The vessel wall cells are immunoreactive with vimentin and smooth muscle actin (SMA; Figure 2-33), whereas the stromal cells are immunoreactive with vimentin only, except in areas of increased fibrosis, where focal SMA may be identified. Desmin may be focally immunoreactive in larger vessels at the periphery of the tumor. Factor VIII–RAg, CD34, and CD31 highlight the endothelium, but not the stromal cells. Stromal and endothelial cells are usually reactive with androgen receptors (75%), while progesterone receptors are occasionally reactive. Other markers, including nuclear staining for β-catenin, CD117, platelet-derived growth factor B, basic fibroblast growth factor, insulin-like

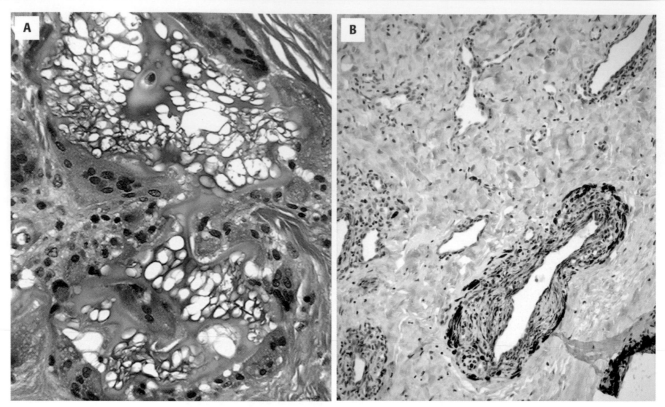

FIGURE 2-33

A, Embolic material surrounded by multinucleated giant cells in this nasopharyngeal angiofibroma. **B,** The smooth muscle can be highlighted with a smooth muscle actin immunohistochemistry, which shows the variability of muscle around the vessels.

growth factor type II, and nerve growth factor are also reactive. Epstein-Barr virus is not identified in these lesions.

DIFFERENTIAL DIAGNOSIS

The main differential diagnoses of NPA include LCH, sinonasal polyps (including antrochoanal type), peripheral nerve sheath tumors, SFT, and desmoid tumor. *LCHs* have a lobular architecture and lack the stromal cells and collagen of angiofibroma. *Polyps* with stromal atypia have inflammatory cells and lack the vascular pattern. *Peripheral nerve sheath tumors* have a fascicular architecture and are S100 protein positive. *SFTs* show increased cellularity, do not have the vascular pattern, and strongly express CD34. A desmoid tumor or *desmoid-type fibromatosis* has long sweeping fascicles and infiltrative borders without the prominent vascularity of NPA.

PROGNOSIS AND THERAPY

This benign tumor is characterized by local aggressive growth, with recurrences in about 20 % of patients (>50 % in older series), most commonly intracranial, and usually within the first 2 years after diagnosis. Mortality has ranged up to 9 % due to hemorrhage and intracranial extension, but this figure has dropped with improved radiographic and surgical techniques. Patients may be managed with selective angiographic embolization or hormonal therapy prior to definitive surgical resection (usually via a lateral rhinotomy). However, most clinicians do not wish to use hormone manipulation in pubertal males. Radiation therapy has been successfully implemented to manage large, intracranial, or recurrent tumors, but surgery is still the therapy of choice. The rare case of malignant transformation represents post radiation sarcoma.

■ ECTOPIC PITUITARY ADENOMA

A benign pituitary gland neoplasm occurring separately from and without involvement of the sella turcica (i.e., with normal anterior pituitary gland) is referred to as ectopic pituitary adenoma. Involvement of the sinonasal tract by pituitary adenomas is encountered more commonly as direct extension of an intrasellar neoplasm, while only rarely as an ectopic neoplasm. It has been estimated that secondary extension into the sinonasal tract is seen in approximately 2 % of intrasellar pituitary adenomas (which account for about 10 % to 15 % of all intracranial tumors). The sphenoid bone and sinus are the most frequent locations for ectopic lesions, although rarely the nasal cavity, nasopharynx, and petrous temporal bone may be affected. Embryologic remnants along the migration path of the Rathke pouch (infrasellar) are presumed to be the source of pituitary adenomas.

CLINICAL FEATURES

Similarly to sellar adenomas, sinonasal pituitary adenomas are more common in females than males (1.3:1), with a mean age at presentation of 54 years (range, 2-84 years). Patients usually have nonspecific complaints such as nasal obstruction, chronic sinusitis, bloody nasal discharge or epistaxis, headaches, and diplopia or other visual field defects. Up to 50% of patients affected will have clinical evidence of hormonal hyperactivity, including Cushing disease, acromegaly (growth hormone), hyperthyroidism (thyroid-stimulating hormone [TSH]), amenorrhea (prolactin, luteinizing hormone [LH], or follicle-stimulating hormone [FSH]), and hirsutism. In endocrinologically silent tumors, the diagnosis is often unsuspected before surgery. The vast majority of tumors involve the sphenoid sinus, although nasopharynx and nasal cavity can be rarely affected. Laboratory tests can be performed to detect hormone production with or without stimulation/suppression testing. Additionally, releasing hormones can also be measured.

RADIOLOGIC FEATURES

CT and MRI studies of ectopic pituitary adenomas define the extent and location of the tumor, characterized by the presence of an irregular sphenoidal or nasal mass with bone destruction in the presence of a normal pituitary gland. Thin slices or high resolution studies are required to show these features. There is usually early, intense heterogeneous enhancement. With MR, T1WI post contrast, show strong enhancement. Upward invasion with sellar involvement may be seen in large ectopic adenomas (Figure 2-34). Tumor size does not seem to correlate with symptom severity.

PATHOLOGIC FEATURES

ECTOPIC PITUITARY ADENOMA—DISEASE FACT SHEET

Definition
- A benign pituitary neoplasm occurring separately from, and without involvement of the sella turcica (a normal anterior pituitary gland)

Incidence and Location
- Rare
- Sphenoid sinus most common location followed by nasal cavity

Morbidity and Mortality
- Morbidity associated with hormonal manifestations and local invasion

Gender, Race, and Age Distribution
- Females > males (1.3:1)
- Mean age, 54 years (range, 2 to 84 years)

Clinical Features
- Nasal obstruction
- Chronic sinusitis
- Bloody nasal discharge or epistaxis
- Headaches
- Visual field defects (diplopia)
- Up to 50% have hormone hyperactivity

Radiographic Features
- CT and MR define extent and location of tumor
- Sella may be involved by upward extension, although usually normal

Prognosis and Treatment
- Excellent prognosis with control of endocrine abnormalities after complete surgical resection
- Recurrence may develop in large tumors
- Malignant transformation exceptionally rare
- Surgery is curative, but only if completely removed
- Drugs (dopamine-agonists, somatostatin analog) and radiation may be used postoperatively for control

---

ECTOPIC PITUITARY ADENOMA—PATHOLOGIC FEATURES

Microscopic Findings
- Submucosal location of unencapsulated tumor
- Tumors arranged in solid, organoid, and trabecular patterns separated by delicate fibrovascular septa
- Monotonous population of round or polygonal epithelial cells with eosinophilic cytoplasm
- Round or oval nuclei with "salt-and-pepper" chromatin and inconspicuous or small nucleoli
- Nuclear pleomorphism and mitoses are rare
- Necrosis can be seen in about one-third of cases
- Lymphovascular and perineural invasion are not identified

Ultrastructural Features
- Intracytoplasmic neurosecretory granules, type dependent on the tumor hormone production

Immunohistochemical Features
- Strong keratin, CD56, chromogranin, synaptophysin, NSE reactivity
- May stain for the hormone peptides, including ACTH, prolactin, TSH, GH, FSH, and LH or pituitary transcription factors

Pathologic Differential Diagnosis
- Olfactory neuroblastoma, neuroendocrine carcinoma, Ewing sarcoma/primitive neuroectodermal tumor, carcinoma, melanoma, lymphoma

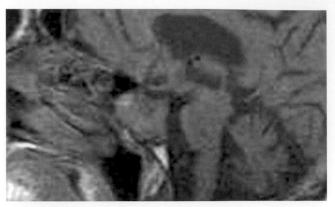

FIGURE 2-34

Large prolactinoma of sphenoidal sinus with secondary invasion of sella. Frequently, a sellar component can be identified clinically or radiographically.

MICROSCOPIC FEATURES

There is usually a polypoid, solitary mass, on average 2.9 cm in greatest dimension. The surface epithelium is usually intact and uninvolved, subtended by the unencapsulated neoplasms (Figure 2-35). Delicate fibrovascular septa separate the tumor into solid, organoid, trabecular, festoon, ribbon or glandular patterns (Figure 2-36). The neoplasms are histologically identical to their intrasellar counterparts. Most neoplasms are composed of a monotonous population of round to oval epithelial cells with

eosinophilic cytoplasm, usually characterized as chromophobe adenomas. The nuclei are round or oval and contain clumped chromatin with inconspicuous or small nucleoli (Figure 2-36). Focal pleomorphism can be seen, as with all endocrine-type neoplasms. Mitotic activity is usually limited (<3 mitoses per 10 high-power fields). Necrosis can be seen in up to one-third of cases. However, perineural and lymphovascular invasion are not seen. Bone remodeling is seen.

ANCILLARY STUDIES

ULTRASTRUCTURAL FEATURES

The identification of intracellular neurosecretory granules confirms the neuroendocrine nature of the process, with number, variable size and shape and type of granules specifically associated with hormone production. There is usually abundant and prominent rough endoplasmic reticulum and a large Golgi apparatus.

IMMUNOHISTOCHEMICAL FEATURES

The tumor cells have strong and diffuse reactions with keratin, chromogranin, synaptophysin (Figure 2-37), CD56, and neuron specific enolase. Specific hormones may be produced by the tumor, and should be sought to

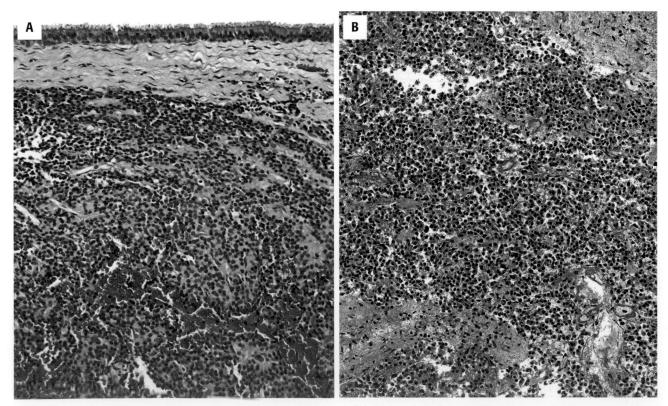

FIGURE 2-35

A, Ectopic pituitary adenoma of the sphenoid sinus underlying respiratory-ciliated mucosa. **B**, The tumor consists of lobules of monotonous epithelial cells with eosinophilic cytoplasm. Note the thin, delicate fibrovascular septa separating the tumor lobules.

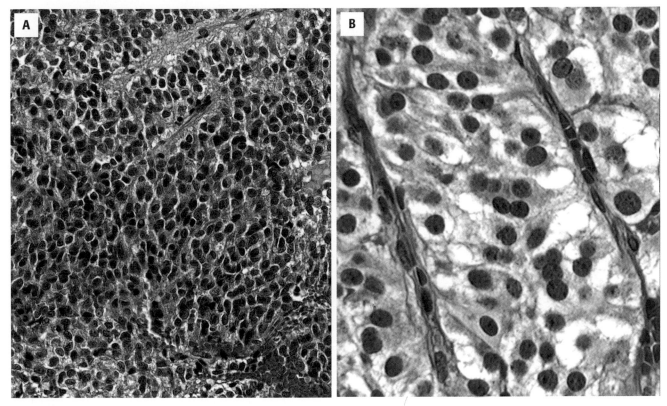

FIGURE 2-36

A, A greater degree of variability is seen in this tumor, with a more plasmacytoid appearance. The nuclear chromatin is more coarse and heavy **B**, Delicate, salt-and-pepper nuclear chromatin distribution. There are delicate fibrovascular septa.

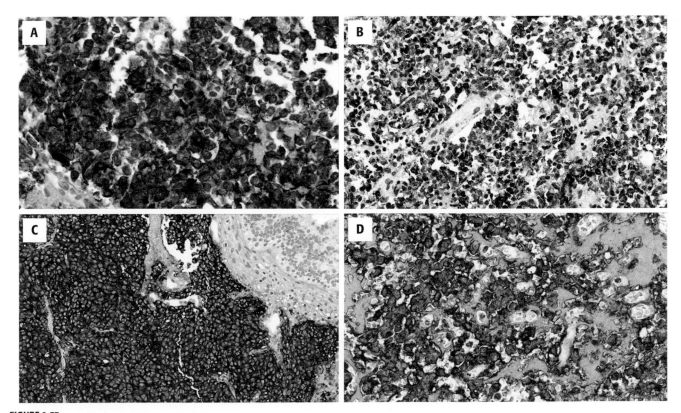

FIGURE 2-37

A, Keratin. **B**, Chromogranin. **C**, Synaptophysin. **D**, This tumor was prolactin immunoreactive. The overall "neuroendocrine" nature of the tumor can be supported by these immunohistochemistry studies.

confirm the diagnosis. These include adrenocortico-tropin (ACTH), prolactin (Figure 2-37), growth hormone, β-TSH, pituitary-specific transcription factor (Pit-1), β-subunit and α-subunit of glycoprotein hormones, soluble fibrin (SF-1), FSH, and LH. The most common immunohistochemically expressed hormones are ACTH and prolactin. Prolactin tumors tend to be chromogranin-A negative, but chromogranin-B positive. Similar to intracranial counterparts, the tumors may be mono-, pluri-, or non-hormonal.

DIFFERENTIAL DIAGNOSIS

Keen attention to the morphologic and immunopheno-typic features is necessary if the diagnosis is to be correct. Anatomic location is a key tip-off to the diagnosis. The differential diagnosis includes olfactory neuroblastoma, low-grade neuroendocrine carcinoma (carcinoid tumor), ES/PNET (Ewing sarcoma/primitive neuroectodermal tumor), carcinoma/NOS (not otherwise specified), melanoma, and lymphoma. Neuroendocrine features alone will not separate these first two lesions, but *olfactory neuroblastoma* involves the ethmoid sinus (cribriform plate), has a neurofibrillary background, rosette formation, and usually S100 protein supporting reaction and negative keratin expression. *ES/PNET* is uncommon in this location and usually has scant cytoplasm with CD99 and FLI-1 immunoreactivity, while a negative reaction with keratin and chromogranin. The separation with *carcinomas* can be extremely difficult, but the lack of lymphovascular invasion and atypical mitoses and the identification of specific pituitary hormones, pituitary transcription factors, or electron microscopy help to resolve this difficulty. *Melanoma* is confirmed by expression of melanocytic markers (HMB45, Melan-A). *Lymphoma* usually has a dispersed architecture and CD45RB immunoreactivity.

PROGNOSIS AND THERAPY

While histologically benign, there is a potential for significant morbidity related to their local mass effects (invasion into bone and cranial cavity) and hormonal manifestations. Recurrences develop, especially if the tumors are large and incompletely excised. Malignant transformation is exceptionally rare. Most tumors are amenable to complete surgical removal, with follow-up drugs or radiation therapy if necessary to control hormone symptoms. These drugs include dopamine-agonists (bromocriptine), somatostatin analogs (octreotide), corticosteroids (hydrocortisone, prednisone), and thyroxin. Stereotactic radioablation is usually employed for larger or incompletely removed tumors.

SUGGESTED READINGS

The complete suggested readings list is available online at www.expertconsult.com.

3

Malignant Neoplasms of the Nasal Cavity, Paranasal Sinuses, and Nasopharynx

■ Lester D. R. Thompson

Malignant sinonasal tract (SNT) tumors comprise <1% of all neoplasms and ~3% of those of the upper aerodigestive tract. Squamous cell carcinoma (SCC) and adenocarcinoma are strongly associated with environmental factors, including tobacco and alcohol, and occupational exposures, such as heavy metal particles (nickel, chromium) and the leather, textile, furniture, and wood industries.

SNT malignancies most commonly affect the maxillary sinus (~60%), followed by the nasal cavity (~22%), ethmoid sinus (~15%), and frontal and sphenoid sinuses (~3%). SNT tumors are diverse, with the majority composed of SCC and its variants (55%), followed by nonepithelial neoplasms (20%), glandular tumors (15%), undifferentiated carcinoma (7%), and miscellaneous tumors (3%).

Carcinoma of the nasopharynx differs in many aspects from that of the nasal cavity and paranasal sinuses and will be discussed separately.

The clinical presentations, radiologic features, and pattern of tumor spread for SCC, adenocarcinoma, and most of the other malignant neoplasms of the SNT are similar. These features will be discussed in detail under the section on SCC and not repeated elsewhere. Gross appearance of the SNT and nasopharyngeal malignancies has limited value in aiding diagnosis, because the initial diagnosis depends on tissue obtained by endoscopy or polypectomy. The treatment of choice for most SNT malignancies, with the exception of nasopharyngeal carcinoma, malignant lymphoma, and rhabdomyosarcoma (RMS), is surgical resection with clear margins. Treatment for SCC will be used as a model.

■ SQUAMOUS CELL CARCINOMA

SCC is a malignant epithelial neoplasm arising from surface epithelium with squamous cell differentiation. Also known as epidermoid carcinoma, Ringertz carcinoma, and cylindrical cell carcinoma, there are two major histologic subtypes: keratinizing and nonkeratinizing. Other variants are also recognized, although less frequently in the SNT. Schneiderian papilloma, inverted type, specifically, may be a precursor lesion in a subset of carcinomas, along with association with human papillomavirus (HPV).

CLINICAL FEATURES

SCC represents ~3% of all head and neck malignancies but is the most common malignant epithelial tumor of the SNT. SCC has a male predilection (2:1), with a peak incidence in the 6th to 7th decades. The location in order of decreasing frequency is the maxillary sinus, nasal cavity (usually lateral wall), ethmoid sinus, frontal sinus, and sphenoid sinus. Early diagnosis is difficult because symptoms and signs are nonspecific and closely resemble those of chronic sinusitis, allergic reactions, and nasal polyposis. Initial symptoms are related to the effects of the mass causing unilateral nasal obstruction. Secondary infection is common, giving rise to a mucoid or purulent rhinorrhea. Epistaxis develops when the mucosa is ulcerated or tumor extends into the sinus wall. Tumors involving the ethmoid, maxillary, or frontal sinuses may cause proptosis, restriction of eye movements, diplopia, or loss of vision. Epiphora results from lacrimal sac or duct obstruction by the tumor. Compression of the nerve at the primary site or perineural space invasion can compromise the function of cranial nerves resulting in numbness, paresthesia, or pain. Teeth loosening or fistula may be identified within the oral cavity. A mass or discolored lesion may be visualized endoscopically and biopsied.

Late manifestations include facial swelling and cheek paresthesia resulting from anterior maxillary extension into the soft tissue and infraorbital nerve involvement, respectively. Inferior extension into the oral cavity forms a visible mass in the palate or alveolar ridge. Posterior extension can cause trismus from pterygoid muscle invasion. Ear symptoms suggest possible involvement of the nasopharynx, eustachian tube, and pterygoid plates. Upward extension into the skull base may lead to cranial nerve involvement and dura invasion. In the initial workup, it is rare to find cervical lymph node metastasis.

RADIOLOGIC FEATURES

Computed tomography (CT) and magnetic resonance imaging (MRI) have largely replaced conventional radiographs in imaging SNT disease and are indispensable in evaluating the extent of disease. CT and MRI complement each other, helping to separate inflammatory disorders and benign and malignant neoplasms and to provide pretreatment information, including location, size, extent, local invasion, and regional and distant metastasis. Of particular interest is tumor extension into the pterygopalatine and infratemporal fossae, and tumor relationship to the blood vessels (especially internal carotid artery and cavernous sinus), nerves, and cranial cavity. CT best highlights bony structures, with bony destruction and soft tissue invasion usually indicative of an aggressive lesion. MRI is superior to CT in its ability to delineate sinus tumors from inflammatory disease and it can better delineate tumor from the adjacent soft tissues. Using MRI, inflamed mucosa, polyps, and noninspissated secretions with a high water content have high signal intensity on T2-weighted images. In contrast, cellular paranasal neoplasms have lesser amounts of water and demonstrate intermediate signal intensities on T2-weighted images. Perineural spread is best demonstrated by a gadolinium-contrasted MRI and T1-weighted images with fat suppression. CT helps detect cervical lymph node metastasis, especially when there are multiple, clustered lymph nodes exceeding 1.0 cm. The status of cervical lymph nodes is best determined by positron emission tomography (PET) using [18]fluorodeoxyglucose ([18]FDG-PET) to detect tissue with increased metabolism (i.e., nodal metastasis).

PATHOLOGIC FEATURES

GROSS FINDINGS

Nasal tumors are usually exophytic/fungating and prone to become friable, necrotic, and ulcerated with increasing tumor size. Sinus tumors may be well circumscribed, filling the sinus cavity in an expansile fashion with erosion of the bone wall, while others are more destructive, inverted, necrotic, and hemorrhagic.

MICROSCOPIC FINDINGS

Most authors use a three-grade system based on (a) extent of keratinization, (b) mitotic activity, and (c) nuclear features. This grading method (well, moderately, poorly differentiated) correlates to some extent with the tumor behavior. In general, SCC of the nasal cavity is well differentiated and keratinizing, whereas sinus counterparts are nonkeratinizing and moderately or poorly differentiated.

As previously mentioned, SCC is subclassified by cell type into keratinizing (80% to 85%) and nonkeratinizing (15% to 20%) subtypes. In keratinizing SCCs, it is not uncommon to see dysplasia of the adjacent or overlying surface epithelium. Tumor cells exhibit

SQUAMOUS CELL CARCINOMA—PATHOLOGIC FEATURES

Gross Findings

- Exophytic, friable, necrotic, and ulcerated mass
- Local soft tissue infiltration and bony destruction

Microscopic Findings

Nasal Cavity
- Well-differentiated, keratinizing (80% to 85%)
- Squamous pearls, intercellular bridges, hyperchromatic nuclei

Paranasal Sinus
- Moderately to poorly differentiated, nonkeratinizing
- Spindle cell, papillary, endophytic, verrucous types recognized

Immunohistochemical Features

- Positive with CK5/6, CK8, CK13, p63
- Negative with CK10

Pathologic Differential Diagnosis

- Pseudoepitheliomatous hyperplasia, Schneiderian papilloma, squamous papilloma, oropharyngeal carcinoma, *NUT* midline carcinoma

keratinization, intercellular bridges, dyskeratosis, and squamous "pearls" (Figure 3-1) and usually have enlarged, hyperchromatic nuclei, with a variable degree of nuclear anaplasia. Mitotic figures are usually easy to find and include atypical forms. Stromal invasion by irregular nests and cords of cells in a desmoplastic stroma is often associated with a chronic inflammatory response. However, in superficial biopsies, the only sign of stromal invasion may be in the form of single cells becoming isolated from the base of rete pegs or the tip of tongue-like protrusions (Figure 3-2).

The nonkeratinizing subtype of SCC forms solid nests of variable sizes, frequently with relatively smooth borders. There is a loss of polarity. Individual tumor cells reveal uniform large, round, or oval nuclei with prominent nucleoli. The cytoplasm varies from pale acidophilic to amphophilic to vacuolated. The cells may have distinct borders. Occasionally, individual cell keratinization may be identified (Figure 3-3). Spindled tumor cells may be seen, and when predominant, they are diagnosed as spindle cell SCC. Papillary and endophytic patterns can be seen. The papillary type has a dysplastic epithelium lining thin fibrovascular cores. The inverted type is often poorly differentiated, referred to as "transitional cell carcinoma" or "Schneiderian carcinoma." The tumor cells are arranged in broad sheets that have smooth borders and are surrounded by basement membrane–like material (Figure 3-3). In superficial or small biopsies, evidence of stromal invasion is usually absent. In these cases, correlation with radiologic evidence of local destruction confirms the invasive nature of the malignancy. Similarly, biopsies of verrucous squamous carcinoma and papillary squamous carcinoma are prone to be underdiagnosed without including the base of the

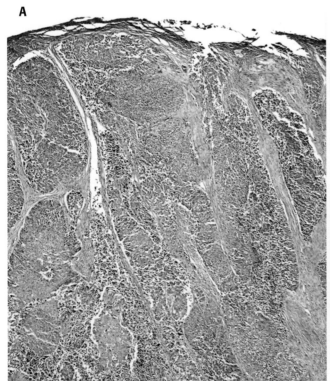
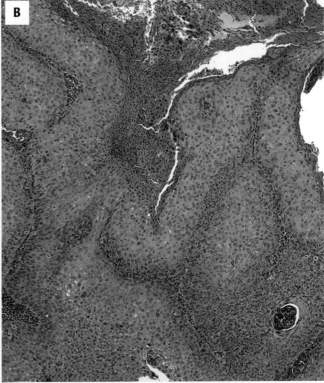

FIGURE 3-1

A, Tumor cells form solid sheets with infiltrative borders and stromal fibrosis in this nonkeratinizing squamous cell carcinoma. **B**, A papillary configuration with remarkable atypia and parakeratosis.

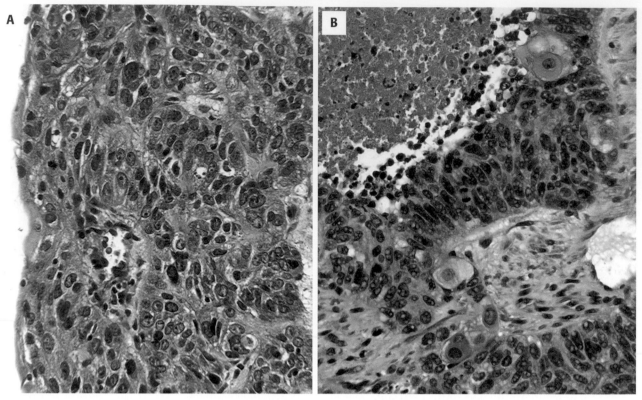

FIGURE 3-2

A, Poorly-differentiated squamous cells show irregular hyperchromatic nuclei, small nucleoli, and a moderate amount of cytoplasm. **B**, Isolated foci of individual cell keratinization in this otherwise basaloid squamous cell carcinoma. Note the area of necrosis (*upper left*).

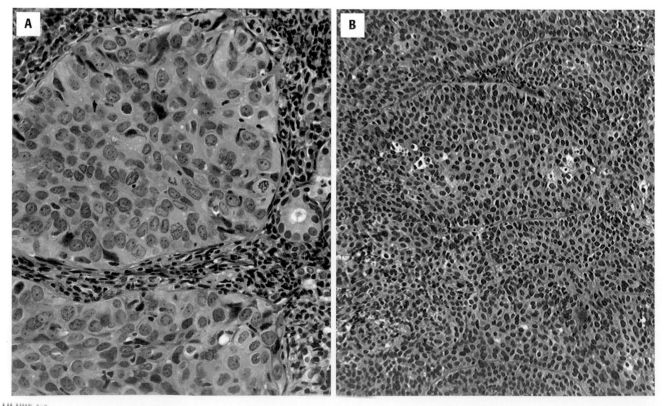

FIGURE 3-3

A, Obvious cytologic atypia and loss of polarity are seen within the invasive tumor nests. There are mitoses. **B**, Sheets of smooth bordered "transitional"-type epithelium comprise this nonkeratinizing squamous cell carcinoma.

lesion. Variants of SCC, such as verrucous carcinoma and basaloid type, are rare in the SNT.

ANCILLARY STUDIES

Although the diagnosis of SCC seldom requires immunohistochemistry, the cells are immunoreactive with CK5/6, CK8, CK13, and p63 but negative with CK10. Some nonkeratinizing SCCs are reported to be p16 positive but are Epstein-Barr virus encoded RNA, or EBER, negative.

DIFFERENTIAL DIAGNOSIS

Pseudoepitheliomatous hyperplasia in the SNT region is most commonly associated with mucosal ulcer with or without prior medical interventions and may be associated with rhinoscleroma, fungal infection, and neoplastic disease (granular cell tumor, lymphoma, and fibrohistiocytic tumors). The elongated and thickened rete pegs extend into the underlying connective tissue and have smooth, sharp, and sometimes pointed borders. There is no desmoplastic stroma. The cells resemble each other and have uniform nuclei without nuclear atypia and rare mitotic figures. *Schneiderian* and *squamous papillomas* may occasionally have malignant transformation, with areas of squamous dysplasia and carcinoma in situ. Schneiderian papillomas have inverted epithelial growth, with admixed mucocytes and intraepithelial inflammatory cysts. They lack desmoplasia, single cell invasion, and atypical mitoses. When broad sheets of cytologically malignant squamous cells are seen in biopsies, the diagnosis of SCC should be considered, even though stromal invasion is not demonstrable. Clinical and radiologic findings should be requested to aid decision making. *Oropharyngeal carcinoma* arises from a different site, may show comedonecrosis with a basaloid pattern and associated lymphoid infiltrate, and usually has a strong p16 or HPV reaction. *NUT midline carcinoma*, defined by the balanced chromosomal translocation t(15;19) resulting in *BRD4-NUT* oncogene, tends to be a poorly differentiated carcinoma with squamous differentiation and CD34 immunoreactivity; however, it requires molecular studies to confirm the diagnosis.

PROGNOSIS AND THERAPY

If SCC is confined to the nasal cavity, the 5-year survival rate is in the range of 80%, dependent on keratinization, tumor grade, and stage. Clinical stage is most important, while nonkeratinizing tumors have a better prognosis than keratinizing carcinomas. Involvement of the paranasal sinuses adversely affects the prognosis. Most treatment failures are related to locally advanced disease and tumor recurrence in areas inaccessible to surgical resection, such as skull base, dura, and brain. Local recurrences are seen in up to 45%, with spread to adjacent structures. Cervical lymph node metastasis develops in up to 20% of patients with uncommon distant metastases. Patients are at a higher risk for the development of a second primary.

Treatment depends on the tumor location and extent. T1 and T2 nasal tumors are treated by surgical resection, while T3 and T4 tumors receive postoperative radiotherapy. Various surgical approaches are employed, matched to the complex anatomy of the region, with cosmetic reconstruction as permitted. Adjuvant radiotherapy is usually employed, with variable protocols based on tumor type. Chemotherapy may be used neoadjuvantly or postoperatively.

■ SINONASAL ADENOCARCINOMA

Malignant glandular neoplasms of the SNT can originate from the respiratory epithelium or the underlying mucoserous glands, with the majority arising from the mucoserous glands (60%). The respiratory epithelial derived tumors tend to develop high in the nasal cavity and ethmoid sinus, while salivary gland neoplasms develop more frequently in the lower nasal cavity and maxillary sinus. SNT adenocarcinomas are separated into salivary gland, intestinal and nonintestinal types. By definition, the intestinal-type adenocarcinomas are malignant epithelial glandular tumors of the SNT that histologically resemble intestinal adenocarcinoma.

CLINICAL FEATURES

SALIVARY GLAND–TYPE ADENOCARCINOMA

The genders are equally affected with a wide age range, although most are older patients (mean, 55 years). The majority develop in the maxillary sinus (~60%) or a combination of sinuses and nasal cavity. Symptoms are nonspecific and include obstructive symptoms, epistaxis, and pain. Palatal swelling may be seen.

NON–SALIVARY GLAND–TYPE ADENOCARCINOMA

These are divided into two major categories: intestinal-type adenocarcinoma and nonintestinal-type adenocarcinoma (also nonenteric or seromucinous adenocarcinoma). The intestinal type has a strong male predominance (about 90%), and tends to affect older

---

SINONASAL TRACT ADENOCARCINOMA—DISEASE FACT SHEET

Definition
- Salivary gland–type adenocarcinoma arising from mucoserous glands (60%)
- Non–salivary gland–type adenocarcinoma arising from respiratory mucosa

Incidence and Location
- Second most common carcinoma of sinonasal tract
- 15% of sinonasal tract carcinomas
- Paranasal sinuses > nasal cavity

Morbidity and Mortality
- Salivary gland–type adenocarcinomas have 40% to 60% mortality
- Non–salivary gland–type adenocarcinomas have ~60% mortality, but grade dependent

Gender and Age Distribution
Salivary Gland–Type Adenocarcinoma
- Equal gender distribution
- 3rd to 8th decades, mean: 55 years

Non–Salivary Gland–Type Adenocarcinoma
- Male >>> female (specifically with industrial exposure)
- 5th to 7th decades (low grade: 6th decade; high grade: 7th decade)

Clinical Features
- Unilateral nasal obstruction
- Epistaxis
- Purulent or clear rhinorrhea
- Pain or visual disturbances if large
- Intestinal-type has very strong association with wood workers and leather workers (500× increased incidence)

Radiographic Findings
- CT and MRI define extent of the tumor and identify invasion

Prognosis and Treatment
Salivary Gland–Type Adenocarcinoma
- Prognosis depends on stage and tumor type (~50% 10-year survival for adenoid cystic carcinoma)
- Recurrences common (60%)
- Complete surgical resection with optional radiation

Non–Salivary Gland–Type Adenocarcinoma (Intestinal Type)
- 80% 5-year survival for papillary intestinal-type adenocarcinoma, but 40% overall survival for poorly differentiated carcinoma (histologic grade dependent)
- Recurrence in 50% of patients
- Complete surgical resection with radiation

---

aged males (mean, 5th to 7th decades). There is a well-known occupational exposure, specifically in wood workers and leather workers. While the carcinogenic substance is unknown, it is thought to be particulate in nature, as spouses of these workers also have an increased risk. Prolonged occupational exposure, frequently over decades, is necessary for development These tumors tend to occur in the ethmoid sinus and

nasal cavity, specifically the lower and middle turbinate in the latter. Unilateral obstruction, rhinorrhea, and epistaxis are the most common symptoms.

The nonintestinal-type adenocarcinomas are separated into low- and high-grade adenocarcinoma. Tumors tend to develop in men slightly more commonly, although high-grade tumors are much more common in men than in women. There is a wide age range, although low-grade tumors tend to occur in patients about a decade younger than those with high-grade tumors (54 years vs. 63 years, respectively). The nasal cavity and ethmoid sinus tend to be affected more commonly than other sites.

PATHOLOGIC FEATURES

GROSS FINDINGS

Salivary gland–type adenocarcinomas tend to be large, firm, solid masses, extensively infiltrative at the time of diagnosis. Intestinal-type adenocarcinomas tend to be fungating, with an ulcerated friable surface. Cut surface reveals gray, translucent, mucoid parenchyma.

SINONASAL TRACT ADENOCARCINOMA—PATHOLOGIC FEATURES

Gross Findings
Salivary Gland–Type Adenocarcinoma
- Large, firm, solid, submucosal mass

Non–Salivary Gland–Type Adenocarcinoma
- Fungating, ulcerated, and friable mass, often mucoid to translucent

Microscopic Findings
Salivary Gland–Type Adenocarcinoma
- Adenoid cystic carcinoma most common, with cribriform and cystic pattern, small basaloid cells with hyperchromatic nuclei

Non–Salivary Gland–Type Adenocarcinoma
- Intestinal and nonintestinal types
- Papillary, colonic, solid, mucinous, and mixed types
- Usually tall, nonciliated, columnar cells, mucin producing
- Tumor grade determines nuclear features
- Frequently have background of necrosis and inflammation

Immunohistochemical Features
- **Intestinal types** are CK7, CK20, CDX-2, villin, mCEA, MUC2, MUC5, BRST-1, and B72.3 positive
- **Nonintestinal types** are CK7 and S100 positive, but negative for CK20, CDX-2, villin, and MUCs
- p53, EGFR, c-erbB-2 expression, and *RAS* mutation provide prognostic value

Pathologic Differential Diagnosis
- Schneiderian papilloma, hamartoma, metastatic colon carcinoma, lymphoma, olfactory neuroblastoma

MICROSCOPIC FINDINGS

Salivary Gland–Type Adenocarcinoma

Adenoid cystic carcinoma (ACC) is the most common salivary gland–type adenocarcinoma to occur in the SNT. Other salivary gland–type tumors, such as mucoepidermoid carcinoma, acinic cell carcinoma, and low-grade papillary adenocarcinoma, rarely involve this region. ACC is invasive with perineural and bone invasion, composed of small basaloid cells with hyperchromatic nuclei and scant cytoplasm arranged in tubules, cribriform glands, and solid sheets. Reduplicated basement membrane material and bluish glycosaminoglycan material within the spaces are common (Figure 3-4). Predominantly solid ACC can be distinguished from undifferentiated small cell carcinomas and basaloid SCC by its lower mitotic activity and the presence of myoepithelial cell differentiation by immunohistochemistry.

Non–Salivary Gland–Type Adenocarcinoma

This is a heterogeneous group of tumors that is divided into intestinal and nonintestinal types, with the intestinal type further separated into papillary (~25%), colonic (~45%), solid (~18%), mucinous/colloid (5%), and mixed (7%) types (Barnes classification).

Intestinal-Type Adenocarcinoma

Intestinal-type adenocarcinoma is made up of absorptive cells and goblet cells forming glands, nests, and mucin. The degree of differentiation varies. Some are extremely well differentiated, having the appearance of colonic tubular and villous adenomas, with nuclear stratification and mild nuclear atypia (Figure 3-5). Some tumors contain small intestinal-type cells, such as Paneth cells and enterochromaffin cells (Figure 3-6). Occurring at the base of glands are a few layers of smooth muscle cells simulating muscularis mucosae. Other tumors resemble moderately differentiated colonic adenocarcinoma with confluent glands (Figure 3-7), nuclear pleomorphism, prominent nucleoli, and increased mitotic activity. Some tumor cells produce abundant mucinous material (Figure 3-7), while others have signet-ring formation. Necrosis is common, while multinucleated giant cells may be seen reacting to extravasated mucin. Papillary and solid patterns are recognized (Figure 3-7). In biopsies, the presence of mucous pools and necrotic debris dissecting between the stroma creating an alveolar pattern should raise the suspicion of the possibility of malignancy. In all cases, the patient should be examined for evidence of intestinal tumor before the neoplasm is accepted as a primary lesion of the upper respiratory tract.

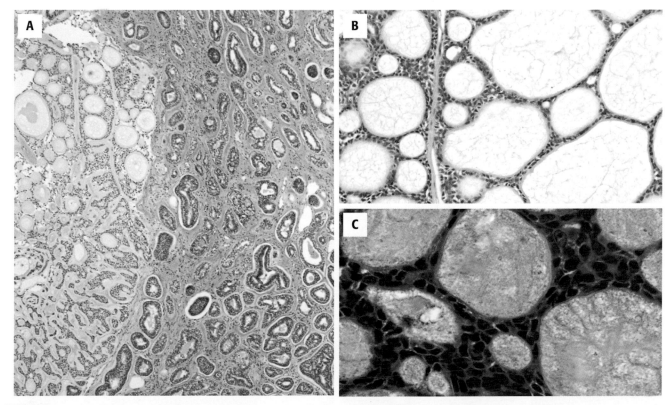

FIGURE 3-4

Adenoid cystic carcinoma. **A**, Tumor cells predominantly form tubules with abundant hyalinized stroma. Some cribriforming is present. **B** and **C**, Small cells with hyperchromatic, angular nuclei surround blue mucinous or pale material.

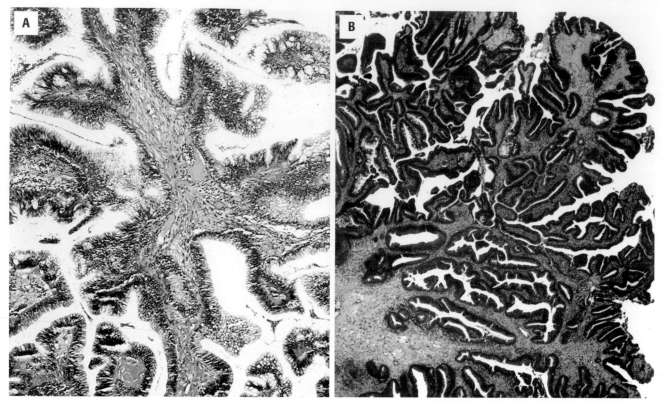

FIGURE 3-5

A and **B**, This intestinal-type adenocarcinoma resembles villous adenoma of colon with multiple papillary projections, smooth muscle within the septa, and nuclear stratification.

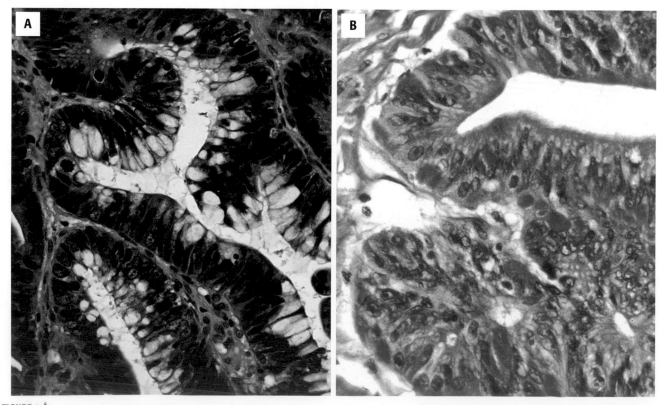

FIGURE 3-6

A, Tumor cells within an intestinal-type adenocarcinoma (ITAC) demonstrate stratification, elongation, hyperchromasia, and mucinous differentiation. Note the mitoses. **B**, Stratified nuclei with mild nuclear atypia and Paneth cells (showing abundant granular eosinophilic cytoplasm) in an ITAC.

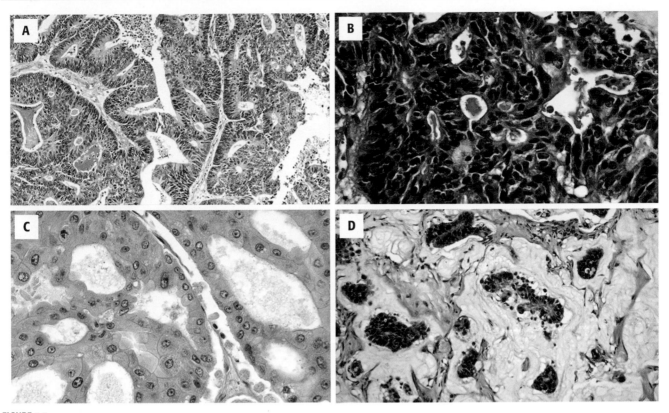

FIGURE 3-7

Intestinal-type adenocarcinomas can have a variety of different appearances, including moderately differentiated adenocarcinoma with cribriform glands with central comedonecrosis (**A**); more poorly differentiated glands and nuclear stratification (**B**); an oncocytic appearance with mitoses (**C**); and neoplastic glands producing and floating in abundant mucin (**D**).

Nonintestinal-Type Adenocarcinoma

The nonintestinal-type adenocarcinomas are also divided into low grade and high grade, based on architecture, nuclear features, and mitotic activity. Low-grade adenocarcinomas are submucosal, unencapsulated proliferation of uniform cells arranged in compact acini, back-to-back, confluent glands, cystic spaces, and papillae (Figure 3-8). They maintain nonciliated tall columnar to cuboidal configuration and are arranged in a single layer with basal nuclei lacking nuclear stratification. The cytoplasm is abundant, but variable in appearance, eosinophilic (Figure 3-8), basophilic, granular, or clear-mucinous. The nuclear atypia is mild to moderate. Nucleoli may be prominent. The mitotic activity is generally low. High-grade adenocarcinomas are usually invasive, with angioinvasion, neurotropism, and bone destruction. They are often solid, demonstrating necrosis, nuclear pleomorphism, prominent nucleoli, and high mitotic activity. Some contain abundant signet-ring cells. Special stains are helpful to identify mucus secretion.

ANCILLARY STUDIES

Mucicarmine positive material is usually easily identified both intracytoplasmic and intraluminal. Most adenocarcinomas do not require immunohistochemical stains. *ACC* is keratin, CK7, S100 protein, calponin, and p63 positive. *Intestinal-type adenocarcinomas* show keratin, CK20 (up to 86%; Figure 3-9), CDX-2 (Figure 3-9), villin, CK7, EMA, B72.3, BRST-1, mCEA, and MUC2 and MUC5 immunoreactivity. Various neuroendocrine markers may also be present (chromogranin, synaptophysin, CD56). p53, epidermal growth factor receptor (EGFR), and c-erbB-2 may provide prognostic information. There may be an increased proliferation rate with Ki-67. *K-* or *H-RAS* point mutations tend to be associated with a poor prognosis. The *nonintestinal-type adenocarcinomas* are positive with keratins, including CK7 (Figure 3-9) and even S100 protein, but are negative with CK20, CDX-2, villin, and MUCs. Myoepithelial markers (p63, calponin) are negative, as are neuroendocrine markers.

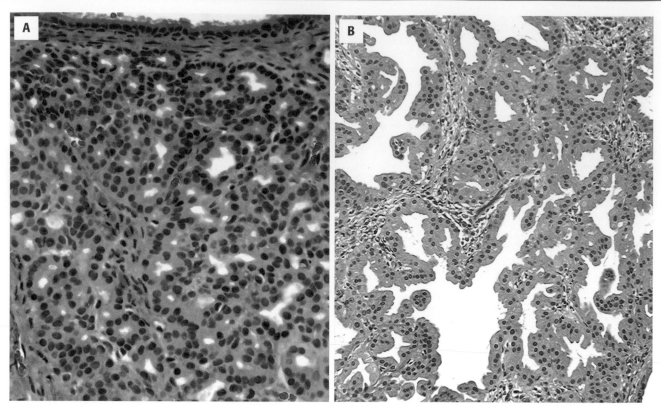

FIGURE 3-8

A, This nonintestinal-type low-grade adenocarcinoma shows complex glands with nuclear atypia, but no stratification. There is an intact overlying respiratory epithelium. **B**, A complex papillary architecture, lined by cuboidal cells with low nuclear atypia.

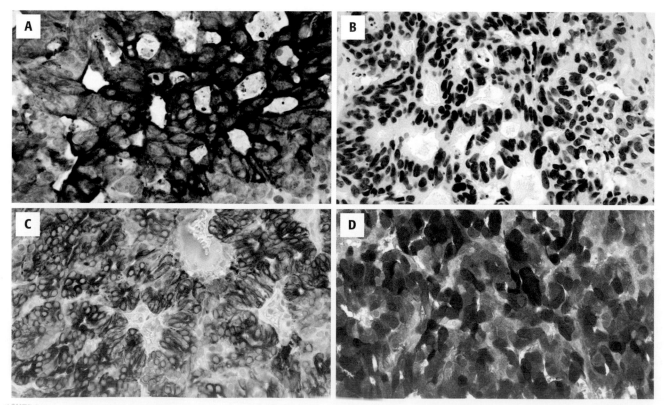

FIGURE 3-9

Intestinal-type adenocarcinomas will be positive with selected immunohistochemistry studies including CK20 (**A**) and CDX-2 (**B**). Nonintestinal adenocarcinomas are positive with CK7 (**C**) and may show a strong reaction with S100 protein (**D**).

DIFFERENTIAL DIAGNOSIS

Adenoid cystic carcinoma must be separated from high-grade carcinomas, lymphoma, and olfactory neuroblastoma. *Schneiderian papilloma* (oncocytic variant specifically) with their complex back-to-back, confluent glands and papillary architecture may be overdiagnosed as low-grade adenocarcinoma or mucoepidermoid carcinoma, but the cells are cytologically benign. *Papillary sinusitis* lacks dysplasia and infiltration. *Hamartomas* have widely separated glands with ciliated, stratified nuclei and thick basement membranes. *Metastatic adenocarcinoma* of gastrointestinal origin and clear cell tumors of any site must be excluded.

PROGNOSIS AND THERAPY

The overall 10-year survival rate for ACC is 40% to 60%. Aggressive local therapy is warranted even in patients with distant metastases, since a significant number of patients will live for many years with their disease. Recurrences are common (up to 60%). The treatment of choice for ACC is surgical resection with clear margins often accompanied by postoperative radiotherapy to improve local control, especially in cases with positive or close margins. The propensity for perineural spread makes obtaining clear margins difficult.

Among patients with non–salivary gland–type adenocarcinoma, histologic grade affects outcome. Well-differentiated tumors with predominantly papillary and tubular structures have better prognosis (80% 5-year survival) than their poorly differentiated counterparts (40% 5-year survival). Patients with industrial exposure have a better outcome than the sporadic cases, but perhaps because they are detected earlier due to regular surveillance. Recurrences develop in ~50% of patients with distant metastasis in ~15%. Overall survival is ~40%, with death in ~3 years. Treatment is radical surgical resection with postoperative radiotherapy.

■ SINONASAL UNDIFFERENTIATED CARCINOMA

Sinonasal undifferentiated carcinoma (SNUC) is a rare and highly aggressive undifferentiated carcinoma, showing extensive local destruction, histologic pleomorphism, and necrosis, separate from olfactory neuroblastoma. The taxonomy is not well developed or accepted, but it is considered a distinctive carcinoma of the SNT of uncertain histogenesis lacking squamous or glandular differentiation. There is no known etiology, although isolated EBER-positive cases are reported in Asians.

CLINICAL FEATURES

SINONASAL UNDIFFERENTIATED CARCINOMA—DISEASE FACT SHEET

Definition
- High-grade aggressive undifferentiated carcinoma with extensive local disease, lacking squamous and glandular differentiation

Incidence and Location
- Rare
- Nasal cavity, maxillary sinus, ethmoid sinus, often combined

Morbidity and Mortality
- Mortality of 80% in 5 years

Gender And Age Distribution
- Male > female (2 to 3:1)
- Wide age range (20 to 76 years); mean: 6th decade

Clinical Features
- Nasal obstruction and/or epistaxis of short duration
- Proptosis, periorbital swelling, and facial pain
- Destructive lesion
- May have cranial nerve involvement

Prognosis and Treatment
- Median survival is <18 months
- About 30% have cervical lymph node metastasis
- Combination multimodality therapy (surgery, chemotherapy, radiation)

This type of undifferentiated carcinoma is a distinct clinicopathologic entity. The majority of patients present with locally advanced disease with frequent bony, cranial, or orbital involvement at diagnosis. The median age is in the 6th decade with a male predominance (2 to 3:1). Previous radiation may be an etiologic factor. Patients have nonspecific symptoms, indistinguishable from other SNT tumors, but the symptoms are usually of short duration (rapid onset of symptoms). The nasal cavity, maxillary sinus, and ethmoid sinus are usually involved, frequently showing spread into directly contiguous sites (Figure 3-10).

PATHOLOGIC FEATURES

GROSS FINDINGS

Tumors are usually large (>4 cm) and fungating with poorly defined margins and show bony destruction (Figure 3-11).

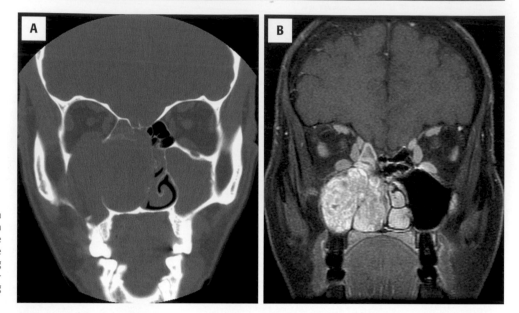

FIGURE 3-10

A, A computed tomography scan shows a large, destructive mass within the right maxillary sinus, filling the nasal cavity, and expanding into the orbit. **B**, Magnetic resonance imaging of the same patient shows the significant extent of the tumor, highlighting the soft tissue component.

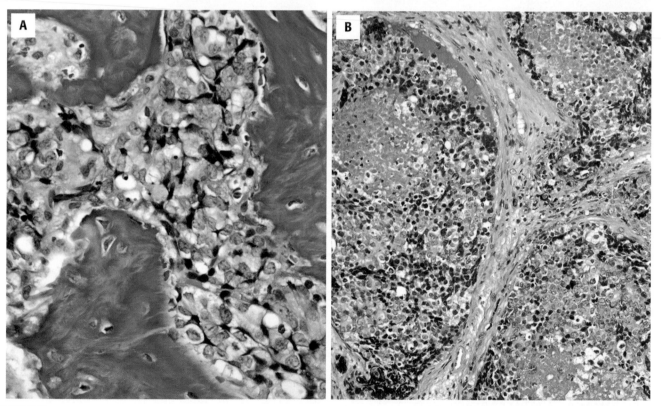

FIGURE 3-11

A, Bone invasion by the undifferentiated neoplastic epithelial cells of sinonasal undifferentiated carcinoma. **B**, There is often a lobular architecture, showing central comedonecrosis.

MICROSCOPIC FEATURES

The tumor is hypercellular, arranged in nests, lobules (Figure 3-11), trabecular, and sheets, without any squamous or glandular differentiation. Surface involvement is rare, but ulceration may preclude such a determination. The large polygonal cells have a high nuclear:cytoplasmic ratio with medium-size to large nuclei surrounded by scant eosinophilic cytoplasm (Figure 3-12). The chromatin may be hyperchromatic to hypochromatic, with inconspicuous to prominent single nucleoli. Necrosis, including comedonecrosis, is common. Mitotic figures are increased. Lymphovascular invasion and neurotropism are common findings. Three cell types are described, but they do not alter the diagnosis.

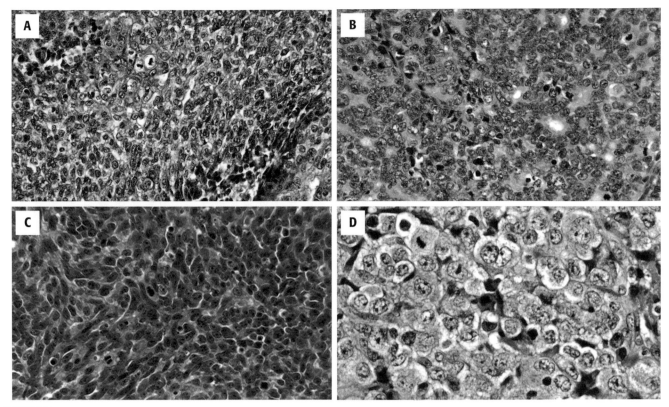

FIGURE 3-12

A number of different patterns of growth and cytologic appearances can be seen in sinonasal undifferentiated carcinoma (SNUC). **A**, A sheet of malignant small tumor cells reveals nuclear molding, resulting from high nuclear:cytoplasmic ratios. There is a "suggestion" of squamous differentiation. **B**, A number of rosettes can be seen in SNUC. **C**, The neoplastic cells have a molded appearance, single nucleolus, and increased mitoses. **D**, Vesicular open nuclear chromatin with prominent nucleoli. Note the lack of an inflammatory infiltrate.

SINONASAL UNDIFFERENTIATED CARCINOMA—PATHOLOGIC FEATURES

Gross Findings

- Large fungating mass (>4 cm) with bone destruction/invasion

Microscopic Findings

- Hypercellular tumor arranged in nests, lobules, and sheets of undifferentiated cells (no squamous or glandular differentiation)
- Polygonal cells with high nuclear:cytoplasmic ratio with medium to large nuclei and single, variable nucleoli
- High mitotic activity
- Tumor necrosis, lymphovascular invasion, perineural invasion are common

Immunohistochemical Features

- Usually pan-keratin, CK7, CK8, CK19 positive
- Occasionally EMA, NSE, p53, p63, chromogranin/synaptophysin positive
- Rarely is S100 protein and CD99 positive

Pathologic Differential Diagnosis

- Olfactory neuroblastoma, neuroendocrine carcinoma, lymphoma, melanoma, rhabdomyosarcoma, Ewing sarcoma/primitive neuroectodermal tumor, *NUT* midline carcinoma

ANCILLARY STUDIES

The majority of tumors react with keratins (simple keratins, especially CK7, CK8, and CK19). Epithelial membrane antigen (EMA), neuron-specific enolase (NSE), and p53 may be positive. Chromogranin and synaptophysin are occasionally positive, as is p63. CK5/6, CK13, and CK14 are negative, as is EBER (in Western patients).

DIFFERENTIAL DIAGNOSIS

Separation of SNUC from olfactory neuroblastoma (ONB) and neuroendocrine carcinoma remains controversial. *ONB* has a specific anatomic site of involvement, lobular architecture, and neural features and is typically keratin negative. *Neuroendocrine carcinomas* may overlap with SNUC, a separation that at present does not have clinical implications. Immunohistochemical stains are valuable to diagnose nasopharyngeal carcinoma, lymphoma, melanoma, RMS, and Ewing sarcoma/primitive neuroectodermal tumor (ES/PNET) (Table 3-1). A *NUT midline carcinoma* may appear undifferentiated, showing abrupt keratinization and CD34 immunoreactivity, along with t(15;19) fusion gene *BRD4-NUT*.

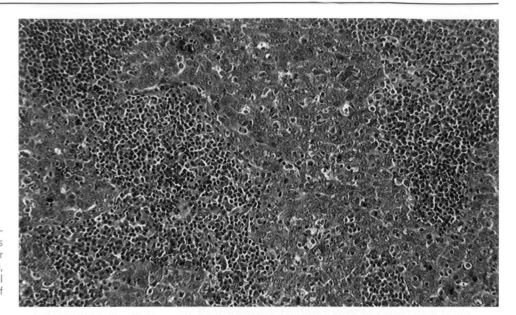

FIGURE 3-13

Loosely cohesive tumor cells are inter-mingled with small lymphocytes in this nonkeratinizing carcinoma. The tumor cells have large round to oval nuclei, prominent nucleoli, and ill-defined cell borders. There is a nearly 1:1 ratio of lymphoid cells to epithelial cells.

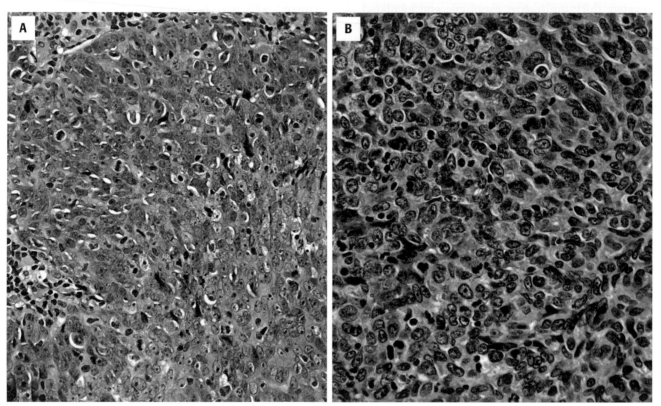

FIGURE 3-14

A, A syncytium of neoplastic cells with very high nuclear:cytoplasmic ratio. Note the prominent nucleoli within vesicular nuclei. **B**, The epithelial cells may be polygonal to spindled, usually associated with inflammatory cells.

ANCILLARY STUDIES

NPCs as a group show strong and diffuse reactions with pan keratin, often highlighting wisps of cyto-plasm in a reticular pattern as they surround lympho-cytes (Figure 3-16). High-molecular-weight keratins

(CK5/6 [Figure 3-16], 34βE12) are positive, while CK7 and CK20 are negative. p63 shows a strong nuclear reaction (Figure 3-16), while p16 is negative. EBV is found in nearly 100% of tumors, but the technique and antigen sought influence the positivity rate: EBV latent membrane protein 1 (LMP1) is weak, patchy,

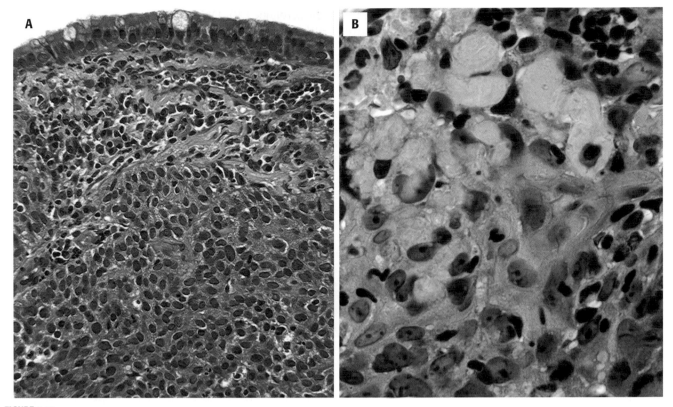

FIGURE 3-15

A, This is a more "differentiated" appearance to nasopharyngeal nonkeratinizing carcinoma. Note the intact respiratory epithelium. Inflammatory cells are present at the periphery. **B**, In a few cases, amyloid deposits may be seen, usually immediately adjacent to the malignant epithelial cells.

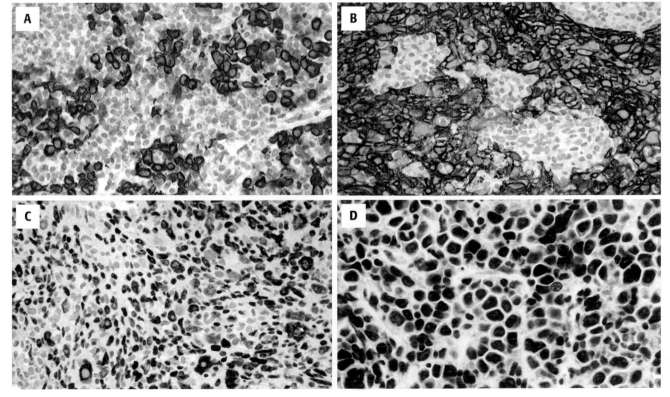

FIGURE 3-16

Nasopharyngeal carcinoma usually reacts with a variety of different immunohistochemical studies, including pan-keratin (**A**); CK5/6, which reveals strong membrane reaction (**B**); p63 nuclear stain in the epithelial component (**C**); and strong and diffuse nuclear Epstein-Barr encoded RNA (EBER) reaction (**D**).

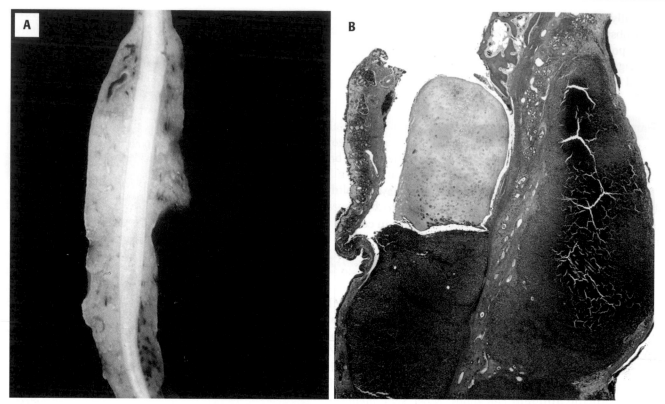

FIGURE 3-18

A, A black polypoid mass on the nasal septal cartilage was histologically a melanoma. **B**, Note the destruction of the cartilage on this low-power view of a malignant mucosal melanoma. There is surface ulceration.

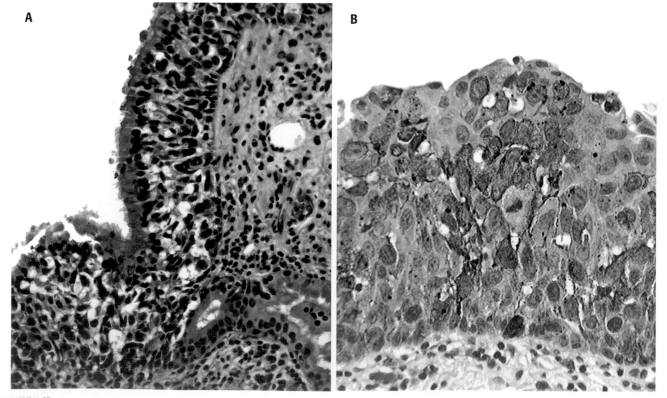

FIGURE 3-19

A, The surface respiratory epithelium shows an increased number of atypical melanocytes, a finding helpful in the diagnosis of a primary malignant mucosal melanoma. **B**, A melanoma in situ shows full thickness involvement by the pigmented neoplastic melanocytes.

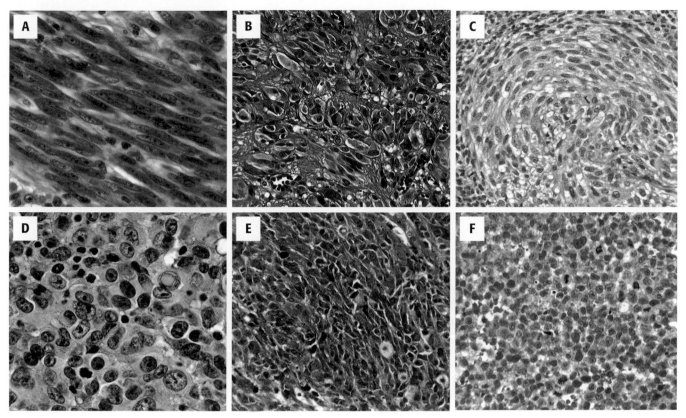

FIGURE 3-20

Malignant mucosal melanomas can be arranged in a number of different patterns as well as showing a number of different cell types. **A**, Tight fascicles of spindle cells comprise this melanoma. **B**, A polygonal epithelioid appearance to this melanoma. **C**, A whorled to meningothelial pattern with mitotic figure. **D**, Pleomorphic plasmacytoid cells with intranuclear cytoplasmic inclusions. **E**, Pigment can be seen, present in a spindle cell type. **F**, An undifferentiated solid sheet of cells comprises this melanoma.

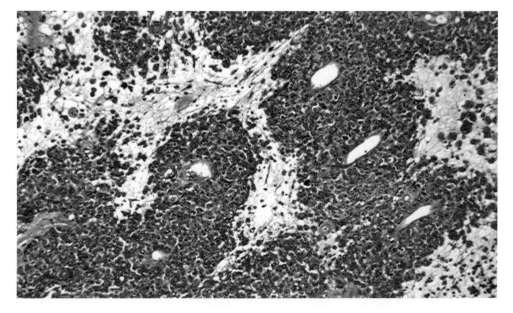

FIGURE 3-21

A peritheliomatous arrangement of the neoplastic cells is unique to melanoma of the sinonasal tract.

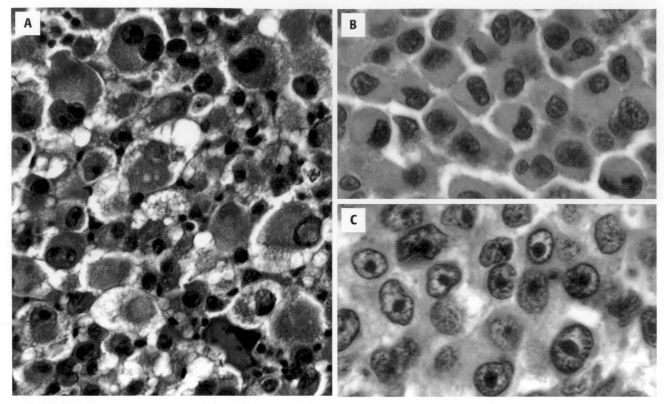

FIGURE 3-22

A, Remarkably plasmacytoid differentiation in this melanoma, showing binucleation and intranuclear inclusions. **B**, Rhabdoid cells with abundant, opaque eosinophilic cytoplasm are seen in this melanoma. **C**, Prominent, eosinophilic nucleoli.

ANCILLARY STUDIES

ULTRASTRUCTURAL FEATURES

The presence of premelanosomes and melanosomes confirms a melanocytic origin.

IMMUNOHISTOCHEMICAL FEATURES

The neoplastic cells are immunoreactive with S100 protein, HMB45, Melan A, microphthalmia transcription factor, tyrosinase, and vimentin (Figure 3-23). p16 is usually lost in MMM. *BRAF* mutations are frequently identified.

DIFFERENTIAL DIAGNOSIS

The wide morphologic diversity includes many malignant neoplasms such as sinonasal undifferentiated carcinoma, lymphoma, olfactory neuroblastoma, melanotic neuroectodermal tumor of infancy (Figure 3-24),

rhabdomyosarcoma (RMS), leiomyosarcoma (LMS), fibrosarcoma, mesenchymal chondrosarcoma, plasmacytoma, angiosarcoma, and, rarely, metastatic melanoma to the SNT (Table 3-1). Pertinent immunohistochemical studies allow for appropriate separation. Metastatic melanoma to the SNT, if it develops, is usually a late event and part of systemic disease.

PROGNOSIS AND THERAPY

The overall prognosis for SNT melanoma is poor, with a 5-year survival ranging from 17% to 47%. Recurrences are common, with a poor prognosis associated with advanced stage, obstructive symptoms, tumor ≥3 cm, mixed anatomic sites of involvement, undifferentiated histology, high mitotic index, and vascular invasion. Matrix metalloproteinase (MMP) expression is associated with patient outcome (MMP14 expression associated with poor prognosis). Wide local excision is the treatment of choice, with radiation providing only palliation.

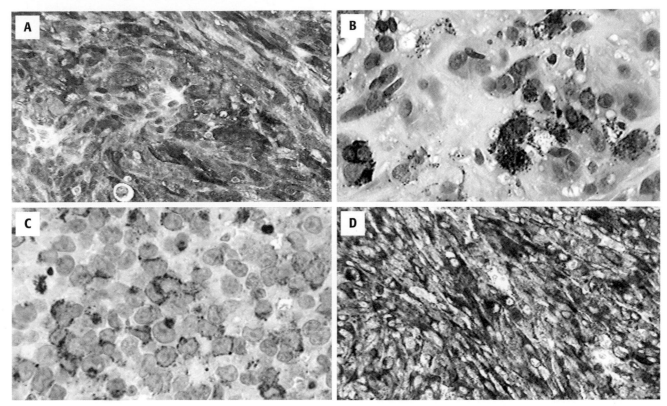

FIGURE 3-23

The neoplastic cells are reactive with S100 protein (**A**), Melan A (**B**), and HMB45 (**C** and **D**) to a variable degree, ranging from strong, diffuse, and heavy reactions to light, granular, and sparse reactivity.

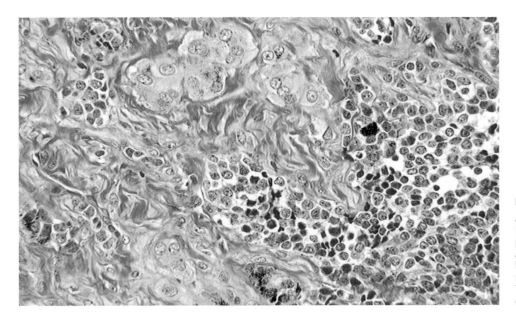

FIGURE 3-24

A melanocytic neuroectodermal tumor of infancy has a dual population of large, pigmented cells with small, primitive cells. A dense fibrous stroma separates the biphasic populations. There is little pleomorphism and mitotic activity is scarce. The young age at presentation helps with clinical separation from melanoma.

■ OLFACTORY NEUROBLASTOMA

Olfactory neuroblastoma (ONB; esthesioneuroblastoma) is a malignant neoplasm thought to arise from the specialized sensory neuroepithelial (neuroectodermal) olfactory cells (bipolar neurons) normally found in the upper part of the nasal cavity, including the superior nasal concha, the upper part of the septum, the roof of the nose, and the cribriform plate of the ethmoid sinus. Olfactory epithelium contains three cell types (basal cells, olfactory neurosensory cells, and sustentacular supporting cells), all of which are also in the tumor.

CLINICAL FEATURES

OLFACTORY NEUROBLASTOMA—DISEASE FACT SHEET

Definition
- Malignant neuroectodermal neoplasm arising from olfactory epithelium

Incidence and Location
- Approximately 2% to 3% of sinonasal tract malignancies
- About 0.4/1,000,000 population
- Encompasses cribriform plate

Morbidity and Mortality
- Stage-dependent mortality, overall ~60% 5-year survival

Gender and Age Distribution
- Equal gender distribution
- Bimodal distribution: peak at 11 to 20 and 51 to 60 years, respectively

Clinical Features
- Unilateral nasal obstruction and epistaxis most common
- Anosmia, headaches, pain, and ocular disturbances
- Often slow growing
- Anosmia is uncommon (<5% of patients)

Radiographic Features
- Dumbbell-shaped mass on either side of the cribriform plate
- MRI: intense enhancement on T1-weighted imaging with gadolinium contrast

Prognosis and Treatment
- Prognosis is stage and grade dependent:
- 75% to 90% 5-year survival (stage A) to 45% (stage C)
- 80% low grade vs. 25% high grade
- Approximately 30% recurrence rate, usually within 2 years
- Metastasis develops in lymph nodes (up to 35%)
- Meticulous surgical eradication with postoperative radiotherapy
- Chemotherapy and bone marrow transplantation show promise

ONBs account for approximately 2% to 3% of SNT malignancies (0.4/1,000,000 population/year). There is a slight male predilection (1.2:1). The tumor may occur at any age, with a bimodal age distribution peak at 11 to 20 years and 51 to 60 years. These slow growing tumors most commonly cause unilateral nasal obstruction (70%), epistaxis (50%), headaches, pain, rhinorrhea, visual disturbances, and a mass high in the nasal cavity and ethmoid region. Anosmia is uncommon (<5% of patients).

RADIOGRAPHIC FEATURES

The classic presentation is with a "dumbbell-shaped" mass encompassing the cribriform plate of the ethmoid sinus (as the "waist"; Figure 3-25), with expansion into the intracranial and nasal cavity areas. Peripheral tumor cysts in the intracranial portion are very suggestive of ONB. MRI demonstrates remarkable tumor enhancement on T1-weighted images with gadolinium contrast. Calcifications may be identified, generally best seen on CT studies.

PATHOLOGIC FEATURES

OLFACTORY NEUROBLASTOMA—PATHOLOGIC FEATURES

Gross Findings
- Polypoid, glistening, soft, vascular masses high in the nasal cavity and ethmoid region

Microscopic Findings
- Circumscribed lobule separated by vascularized stroma is maintained to some degree in all grades
- Tumor cells form solid nests, Homer Wright pseudorosettes with neurofibrillar matrix (30%), and Flexner-Wintersteiner–type true rosettes with glandular lumen (5%)
- Cells are syncytial, uniform and small, with round nuclei and "salt-and-pepper" nuclear chromatin
- High-grade tumors have larger tumor cells, nuclear pleomorphism, and increased mitotic activity; neurofibrillary matrix is scant or absent

Immunohistochemical Features
- Neuron-specific enolase, chromogranin, synaptophysin, CD56 positive in 80% of tumors
- S100 protein–positive cells confined to the periphery of tumor nests

Pathologic Differential Diagnosis
- Sinonasal undifferentiated carcinoma, lymphoma, plasmacytoma, NUT midline carcinoma, rhabdomyosarcoma, melanoma, neuroendocrine carcinoma, Ewing sarcoma/primitive neuroectodermal tumor, pituitary adenoma

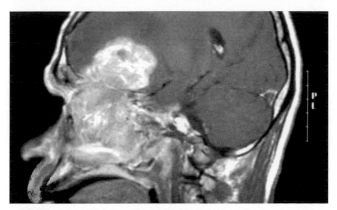

FIGURE 3-25

A T1-weighted gadolinium-contrast magnetic resonance image shows a dumbbell-shaped mass extending through the cribriform plate and filling the nasal vault and the intracranial cavity.

GROSS FINDINGS

The excised tumors vary from small polypoid nodules to large masses involving the bilateral ethmoids and nasal cavity with extension into the adjacent paranasal sinuses, superior nasal concha, turbinates, and upper septum. The cut surface appears glistening, gray-tan to pink-red, and hypervascular.

MICROSCOPIC FINDINGS

The histologic appearance of olfactory neuroblastoma varies by degree of differentiation, although a semblance of lobular architecture is maintained throughout (Figure 3-26). The tumor cells are identified below an intact mucosa, often immediately subtending the olfactory epithelium. In situ tumor is rare. Low-grade tumors contain cellular nests surrounded by fine fibrovascular septa in an organoid fashion. Sustentacular

supporting cells line these lobules or nests. The primitive neuroblastoma cells are relatively uniform, slightly larger than lymphocytes, and lie in a finely fibrillar neuronal stroma (Figure 3-27). The syncytium of cells have a very high nuclear:cytoplasmic ratio, small, round to oval nuclei with uniformly distributed fine or coarse nuclear chromatin (Figure 3-28). Homer Wright pseudorosettes (seen in up to 30% of cases) are characterized by palisaded or cuffed neoplastic cells with finely fibrillar or granular material in the center (Figure 3-29). True Flexner-Wintersteiner rosettes (seen in ~5% of cases) form duct-like spaces lined by nonciliated columnar cells with basally placed nuclei, but are only identified in higher grade tumors (Figure 3-29). Calcification (psammomatous or concretion) may be seen. Rarely, ganglion cells, melanin-containing cells, and rhabdomyoblastic cells may be seen.

As the olfactory neuroblastomas become higher grade (less differentiated), pseudorosettes and fibrillar stroma are less common. The nuclei become more pleomorphic, chromatin is more coarse, mitotic figures increase, and tumor necrosis is present (Figures 3-27 and 3-30). Tumors are graded based on the degree of differentiation, presence of neural stroma, mitotic figures, and necrosis from grade 1 to 4 (Table 3-2). The grade correlates with prognosis, although not as sensitively as tumor stage. Kadish staging (groups A, B, and C) is based on the clinical extent of disease.

ANCILLARY STUDIES

ULTRASTRUCTURAL FEATURES

Membrane-bound dense core neurosecretory granules are present in the cytoplasm and in nerve processes, which additionally contain neurotubules and

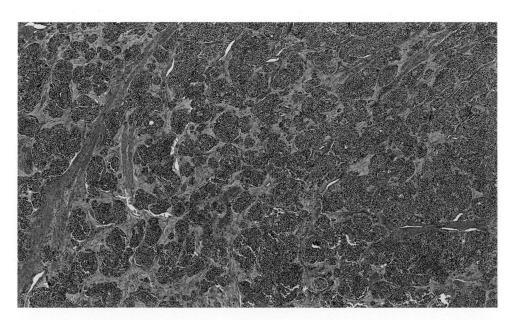

FIGURE 3-26

Well-formed lobules of closely packed cells separated by a highly vascularized stroma make up this olfactory neuroblastoma.

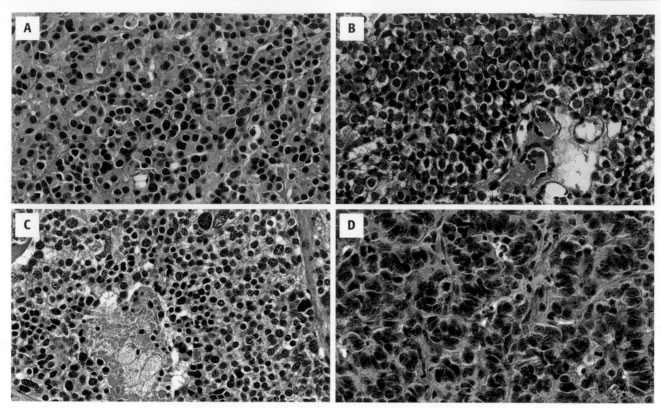

FIGURE 3-27

The neoplastic cells of olfactory neuroblastoma vary depending on the grade of the tumor. The tumor cells become progressively larger, more pleomorphic, with more mitotic figures, less stroma, and necrosis as one moves from **A**, grade 1, **B**, grade 2, **C**, grade 3, to **D**, grade 4 tumors.

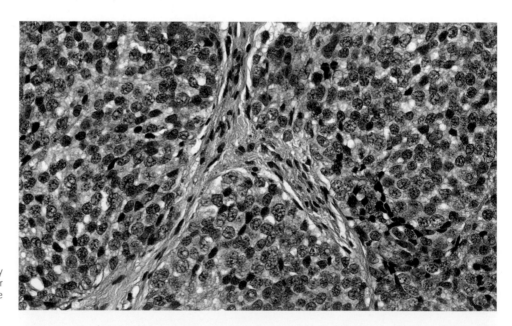

FIGURE 3-28

The lobules of tumor are separated by fibrosis. Note the slightly more granular nuclear chromatin that is seen in a grade 2 tumor.

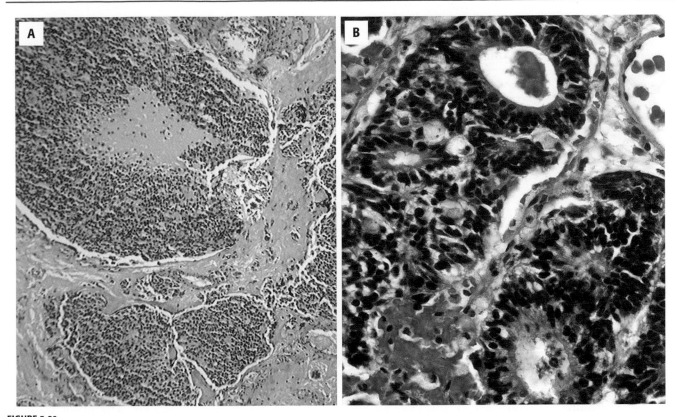

FIGURE 3-29

A, A large pseudorosette (Homer Wright) shows a central area of neurofibrillary matrix. **B**, The columnar tumor cells form the glandular spaces of a true Flexner-Wintersteiner rosette.

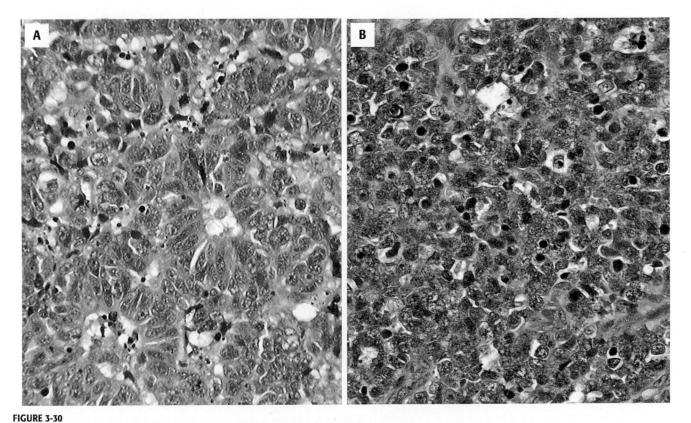

FIGURE 3-30

A, A grade 3 olfactory neuroblastoma showing a true Flexner-Wintersteiner rosette and increased mitotic figures. **B**, More of a sheet-like proliferation, with pleomorphism, increased mitoses and a near complete absence of neural matrix.

TABLE 3-2

Hyams' Grading System for Olfactory Neuroblastoma

Feature	Grade 1	Grade 2	Grade 3	Grade 4
Architecture	Lobular	Lobular	Lobular	Lobular
Mitotic activity	Absent	Present	Prominent	Marked
Nuclear pleomorphism	Absent	Moderate	Prominent	Marked
Fibrillary matrix	Prominent	Present	Minimal	Absent
Rosettes	Homer Wright	Homer Wright	Flexner-Wintersteiner	Flexner-Wintersteiner
Necrosis	Absent	Absent	Present	Common

neurofilaments. The diameter of the granules is from 50 to 250 nm. Olfactory differentiation with olfactory vesicles and microvilli on apical borders may be seen in Flexner-Wintersteiner rosettes.

HISTOCHEMISTRY

Silver stains highlight neurosecretory granules, and include Grimelius, Bodian, and Churukian-Schenk stains.

IMMUNOHISTOCHEMICAL FEATURES

NSE, chromogranin, synaptophysin, and CD56 are expressed in a diffuse pattern in ~80% of tumors (Figure 3-31). A small number of cells at the periphery of tumor nests react with the antibodies against S100 protein and glial fibrillary acidic protein (GFAP) to suggest Schwann cell differentiation (Figure 3-31). Keratins are rarely positive, and usually only in isolated cells. The tumor cells are negative with CD45RB, HMB45, desmin, and CD99.

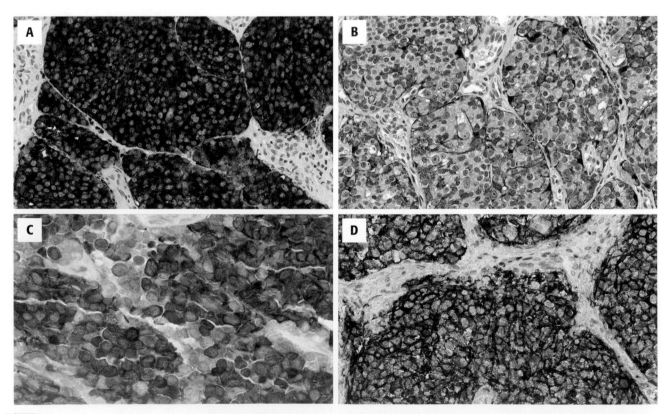

FIGURE 3-31

The neoplastic cells of olfactory neuroblastoma show a variety of different reactions. **A**, A diffuse expression with synaptophysin. **B**, S100 protein immunohistochemistry is only positive in cells at the periphery of tumor nests, indicative of Schwannian cell differentiation. **C**, Strong and diffuse neuron-specific enolase. **D**, CD56 highlights nearly all of the cells in a membranous distribution.

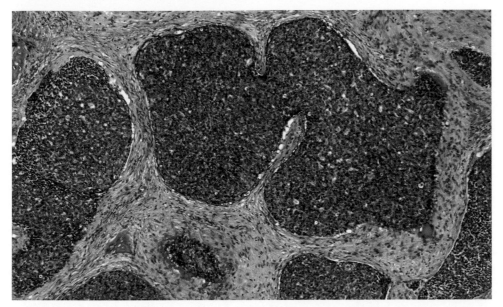

FIGURE 3-32

The solid, lobular pattern of growth in this adenoid cystic carcinoma can mimic an olfactory neuroblastoma. However, note the palisading at the periphery and the reduplicated basement membrane material.

DIFFERENTIAL DIAGNOSIS

The small, round blue cell neoplasm group of the SNT includes sinonasal undifferentiated carcinoma, *NUT* midline carcinoma, ACC (Figure 3-32), lymphoma, plasmacytoma, RMS, melanoma, neuroendocrine carcinoma, pituitary adenoma, and ES/PNET (Table 3-1). In a small biopsy with crush artifact, misinterpretation is common, especially as edge effect and diffusion artifacts with immunohistochemistry may not resolve the differential. Carcinomas tend to have higher mitotic activity, larger nucleoli, and obvious necrosis. A targeted immunohistochemistry panel may need to be expanded to encompass the differential, especially if the lesion is high in the nasal cavity.

PROGNOSIS AND THERAPY

The prognosis is both stage and grade dependent, with stage A tumors experiencing a 75% to 90% 5-year survival, while stage C has a 45% survival. Likewise, low-grade tumors have an 80% survival, while high-grade tumors have a 25% 5-year survival. Recurrence is common (~30%), usually within 2 years of the initial presentation. Metastasis develops in up to 35% of cases (lymph nodes), while distant metastasis occurs in ~10% of patients (lung, bone, liver, skin). En bloc resection of the tumor and cribriform plate with clear margin via a trephination and bicraniofacial approach is the treatment of choice for these tumors, although endoscopic methods are gaining popularity. Postoperative radiation is given to most patients to improve local control. Patients with advanced tumor or poorly differentiated tumor usually receive multimodality

treatment, including high-dose chemotherapy and bone marrow transplantation. Poor prognostic indicators include high-grade tumor, high stage, metastases, females, age <20 or >50 years at presentation, intracranial spread, high proliferation, and polyploidy/aneuploidy.

■ EXTRANODAL NK/T-CELL LYMPHOMA, NASAL TYPE

Lymphoma is the most common malignant nonepithelial neoplasm found in the upper respiratory tract and most commonly involves the nasal cavity, the maxillary sinus, nasopharynx, and salivary gland. This discussion will be limited to extranodal NK/T-cell lymphoma, nasal type (NK/T LNT), which is more common in the sinonasal region, although B-cell lymphomas tend to be more common in the nasopharynx, Waldeyer ring, and the sinuses (Figure 3-33). Hodgkin lymphoma is uncommon in either location. Additionally, there are geographic differences, where Asian and South American patients have a much higher frequency of SNT lymphoma (~7% of lymphomas), with the majority NK/T LNT, while in Western countries, SNT lymphomas account for <2% of lymphomas, with B-cell types predominating.

There are a number of differences between the types of lymphoid lesions that affect each of these locations, most closely related to the function of tissues affected. For example, the SNT does not normally contain lymphoid tissue; therefore, EBV-associated NK/T LNT tends to be more common. The nasopharynx, by contrast, has a rich lymphoid tissue, which can be affected by follicular hyperplasia or by B-cell lymphomas, most specifically, mantle cell lymphoma. The distinction of

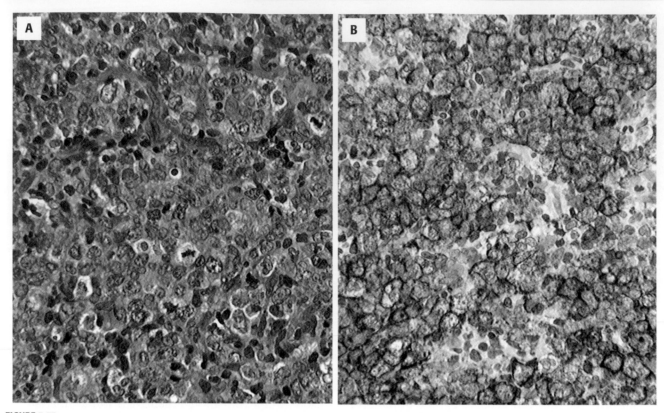

FIGURE 3-33

A, A diffuse large B-cell lymphoma of the maxillary sinus with large, atypical lymphoid cells. **B**, The neoplastic cells show a strong cytoplasmic reaction with CD20.

NK/T LNT from other diseases that give the clinical picture of midline destructive disease cannot be overstressed. The differences in treatment and patient outcome are diametrically opposite in many cases. Unfortunately, the diagnosis of NK/T LNT is often very challenging in the initial stages of presentation, requiring very close clinical correlation between the pathologist, otorhinolaryngologist, oncologist, and radiation therapist.

Many different names have been used for this disorder in the past: angiocentric NK/T cell lymphoma, polymorphic reticulosis, lethal midline granuloma, Stewart granuloma, and peripheral NK/T cell lymphoma, to name just a few. It is wisest to use the current WHO criteria since it incorporates clinical, histologic, immunophenotypic, molecular, and treatment considerations into the classification scheme.

CLINICAL FEATURES

Peripheral T-cell lymphomas are uncommon, accounting for 10% to 15% of all non-Hodgkin lymphomas. The tumors are much more common in Asia and South and Central America than in Western countries. All ages can be affected, but patients usually present in the 5th to 6th decades, although there is a rare hydroa vacciniforme–like

lymphoma in children, which is also EBV positive. In general, men are more commonly affected than women (3:1). The most frequent initial clinical presentation is nonspecific, with nasal discharge, sinusitis, headaches, facial and periorbital swelling, and epistaxis. As the tumor develops, the more destructive nature of the neoplasm is manifest through midline destruction (i.e., nasal cavity ulceration, paranasal sinus necrosis [frequently bilateral]), with palatal extension and fistula formation, orbital swelling (Figure 3-34), and a prominent edema (often with erythematous and "warm" skin overlying these structures). Pain and paresthesias develop with further destruction of the tissues. Systemic manifestations of weight loss, fever, fatigue, and profound night sweating can also be seen, especially if the stage of the lymphoma results in involvement of extra-SNT sites (skin, soft tissues, gastrointestinal tract). Most patients have stage IE or IIE disease at presentation (E: extranodal). Therefore, this particular type of lymphoma may be indolent or aggressive, depending on the overall morphology and the stage of lymphoma. There is a very strong association with EBV in both the endemic and nonendemic populations. Patients who are immunosuppressed (especially after organ transplantation) may develop the lymphoma more often. A few cases will have a hematophagocytic syndrome with pancytopenia or hyper-IgE syndrome (Job syndrome). Serum EBV-DNA copy number may be a useful tumor marker.

EXTRANODAL NK/T-CELL LYMPHOMA, NASAL TYPE—DISEASE FACT SHEET

Definition
- Malignant NK/T-cell lymphoma with the bulk of the disease in the sinonasal tract

Incidence and Location
- Most common nonepithelial malignancy of the sinonasal tract
- About 10% to 15% of all non-Hodgkin lymphomas
- Nasal cavity and paranasal sinuses concurrently affected

Morbidity and Mortality
- Mortality in 50% to 70% of patients

Gender, Race, and Age Distribution
- Male > female (3:1)
- Endemic in Asians, Central and Latin Americans
- Peak in 6th decade

Clinical Features
- Early disease difficult to detect with nonspecific symptoms
- Nasal obstruction, epistaxis, nasal discharge, and swelling
- Septal perforation and bone destruction later in course
- Uncommonly have fever and weight loss
- Most patients present with low-stage disease (stage I/IIE)
- Very strong association with Epstein-Barr virus

Prognosis and Treatment
- Overall prognosis is 30% to 50%
- Relapse/recurrences develop in up to 50%
- Advanced stage, bulky disease, and systemic symptoms yield a worse prognosis
- Combined radiotherapy and chemotherapy

EXTRANODAL NK/T-CELL LYMPHOMA, NASAL TYPE—PATHOLOGIC FEATURES

Microscopic Findings
- Early disease difficult to detect in background reactive lymphoid infiltrate
- Diffuse infiltrate that is frequently angiocentric and angioinvasive associated with tumor necrosis
- Variable, mixed small and large lymphoid cells
- May occasionally have extensive pseudoepitheliomatous hyperplasia of the epithelium

Immunohistochemical Features
- Positive: CD2, cytoplasmic CD3ϵ, CD56, perforin, TIA1, granzyme B, and EBER
- CD5, CD16, CD57 are usually negative

Pathologic Differential Diagnosis
- Reactive/inflammatory infiltrate, Wegener granulomatosis, lymphomatoid granulomatosis, olfactory neuroblastoma, Ewing sarcoma/primitive neuroectodermal tumor, carcinoma, melanoma

PATHOLOGIC FEATURES

GROSS FINDINGS

A raised polypoid unilateral lesion usually within the nasal cavity in the early stage develops progressively into an ulcerated and necrotic mass, which may become bilateral. The cut surface reveals gray-white, friable, homogeneous tissue.

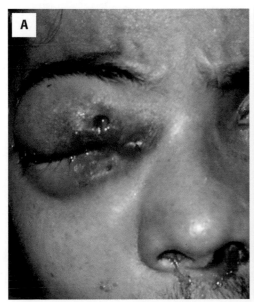 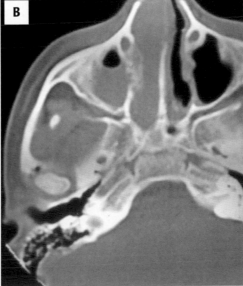

FIGURE 3-34

A, A 19-year-old presented with a large destructive lesion of the nasal cavity, maxillary sinus and orbit, showing marked orbital edema, erythema, and crusting. **B**, The medial wall of the maxillary sinus is destroyed with a mass filling the maxillary sinus and nasal cavity in this computed tomography image. (**A**, *Courtesy of Dr. R. Carlos.*)

MICROSCOPIC FINDINGS

NK/T LNT is a polymorphic neoplastic infiltrate with angioinvasion and/or angiodestruction with strong EBV association. In contrast to the nasopharynx and tonsils, NK/T LNT is much more common than B-cell lymphomas in the nasal cavity. There is a developmental arc associated with disease progression. Initially, there is a subepithelial, diffuse, and polymorphous cellular infiltrate composed of normal appearing lymphocytes, histiocytes, immunoblasts, eosinophils, and plasma cells. Within this milieu are a number of atypical lymphoid cells, increasing in number as the disease progresses. These neoplastic cells have a broad cytomorphologic pattern, ranging in size from small to large, the latter usually remarkably atypical. These hyperchromatic cells have irregular, pleomorphic nuclei with prominent nucleoli. Tumor cell folding, cleaving, and grooving are characteristic for an NK/T-cell lymphoma. This intermixed population of atypical NK/T cells interspersed throughout the specimen is often exceedingly difficult to identify, even with ancillary techniques (Figure 3-35). However, the presence of EBV-positive cells is strong supportive evidence of a neoplasm. The prominent background inflammatory component may completely obscure the underlying neoplasm, simulating an infectious or inflammatory condition. When the vascular walls are invaded by the neoplastic cells to the point that they occlude the lumen of the vessel, the presence of profound necrosis brings to mind the possibility of a neoplasm (Figure 3-36). Angiocentricity and angioinvasion with necrosis are seen in ~50% to 60% of NK/T LNT cases (Figure 3-37). Due to a lack of ubiquitous angioinvasion and destruction, the WHO proposed the term *extranodal NK/T-cell lymphoma, nasal type*, instead of angiocentric NK-T cell lymphoma. Necrosis of the coagulative or ischemic (geographic) type may be widespread, however, further limiting interpretation, especially on small biopsies. Occasionally, pseudoepitheliomatous hyperplasia and epitheliotropism may simulate an epithelial malignancy. Multiple and repeat biopsies are often required to render a definitive diagnosis, frequently in a patient who is deteriorating clinically!

ANCILLARY STUDIES

HISTOCHEMISTRY

Elastic stains may be useful in identifying disruption of the elastic membrane of the vessel walls.

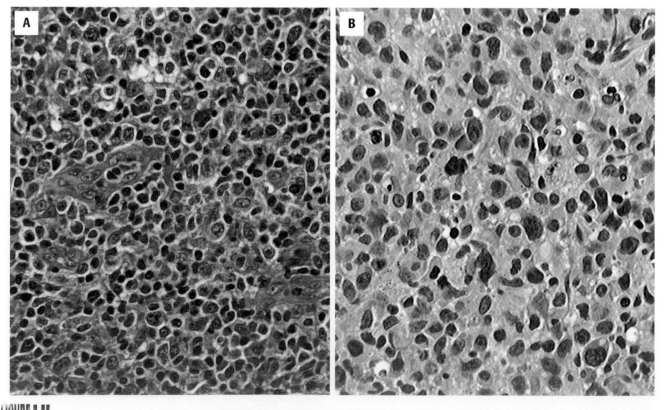

FIGURE 3-35

A, A mixed population of inflammatory cells harboring the atypical lymphoid elements. **B,** More cytologically atypical lymphoid cells, easier to identify after the disease has progressed.

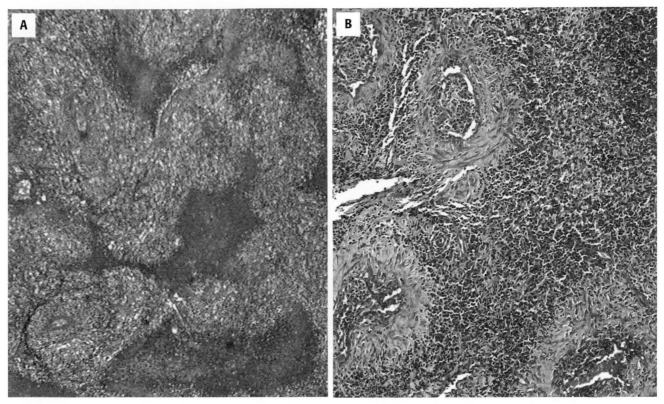

FIGURE 3-36

A, Necrosis is noted between islands of atypical lymphoid cells and prominent arteries. **B**, Arteries are invaded and surrounded by atypical lymphoid cells.

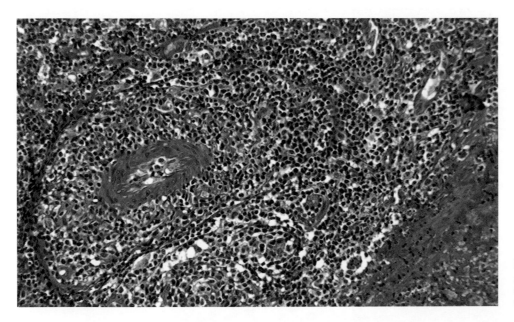

FIGURE 3-37

A vessel is surrounded and invaded by atypical lymphoid cells; necrosis is present in the lower right.

IMMUNOHISTOCHEMISTRY

By in situ hybridization, nearly 100% of NK/T LNT have detectable EBER, better developed in Asian patients but also present in Western patients (Figure 3-38). NK-cell lineage is seen most commonly (up to 75%), while T-cell lineage is seen in ~25% to 35% of cases. The neoplastic cells are positive with T-cell (CD3ϵ [Figure 3-38], CD2, CD5, CD8[±], CD56, CD94) and natural killer cell/cytotoxic-related markers (perforin, TIA1, granzyme B) (Figure 3-38). CD43 and CD45RO may be positive. Vimentin is positive, while p63 is occasionally positive. However, CD5, CD16, and CD57 are usually negative.

MOLECULAR GENETICS

T-cell receptor (TCR) gene rearrangement will be present in T-cell tumors, but it is germline. Further, NK-cell tumors do not carry TCR gene rearrangements.

DIFFERENTIAL DIAGNOSIS

Inflammatory (chronic rhinosinusitis), infectious lesions, and Wegener granulomatosis are key considerations when faced with a lymphoid process. In benign conditions, nuclear atypia and mitotic activity are absent or minimal. Biocollagenolytic necrosis is usually absent in lymphoma, while antineutrophil cytoplasmic antibodies (ANCA) and proteinase 3 (PR3) will be positive in *Wegener granulomatosis*. Carcinoma, melanoma, RMS, ES/PNET, and olfactory neuroblastoma have unique patterns of growth and immunohistochemistry profiles. Immunohistochemical stains and in situ hybridization for EBER are helpful to confirm NK/T LNT. Separation from *lymphomatoid granulomatosis* (LYG) may be nearly impossible, as the latter diagnosis significantly overlaps the clinical, morphologic, and immunophenotype features of NK/T LNT. LYG may be a T-cell–rich EBV-related B-cell lymphoproliferative disease, in which T cells are abundant and reactive in nature. In contrast, NK/T LNT is a T-cell lymphoproliferative disorder, in which EBV occurs in T and NK cells. Separation from other "small round blue cell tumors" can usually be achieved with pertinent immunohistochemistry (Table 3-1).

PROGNOSIS AND THERAPY

The overall prognosis for NK/T LNT ranges from 30% to 50%, with relapses or recurrences developing in up

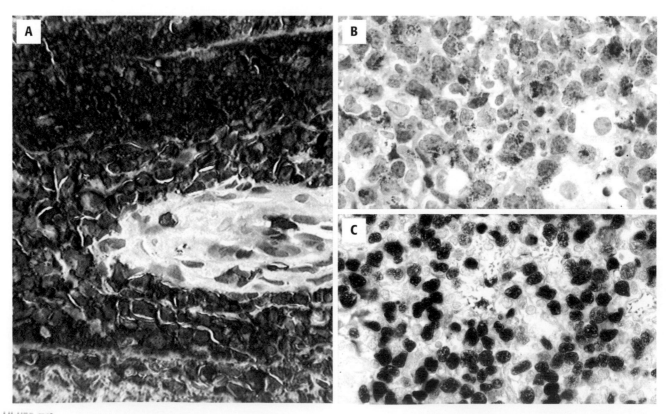

FIGURE 3-38

A, The neoplastic cells within this vessel are strongly and diffusely immunoreactive with CD3ϵ. **B,** The neoplastic cells show a positive granzyme reaction. **C,** Nearly all of the cells are strongly and diffusely positive with EBER by in situ hybridization. (*B and C, Courtesy of Dr. J. R. L. Chan.*)

to 50% of patients. Prognosis is determined by stage, bulky disease, and whether systemic symptoms are present (stage IE: 70%; stage IIE: 40% at 5 years). Most patients present with stage I or II disease. Systemic disease development is common. A worse prognosis is experienced in patients with bulky disease, advanced stage, multiple sites of involvement, and older age. Treatment for localized disease is radiotherapy with or without chemotherapy (specific to NK/T cell phenotype). Early radiation is advocated, especially in low-stage disease. Stem cell transplantation may be beneficial. It must be stressed again that diffuse large B-cell lymphomas are managed differently, although also showing a 5-year survival of 40% to 60%.

■ MESENCHYMAL MALIGNANCIES

SARCOMA—DISEASE FACT SHEET

Rhabdomyosarcoma

- Malignant neoplasm with skeletal muscle phenotype
- About 20% of rhabdomyosarcomas involve sinonasal tract
- Nasopharynx more commonly involved than sinonasal tract
- Age: childhood/young adults (embryonal subtype); adults (alveolar subtype)
- Difficulty breathing, epistaxis, facial swelling, sinusitis
- Overall mortality between 44% and 69%, depending on age, histologic subtype, and stage
- Combined multimodality therapy (chemotherapy, radiotherapy, surgery)
- Gross: large, bulky, fleshy, polypoid, grape-like masses, simulating polyps
- **Embryonal type (80%):** round to spindled primitive mesenchymal cells with hyperchromatic nuclei; rhabdomyoblasts with cross-striations rare; myxoid stroma may be present, occasionally abundant
- **Alveolar type (20%):** fibrous septa separating loosely cohesive rhabdomyoblasts into alveolar spaces; multinucleated giant cells may be present
- **IHC:** desmin, myoglobin, myogenin, MYOD1, SMA positive
- **Differential diagnosis:** lymphoma, polyps with stromal atypia, carcinoma, Ewing sarcoma/primitive neuroectodermal tumor, olfactory neuroblastoma, melanoma

---

Fibrosarcoma

- Malignant neoplasm with only fibroblastic/myofibroblastic differentiation
- Uncommon, usually with a paranasal sinus location
- Female > male (3:2), with a peak in 5th to 6th decades
- Nasal obstruction and epistaxis most common
- Prognosis generally good with 75% survival, although up to 60% recurrence
- Surgery is treatment of choice with adjuvant radiation
- Smooth, nodular, polypoid, fleshy mass, with necrosis and hemorrhage in higher grade tumors
- Surface epithelial invagination common
- Spindle cells arranged in short, compact fascicles at acute angles (herringbone)
- Cellularity is variable

- Fusiform cells with centrally placed hyperchromatic, needle-like nuclei and tapering cytoplasm
- Mitotic figures are variable
- Bizarre, pleomorphic cells are usually absent
- **IHC:** vimentin, and rarely, focal actin positivity
- **Differential diagnosis:** fibromatosis, glomangiopericytoma, inflammatory myofibroblastic tumor, solitary fibrous tumor, peripheral nerve sheath tumors, benign and malignant fibrous histiocytoma, synovial sarcoma, rhabdomyosarcoma, spindle cell melanoma, spindle cell squamous cell carcinoma

---

Leiomyosarcoma

- Malignant tumor of smooth muscle phenotype
- Arises from the vascular structures of the sinonasal tract
- All ages, although younger if Epstein-Barr virus associated
- Radical resection, with prognosis based on stage and site; recurrences are common
- Infiltrative, interlacing fascicles to storiform bundles of spindled cells
- Centrally located, blunt-ended to cigar-shaped nuclei with a perinuclear vacuole
- Increased mitoses and necrosis help confirm the diagnosis
- **IHC:** positive with vimentin, actins, and variably with desmin
- **Differential diagnosis:** leiomyoma, spindle cell squamous cell carcinoma, malignant peripheral nerve sheath tumor, fibrosarcoma, rhabdomyosarcoma

---

Angiosarcoma

- Uncommon, high-grade malignant vascular neoplasm, occasionally associated with radiation
- Patients are usually middle aged, with males > females (2:1)
- Epistaxis is the most common symptom, followed by obstruction and discharge
- Combination therapy yields best outcome, although 60% die <2 years
- Large, nodular, polypoid mass with soft-friable, hemorrhagic cut surfaces
- Freely anastomosing vascular channels, irregular, cleft-like with small to large spaces, lined by atypical, enlarged, spindled to epithelioid endothelial cells
- Extravasated erythrocytes and neolumen formation
- Mitoses and necrosis are common
- **IHC:** positive with CD34, CD31, factor VIII–RAg, vimentin, podoplanin
- **Differential diagnosis:** granulation tissue, lobular capillary hemangioma, angiofibroma, juvenile nasopharyngeal angiofibroma, epithelioid hemangioma, glomangiopericytoma, Kaposi sarcoma, Masson vegetant endothelial hyperplasia, intravascular papillary endothelial hyperplasia

---

RHABDOMYOSARCOMA

RMS is a primitive malignant soft tissue tumor with histologic and phenotypic features of embryonic skeletal muscle. About 40% of all RMSs develop in the head and neck, ~20% of which involve the SNT and nasopharynx. RMS is the most common childhood sarcoma and is subtyped, specifically in the SNT, into the following categories: embryonal (80%) and alveolar (20%). RMS has a peak incidence during the 1st and 2nd decades of life, with a slight male predominance (1.2:1). The embryonal type predominates in childhood, while the alveolar type predominates in adults. Patients present with difficulty breathing, epistaxis, facial swelling, visual disturbances, and sinusitis, often of a short duration. Within the head and neck, the orbit, oropharynx, ear, and temporal bone, specifically, are affected more often than the nasopharynx and SNT. CT and MRI delineate the size and extent of the tumor (Figure 3-39). Tumors produce bulky, fleshy, polypoid masses simulating multiple nasal polyps (Figure 3-39). The botryoid variant has a "grape-like" appearance, as the name implies. The surface epithelium is usually intact.

Embryonal RMS is made up of round to spindled cells with elongated to round hyperchromatic nuclei (Figure 3-40). The tumor has a distinct accumulation of primitive cells and rhabdomyoblasts beneath the squamous or respiratory mucosa, imparting a distinctive appearance referred to as a "cambium layer" (Figure 3-41). In the deeper parts of the tumor, primitive cells predominate and admix with a varying number of rhabdomyoblasts (Figure 3-42). Rhabdomyoblasts have many different appearances ranging from elongated strap-shaped cells to small, round "tadpole" cells, both having densely eosinophilic cytoplasm. Cross-striations are rare (Figure 3-43). A myxoid stroma may be present, occasionally abundant.

Alveolar RMS shows loosely cohesive groups of small to medium cells separated into clusters by fibrous septa, simulating a glandular neoplasm (Figure 3-44). Multinucleated giant cells may be seen. While most

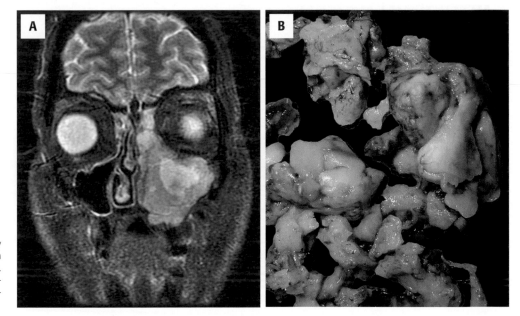

FIGURE 3-39

A, Magnetic resonance imaging study shows the extent of the tumor within the maxillary and ethmoid sinuses. **B**, This macroscopic image demonstrates the similarity between sinonasal polyps and rhabdomyosarcoma.

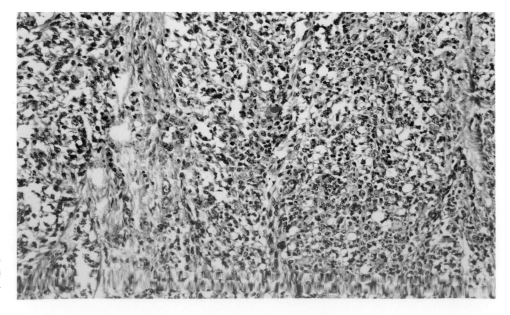

FIGURE 3-40

There is a hypercellular tumor composed of primitive mesenchymal cells and rhabdomyoblasts. Note the pink cytoplasm.

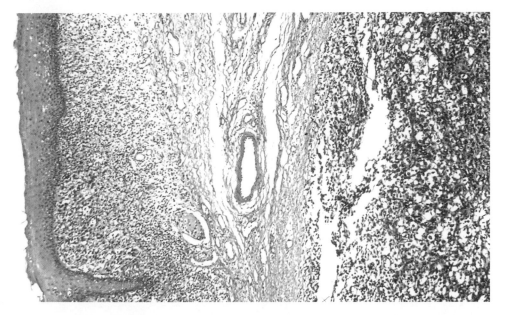

FIGURE 3-41

The sarcoma botryoid type is characterized by three distinct zones: hypercellular, cambium layer beneath the squamous mucosa; a second underlying zone of hypocellular myxoid stroma; and a third zone of predominantly primitive mesenchymal cells. *(Courtesy of Dr. Yao S. Fu.)*

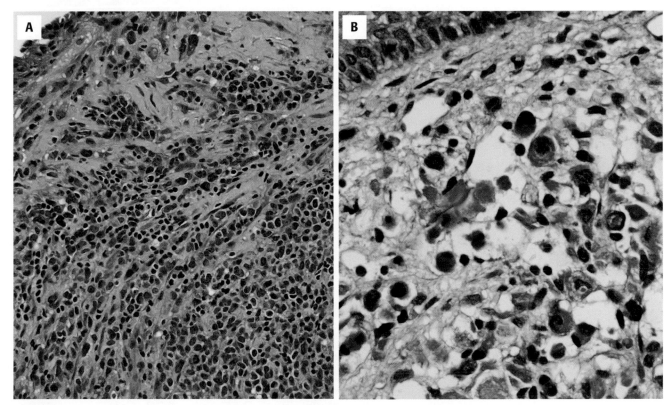

FIGURE 3-42

A, A respiratory epithelium overlying a diffuse atypical small, blue, round cell proliferation. **B**, A squamous mucosa overlying rhabdomyoblasts with eosinophilic cytoplasm.

rhabdomyoblasts have eosinophilic cytoplasm, some have vacuolated/cleared cytoplasm. Glycogen is easily identified.

RMS expresses desmin, myogenin, MYOD1, muscle-specific actin, smooth muscle actin, myoglobin, fast myosin, MITF, and CD56 (Figure 3-45). CD99 and keratin may be positive (~5%). *FKHR* may show gain of function mutations when fused with PAX3 or PAX7 in alveolar RMS, detected by fluorescence in situ hybridization (FISH). RMS should be separated from other small, round blue cell tumors (Table 3-1). These tumors can be excluded by the use of a panel of appropriate immunohistochemical stains.

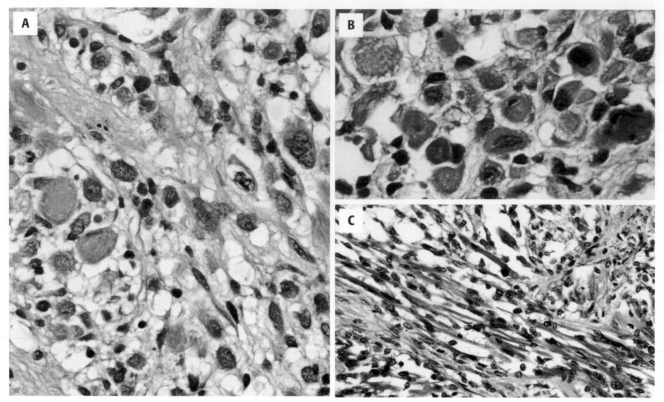

FIGURE 3-43

A, Rhabdomyoblasts with elongated and spindled cells. **B**, Predominantly primitive appearing cells with abundant, eccentrically placed eosinophilic cytoplasm. **C**, Strap cells with cross striations are very uncommon.

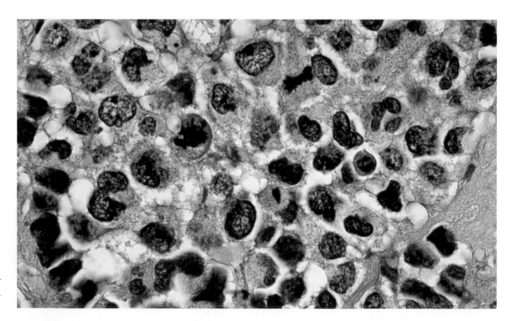

FIGURE 3-44

Alveolar rhabdomyosarcoma has tumor cells that form dilated alveolar spaces. Note the dilapidated wall appearance.

SNT polyps with stromal atypia have inflammatory cells, lack the cellularity of an RMS, and usually have different clinical findings. The atypical spindle cells (Figure 3-46) are myofibroblasts and so may have a similar immunoreactivity with actins. The overall prognosis is determined by age, histologic subtype, and the clinical stage at presentation (considered highly aggressive and systemic tumors, by definition). A better prognosis is seen in children and in patients with the botryoid type. Overall survival is 44% to 69% but can be as high as 90% for stage I tumors. The 5-year overall survival for children and adults is 60% and 10%,

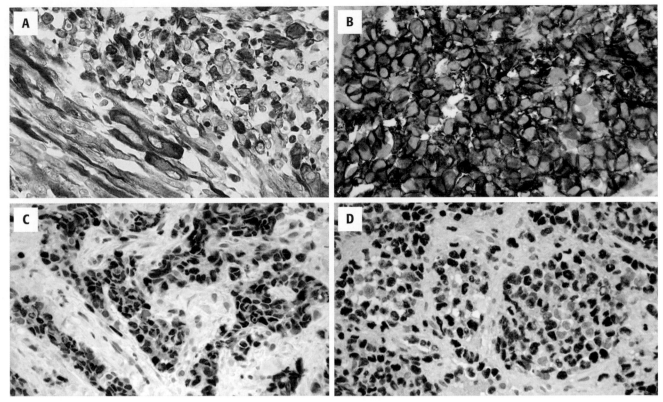

FIGURE 3-45

A, A strong desmin immunoreaction is noted in the cytoplasm of this embryonal type rhabdomyosarcoma in both spindled and epithelioid areas. **B**, CD56 shows a strong and diffuse membranous reaction. **C**, MYOD1 stains nearly all tumor nuclei strongly. **D**, Myogenin stains the nuclei in this alveolar rhabdomyosarcoma.

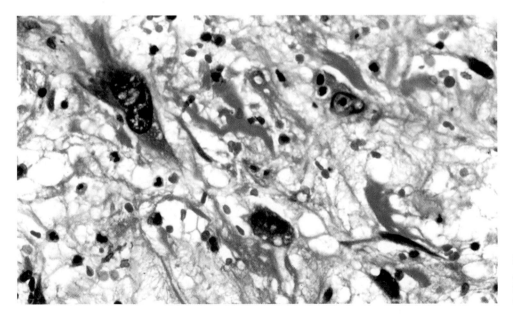

FIGURE 3-46

Atypical stromal cells are in isolation in this sinonasal polyp with myofibroblastic atypia.

respectively. Treatment encompasses a multimodality approach (chemotherapy, radiation, and surgery).

FIBROSARCOMA

Fibrosarcoma is defined as a malignant neoplasm showing fibroblastic and/or myofibroblastic differentiation. Tumors having pleomorphic, bizarre cells are excluded from fibrosarcoma and placed in the undifferentiated pleomorphic sarcoma category (Figure 3-47). This uncommon tumor (<3% of all SNT malignancies) may have prior radiation exposure as an etiologic factor. Females are affected slightly more commonly than males (3:2), with a peak in the 5th to 6th decades. Patients have nasal obstruction, often associated with epistaxis. Pain, sinusitis, nasal discharge, swelling, and anosmia are less common.

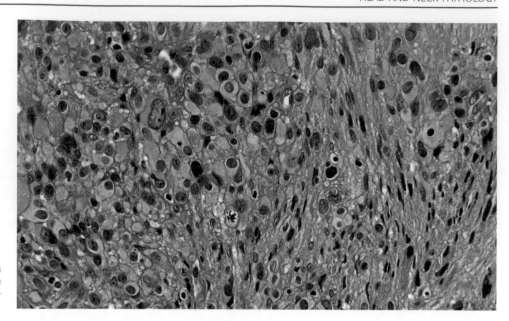

FIGURE 3-47

This highly pleomorphic neoplasm with increased mitotic figures and a storiform pattern would be placed in the undifferentiated pleomorphic sarcoma category.

Fibrosarcoma of the SNT occurs most frequently in the maxillary sinus, nasal cavity, and ethmoid region and is uncommonly confined to the nasal cavity alone.

In resection specimens, the tumor varies from 2 to 8 cm and has a smooth, polypoid, fleshy, white, homogeneous appearance. Necrosis and hemorrhage may be seen in higher grade tumors. Tumors are unencapsulated, with infiltration into the bone and occasional surface ulceration. Calcification may be seen. There is proliferation and entrapment of surface respiratory mucosa simulating inverted papilloma in up to one-third of fibrosarcomas (Figure 3-48). The stroma may be vascular with scattered capillaries mimicking hemangiopericytoma or may show delicate to dense bands of collagen. The cellularity is high, with the spindled cells arranged in a distinct herringbone (chevron) pattern (Figure 3-49) of short, compact fascicles at acute angles. Occasionally a subtle fasciculation is noted, but not a storiform pattern. Although the elongated nuclei are relatively uniform in size and needle shape, there is evidence of nuclear atypia, altered chromatin patterns, small nucleoli, and usually increased mitotic activity in some part of the tumor (Figure 3-50). A low mitotic activity combined with mild nuclear atypia contributes to the misdiagnosis of fibrosarcoma as fibromatosis or peripheral nerve sheath tumor. Poorly differentiated fibrosarcoma is diagnosed when there is nuclear anaplasia, high mitotic activity, scant collagenous stroma, necrosis, and hemorrhage. The majority of SNT fibrosarcomas, however, are well differentiated. By definition, the neoplastic cells are positive with vimentin only, although occasionally

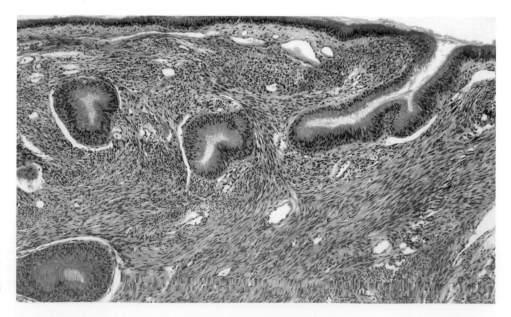

FIGURE 3-48

Sweeping fascicles of minimally pleomorphic spindled cells can occasionally be seen. The overlying and entrapped surface epithelium is unremarkable, including the presence of cilia.

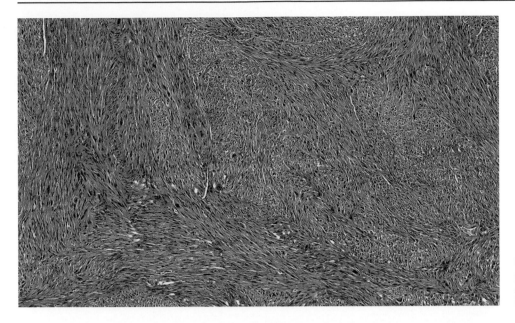

FIGURE 3-49

Short, angular intersections (herringbone or chevron) are most characteristic of a fibrosarcoma. Note the increased cellularity.

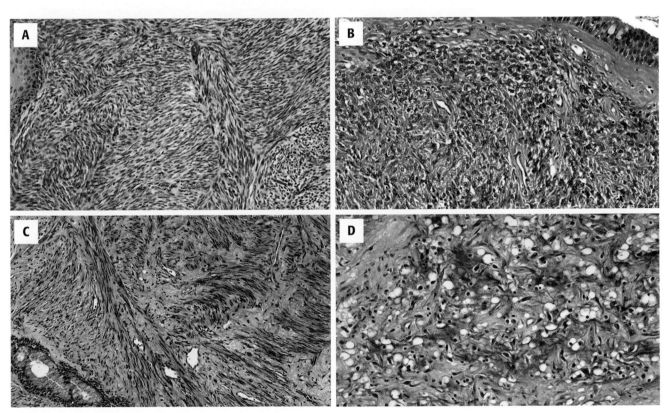

FIGURE 3-50

The tumor cells of fibrosarcoma can have a variety of different patterns and cell types. **A**, Short, compact, acute angle fascicles. There is mild nuclear pleomorphism. **B**, More of an epithelioid appearance to the spindled cells set within collagen. **C**, A hypocellular tumor, showing spindled cells (normal respiratory epithelium present). **D**, This myxoid fibrosarcoma shows abundant bluish myxoid matrix, increased vessels, and spindled tumor cells.

there may be focal, weak actin reactivity. The differential diagnosis includes a variety of spindled cell reactive and neoplastic conditions, including malignant fibrous histiocytoma (Figure 3-47), spindle cell SCC, spindle cell melanoma, malignant peripheral nerve sheath tumor (Figure 3-51), synovial sarcoma, RMS, glomangiopericytoma, inflammatory myofibroblastic tumor, solitary fibrous tumor, and fibromatosis (desmoid type; Figure 3-52). In general, the specific architectural pattern, histologic appearance, and immunophenotype findings allow for separation. Most SNT fibrosarcomas are associated with a favorable outcome

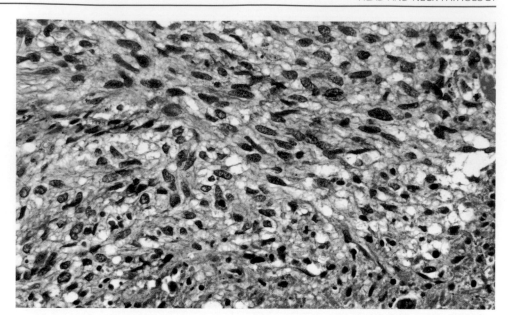

FIGURE 3-51

A malignant peripheral nerve sheath tumor is cellular, has necrosis, and will show epithelioid or fascicular growth. Mitotic activity and pleomorphism are readily identified.

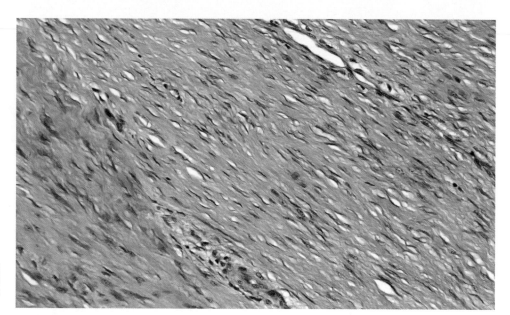

FIGURE 3-52

Heavy keloid-like collagen is deposited between the elongated and bland nuclei. Parallel vessels are noted in this fibromatosis.

(75 % 5-year survival). However, recurrences are common (up to 60 %), probably due to difficulty with obtaining clear surgical margins in the anatomic complexity of the SNT. Distant metastasis is uncommon (15 %), involving the lung and bones most commonly. A poor prognosis is related to male patients, large tumors, advanced tumor stage (multiple sites involved), a high histologic grade, and positive surgical margins. The best prognosis is achieved with complete resection. Adjuvant radiation has been used with mixed results.

LEIOMYOSARCOMA

LMS is a malignant tumor of smooth muscle differentiation. There is a link between EBV infection in immunocompromised patients and the development of LMS. The tumor seems to arise from vascular structures in the SNT. Although any age can be affected, immunocompromise-associated LMS seems to develop in children or young adults, while LMS usually develops in the 6th decade or older. Patients have a nonspecific presentation, such as nasal obstruction, pain, and epistaxis. Radical resection is the treatment of choice, with prognosis dependent on site and stage rather than histology. Recurrences are common (up to 70 %), with late distant metastasis. Tumors are large (>5 cm), nonencapsulated, tan-white, and rubbery to firm, with possible ulceration and necrosis. Histologically, the tumors are infiltrative, with a richly vascularized to myxomatous stroma. The tumor cells are arranged in interlacing fascicular to storiform bundles of spindle-shaped cells, often intersecting at right angles. The tumor cells are spindled with centrally located, blunt-ended to cigar shaped nuclei (Figure 3-53). A perinuclear vacuole or

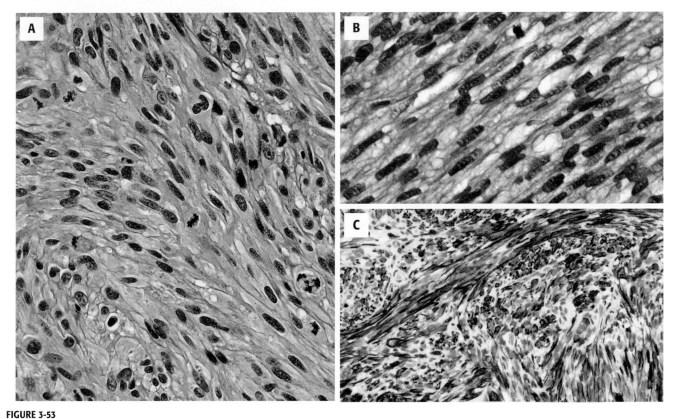

FIGURE 3-53

A, A pleomorphic spindled cell population with numerous mitotic figures is shown as part of this leiomyosarcoma. **B**, Note the perinuclear vacuole or clear halo. A mitotic figure is present. **C**, Strong and diffuse desmin reactivity in this leiomyosarcoma.

clear halo is helpful, making the nucleus appear indented or concave. Nuclei are variably pleomorphic, with nuclear hyperchromasia and increased mitotic activity, including atypical forms. In general, >2 mitoses/10 high-power fields (HPFs) is worrisome for an LMS, while >4 is nearly always LMS. It is not uncommon to see multinucleated giant cells. Epithelioid cells may occasionally predominate. PAS with diastase will highlight intracellular glycogen. Tumor cells will be strongly and diffusely reactive with vimentin and actins (smooth muscle, muscle-specific), while variably positive for desmin (Figure 3-53). Perinuclear keratin is rare. Separation needs to be made between LMS and leiomyoma, spindle cell SCC, malignant peripheral nerve sheath tumor, fibrosarcoma, and RMS.

ANGIOSARCOMA

Angiosarcoma is a very uncommon high-grade malignant vascular neoplasm, which may be associated with radiation. Nearly 50% of all angiosarcomas develop in the head and neck, although the scalp and soft tissues are more common. Most patients are middle aged (mean, 47 years), with more males than females (2:1). Patients present with involvement of the paranasal sinuses or nasal cavity alone. Epistaxis is the most common symptom, followed by nasal discharge and obstruction. The best outcome is achieved with a combination of surgery,

radiation, and chemotherapy, although in general the prognosis is poor (60% die from disease in <2 years). Recurrences are common. A poor prognosis is associated with female sex, age >60 years, large tumors, tumors with metastasis, and tumors with a specific etiology (radiation). Angiography identifies the extent of tumor growth and shows feeder vessel(s), allowing for presurgical angiographic embolization, if desired.

Tumors are large (mean, 4 cm), usually nodular to polypoid masses, with soft-friable cut surfaces showing hemorrhage with clots and necrosis. Tumors show ulcerated surface epithelium with associated necrosis and hemorrhage. The tumors are usually infiltrative into the adjacent soft tissues. Extravasated erythrocytes are noted throughout with freely anastomosing vascular channels. The cleft-like, irregular, small to large spaces are lined by atypical, enlarged, spindled to epithelioid endothelial cells (Figure 3-54). The atypical endothelial cells may be single, multilayered, or papillary/tufted. The cells have intracytoplasmic vacuoles or neolumen, which frequently contain erythrocytes (Figure 3-54). Nuclear chromatin is heavy and coarse, with irregular nuclear contours. Mitoses and necrosis are usually easily identified. Extracellular eosinophilic hyaline globules are absent. The tumor cells are positive with vimentin, CD34, CD31, and factor VIII–RAg. The differential includes granulation tissue, lobular capillary hemangioma, juvenile nasopharyngeal angiofibroma,

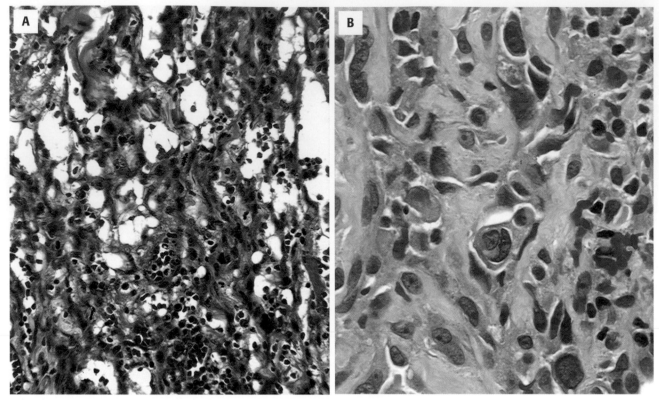

FIGURE 3-54

A, Angiosarcoma shows a richly vascularized tumor with open vascular channels and mitotic figures. **B**, There is remarkable pleomorphism in this angiosarcoma. Note the large endothelial cells with large, irregular nuclei. There are red cells within a neolumen.

epithelioid hemangioma, glomangiopericytoma, Kaposi sarcoma, and Masson vegetant endothelial hyperplasia or intravascular papillary endothelial hyperplasia.

■ EWING SARCOMA

ES and PNET are closely related high-grade, primitive, small round blue cell tumors with a neuroectodermal phenotype. These tumors are considered as a morphologic spectrum, with both expressing similar genetic alterations. There is a worldwide overall tumor incidence of 2/1,000,000 children per year, with ~20% developing in the head and neck and 20% of these cases in the SNT. There is an association of SNT cases with retinoblastoma.

CLINICAL FEATURES

There is a slight male predominance. The tumor is most common in children and young adults (80% of cases) who present with pain, mass, and obstruction. Elevated serum lactate dehydrogenase helps in detecting recurrence. Radiographically, there is a destructive osteolytic lesion with bony erosion and a periosteal reaction ("onion skin").

EWING SARCOMA—DISEASE FACT SHEET

Definition
- High-grade, primitive neuroectodermal neoplasm

Incidence and Location
- Rare (2/1,000,000 children/year)
- About 20% occur in head and neck with ~20% arising in sinonasal tract
- Maxillary sinus > nasal fossa

Morbidity and Mortality
- Better prognosis in head and neck, with ~30% mortality

Gender and age Distribution
- Slight male predominance
- Most common in children and young adults

Clinical Features
- Pain, mass, and obstruction

Prognosis and Treatment
- Size and stage dependent, although sinonasal tract location has better prognosis than thoracoabdominal disease
- Better prognosis when *EWS/FLI1* fusion is present
- Overall 60% to 70% 5-year survival
- Multimodality therapy

PATHOLOGIC FEATURES

GROSS FINDINGS

The tumors, which measure up to 6 cm, are often polypoid and multilobular, gray-white, and glistening, and often associated with ulceration and hemorrhage. Bone erosion is common. Tumors of the head and neck are much smaller at presentation than those of other anatomic sites. Tumors are seen most commonly in the maxillary sinus, followed by the nasal cavity.

MICROSCOPIC FINDINGS

Diffuse, densely cellular, sheets and nests of uniform, small- to medium-sized round cells with scant vacuolated cytoplasm (high nuclear:cytoplasmic ratio) make up this neoplasm. The cell borders are indistinct. The nuclei are round with fine chromatin distribution and small nucleoli (Figure 3-55). Mitotic figures are common. Coagulative necrosis is frequently identified (Figure 3-56), while there is peritheliomatous tumor sparing. Occasionally there is a greater degree of chromatin clumping and nuclear pleomorphism, as well as the presence of true rosettes and pseudorosettes. Atypical forms have a more lobular architecture, increased extracellular matrix, an alveolar pattern, pleomorphism, increased spindle cells, and increased mitoses.

EWING SARCOMA—PATHOLOGIC FEATURES

Gross Findings

- Often polypoid and multilobular, gray-white, glistening tumor with ulceration and hemorrhage
- Bone erosion/destruction is common in this large tumor (up to 6 cm)

Microscopic Findings

- Dense, solid sheets of small- to medium-sized monotonous cells
- High nuclear to cytoplasmic ratio with round nuclei
- Fine nuclear chromatin distribution, small nucleoli
- Mitotic activity is high with coagulative tumor necrosis common
- Occasionally may have neural differentiation

Immunohistochemical Features

- Positive: FLI1 (nuclear), CD99, vimentin; rarely keratin
- May react with other neural markers (NSE, synaptophysin, S100 protein, NFP, GFAP, chromogranin)

Molecular Features

- t(11;22)(q24;q12) or t(21;22)(q22;q12) most common
- FISH (fusion or break-apart probe) or PCR detection

Pathologic Differential Diagnosis

- Lymphoma, rhabdomyosarcoma, olfactory neuroblastoma, melanoma, sinonasal undifferentiated carcinoma, pituitary adenoma, NUT midline carcinoma, melanotic neuroectodermal tumor of infancy, mesenchymal chondrosarcoma, small cell osteosarcoma, small cell carcinoma

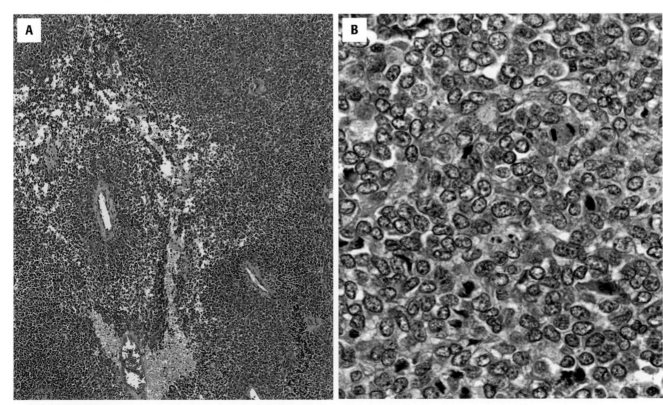

FIGURE 3-55
A, Sheets of medium-sized cells without a specific pattern. **B**, Fine chromatin and small nucleoli are noted, along with a mitosis.

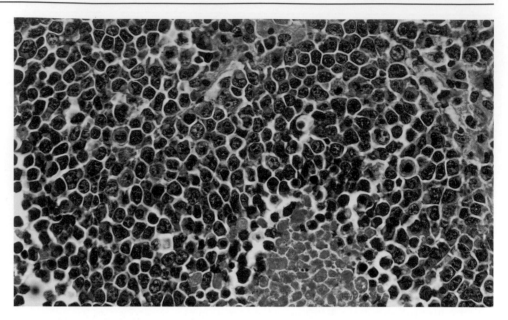

FIGURE 3-56

The sheet of medium cells with scant cytoplasm demonstrates coagulative necrosis.

ANCILLARY STUDIES

HISTOCHEMICAL STUDIES

By periodic acid–Schiff (PAS) stains, glycogen is present in the cytoplasm.

IMMUNOHISTOCHEMICAL FEATURES

CD99 (MIC2) represents the monoclonal antibody to *EWS/FLI1* fusion product. FLI1 yields a strong nuclear stain, while vimentin is expressed in nearly all ES/PNET tumors. NSE and synaptophysin are expressed less commonly. Uncommonly, S100 protein, GFAP, and keratin will also be expressed.

MOLECULAR GENETICS

The chromosomal translocation at t(11;22)(q24;q12) or t(21;22)(q22;q12) can be identified by PCR or FISH with either a fusion method or a dual-color break-apart probe (detected in ~95% of cases). Many chimeric *EWS* transcripts, representing different combinations of exons from *EWS* with other partner genes, are known (ERG, ETV1, ETV4 [E1A-F], FEV, ZSG).

DIFFERENTIAL DIAGNOSIS

The differential diagnosis includes all the malignant small round blue cell tumors, such as lymphoma, RMS, olfactory neuroblastoma, mesenchymal chondrosarcoma, small cell osteosarcoma, sinonasal undifferentiated carcinoma, melanotic neuroectodermal tumor of infancy, melanoma, small cell carcinoma, *NUT* midline carcinoma, and pituitary adenoma (Table 3-1). Their distinct clinical presentations, patterns of growth, and immunohistochemical profiles allow for separation.

PROGNOSIS AND THERAPY

ES/PNET is considered to be a highly aggressive neoplasm, often spreading into the adjacent paranasal sinuses. Staging according to the Clinical Groups of the Intergroup Rhabdomyosarcoma Study allows for a unified approach to the tumor. SNT lesions tend to have a slightly better prognosis (60% to 70% 5-year survival) than their thoracoabdominal counterparts, probably due to a smaller size at presentation (size and stage are important prognostic indicators). Patients with the *EWSR1/FLI1* fusion tend to have a better prognosis. Metastasis, seen in up to 30% of patients, is usually to lungs, bone marrow, bone, brain, and lymph nodes. Multimodality therapy (chemotherapy, radiation, and surgery) achieves the best outcome, with autologous bone marrow or peripheral blood stem cell rescue. Poor prognostic factors include large size (tumor >8 cm), elevated white blood cell and sedimentation rates, filigree microscopic pattern, and lack of response to chemotherapy prior to resection.

■ TERATOCARCINOSARCOMA

This rare complex malignant neoplasm of SNT consists of various carcinomatous and sarcomatous elements, including immature epithelial, neuroepithelial, and mesenchymal tissues resembling immature teratoma.

By definition, germ cell tumors are not included (embryonal carcinoma, choriocarcinoma, seminoma). Although unknown, the tumor is thought to arise from the primitive cells in the olfactory membrane that possess the capacity to show multilineage differentiation.

CLINICAL FEATURES

Men are affected much more commonly than women, with a mean age of 60 years at presentation. Similar to other malignant SNT neoplasms, nasal obstruction and epistaxis are the most common complaints, usually of a short duration. The tumor occurs most commonly high in the nasal cavity, ethmoid sinus, and maxillary sinus, frequently involving more than one location. Vasopressin may be ectopically or inappropriately elevated.

PATHOLOGIC FEATURES

GROSS FINDINGS

The tumors are large (generally >4 cm), bulky, polypoid friable to fleshy with necrosis (Figure 3-57).

MICROSCOPIC FINDINGS

Teratocarcinosarcoma is a heterogeneous neoplasm containing intermingled carcinomatous and sarcomatous tissues, along with teratoma-like elements (Figure 3-58). Elements from all three germ cell layers may be present, but the components may be either benign or malignant and are topographically mixed, with transitions between the tumor elements. The carcinoma may be squamous or adenocarcinoma. The stromal elements include hypercellular immature tissue with spindle cells embedded in a myxoid matrix, islands of cartilage and bone, smooth muscle, and skeletal muscle in varying degrees of maturation (Figure 3-59). Primitive neuroepithelial elements with blastomatous cells, rosettes, pseudorosettes, or neurofibrillary matrix often predominate in these tumors (Figures 3-60 and 3-61).

ANCILLARY STUDIES

Immunohistochemistry will highlight the various constituent elements accordingly: neuroepithelial elements are usually positive with NSE, chromogranin, synaptophysin, CD56, S100 protein, and CD99; spindle cell elements express vimentin, GFAP, desmin, myogenin, calponin and/or actins; and epithelial elements are positive for cytokeratins and EMA.

TERATOCARCINOSARCOMA—DISEASE FACT SHEET

Definition
- A complex malignant neoplasm with immature and malignant endodermal, mesodermal, and neuroepithelial elements

Incidence and Location
- Extremely rare
- Ethmoid and maxillary antrum

Morbidity and Mortality
- 60% of patients die within 3 years

Gender and Age Distribution
- Male >> female
- Mean, 60 years (adults)

Clinical Features
- Nasal obstruction and epistaxis of short duration

Prognosis and Treatment
- Poor prognosis with highly aggressive behavior
- Overall, 60% die within 3 years
- Recurrences are common usually in <3 years
- Multimodality therapy does not seem to alter prognosis

TERATOCARCINOSARCOMA—PATHOLOGIC FEATURES

Gross Findings
- Large (>4 cm), bulky, polypoid friable masses, with necrosis

Microscopic Findings
- Carcinomatous and sarcomatous component, mingled with multiple mature and immature tissues from all germ cell layers
- Carcinoma can be squamous or adenocarcinoma
- Neural elements show prominent rosettes and blastema-like cells
- Cartilage, bone, or muscle may comprise sarcoma

Immunohistochemical Features
- Neuroepithelial elements positive: NSE, chromogranin, synaptophysin, CD56, CD99, S100 protein
- Spindle cells positive: vimentin, GFAP, desmin, myogenin, calponin and/or actins
- Epithelial elements positive: cytokeratins and EMA

Pathologic Differential Diagnosis
- Olfactory neuroblastoma, rhabdomyosarcoma, carcinoma (adenocarcinoma and sinonasal undifferentiated carcinoma)

DIFFERENTIAL DIAGNOSIS

Depending on the cellular elements present in the biopsy, considerations include olfactory neuroblastoma, RMS, and carcinoma (sinonasal undifferentiated carcinoma and adenocarcinoma). A germ cell tumor usually

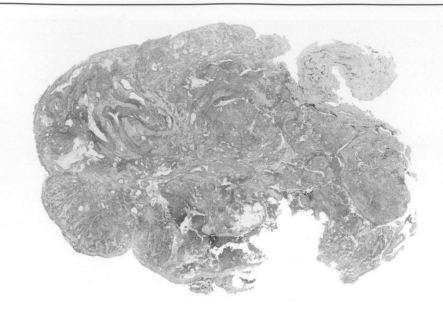

FIGURE 3-57

This polypoid tumor shows a variety of different patterns of growth and different cellular compartments, including epithelial, mesenchymal, and teratomatous.

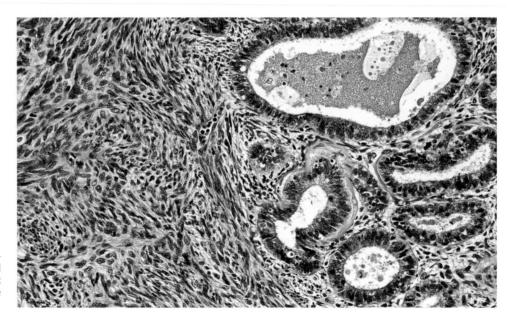

FIGURE 3-58

The adenocarcinoma is intimately associated with the sarcomatous portion, arranged in a "teratoma-like" distribution. Cytologic atypia is present in both constituents of the neoplasm.

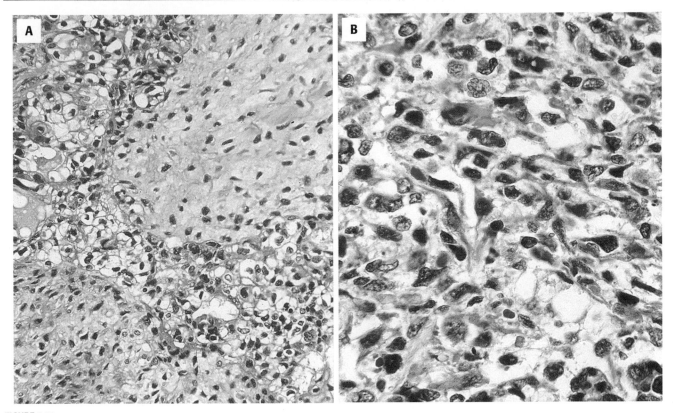

FIGURE 3-59
A, Immature cartilage and spindle cells in a teratocarcinosarcoma. **B**, Rhabdomyoblasts have elongated nuclei and eosinophilic cytoplasm. *(Courtesy of Dr. Yao S. Fu.)*

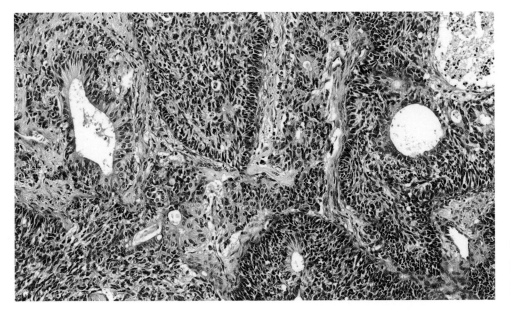

FIGURE 3-60

A primitive blastema-like component is immediately adjacent to a malignant glandular element that is juxtaposed with a malignant, cellular spindle cell component.

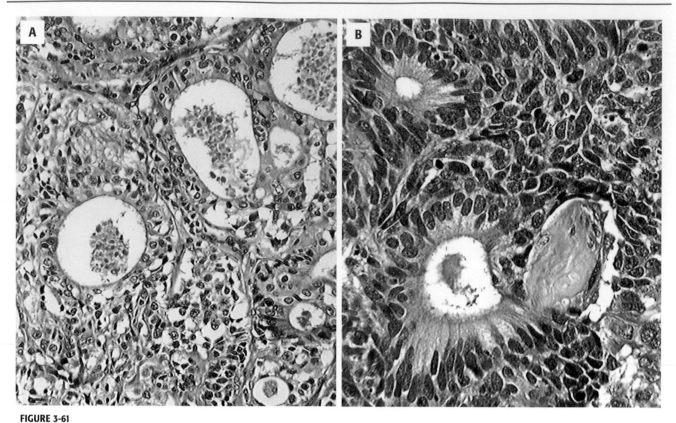

FIGURE 3-61
A, An adenocarcinoma adjacent to primitive blastema-like cells. **B**, The primitive cells can sometimes be arranged in a true rosette, similar to a teratoma.

has distinct features of embryonal, yolk sac, and semi-noma. The presence of all three elements usually confirms the diagnosis.

PROGNOSIS AND THERAPY

This is a highly aggressive neoplasm with a poor prognosis. Most patients (60%) die within 3 years. Recurrences are common (up to 70%), often with intracranial extension, usually developing within 2 years of diagnosis. Cervical lymph node metastasis is seen in ~30% of patients. Aggressive multimodality therapy (surgery, chemotherapy, radiation) does not seem to alter the prognosis.

SUGGESTED READINGS

The complete suggested readings list is available online at www.expertconsult.com.

4

Non-Neoplastic Lesions of the Larynx, Hypopharynx, and Trachea

■ Lester D. R. Thompson

■ VOCAL CORD POLYPS AND NODULES

Vocal cord polyps and nodules represent reactive changes of laryngeal mucosa and adjacent stroma that result in a benign polypoid or nodular growth. The etiology is multifactorial, including laryngeal trauma (accidents or surgery), excessive and improper use of voice (vocal abuse), iatrogenic or functional lesions, infection, hypothyroidism, and smoking.

CLINICAL FEATURES

"Nodule" and "polyp" are not clinically synonymous terms, although they are frequently used interchangeably in the pathology community. About 1.5 % of the general population has hoarseness and the presence of a polyp/nodule is one of the most frequent significant causes. Nearly 2.5 % of children have nodules, with boys affected more often than girls (2:1). Among young adults, nodules are more frequent in young women. In contrast, polyps occur in any age group with an equal gender distribution. For both types of lesions, vocal changes and hoarseness are the most frequent presenting symptoms. The speaking voices of singers, actors, public speakers, lecturers, and coaches are affected by excessive (overuse) and improper (abuse) use of voice. Interestingly, extroverted patients are more likely to develop vocal cord polyps and nodules.

PATHOLOGIC FEATURES

VOCAL CORD POLYPS AND NODULES—DISEASE FACT SHEET

Definition
- Reactive changes of the laryngeal mucosa and adjacent stroma that result in a benign polypoid or nodular growth

Incidence and Location
- Infrequent (<1% of population)
- ~2.5% of children (boys > girls; 2:1)

Gender and Age Distribution
- Nodule is more common in young women
- Polyps occur at any age and in both genders equally

Clinical Features
- Vocal abuse or overuse, phonation changes, hoarseness
- Other causes include infection, smoking, and hypothyroidism

Prognosis and Treatment
- Excellent
- Voice or speech therapy, behavior modification, vocal hygiene, and medical management before surgery

---

VOCAL CORD POLYPS AND NODULES—PATHOLOGIC FEATURES

Gross Findings
- Nodules are bilateral, edematous to gelatinous, on opposing surfaces usually in the middle third of vocal cord (<0.5 cm)
- Polyps are unilateral, involve ventricular or Reinke space, and are a pedunculated soft, rubbery translucent to red mass (up to 3 cm)

Microscopic Findings
- Arc of development
- Edematous with proteinaceous material within interstitium
- Vascularized stroma with hemorrhage in loose myxoid stroma
- Myxoid stroma (pale blue-pink matrix material)
- Hyaline (fibrin-type material adjacent to vessels)
- Fibrous (spindle cells in dense stroma)
- Scant inflammation

Pathologic Differential
- Amyloidosis, myxoma, contact ulcer, ligneous conjunctivitis, granular cell tumor, diagnosis spindle cell (sarcomatoid) squamous cell carcinoma

GROSS FINDINGS

Grossly, nodules are almost always bilateral, affecting the anterior to middle third of the true vocal cord and presenting as an edematous, gelatinous, or hemorrhagic mass, typically a few millimeters in size (Figure 4-1). By contrast, a polyp is unilateral (>90%), affecting the aryepiglottic fold, ventricular space, vocal fold, or Reinke space, as a sessile, raspberry-like to pedunculated soft, rubbery, translucent (edematous) to erythematous mass (Figure 4-2) up to a few centimeters in greatest dimension.

MICROSCOPIC FINDINGS

There is no definitive histologic distinction between laryngeal nodules and polyp, as they represent different

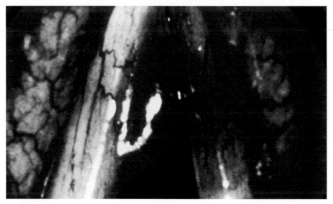

FIGURE 4-1
Bilaterally edematous nodules on opposing surfaces of the vocal cords.

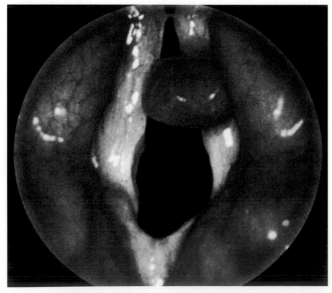

FIGURE 4-2
A polyp projects from the vocal cord on one side only.

stages of an arc of development. In the early stages, there is edema and deposition of proteinaceous material in the subepithelium and interstitium (Figure 4-3). There is increased vascularization with subsequent hemorrhage (Figure 4-4). Inflammation is scant to absent, but dilated vessels (telangiectasia) and granulation-type tissue may occasionally be seen. Myxoid stroma (pale blue-pink matrix material; Figure 4-5) tends to be an intermediate phase as the lesion progresses to more mature variants: a hyaline type, with fibrin-type material closely opposed to vascular spaces (Figure 4-6); or a fibrous type, with spindle cells in a dense fibrous stroma (Figure 4-7). However, any or all of these changes may be seen within the same polyp. Therefore, the designations of edematous, vascular, myxoid, hyaline or fibrous type are not important, as they represent degrees of development. By convention, however, the dominant histologic pattern determines the type. The surface epithelium may become metaplastic, atrophic, keratotic, and hyperplastic. Crystals can be seen in some polyps.

DIFFERENTIAL DIAGNOSIS

The differential diagnosis includes amyloidosis, myxoma, contact ulcer, ligneous conjunctivitis, and, rarely, neoplasms (granular cell tumor, spindle cell [sarcomatoid] squamous cell carcinoma [SCSCC]). Amyloidosis shows a perivascular or periglandular accentuation of an acellular, extracellular eosinophilic matrix material. Myxoma, uncommon at this site, is an avascular, hypocellular lesion with occasional stellate spindle cells in an abundant basophilic, gelatinous matrix. Contact ulcer shows surface ulceration with fibrinoid necrosis and primarily affects opposing surfaces of the posterior true vocal cords. Ligneous ("woody") conjunctivitis, a rare chronic condition affecting mucous membranes, results in firm, clotted fibrin-rich matrix material deposition that creates a hard, subepithelial nodule. In general, the neoplasms can be easily separated on the basis of their characteristic histologic findings.

PROGNOSIS AND THERAPY

Voice or speech therapy, behavior modification, and vocal hygiene are first-line treatments for polyps and nodules. Drug therapy may also help select underlying conditions, such as hypothyroidism. Surgery usually has limited value because it is the underlying cause that needs to be managed.

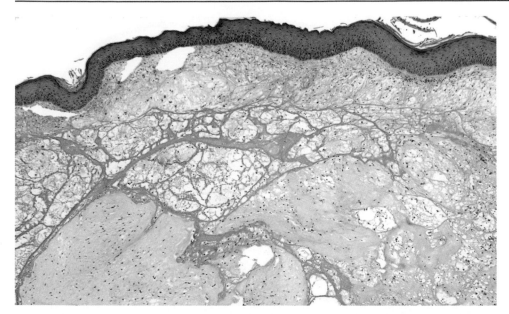

FIGURE 4-3

The surface epithelium of a polyp is unremarkable, covering the hypocellular, edematous stroma.

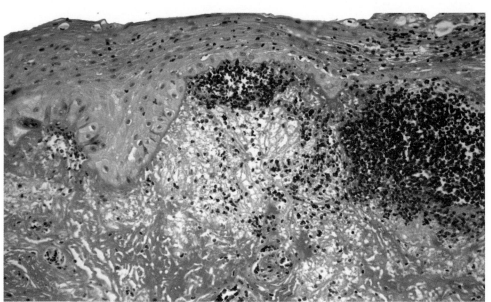

FIGURE 4-4

Below an intact, inflamed squamous mucosa is an area of edema, vascular proliferation, and degeneration seen within a polyp.

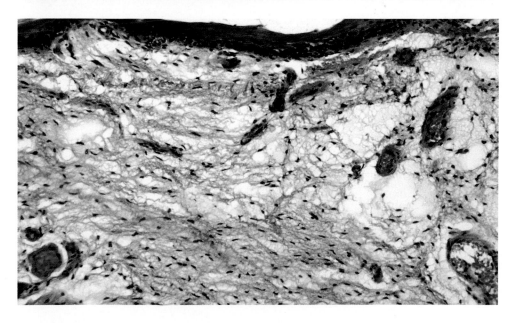

FIGURE 4-5

Basophilic myxoid material separates small stellate cells without cytologic atypia. The surface epithelium is intact and uninvolved.

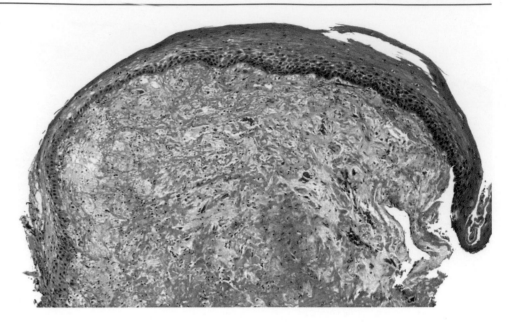

FIGURE 4-6

Hyaline change in a polyp with fibrin-type material and edematous change.

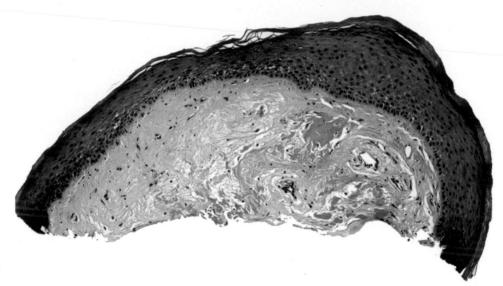

FIGURE 4-7

Fibrous connective tissue deposition beneath a keratotic epithelium. Note a small area of fibrinoid material.

■ CONTACT ULCER

CLINICAL FEATURES

Also known as pyogenic granuloma, this frequent benign reactive epithelial response to injury is generally associated with acid regurgitation, vocal abuse, and intubation. Gastric-laryngeal reflux or gastroesophageal reflux disease (GERD) is frequently missed as the patient is unaware of the underlying cause (hiatal hernia), although the patient may report heartburn and/or belching as a result of the acid reflux. Interestingly, pepsin is thought to be the injurious agent and not the hydrochloric acid. As a result of intubation, female patients

are affected more commonly, especially in the emergent setting when an inappropriately sized endotracheal tube has been selected. Otherwise, contact ulcer occurs more frequently in adult men, who present with hoarseness, cough, sore throat, chronic throat clearing, habitual coughing, or pain.

PATHOLOGIC FEATURES

GROSS FINDINGS

Contact ulcer usually presents as a bilateral, polypoid or nodular mass (Figure 4-8), up to 3 cm in size, most frequently affecting the posterior larynx. There is

CONTACT ULCER–DISEASE FACT SHEET

Definition

- Benign reactive epithelial response to an injury usually in the posterior larynx

Incidence and Location

- Frequent, especially in patients with gastroesophageal reflux disease or vocal abuse
- Posterior larynx is most common site

Gender, Race, and Age

- Male > female (except in postintubation distribution setting)
- Adults > children

Clinical Features

- Hoarseness, cough, sore throat, and pain
- Chronic throat clearing and habitual coughing
- Vocal abuse/misuse
- Gastrolaryngeal reflux disease symptoms (heartburn, belching)

Prognosis and Treatment

- Excellent
- Control gastroesophageal reflux disease, vocal rehabilitation, and then perhaps surgery

CONTACT ULCER–PATHOLOGIC FEATURES

Gross Findings

- Bilateral, ulcerated, polypoid to nodular mass
- Posterior larynx with kissing ulcer on contralateral cord
- Up to 3 cm

Microscopic Findings

- Surface ulceration with fibrinoid necrosis
- Exuberant granulation tissue, with vessels aligned perpendicular to surface
- Central areas may have hemosiderin-laden macrophages
- Reactive and plump endothelial cells (without atypia)
- May have surface reepithelialization with time but fibrinoid necrosis usually remains; prominent fibrosis may develop

Pathologic Differential Diagnosis

- Infectious agents
- Inflammatory conditions (Wegener granulomatosis)
- Vascular lesions (Kaposi sarcoma and angiosarcoma)
- Epithelial neoplasms, specifically spindle cell (sarcomatoid) squamous cell carcinoma

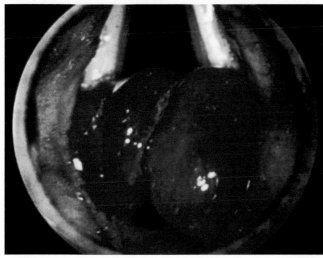

FIGURE 4-8

A laryngoscopic view of contact ulcer shows a polypoid, bilateral, beefy red mass involving the posterior vocal cords. A "kissing ulcer" is characteristic.

usually a "kissing ulcer" on the contralateral cord, with a red to beefy appearance.

MICROSCOPIC FINDINGS

Histologic sections reveal extensive surface ulceration, covered by fibrin and/or fibrinoid necrosis, overlying exuberant granulation tissue (Figures 4-9 and 4-10). Vessels in the granulation tissue, often arranged perpendicular to the surface, are lined by plump reactive

endothelial cells without atypia and are surrounded by marked acute and chronic inflammation, including plasma cells, histiocytes, and giant cells (Figure 4-10). Hemosiderin-laden macrophages may be seen at the base of the polyp, especially in lesions of long clinical duration (Figure 4-9). Surface bacterial or fungal colonization is frequently identified. In the early stages, surface ulceration without granulation tissue may be identified. Over time, the lesion may demonstrate an irregular hyperplastic epithelium secondary to regenerative surface reepithelialization, although a residuum of fibrinoid necrosis is usually identified below the surface (Figure 4-11). These changes characterize the chronic phase of the disease, which may also show prominent stromal fibrosis.

DIFFERENTIAL DIAGNOSIS

The diagnosis of contact ulcer is usually a clinical pathologic correlation, since the histologic findings are largely nonspecific. In light of this, the morphologic differential diagnosis includes a variety of infectious agents, inflammatory conditions (Wegener granulomatosis, inflammatory myofibroblastic tumor), vascular lesions (Kaposi sarcoma [KS], angiosarcoma), and epithelial neoplasms (SCC, SCSCC). Special stains (Gomori methenamine silver [GMS], periodic acid–Schiff [PAS], Brown-Hopps [tissue Gram stain], Warthin-Starry) and culture should confirm an infectious agent. Wegener granulomatosis has geographic biocollagenolytic blue, granular necrosis, genuine vasculitis, and

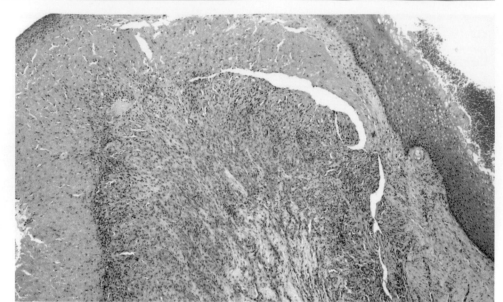

FIGURE 4-9

A polypoid nodule has most of the surface epithelium denuded and replaced by fibrinoid necrosis. The vessels are arranged perpendicular to the surface and are surrounded by a rich granulation-type tissue, including hemosiderin-laden macrophages.

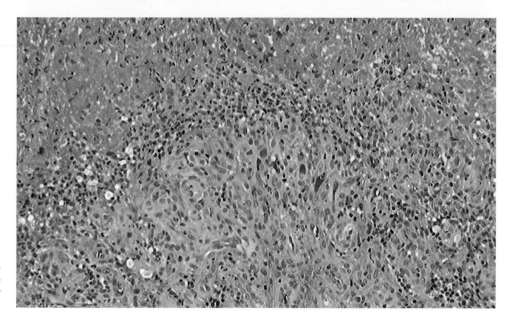

FIGURE 4-10

The fibrinoid necrosis replaces the surface epithelium and directly covers the granulation-type tissue. Inflammatory elements are prominent.

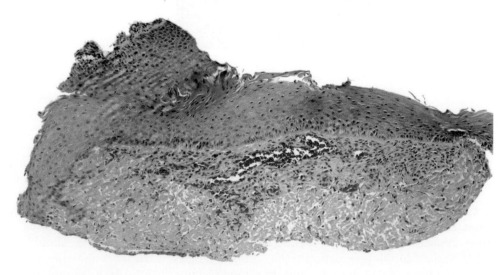

FIGURE 4-11

The surface epithelium has grown over the defect, but the fibrinoid necrosis is still present to give a hint of the previous damage.

helpful laboratory findings (antineutrophil cytoplasmic antibodies titers). KS and angiosarcoma are rare in the larynx but show slit-like spaces with pleomorphic cells, freely anastomosing vascular channels, intracellular spheroid hyaline globules (KS), and atypical mitotic figures.

PROGNOSIS AND THERAPY

Once the correct diagnosis of contact ulcer is made, appropriate identification and removal of the specific inciting factor can eliminate the morbidity associated with surgery. Medical management includes aggressive acid-suppressive therapy to control GERD. In addition, vocal rehabilitation and behavioral modifications to minimize shouting, habitual coughing, and/or throat clearing are helpful in controlling the disease.

■ AMYLOIDOSIS

Amyloidosis (amyloidoma) encompasses a family of different types of benign accumulations of extracellular, acellular, fibrillar, insoluble protein deposits. Laryngeal amyloidosis is commonly both localized and primary and is the most common site of localized disease, although

rare, accounting for <1% of benign laryngeal tumors. Multifocal disease is present in up to 15 % of patients. It may be part of mucosa-associated lymphoid tissue (MALT) or a neuroendocrine tumor product. In fact, this mucosal association implies that at least a few laryngeal amyloid cases may be the result of a lymphoproliferative disorder with an origin from MALT (MALT lymphoma). Moreover, the monoclonal nature of the associated lymphoplasmacytic infiltrate in some cases, and the association with a systemic plasma cell dyscrasia, suggests a pathogenesis from an immunocyte dyscrasia.

There are a variety of classifications of amyloidosis, according to its distribution (localization), clinical type, by the presence or absence of underlying disease, its precursor protein (immunocytochemical nature), and patterns of extracellular deposition. Different sources of amyloidosis are recognized, with immunoglobulin light chains most common in the larynx.

CLINICAL FEATURES

Almost all patients experience hoarseness or voice changes, usually caused by mechanical factors, conditioned by the size and location of the amyloid. Patients usually present as adults, although children can rarely be affected, and there is no gender predilection.

PATHOLOGIC FEATURES

AMYLOIDOSIS—DISEASE FACT SHEET

Definition
- Benign accumulation of extracellular, fibrillar insoluble protein deposits of amyloid

Incidence and Location
- <1% of all laryngeal neoplasms
- Usually in false vocal cord, but can be multifocal (15%)

Morbidity and Mortality
- Depends on primary or systemic disease and whether single or multifocal
- May be slowly progressive

Gender, Race, and Age Distribution
- Equal gender distribution
- Usually adults, but rarely children are affected

Clinical Features
- Hoarseness and voice changes

Prognosis and Treatment
- Good, although dependent on localized or systemic disease and whether primary or secondary
- Surgery is the treatment of choice
- Must exclude systemic disease with clinical, radiographic, and laboratory workup

---

AMYLOIDOSIS—PATHOLOGIC FEATURES

Gross Findings
- Firm, starch-like, waxy translucent cut surface
- Up to 4 cm

Microscopic Findings
- Subepithelial deposits
- Acellular, extracellular, eosinophilic, homogeneous matrix material
- Perivascular and periglandular predilection (compression atrophy may result)
- Lymphoplasmacytic infiltrate (may be light chain restricted)
- Foreign body giant cell reaction can be seen

Special Studies
- "Apple-green" birefringence with polarized light using a Congo red stain (metachromatic with methyl violet)
- May show κ or λ light chain restriction and positive amyloid P immunoreactivity

Pathologic Differential Diagnosis
- MALT lymphoma, vocal cord polyps, ligneous conjunctivitis, lipoid proteinosis, component of multiple myeloma, neuroendocrine carcinoma, and medullary thyroid carcinoma

GROSS FINDINGS

Although there are conflicting data, the false vocal cord seems to be more frequently affected, showing a firm, "starch-like," waxy, translucent cut surface, measuring up to 4 cm in greatest dimension. Multifocal disease elsewhere in the upper aerodigestive tract can be seen in up to 15% of patients.

MICROSCOPIC FINDINGS

Amyloid consists histologically (irrespective of any associated findings) of a subepithelial, extracellular, acellular, hyaline-like, homogeneous, eosinophilic matrix material dispersed randomly throughout the stroma (Figure 4-12), although revealing a predilection for vessels or mucoserous glands (Figure 4-13).

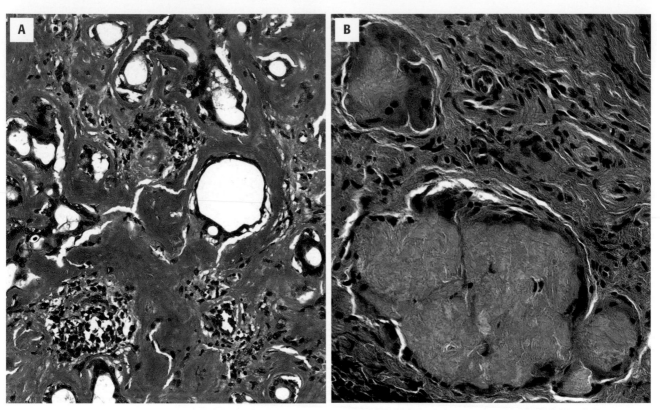

FIGURE 4-12

A, Periductal deposition with compression atrophy is characteristic for amyloid. **B**, Fragments of amorphous, acellular, eosinophilic amyloid material is found in the stroma, with a foreign body giant cell reaction.

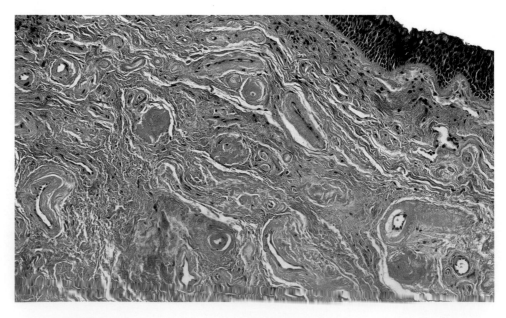

FIGURE 4-13

The respiratory type epithelium overlies a stroma in which there are periductal and perivascular deposits of eosinophilic hyaline amyloid material.

A sparse inflammatory infiltrate composed of lymphocytes and plasma cells (Figure 4-14) may be seen; however, significant cytologic atypia of this lymphoplasmacytic infiltrate is not appreciated. Occasional histiocytes and giant cells may be either at the peripheral margin of or enclosed within the amyloid (Figure 4-12). The amyloidosis of the larynx is composed of a protein that is immunologically identical to the variable region of the light chain fragment of immunoglobulin.

ANCILLARY STUDIES

ELECTRON MICROSCOPY

Electron microscopy reveals the characteristic loose, interlacing meshwork of nonbranching, irregular fibrils of indefinite length as the protein arranges itself into β-pleated sheets (appreciated by x-ray crystallography).

SPECIAL STAINS

Amyloid can be confirmed with histochemical techniques (Congo red, methyl violet [metachromatic pink-violet staining]), with the characteristic apple-green birefringence seen under polarized light with Congo red (Figure 4-15) proving to be the most reliable and easy-to-interpret.

IMMUNOHISTOCHEMICAL FEATURES

CD20 and CD3 highlight the admixture of B and T cells in the sparse lymphoplasmacytic infiltrate, respectively, although T cells tend to predominate, especially at the periphery of the amyloid deposits. Immunoreactivity

with amyloid P and light chains (κ and λ) is more variable, although light chain restriction of the plasma cells can be seen in some cases.

DIFFERENTIAL DIAGNOSIS

The differential diagnosis is limited and includes hyalinized vocal cord polyps (usually lacks an associated lymphoplasmacytic infiltrate), ligneous conjunctivitis (fibrin-rich nodular deposits), and lipoid proteinosis (amorphous hyaline deposits), all of which are negative for amyloid studies.

It is important to note that amyloid may occur in association with multiple myeloma, laryngeal neuroendocrine tumors (atypical carcinoid, small cell carcinoma), and medullary thyroid carcinoma. In the latter scenario, the determination of a serum calcitonin level can help to distinguish between a primary laryngeal neuroendocrine tumor (serum elevation absent) versus a metastatic/invasive medullary thyroid carcinoma (serum elevation present).

PROGNOSIS AND THERAPY

Excision is usually the treatment of choice. There is a difference, however, in the biologic behavior and clinical management between isolated laryngeal amyloidosis and other forms of amyloidosis. Multifocal or systemic disease must be ruled out by clinical, radiographic, and laboratory investigation (including quantitative immunoglobulin assay, serologic test for rheumatoid arthritis and/or other chronic inflammatory

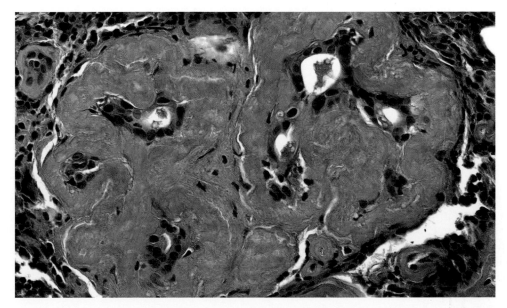

FIGURE 4-14

A sparse inflammatory infiltrate of mature lymphocytes and plasma cells is seen immediately around an amyloid deposit that surrounds mucoserous glands and ducts.

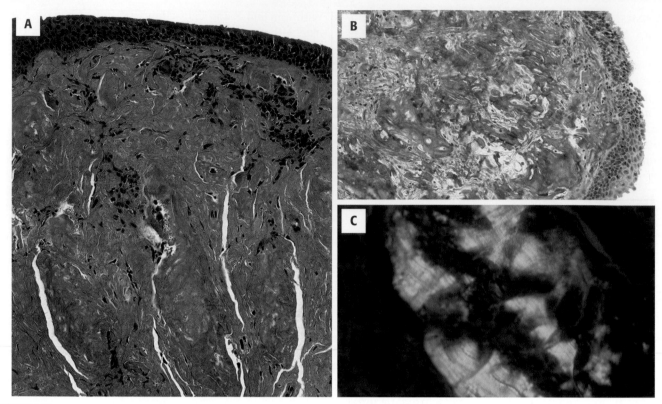

FIGURE 4-15

A, The acellular, eosinophilic, opaque amyloid deposition is noted below an intact surface epithelium with focal inflammation. **B**, Congo red stain highlights the amyloid. **C**, "Apple-green" birefringence when viewed under polarized light of a Congo red stain.

conditions, urine and/or serum electrophoresis, Bence-Jones protein analysis) that should be tailored to the individual patient. Prognosis depends on localized versus systemic, and primary versus secondary, disease. The prognosis for isolated laryngeal amyloidosis is excellent as the "tumors" are slow growing, although repeated surgeries (endoscopic) may be necessary for recurrent disease. There does not appear to be any prognostic significance of amyloid deposition in association with other tumors. In these cases, the prognosis is determined by the specific tumor type/morphology itself.

■ CYSTS OF THE LARYNX (INCLUDING LARYNGOCELE)

Cysts of the larynx may be filled with fluid or air and may be lined by different epithelia, each of which has a different name based on anatomic site as well as histologic appearance. Benign cysts (saccular, ductal, oncocytic, tonsillar) are usually distinct from laryngocele, which is usually a clinical/radiographic finding. These lesions may result from repeated increases of intralaryngeal pressure, infection, trauma, or in association with tumors.

CLINICAL FEATURES

CYSTS OF THE LARYNX (INCLUDING LARYNGOCELE)— DISEASE FACT SHEET

Definition
- Outpouchings of the laryngeal ventricle and saccule are called laryngoceles
- Saccular, ductal, oncocytic, and tonsillar cysts are benign epithelial cysts within specific anatomic sites of the larynx

Incidence and Location
- Uncommon, although more frequent in younger patients

Gender and Age Distribution
- Laryngocele: males > females; all ages are affected
- Cysts: equal gender distribution; usually older adults (50 to 60 years)

Clinical Features
- Divided into internal or external laryngocele
- Symptoms are variable and nonspecific with airway obstruction, hoarseness, mass, and foreign body sensation

Prognosis and Treatment
- Excellent
- Marsupialization (laryngocele) or surgery for cysts

Outpouchings from the laryngeal ventricle and saccule of the normal laryngeal mucosa result in a laryngocele. Laryngoceles are rare (1 in 2.5 million), develop in men more often than in women, appear across all ages, and are divided clinically into internal (expansion into the false vocal fold) and external (extension through the thyrohyoid membrane into the soft tissues of the neck). The vast majority present with an internal unilateral mass. Symptoms are variable and include airway obstruction, hoarseness, mass, or foreign body sensation; however, symptoms may spontaneously resolve when the expelled air decompresses the mass.

In general, the symptoms for patients with cysts are nonspecific and heavily overlap those of laryngocele. The most common laryngeal cysts are ductal cysts (75 %), followed by saccular cysts (located between true and false cords). Tonsillar cysts show a predilection for the epiglottis, while ductal and oncocytic cysts predilect to the ventricular folds and ventricle of Morgagni. Patients are usually older adults (50 to 60 years), with an equal gender distribution.

PATHOLOGIC FEATURES

GROSS FINDINGS

The gross appearance of laryngeal cysts is determined by the point of origin in the larynx and the type of cyst (saccular, ductal, oncocytic, tonsillar). The cyst can be considered to be either external or internal to the larynx based on the degree of compression by the cyst and the extent of disease within the larynx. Cysts generally do not communicate with the interior of the larynx, while a laryngocele is an air-filled herniation or dilatation of the saccule, either internal or external to the

CYSTS OF THE LARYNX (INCLUDING LARYNGOCELE)— PATHOLOGIC FEATURES

Gross Findings

- Point of origin and type of cyst determine the macroscopic appearance
- Internal or external to the larynx
- Cysts do not generally communicate with the lumen
- Saccular cysts (submucosal) filled with mucus, affect the false cord
- Retention cysts (tonsillar) affect epiglottis
- Traumatic cysts affect the arytenoid region
- Size ranges from 0.5 to 8 cm

Microscopic Findings

- Cysts are surrounded by fibrous connective tissue
- Squamous or respiratory epithelium
- Vascular elements seen in vascular cysts
- Oncocytic epithelium may line the cysts
- Inflammation within wall in tonsillar cysts

Pathologic Differential Diagnosis

- External jugular phlebectasia, prolapse, branchial cleft cyst, thyroglossal duct cyst, dermoid cyst, teratoma, laryngeal webs

larynx, but communicating with the lumen (Figure 4-16). Saccular cysts (anterior or lateral) are submucosal and do not communicate with the lumen but are instead filled with mucus or acute inflammatory elements. As air and fluid are forced into a laryngocele, the distinction between a laryngocele and other laryngeal cysts may be impossible. The size of these cysts ranges from 0.5 to 8 cm, depending on the location. Eversion and prolapse occur, further complicating the classification of cysts of the larynx. The cysts are variably filled with thin serous fluid to tenacious, thick, mucinous, gelatinous, or bloody fluid.

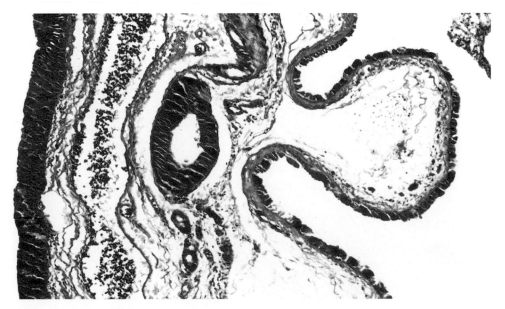

FIGURE 4-16

An intact mucosa is seen on the left, while an outpouching of oncocytic epithelium on the right is part of an external laryngocele.

MICROSCOPIC FINDINGS

Histologic examination, while unnecessary for diagnosis of a laryngocele, will show an epithelium-lined cyst, containing respiratory or squamous mucosa.

Cysts have a variably thick surrounding wall of fibrous connective tissue. The lining of the cysts helps to differentiate them into a variety of subtypes. Most of the cysts are lined with squamous or respiratory epithelium (retention and saccular) (Figure 4-17), while a few are lined with fibrous connective tissue. A cyst in which there is an admixture of both mesodermal and endodermal layers qualifies as a *congenital* or *embryonal cyst*. This type of cyst contains squamous or respiratory epithelium along with some other mesodermal element, intimately associated with the epithelial component. The *traumatic cyst* is not common but is more frequently described as surgical intervention in the larynx has increased. Small islands of tissue are implanted deep into the stroma and undergo cystic degeneration. A *saccular cyst* is lined by ciliated respiratory epithelium with increased numbers of goblet cells and a partially or completely metaplastic squamous or oncocytic epithelium (Figure 4-18). A *ductal cyst* (which results from obstruction of intramucosal ducts of seromucinous glands) shows a double-layered cylindrical, cuboidal, or flattened ductal epithelium with squamous or oncocytic metaplasia. A *tonsillar cyst* resembles tonsillar crypt epithelium with squamous epithelium, keratin, and lymphoid tissue in the wall (Figure 4-19). Any of these cysts can become infected and, when infected, are referred to as a pyocele, although they are still classified by the original cyst type. The larger the ventricular appendix, the more predisposed the individual is to infection or inflammation.

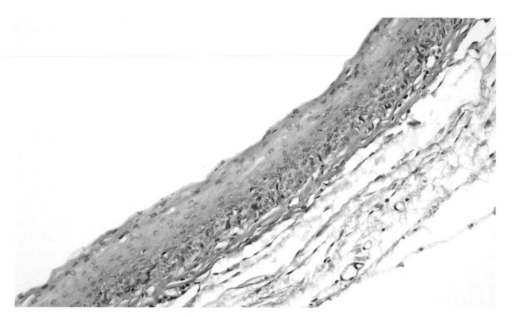

FIGURE 4-17

A metaplastic squamous mucosa is identified within this laryngeal cyst.

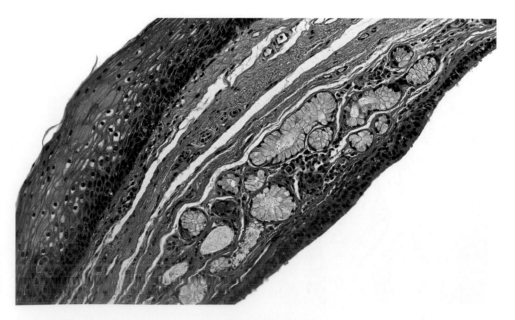

FIGURE 4-18

A saccular cyst shows a respiratory, oncocytic epithelium lining a space surrounded by mucoserous glands. The squamous mucosa (far left) is the lining of the larynx mucosa.

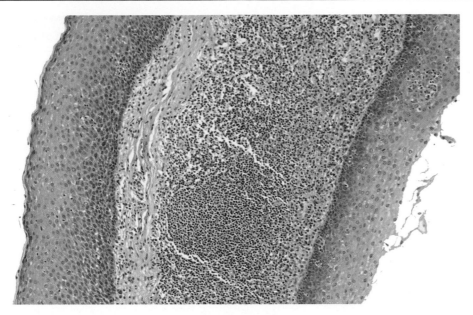

FIGURE 4-19

A tonsillar cyst shows squamous epithelium associated with a lymphoid infiltrate of the wall, resembling tonsillar epithelium.

Oncocytes can be present within a wide variety of lesions in the larynx, including, but not limited to, oncocytic papillary cystadenoma, oncocytic cyst (Figure 4-20), oncocytoma, oxyphilic adenoma, eosinophilic papillary cystadenoma, and oncocytic hyperplasia. Oncocytic metaplasia and/or hyperplasia is most likely an aging phenomenon with an aggregation of mitochondria within the cytoplasm of the lesional cells. The separation from a cyst may be difficult, although oncocytic metaplasia and/or hyperplasia should be multifocal or diffusely present within the larynx. The cells are polyhedral to round with distinct cell borders, characteristically abundant cytoplasm containing a varying number of fine to coarse, eosinophilic granules, and small, round, centrally situated, pyknotic to vesicular nuclei.

DIFFERENTIAL DIAGNOSIS

The differential diagnosis is often limited histologically but may be quite broad clinically. For example, *external jugular phlebectasia* (a congenital dilatation of the jugular vein) frequently presents as a neck mass, particularly during straining or crying (Valsalva maneuver) similar to a laryngocele. However, it does not require surgery, although surgery is often performed for cosmetic purposes. The histologic appearance is of a dilated vascular space and is different from that of laryngocele or other laryngeal cysts. Therefore, histologic confirmation of the lesion is mandatory to help define the type of cyst. *Prolapse* of the ventricle can sometimes resemble

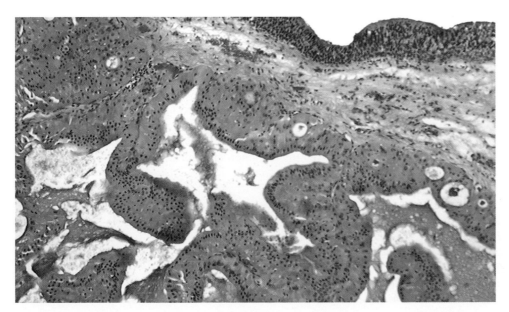

FIGURE 4-20

A papillary oncocytic proliferation within the larynx, composed of enlarged, polyhedral cells with abundant, opaque, oxyphilic cytoplasm. The nuclei are small and hyperchromatic cells.

a cyst on gross examination. However, prolapse can be "put back" to restore normal anatomy, while cysts cannot. *Large branchial cleft cysts* and *thyroglossal duct cysts* may push into the laryngeal spaces, thereby creating the illusion of a primary cyst of the larynx. Histologic examination, combined with the clinical site of origin, should help in distinguishing these from other cysts of the region. A true *teratoma* has tissue from all three layers and is different from the developmental cysts of the larynx. Other clinical entities include laryngeal webs, vascular rings, hemangiomas, and foreign bodies. These entities can usually be excluded clinically or by biopsy. *Squamous cell carcinoma* (SCC), usually supraglottic, can be associated with laryngeal cysts, perhaps induced by the carcinoma.

PROGNOSIS AND THERAPY

Surgical marsupialization is the treatment of choice for a laryngocele, while benign cysts can be managed symptomatically, with aspiration or endoscopic removal only as clinically necessary to maintain a patent airway. Airway obstruction, infection (laryngopyocele), or recurrences are possible complications.

■ REACTIVE EPITHELIAL CHANGES

There is a lack of uniformity and an inconsistency of terminology used to describe reactive, hyperplastic, and "precancerous" epithelial lesions of the larynx, both clinically and histopathologically. This results in a lack of concordance with the term used and the biology of the lesion. Dozens of classification schemes have been proposed, but none has gained substantial support in either the clinical or pathology communities. No matter which system is used, it is imperative that the term clearly convey to the clinician the potential biologic risk for the development of a malignant tumor.

CLINICAL FEATURES

The spectrum of laryngeal reactive epithelial lesions is usually seen in adults, especially after age 50, and more frequently in men. The incidence varies but is correlated with the same "carcinogenic" factors that result in carcinoma, including smoking, alcohol use/abuse, chronic irritation, air pollution, vocal abuse, chronic laryngitis (including infectious agents), habitual throat clearing, industrial pollution, and/or occupational exposure to specific agents (including radiation). Most of the lesions of the larynx present with symptoms of hoarseness,

---

---

cough, airway obstruction, dysphagia, changes in phonation, and sore throat, all of which are indistinguishable from those of carcinoma. Asymptomatic patients are occasionally identified. Leukoplakia, pachydermia, hyperplasia, pseudoepitheliomatous hyperplasia (PEH), metaplasia, keratosis, and contact ulcer are clinical and histologic terms that overlap with one another as well as with a number of distinctly different histologic lesions. For example, leukoplakia, used clinically, is a descriptive term designating a white patch or plaque, but histopathologically may describe keratosis, PEH, dysplasia, and SCC in situ. Therefore, these clinically macroscopic and microscopically morphologic diagnoses must be taken in context. Finally, there is a small but well-accepted risk of certain "reactive" lesions representing preneoplastic processes, which left untreated may develop into carcinoma. Therefore, it is imperative to recognize these various epithelial processes and to place them in a teleologic arc of development when appropriate.

PATHOLOGIC FEATURES

GROSS FINDINGS

All of these epithelial reactions can be ulcerated, flat, polypoid, papillary, or verrucous in gross appearance,

REACTIVE EPITHELIAL CHANGES—PATHOLOGIC FEATURES

Gross Findings

- Variable and include ulcerated, flat, polypoid, papillary, verrucous, red, or white lesions
- Frequently bilateral and usually along the vocal cords

Microscopic Findings

- Aggregate of findings are necessary before a precancerous lesion is diagnosed
- **Hyperplasia** is an increase in cell number or cell layer
- **Verrucous hyperplasia** has hyperplastic epithelium with verrucous projections, hyperkeratosis, and sharp interface with stroma
- **Pseudoepitheliomatous hyperplasia** is exuberant, large, bulbous projections of epithelium contained by an intact basement membrane without cytologic atypia
- **Metaplasia** is transformation to a simpler epithelium
- **Koilocytosis** has crenated nucleus, perinuclear halo, prominent, thick cell walls (usually in papilloma)
- **Keratosis** is an increased amount of keratin production
- **Parakeratosis** has flat nuclei with the keratosis
- **Dyskeratosis** is abnormal keratinization, usually close to the basal zone
- **Radiation changes** include nuclear enlargement but in cells with a low nuclear to cytoplasmic ratio, cytoplasmic vacuolization, and cellular atrophy, along with vascular proliferation
- **Necrotizing sialometaplasia** is a lobular arrangement of destroyed glands with metaplastic squamous epithelium growing through the mucoserous gland structures

Pathologic Differential Diagnosis

- Reactive and hyperplastic lesions, dysplasia, squamous cell carcinoma

ranging from red (erythroplakic) to white (leukoplakic), and can involve a microscopic area or the entire larynx (pachyderma laryngis), thus mimicking neoplasia clinically. Keratosis, PEH, and Teflon granuloma generally affect the true vocal folds/cords, while the posterior cords and subglottis are affected by granular cell tumor and PEH; any area can be affected by radiation. However, most of these reactive lesions occur along the true vocal cords, are frequently bilateral, and rarely involve the commissures. The lesions range from a circumscribed thickening of the mucosa to an ill-defined plaque, often exhibiting a rough surface. Late radiation changes induce atrophy with glottic stenosis, while foreign body material is usually a firm, polypoid lesion. Unfortunately, no clinical appearance has been consistently correlated to a particular underlying histology.

MICROSCOPIC FINDINGS

It is important to remember that the overlying mucosa varies in epithelial type across the larynx, ranging from squamous epithelium on the epiglottis, transitional epithelium in the glottis, and respiratory-type epithelium in the supraglottic and infraglottic portions of the larynx.

The areas of transition are normal, but in diseased states, the overall histology can vary considerably.

The histologic findings may be focal or diffuse, with the overall degree or quantity influencing the diagnosis, since the characteristics become more "atypical" in aggregate. The degree of each of these changes takes on importance, especially because of their known association with SCC. Critical judgment, including expert consultation or multiple biopsy sample taken sequentially over time, is essential to an accurate diagnosis. The presence alone of any one of these reactive epithelial changes is just a morphologic diagnosis and does not necessarily equate to a specific pathologic condition. The histologic appearance is variable, with architecture and histology used simultaneously to evaluate these lesions.

Reactive lesions include hyperplasia, which is an absolute increase in the number of cells or cell layers (Figure 4-21). This process may involve the surface or the deep, basal (Figure 4-22), and parabasal cell layers. There is no cytologic atypia; *atypia* is used here in the context of inflammatory and regenerative changes particularly referring to cytologic features. This is not considered a precancerous lesion.

Verrucous hyperplasia and verrucous squamous cell carcinoma are very difficult to separate, and some have suggested that they vary only in stage and size, the lesions representing a developmental spectrum. The distinction based on histologic features alone, even when specialized studies have been performed (including DNA analysis), is often not possible. However, true verrucous hyperplasia shows a hyperplastic squamous epithelium with regularly spaced, verrucous projections with hyperkeratosis and is sharply defined at the epithelial–stromal interface (Figure 4-23). Parakeratotic crypting is not usually present. There is considerable overlap with verrucous carcinoma, which may require a larger biopsy sample coupled with clinical correlation via excellent communication between the pathologist and surgeon.

PEH represents an exuberant reactive overgrowth of the prickle cell layer of squamous epithelium without cytologic atypia, often with large, bulbous projections into the underlying stroma, but always respecting the basement membrane (Figure 4-24). It is associated with fungal and mycobacterial infections, as well as granular cell tumor (Figure 4-25), and is frequently confused with SCC.

Metaplasia results when there is a change from a specialized respiratory epithelium to a more simple squamous epithelium and can occur anywhere within the larynx.

Koilocytosis is defined by a centrally placed crenated nucleus surrounded by clear cytoplasm, which forms a "halo," and prominent, thick cell walls/borders ("cookie cutter" appearance). Koilocytosis is generally identified as part of a papilloma (Figure 4-26) or carcinoma but is not identified in isolation, although glycogenation can sometimes cause diagnostic confusion.

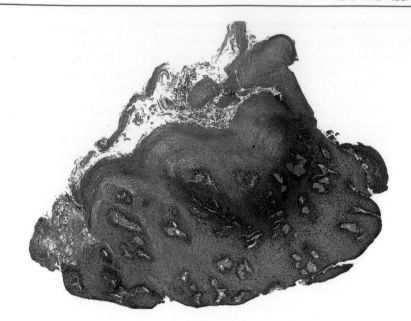

FIGURE 4-21

An increase in the number of layers of squamous epithelium is called hyperplasia, with the overlying increase in keratin termed keratosis.

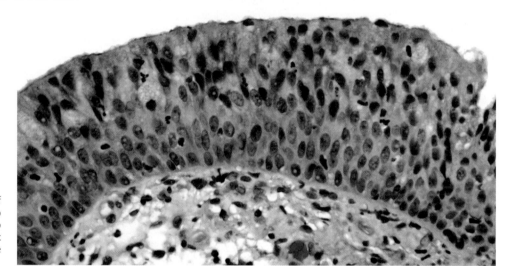

FIGURE 4-22

There is an increase of the number of cells in the basal zone, extending up to the middle one-third, where it comes to an abrupt stop. There is no cytologic atypia in this example of basal zone hyperplasia.

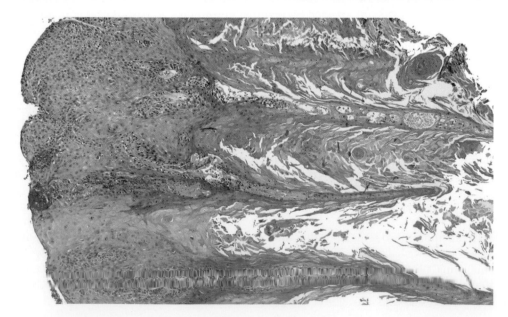

FIGURE 4-23

Verrucous hyperplasia with papillary fronds of squamous epithelium covered with keratin and lacking architectural and cytologic features of malignancy. The base is smooth, although an interface is lacking.

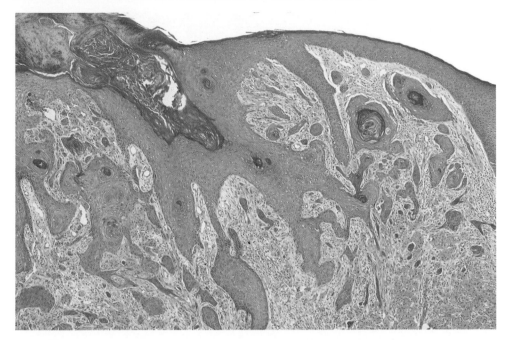

FIGURE 4-24

Pseudoepitheliomatous hyperplasia has a rounded type of growth into the underlying stroma, without cellular pleomorphism. Keratinization is frequent. Note the granular cell tumor.

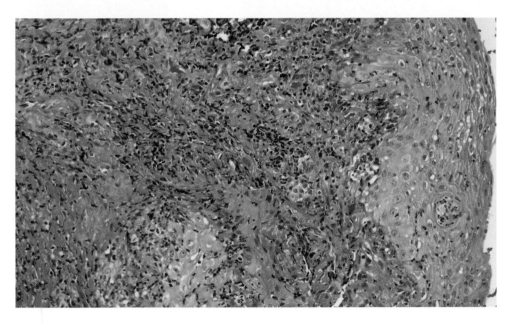

FIGURE 4-25

This example of pseudoepitheliomatous hyperplasia shows an irregular proliferation of the squamous epithelium. Cryptococcus organisms were identified with special stains.

Keratosis is separated from the other reactive and hyperplastic lesions because it may be part of all of them, and so is described in a little more depth. Keratosis is an abnormal production and accumulation of keratin at the surface of the laryngeal mucosa in which the nuclei are lost and the surface epithelial cells are completely replaced by keratin (Figure 4-27). There may be an accentuated granular layer or an irregularly hyperplastic spinous layer. The keratin is often present in an exophytic pattern. Nuclear atypia or pleomorphism is not implied by "keratosis," although keratosis can have atypia (*atypia* is not synonymous with *pleomorphism*). When the nuclei remain with incomplete keratinization, *parakeratosis* is the preferred term (Figure 4-28).

Keratosis is part of the complex response seen in the larynx and does not have any prognostic significance on its own. However, keratosis has been shown to have alterations in oncogenes and tumor suppressor genes (retinoblastoma protein, p53, p21, cyclin D1, Mcm-2, pTEN, tenascin, fibronectin) but not to the extent seen in dysplasia and carcinoma. This suggests there is an insufficient accumulation of the multiple genetic alterations known to result in the very early sequential transformation to carcinoma. There is an ~4% risk of subsequently identifying carcinoma in patients with an initial diagnosis of keratosis. Furthermore, when keratinizing dysplasia is identified, there is a strong association with abnormalities of DNA, to a much greater extent than

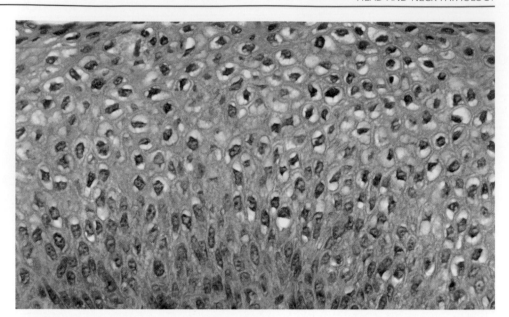

FIGURE 4-26

"Koilocytic" change (nuclear chromatin condensation, perinuclear halo and accentuation of the cell borders) seen in a papilloma.

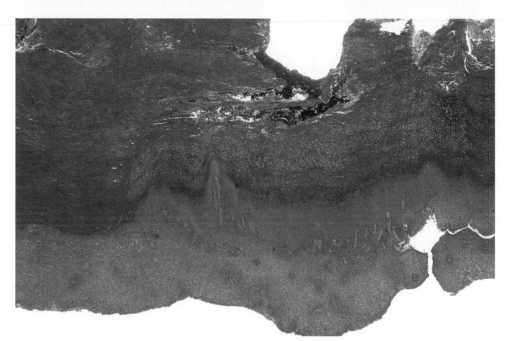

FIGURE 4-27

Keratosis is an accumulation of keratin at the surface.

is seen in nonkeratinizing dysplasias, suggesting abnormal keratinization may be associated with a greater degree of DNA abnormalities.

Reactive epithelial changes can also be associated with radiation-induced changes. These changes are long-lasting or life-persistent morphologic changes affecting the surface epithelium, minor salivary glands, fibrous tissue, vessels, and cartilages. Stages of development (acute, chronic) are recognized, although the acute necrotizing inflammation of the acute stage is seldom biopsied. Features include nuclear enlargement (within epithelial, endothelial, muscle, or stromal cells, which have a maintained nuclear cytoplasmic ratio), multinucleation, cytoplasmic vacuolization, cellular atrophy,

and vascular proliferation; but there are no readily identifiable changes of malignancy (recurrent or residual) (Figure 4-29). Surface erosion and atrophy of the epithelium and minor salivary glands are common. The antecedent-inciting event (radiation) is generally known, and the difficulty generally arises in ruling out recurrent or residual disease rather than separation from a benign reactive epithelial response.

Necrotizing sialometaplasia (NS) is a benign, self-limited, reactive inflammatory process involving minor mucoserous salivary glands. The hallmark feature of this disease is the maintenance of smoothly contoured lobular architecture of the minor mucoserous glands despite necrosis (Figure 4-30). In an attempt at reepithelialization,

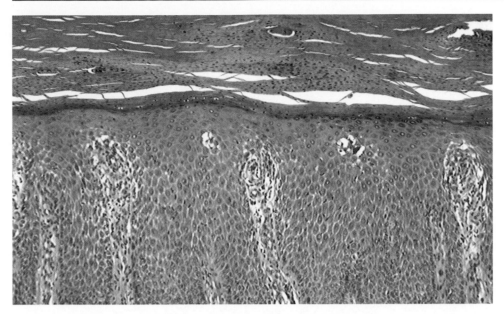

FIGURE 4-28

Keratin accumulation with nuclei, referred to as parakeratosis.

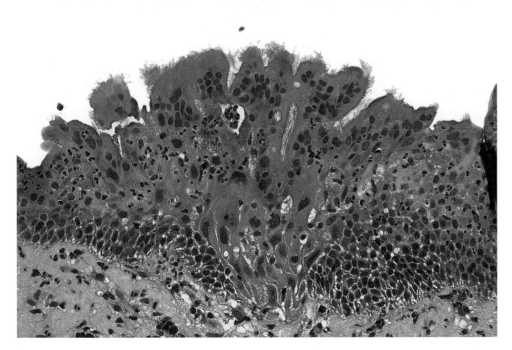

FIGURE 4-29

An area of papillary projection is composed of remarkably enlarged cells with a low nuclear:cytoplasmic ratio and showing nuclear hyperchromasia and irregularity. Acute inflammation can be seen in this example of radiation injury.

there is squamous metaplasia of the residual glands and acini (Figure 4-31). In the immediate area, remnants of uninvolved acini and ducts can be seen along with mucin-producing cells. There is frequently an associated acute and chronic inflammation related to necrosis of the duct or acinar epithelium, in addition to mucus extravasation. Therefore, the lobules of the mucoserous glands remain smooth in contour, now lined by a metaplastic squamous epithelium that is bland in overall appearance. However, as with any reparative or regenerative epithelium, enlarged nuclei, prominent nucleoli, apoptosis, and mitotic figures can be seen (Figure 4-32). Distinguishing between NS and carcinomas is especially difficult when the biopsy is small. With deeper sections and sometimes a larger biopsy, the true nature of the lesion will become apparent.

Teflon granuloma is a foreign body granuloma caused by iatrogenic injection of Teflon paste (used to treat vocal cord paralysis). Teflon is a polarizable, birefringent foreign material with foreign body giant cell reaction in fibrous stroma.

ANCILLARY STUDIES

Immunohistochemical reactions for the subtypes of keratins have been proposed as a means for distinguishing between reactive epithelial changes and carcinoma (CK13 is expressed in normal or reactive conditions, but is decreased or absent in dysplasia and carcinoma,

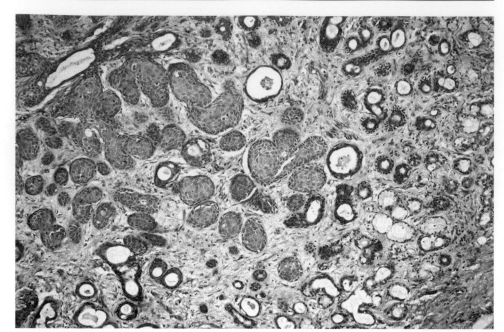

FIGURE 4-30

Necrotizing sialometaplasia is a lobular process, with areas of squamous metaplasia confined to the previous lobular architecture of a mucoserous gland. Uninvolved mucoserous glands can be identified at the periphery.

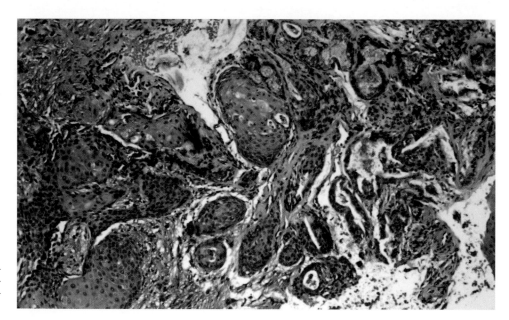

FIGURE 4-31

Extensive squamous metaplasia associated within a lobular architecture, showing mucus-producing glands at the periphery (top).

respectively), but from a practical standpoint, these reactions are insufficiently reliable to be used in a clinical setting. p53 tends to be expressed at higher levels in premalignant lesions than in benign reactive conditions.

DIFFERENTIAL DIAGNOSIS

The differential diagnosis encompasses different lesions within the reactive and hyperplastic category as well as separation from dysplasia and carcinoma. It is well accepted that dysplasia (squamous intraepithelial lesion,

squamous intraepithelial neoplasia) is a precancerous lesion, but the issue of how much *atypia* or *pleomorphism* makes a lesion dysplastic is not well established and poorly reproducible between practitioners. Since there is a sequential continuum, it is nearly impossible to rigidly place a lesion into reactive versus neoplastic, as no single combination of features consistently or accurately separates reactive from dysplastic. Therefore, degrees of atypia and subtle changes often portend the impending carcinoma transformation but may at that time not represent a true "carcinoma." Markers of dysplasia not seen in benign reactive conditions to any significant degree include dyskeratosis, a lack of maturity

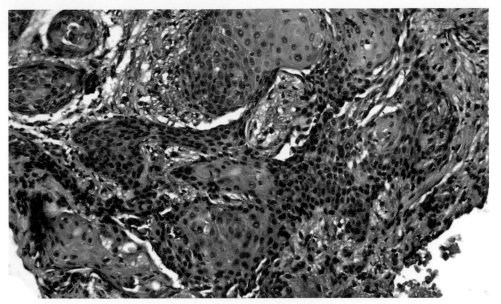

FIGURE 4-32

While well circumscribed and surrounded by an intact basement membrane, there is atypia in the epithelial cells along with dyskeratosis and keratin pearl formation.

or irregular epithelial stratification toward the surface ("basal zone"–type cells identified above the basal zone), anisonucleosis (abnormal nuclear size), anisocytosis (abnormal cell size), pleomorphism (nuclear shape irregularities, chromatin distribution disturbance, nuclear hyperchromasia), changes in nuclear:cytoplasmic ratio, atypical mitotic figures, premature keratinization lower in the proliferating epithelium (toward the basal zone), and increased mitotic figures. It is imperative to underscore that there is a consecutive and cumulative alteration underlying the process of carcinogenesis.

PROGNOSIS AND THERAPY

True hyperplasia and reactive epithelial lesions are self-limiting and reversible, with the majority spontaneously resolving or involuting if the etiologic agent is removed.

However, once moderate to severe dysplasia develops, the persistence and/or progression to carcinoma is a well-established risk. While diagnosis includes a biopsy, the underlying cause of the disorder should be sought and corrected. Due to the relative association of these reactive changes with malignant tumors, clinicopathologic correlation is imperative in identifying the potential risk for malignant transformation and ensuring an excellent long-term prognosis. In hyperplasia, no clinical follow-up is required, but clinical follow-up is vitally important for patients with "dysplasia," since sampling inadequacies and/or the natural progression of the lesion may result in inadequate clinical management.

SUGGESTED READINGS

The complete suggested readings list is available online at
www.expertconsult.com.

5

Benign Neoplasms of the Larynx, Hypopharynx, and Trachea

■ **Nina Gale** ■ **Lester D. R. Thompson**

■ SQUAMOUS PAPILLOMA/PAPILLOMATOSIS

Squamous papillomas (SPs), the most common benign laryngeal tumors, are induced by the human papillomavirus (HPV), most commonly types 6 and 11. Clinically, SPs are usually multiple, with frequent recurrences, especially in children. SPs are thus also referred to as recurrent respiratory papillomatosis (RRP). On the basis of their characteristic bimodal age distribution, SPs have been traditionally divided into juvenile and adult groups. The first incidence peak appears before the age of 5 years, with no gender predominance. The second incidence peak is between 20 to 40 years of age, with a slight male predominance (3:2). The incidence of SPs has been estimated at ~4.3/100,000 in the pediatric population and 2/100,000 among adults.

HPV infection is well documented as a causal agent of SPs but the mechanism by which the virus alters cellular growth and causes papillary lesions has not been fully elucidated. Microtrauma of the laryngeal epithelium enables entrance of HPV into basal epithelial cells. Viral persistence in episomes (extrachromosomal DNA fragments), altered cellular growth, and viral reproduction are the main mechanisms for protraction and spread of the disease. However, each of these phases requires further elucidation, which harbors potential for the development of novel targeted therapies.

It is generally believed that HPV transmission in children occurs in the perinatal period from infected mothers to newborns (vertical transmission). An epidemiologic triad has been proposed: a first-born child, vaginal delivery, and a mother with condylomata during pregnancy. The mode of adult infection remains unclear, although oral sexual practices might be associated with a higher risk of SPs.

CLINICAL FEATURES

Common symptoms at presentation among pediatric patients include dysphonia, hoarseness, and stridor. The clinical course in children is usually characterized by multiple lesions and recurrent and progressive disease, including tracheotomy (14% of patients), a risk of airway obstruction, and a propensity to spread through the aerodigestive tract. Spread to the tracheobronchial tree may be associated with tracheal stenosis, pneumatoceles, and various kinds of infection. The relatively small diameter of airways in children is the most likely explanation for severe respiratory obstruction. The disease is usually not as dramatic in adults, who usually present with dysphonia and hoarseness, although frequent recurrences of multiple lesions with respiratory distress and other complications may also develop. Despite differences in the clinical course between age groups, RRP is now considered a unified biological entity, caused by the same genotypes of HPV. In contrast to RRP, a solitary keratinizing SP (papillary keratosis) in adults is probably not related to HPV infection, or at least not to HPV 6 or 11.

The most common sites of SPs within the larynx are the vocal cords (true and false), Morgagni sinuses, and the subglottic region. Extralaryngeal spread of SPs, found in 30% of children and in 16% of adult patients, most commonly involves the oral cavity, trachea, and bronchi. The squamous–ciliary junction, in particular, is a predisposed site of involvement. Artificially induced squamous metaplasia (possibly as a response to surgical or therapeutic intervention) causes a new iatrogenic squamous–ciliary junction, which consequently provides a setting for further spread of the disease.

SQUAMOUS PAPILLOMA—DISEASE FACT SHEET

Definition

- Benign epithelial tumor, exophytic, composed of branching fronds of squamous epithelium and fibrovascular cores, causally related to HPV infection, usually genotypes 6 and 11

Incidence and Location

- Annual incidence 4.3/100,000 persons in children
- Predominantly larynx; extralaryngeal spread to surrounding aerodigestive areas (children in 30%, adults in 16%)

Morbidity and Mortality

- Overall mortality rate 4% to 14%

Gender and Age Distribution

- Children: no gender predominance
- Adults: male predominance (3:2)
- Bimodal age distribution: first incidence peak before 5 years; second peak in 20 to 40 years

Clinical Features

Children:
- Symptoms include dysphonia, hoarseness, and stridor
- Aggressive course of disease, multiple lesions, rapid recurrences, possible spread to tracheobronchial tree

Adults:
- Symptoms include dysphonia and hoarseness
- Less aggressive course of disease, frequently multiple lesions, less frequent recurrences, and extralaryngeal spread

Prognosis and Treatment

- Clinical course is unpredictable
- Disease in early childhood: increased risk of extralaryngeal spread and likelihood of mortality
- HPV genotypes 11 and 16 related to more aggressive disease, rapid recurrences and progression
- Malignant transformation: previously irradiated patients 14% of cases, nonirradiated patients 2% of cases
- Surgical removal(s) with different types of lasers, microdebriders, and cold knife
- Adjuvant therapy, such as interferon, indol-3-carbinol, and cidofovir, may have potential benefit
- Quadrivalent HPV vaccine might help to achieve a decrease in the incidence of squamous papillomas

SQUAMOUS PAPILLOMA—PATHOLOGIC FEATURES

Gross Findings

- Exophytic, warty, pedunculated or sessile growth, more frequently in clusters than single, fragile, pink to red with finely lobulated surface

Microscopic Findings

- Papillary, branching projections of squamous epithelium overlying fibrovascular cores
- Basal–parabasal cell hyperplasia
- Koilocytosis in superficial zone of squamous epithelium
- Rarely, a mild to moderate degree of pleomorphism

Immunohistochemical Features

- Detection of HPV infection
- In situ hybridization: the most reliable and useful method for routine detection of HPV in tissue specimens

Pathologic Differential Diagnosis

- Adult papillary keratinizing papillomas; verrucous, exophytic, or papillary squamous cell carcinoma

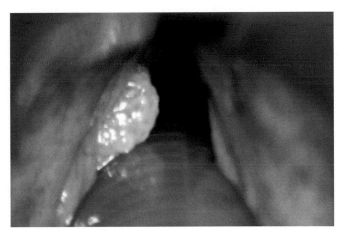

FIGURE 5-1

An endoscopic view of a squamous papilloma located on the left vocal cord.

PATHOLOGIC FEATURES

GROSS FINDINGS

SPs are exophytic, branching, pedunculated or broad-based, pinkish-red lesions with a finely lobular surface, occurring either in clusters or solitary, and measuring up to 10 mm in diameter (Figure 5-1).

MICROSCOPIC FINDINGS

Histologic sections are characterized by exophytic, papillary, mucosal projections consisting of a mainly hyperplastic squamous epithelium overlying thin fibrovascular cores (Figures 5-2 and 5-3). Secondary or tertiary branching papillae are covered by a thinner squamous epithelium. In addition, there is frequent basal and parabasal cell hyperplasia, mostly extending up to the midportion of the epithelium (Figure 5-4), as well as abnormal terminal differentiation. Surface keratosis or parakeratosis is minimal. Mitotic figures are present, mainly within the lower portion of the epithelium. Infrequently, SPs may be lined with both squamous and respiratory epithelia and these lesions are believed to have an increased tendency to recur. In rare cases, SPs may show epithelial changes that are characterized as "atypical" or "dysplastic," including abnormalities in the nuclear and cellular size and shape, increased nuclear:cytoplasmic ratio,

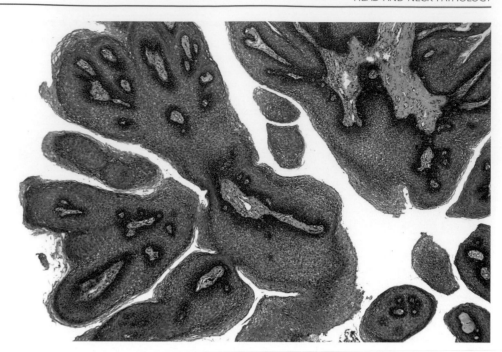

FIGURE 5-2

Branching of exophytic papillary projections consisting of squamous epithelium and thin fibrovascular cores.

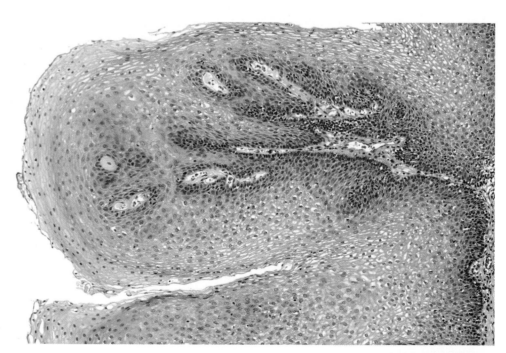

FIGURE 5-3

Papillary branches covered with hyperplastic squamous epithelium.

hyperchromatism, and increased mitoses (Figure 5-5). The most decisive morphologic feature in SPs, together with basal–parabasal cell hyperplasia, is koilocytosis, the only visible cytopathic effect of HPV infection. Koilocytes are characterized by dark, wrinkled, enlarged, or angulated, centrally located nuclei surrounded by a clear area of cytoplasm (perinuclear halos) (Figure 5-4). As a rule, these infected cells are irregularly scattered in the upper and superficial zone of the squamous epithelium, where viral replication takes place.

ANCILLARY STUDIES

Molecular methods are presently considered to be the key tool in the detection of HPV in SPs. These studies can be divided into two groups: (1) those that enable the detection of viral DNA in the context of preserved tissue morphology (e.g., in situ hybridization) and (2) those in which tissue destruction is unavoidable for detection of HPV DNA (e.g., polymerase chain reaction).

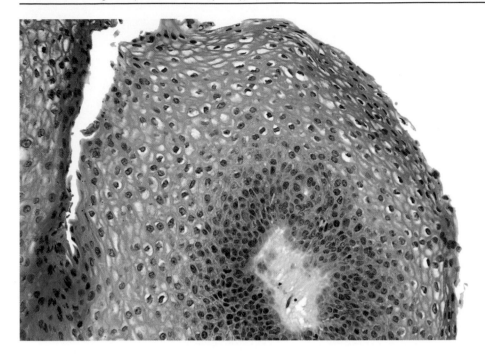

FIGURE 5-4

Covering epithelium of the papillary projections shows incipient basal–parabasal cell hyperplasia. Numerous koilocytes are seen in the upper part of the epithelium.

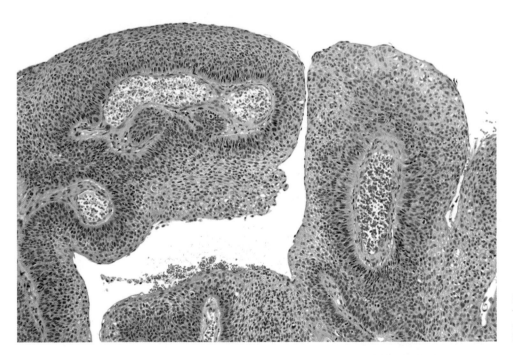

FIGURE 5-5

There are features of nuclear atypia noted within this squamous papilloma, bordering on squamous cell carcinoma.

In situ hybridization (ISH) routinely detects HPV in formalin-fixed, paraffin-embedded tissue specimens. HPV DNA specific ISH signals, usually confined to nuclei of koilocytes (Figure 5-6), are found almost exclusively in the upper middle to superficial squamous epithelium. Improved protocols of ISH have enabled the detection of very low viral copy numbers and even genotyping of HPV.

Polymerase chain reaction is currently the most sensitive method for HPV detection. However, because of frequent contamination problems, it should be applied in diagnostic settings with great caution.

DIFFERENTIAL DIAGNOSIS

Distinguishing various lesions with papillary structures from laryngeal SPs can be a demanding task, especially if the biopsy specimen is small and superficial. An *adult solitary keratinizing SP*, in contrast to HPV-induced RRP, usually shows prominent surface keratinization with keratohyaline granules. There is no evidence of koilocytosis and the hyperplastic epithelium is frequently atypical. *Verrucous squamous cell carcinoma* (VSCC) is covered by a prominent keratotic or parakeratotic layer

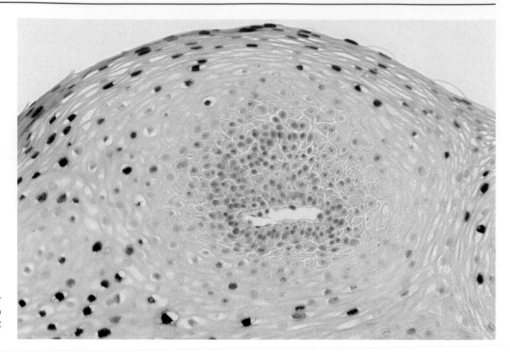

FIGURE 5-6

Positive in situ hybridization signal for human papillomavirus low-risk group (genotypes 6 and 11) in the upper part of the squamous epithelium.

(not a characteristic of SPs), has central keratin pearls, and shows broad epithelial projections infiltrating the underlying tissue in a pushing manner. It lacks koilocytes and does not contain fibrovascular cores within the projections. The *exophytic variant of squamous cell carcinoma* is composed of broad-based projections of the neoplastic epithelium, but without fibrovascular cores, which are characteristically present in SPs. *Papillary squamous carcinoma* resembles the architectural structure of SPs, but the covering epithelium is clearly neoplastic with the absence of maturation, loss of nuclear polarity, and possible evidence of invasive growth.

PROGNOSIS AND THERAPY

The clinical course of patients with SPs is unpredictable and includes periods of active disease and remissions. HPV present in apparently normal laryngeal mucosa seems to be a source of recurrences. Disease progression in early childhood is associated with an increased risk of tracheotomy and eventual progression to the lower respiratory tract with likelihood of mortality. Although SPs are most commonly induced by HPVs 6 and 11, it is serotypes 11 and 16 that are most frequently associated with malignant transformation, which occurs very rarely in adults and exceptionally in children. It seems to develop when additional predisposing factors, such as previous radiation or heavy smoking, are also present. Malignant transformation in children is found preferentially in the tracheobronchial tree and has a very poor prognosis. The overall mortality rate of patients with

SPs ranges from 4% to 14% and is predominantly related to asphyxia, pulmonary extension, and malignant transformation.

Children and adults usually require multiple surgical procedures to maintain a patent airway. Various surgical treatment modalities have been applied, such as different types of lasers, microdebrider, and cold knife. Additional medical therapies have been used to supplement surgery, including therapy with α-interferon, indole-3-carbinol, and cidofovir; however, no adjuvant therapy to date has cured SPs. The recent licensing of prophylactic HPV vaccines, in particular a quadrivalent HPV vaccine, might help to achieve a decrease in the incidence of SPs.

■ GRANULAR CELL TUMOR

Granular cell tumor (GCT) is a benign, slow-growing neoplasm, presumably of Schwann cell origin.

CLINICAL FEATURES

GCT typically appears between the 4th and 5th decades, and very rarely in children. The head and neck region is the most common location, accounting for 30% to 50% of tumors. Although the tongue and subcutaneous tissues are most frequently affected, laryngeal involvement comprises up to 10% of all cases; rare cases have been reported in the trachea. GCT occurs more commonly in black individuals and

GRANULAR CELL TUMOR—DISEASE FACT SHEET

Definition
- Benign tumor of neural (Schwann cell) origin, composed of polygonal to spindle cells with abundant granular cytoplasm, filled with lysosomes

Incidence and Location
- Frequent tumor, with larynx accounting for ~10% of cases
- Predominantly affects skin and mucosal membranes of head and neck, especially tongue and larynx, rarely trachea
- Larynx: posterior area of vocal cords extending to subglottis

Gender, Race, and Age Distribution
- Female preponderance (2:1)
- Predominantly in black patients (two-thirds of cases)
- Peak: 40 to 50 years, rare in children

Clinical Features
- Hoarseness, stridor, airway obstruction
- Laryngoscopic appearance of a smooth, polypoid, sessile lesion, usually <2 cm

Prognosis and Treatment
- Excellent prognosis with low recurrence rate (2% to 8%) after incomplete excision
- Conservative, complete surgical removal

GRANULAR CELL TUMOR—PATHOLOGIC FEATURES

Gross Findings
- Rounded, firm, nonulcerated mass with ill-defined margins, grayish-yellow cut surface

Microscopic Findings
- Unencapsulated lesion
- Pseudoepitheliomatous hyperplasia of overlying squamous epithelium
- Nested and trabecular growth pattern of rounded and polygonal cells giving a syncytial appearance
- Growth around myelinated peripheral nerves
- Cells contain abundant, coarsely granular cytoplasm, with small hyperchromatic to vesicular nuclei
- Aggressive or malignant potential: cytologic atypia, pleomorphism, increased mitoses, and necrosis

Ancillary Studies
- PAS-positive, diastase-resistant cytoplasmic granules
- Positive: S100 protein, vimentin, neuron-specific enolase, and myelin basic protein
- Negative: keratin and muscle markers

Pathologic Differential Diagnosis
- Atypical and malignant variant of granular cell tumor, squamous cell carcinoma, adult-type of rhabdomyoma, paraganglioma

---

shows a female preponderance (2:1). Multiple synchronous or metachronous tumors have been reported. Common presenting symptoms include hoarseness, dysphagia, and cough and, less frequently, stridor and hemoptysis.

RADIOLOGIC FEATURES

Imaging examination, including endoscopy and computed tomography, is usually performed to determine the exact location, extension, and relation to surrounding structures.

PATHOLOGIC FEATURES

GROSS FINDINGS

GCT of the larynx most commonly appears in the posterior region of the vocal cords, with half of reported cases extending into the subglottic area. These are smooth, round, polypoid-sessile, firm, homogeneous lesions, usually <2 cm (Figure 5-7). The overlying surface is usually intact and sectioning reveals a grayish-yellow cut surface with ill-defined margins (Figure 5-8).

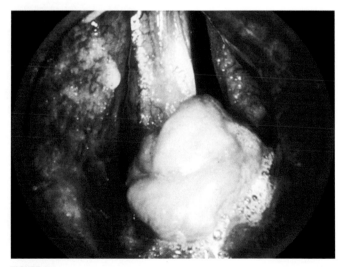

FIGURE 5-7

An endoscopic view of a posterior vocal cord, pale, polypoid mass, histologically confirmed to be a granular cell tumor.

MICROSCOPIC FINDINGS

Morphologically, the tumor consists of clusters and sheets of large rounded, polygonal, or elongated cells with indistinct cellular borders giving a syncytial appearance (Figure 5-9). The periphery is not well delimited, as clusters or individual cells may infiltrate surrounding

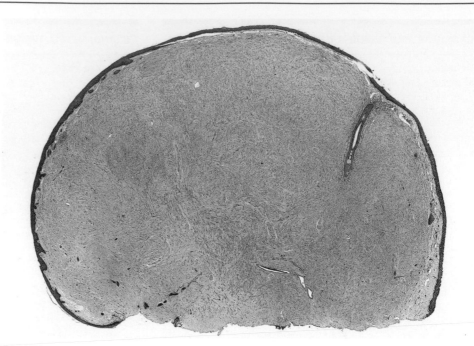

FIGURE 5-8

A polypoid mass with an intact slightly hyperplastic squamous mucosa. The polygonal cell neoplasm fills the stroma below the surface.

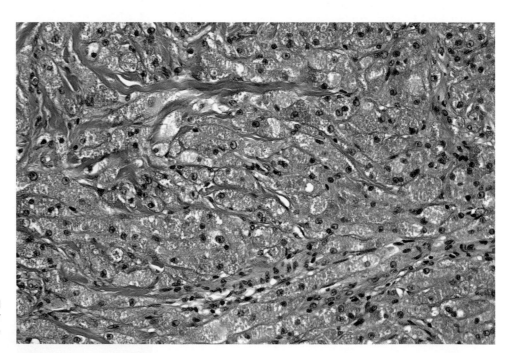

FIGURE 5-9

The tumor consists of rounded and polygonal cells with indistinct cellular borders and characteristically abundant, granular cytoplasm.

structures. If the tumor grows near the epithelial surface, secondary epithelial acanthosis, called pseudoepitheliomatous hyperplasia (PEH), may simulate invasive squamous cell carcinoma (Figure 5-10). In fact, PEH is seen in up to 60% of GCTs of the larynx. Tumor cells show either centrally or eccentrically located small, hyperchromatic to vesicular nuclei, enveloped by characteristically abundant, eosinophilic cytoplasm containing small and regular to larger and coarse granules (Figure 5-11). These granules are periodic

acid–Schiff (PAS) positive and diastase resistant and therefore not composed of glycogen. There is usually no pleomorphism, increased mitoses, or necrosis, which, if present, may indicate more aggressive or even malignant potential. Islands of tumor cells are separated by dense fibrovascular tissue. Abundant desmoplasia, which is often present in older lesions, may mask the presence of granular cells. GCT may grow around myelinated peripheral nerves or even infiltrate nerve fibers (Figure 5-11).

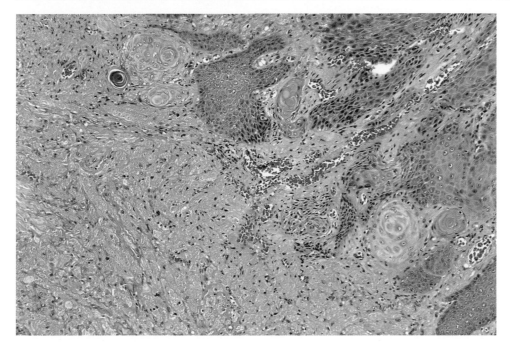

FIGURE 5-10

Pseudoepitheliomatous hyperplasia of the epithelium overlying a granular cell tumor may simulate invasive squamous cell carcinoma, especially in superficial biopsies.

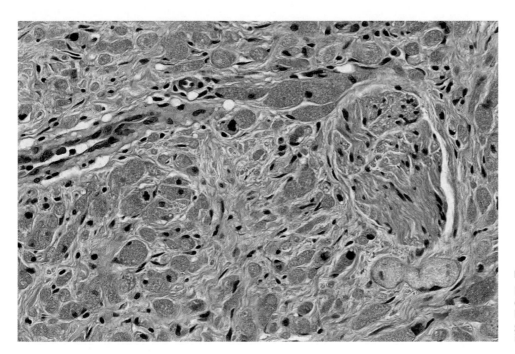

FIGURE 5-11

Nuclei are small, vesicular, and centrally or eccentrically located. Abundant granular cytoplasm is present. Growth of the granular cells around a peripheral nerve is noted (*right*).

ANCILLARY STUDIES

ULTRASTRUCTURAL FEATURES

Ultrastructural examination shows characteristic abundant lysosomes in the cytoplasm in various stages of fragmentation, conferring the granularity seen with light microscopy (Figure 5-12). Lysosomes (0.2 to 0.8 µm) vary from discrete, dense, round bodies with a homogeneous content to large structures with a lamellate appearance. Other organelles, such as mitochondria and cisternae of the endoplasmic reticulum, are scarce. Tumor cells are often surrounded by a basal lamina.

IMMUNOHISTOCHEMICAL FEATURES

GCTs are positive for S100 protein, vimentin, neuron-specific enolase, and myelin basic proteins (Figure 5-13). These findings are in accordance with their suspected Schwann cell origin, which is additionally supported by their lack of immunoreactivity for keratin and muscle

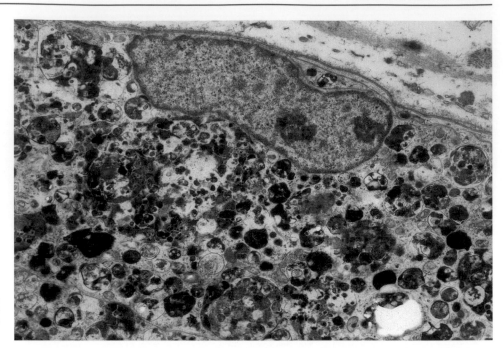

FIGURE 5-12

Electron microscopy reveals the characteristic intracytoplasmic abundance of lysosomal structures in various stages of fragmentation.

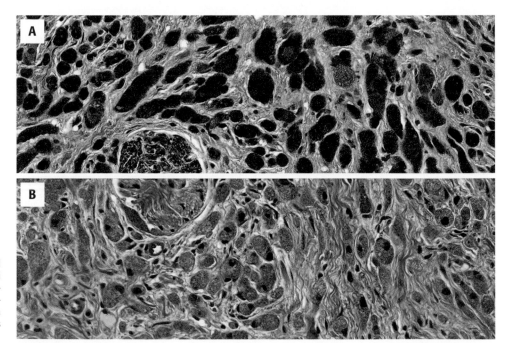

FIGURE 5-13

A, The neoplastic cells are strongly and diffusely immunoreactive in the nuclei and cytoplasm for S100 protein (perineural involvement is noted). **B**, Granular cells are diffusely red with Masson trichrome while the fibrotic stroma is blue.

markers. Positive staining with CD68 is due to the abundance of intracytoplasmic phagolysosomes rather than to a histiocytic lineage of the tumor.

DIFFERENTIAL DIAGNOSIS

GCTs usually have a distinctive histologic appearance and can be identified without further studies. Rapid tumor growth with histologic evidence of pleomorphism and increased mitoses may suggest malignant behavior.

The PEH associated with GCT can be misinterpreted as an invasive *squamous cell carcinoma*. However, the lack of epithelial atypia or increased mitotic activity may help to differentiate between these two entities. An *adult-type rhabdomyoma* shows large, granular, vacuolated cells with an abundance of glycogen and cross-striations (highlighted with phosphotungstic acid–hematoxylin [PTAH] stain) while reacting with immunohistochemical markers for skeletal muscle markers. *Paraganglioma* typically shows an organoid growth pattern (i.e., zellballen) of slightly basophilic granular cells with positive staining for neuroendocrine markers (chromogranin, synaptophysin)

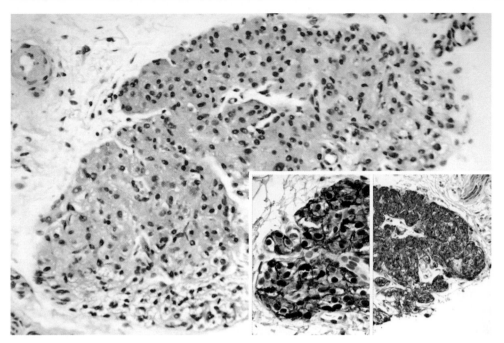

FIGURE 5-14

A paraganglioma shows an organoid architecture of cells with slightly granular cytoplasm. *Inset:* The neoplastic cells show a strong sustentacular cell reaction for S100 protein (*left*) and paraganglia cell chromogranin reaction (*right*).

and a classic peripheral sustentacular (supporting) S100 protein reaction (Figure 5-14).

PROGNOSIS AND THERAPY

Complete excision of the tumor with an attempt to preserve normal structures is the treatment of choice. Larger tumors require a more extensive surgical procedure including laryngofissure or partial laryngectomy. However, the recurrence rate is low even if the surgical margins are positive.

■ ADULT RHABDOMYOMA

Rhabdomyomas are rare benign tumors of striated muscle differentiation. Topographically, they are divided into cardiac and extracardiac types. The latter is less common and additionally classified into adult, fetal, and genital forms according to distinctive clinical and histologic features. Extracardiac rhabdomyomas (ERs) are developmentally linked to the head and neck region (90% of cases), since they arise from the unsegmented mesoderm of the third and fourth branchial arches.

CLINICAL FEATURES

Most cases of adult rhabdomyoma (AR) are found in adults from 16 to 82 years (mean, 52 years). Males are affected three to four times more commonly than females.

The most frequent sites of AR include the hypopharynx, supraglottic or glottic regions of the larynx, and the floor of mouth. Most ARs are solitary, but may be multinodular in the same anatomic location, and usually present as slowly growing masses. The presenting symptoms differ across the affected regions. The majority of patients with laryngeal tumors complain of hoarseness and progressive difficulties of breathing (airway obstruction) and swallowing.

ADULT RHABDOMYOMA—DISEASE FACT SHEET

Definition
- Benign tumor of skeletal muscle differentiation

Incidence and Location
- Very uncommon tumor
- Of extracardiac rhabdomyomas, 90% in head and neck region; most commonly in hypopharynx, larynx, floor of mouth

Gender and Age Distribution
- Male >> female (3 to 4:1)
- Mean, 52 years with wide age range (16 to 82 years)

Clinical Features
- Common symptoms: dysphagia, hoarseness, dyspnea
- Slow-growing, well-demarcated mass without tenderness or pain
- Tumor size: 1.5 to 7.5 cm

Prognosis and Treatment
- Recurrences in up to 42% of cases after incomplete excision usually within 2 to 11 years after diagnosis
- No aggressive or malignant potential
- Complete surgical excision

PATHOLOGIC FEATURES

GROSS FINDINGS

ARs are usually rounded, well-circumscribed, but unencapsulated submucosal lesions, ranging up to 8 cm (mean, 3 cm) in greatest dimension. These are coarsely lobulated, polypoid, or pedunculated masses, grayish red to brown, with a finely granular, soft, and lobulated cut surface.

MICROSCOPIC FINDINGS

Histologically, ARs are composed of sheets, nests, and lobules of large, round to polygonal, closely packed cells, separated by thin fibrovascular stroma (Figure 5-15). Their cytoplasm is abundant, eosinophilic, and characteristically finely granular or vacuolated owing to the presence of glycogen removed during tissue processing (Figure 5-16). An abundance of glycogen (PAS positive, diastase sensitive) may lead to a spider web–like appearance of cells with radially oriented strands of cytoplasm separating the vacuoles. Cytoplasmic cross-striations may be found (Figure 5-17), as well as haphazardly arranged crystalline-like structures called jackstraw inclusions, which are rarely seen. Both structures become intensely visible using PTAH staining (Figure 5-17). The cells of AR contain one or more, peripherally or centrally located, small vesicular nuclei with prominent nucleoli. Mitotic figures are almost always absent.

ADULT RHABDOMYOMA—PATHOLOGIC FEATURES

Gross Findings

- Circumscribed, round or lobular lesion, with red-brown cut surface

Microscopic Findings

- Well-demarcated, unencapsulated lobules
- Closely packed, large polygonal cells
- Tumor cells have small, round nuclei, centrally or peripherally located with prominent nucleoli
- Abundant eosinophilic, granular or vacuolated ("spider web") cytoplasm
- Cytoplasmic cross-striation and haphazardly arranged crystal-like structures

Special Studies

- Cytoplasm is rich in glycogen (PAS positive, diastase sensitive)
- Positivity for myoglobin, muscle-specific actin, desmin, myf4, MYOD1
- Focal positivity for α-smooth muscle actin, vimentin, S100 protein, and Leu-7
- Negative for keratin, EMA, GFAP, and CD68

Pathologic Differential Diagnosis

- Granular cell tumor, paraganglioma, oncocytoma, hibernoma

ANCILLARY STUDIES

ULTRASTRUCTURAL FEATURES

Electron microscopy shows a thin, continuous basal lamina surrounding the individual cells of AR. However, the most important diagnostic criterion is the presence of intracytoplasmic rudimentary myofibrils, found in virtually all cells. These are characterized by alternating thin (actin) and thick (myosin) myofilaments. Apparent condensation of myofibrils is readily identified as Z bands and the intracytoplasmic crystalline-like structures, seen with light microscopy, are considered hypertrophied Z bands. In addition to the intracytoplasmic myofilaments, a variable amount of glycogen and varied number of mitochondria are always seen.

IMMUNOHISTOCHEMICAL FEATURES

The immunohistochemical profile confirms the skeletal muscle origin of this tumor, which is usually positive for desmin, myoglobin, muscle-specific actin (HHF-35), myogenin (myf4), and MYOD1. Focal and weak reactivity may also be detected for smooth muscle actin, S100 protein, and Leu7. Additionally, AR characteristically lacks staining for cytokeratin, epithelial membrane antigen, and CD68.

OTHER ANCILLARY STUDIES

Intracytoplasmic cross-striation and crystalline-like structures are more evident if special stains such as PTAH and trichrome are applied (Figure 5-17). Cytogenetic studies reveal a reciprocal translocation between chromosomes 15 and 17 and/or miscellaneous changes in the long arm of chromosome 10, which seem to support a neoplastic origin, rather than a hamartoma or hyperplasia.

DIFFERENTIAL DIAGNOSIS

The differential diagnosis of AR includes benign and malignant tumors with distinctive abundant eosinophilic, granular, or vacuolated cytoplasm: GCT, paraganglioma, oncocytoma, and hibernoma. *GCT* consists of a syncytium of large polygonal cells with abundant granular cytoplasm, without vacuolization, and showing S100 protein immunoreactivity. *Paraganglioma* is composed of polyhedral cells organized in an organoid (zellballen) pattern that react with neuroendocrine markers (chromogranin and synaptophysin), while peripherally located sustentacular cells stain positively

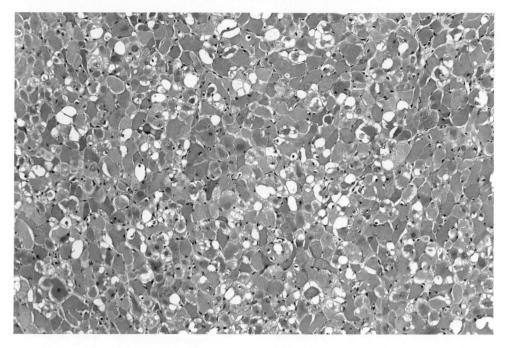

FIGURE 5-15

At low power, there is a diffuse infiltration of polygonal cells with abundant, vacuolated cytoplasm and small nuclei in this adult rhabdomyoma.

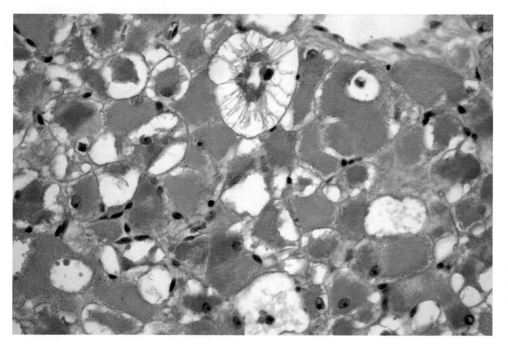

FIGURE 5-16

Characteristic polygonal cells of variable size, with eosinophilic, vacuolated, granular cytoplasm, and mainly peripherally located small hyperchromatic nuclei. A "spider web"–like appearance is noted.

for S100 protein (Figure 5-14). *Oncocytoma* is composed of large cells with abundant granular, eosinophilic cytoplasm that can be confirmed with histochemistry (PAS, PTAH) and electron microscopy (abundant abnormal mitochondria). Hibernoma, exceedingly rare in the larynx, shows tightly packed round to oval cells with a variable degree of cytoplasmic vacuolization and strong cytoplasmic positivity for S100 protein.

PROGNOSIS AND THERAPY

AR is a benign tumor that lacks aggressive behavior or malignant potential. The treatment of choice is surgery, including endoscopic removal. Recurrences have been reported in up to 42 % of cases, usually months to years after an incomplete excision. One should be aware of possible multicentric AR occurring in either the same or a separate location.

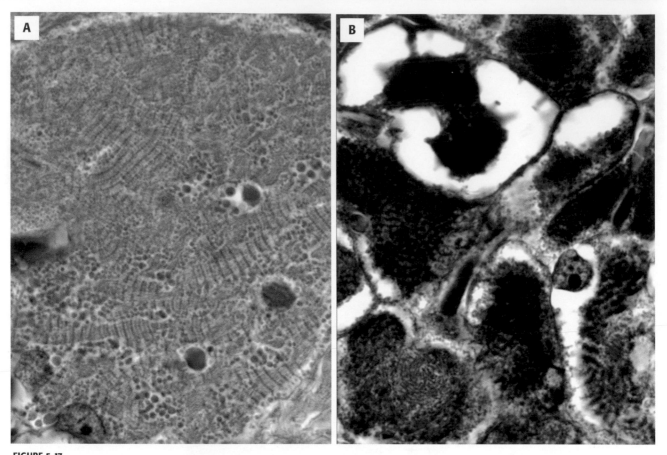

FIGURE 5-17
Crystalline-like structures and cross-striations in the cytoplasm of the rhabdomyocytes in an adult rhabdomyoma (**A**) are highlighted by a PTAH stain (**B**).

■ CHONDROMA

Chondroma is an exceedingly rare benign mesenchymal tumor arising from the cartilaginous structures of the larynx and trachea.

CLINICAL FEATURES

This lesion occurs more commonly in men (2:1) and has a broad age range, from 24 to 79 years old, with a mean (56 years) slightly younger than that for chondrosarcoma. The tumor is typically a slowly growing endolaryngeal mass (Figure 5-18), although involvement of the thyroid cartilage may rarely produce a neck mass. Clinical presentation depends on location and size. Subglottic lesions usually produce dyspnea, hoarseness, and stridor, while supraglottic lesions produce hoarseness, dyspnea, dysphagia, and odynophagia. The most common localization is the posterior lamina of the cricoid cartilage, followed by the thyroid, epiglottis, arytenoids, and tracheal cartilages, in decreasing order.

CHONDROMA—DISEASE FACT SHEET

Definition
- Benign tumor of mature hyaline cartilage

Incidence and Location
- Extremely unusual in larynx and trachea
- Most common: cricoid and thyroid cartilages

Gender and Age Distribution
- Male > female (2:1)
- Peak in 6th decade (wide age distribution, 24 to 79 years)

Clinical Features
- Symptoms include hoarseness and dyspnea, rarely neck mass in extralaryngeal spread
- Slow-growing endolaryngeal lesion, symptoms directly depend on location and size
- May be incidental finding

Prognosis and Treatment
- Excellent prognosis after conservative surgical excision
- Malignant transformation in 7% of cases
- Any recurrence of laryngeal cartilage tumor is considered chondrosarcoma

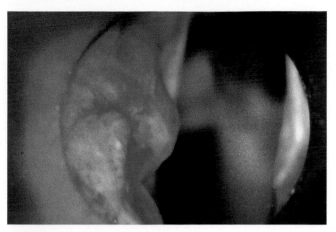

FIGURE 5-18
An endoscopic view of a chondroma shows a smooth endolaryngeal sessile mass in the left supraglottic region.

PATHOLOGIC FEATURES

CHONDROMA—PATHOLOGIC FEATURES

Gross Findings
- Firm submucosal mass, <2 cm, involving laryngeal cartilage
- Well-circumscribed, hard tumor; translucent, gray-blue cut surface

Microscopic Findings
- Lobular growth of benign, bland-looking chondrocytes, resembling normal cartilage
- Monotonous appearance with low cellularity
- Single nucleus per lacuna

Pathologic Differential Diagnosis
- Low-grade chondrosarcoma, chondrometaplasia of the vocal cord, tracheopathia osteoplastica, pleomorphic adenoma

RADIOLOGIC FEATURES

A plain anteroposterior radiograph usually shows a mucosa-covered lesion arising from the laryngeal cartilage. CT further reveals a hypodense, well-circumscribed lesion with regular margins and minimal calcium deposits. The tumor–soft tissue relationship and extent of the lesion can be more sensitively delineated with magnetic resonance imaging. However, radiologic features alone cannot distinguish between chondroma and its malignant counterpart, chondrosarcoma. (Similarly, an apparent chondroma by histology requires radiographic correlation to rule out a well-differentiated chondrosarcoma.)

GROSS FINDINGS

Grossly, chondromas usually measure less than 2 cm in diameter and appear as firm, characteristically glassy, blue-white lesions on cut surface.

MICROSCOPIC FINDINGS

Histologically, a well-defined lobular pattern of the mature hyaline cartilage, confined by perichondrium is seen below an intact squamous mucosa (Figure 5-19). This mature cartilage is characterized as hypocellular with evenly distributed bland-looking chondrocytes in

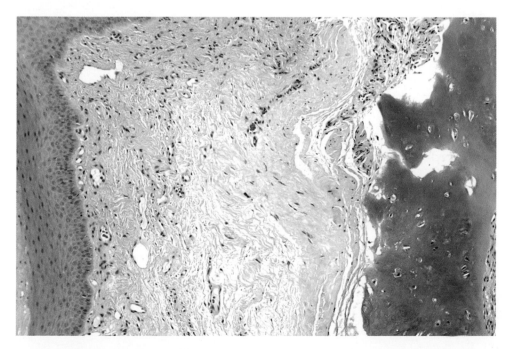

FIGURE 5-19
At low power, the mature hyaline cartilage with characteristic low cellularity is noted below an intact squamous mucosa.

a background of abundant basophilic matrix. Generally, only one chondrocyte is seen within lacunae. These cells contain small, uniform, single, hyperchromatic nuclei, surrounded by clear to eosinophilic cytoplasm (Figure 5-20). Pleomorphism and mitoses are absent. Areas of scattered calcification and ossification may be seen. Myxoid degeneration may also be evident as blue granular material in the cytoplasm and surrounding stroma.

DIFFERENTIAL DIAGNOSIS

Distinguishing chondroma from *low-grade chondrosarcoma* is difficult and fraught with controversy in the medical literature. A small biopsy of a cartilaginous tumor resembling chondroma should be reported with caution. Meticulous examination of the whole specimen is required to avoid an incorrect diagnosis. Histologically, reliable features of chondrosarcoma include bone invasion/destruction, increased cellularity, loss of organization (nonlobular pattern), pleomorphism, multinucleation, increased mitotic activity, and necrosis.

Other benign lesions in the differential include *chondrometaplasia*, characterized by an elastic-rich cartilage nodule, usually located on the vocal cord, with no relation to the laryngeal cartilages, and *tracheopathia osteoplastica*, which can be identified radiographically and laryngoscopically displaying multiple submucosal nodules usually attached to the cartilages (Figure 5-21). *Pleomorphic adenoma* can be easily differentiated by the presence of epithelial and myoepithelial components, which are incorporated in a myxochondroid stroma (Figure 5-22).

PROGNOSIS AND THERAPY

Surgical excision of the tumor with preservation of the larynx is the treatment of choice. The chondroma recurrence rate has been published to be 10%, with a mean time to recurrence of 9 years. Any recurrence, however, should raise the question of an originally underdiagnosed low-grade chondrosarcoma. Transformation to chondrosarcoma is seen in about 7% of cases. Furthermore, many chondrosarcomas (up to 60%) are superimposed on preexisting chondromas which have undergone ischemic change.

SUGGESTED READINGS

The complete suggested readings list is available online at www.expertconsult.com.

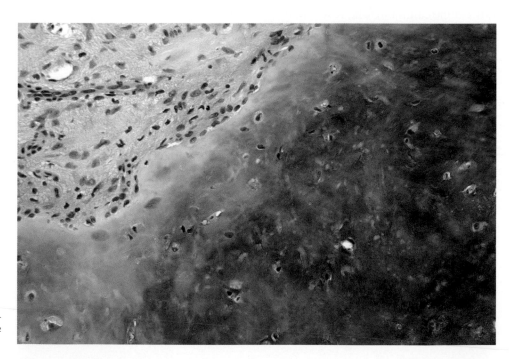

FIGURE 5-20

A well-defined border of the hypocellular cartilaginous neoplasm with the surrounding stroma in a chondroma.

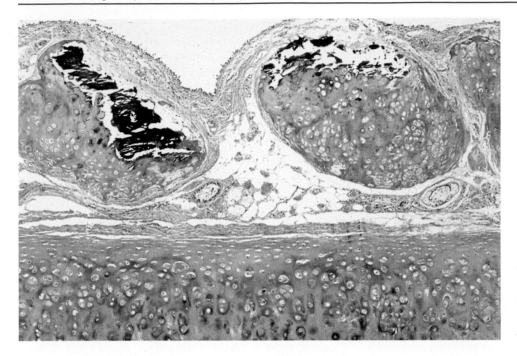

FIGURE 5-21

Submucosal bone deposition or metaplasia is identified separately from the cartilage. This finding, combined with the clinical presentation, is distinctive for tracheopathia osteoplastica.

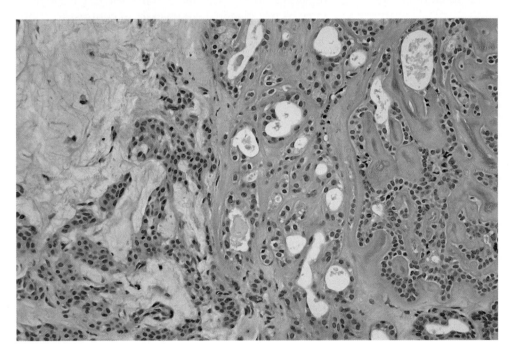

FIGURE 5-22

There is an epithelial and myoepithelial proliferation of a pleomorphic adenoma set within a variably cellular stroma. Note the sclerosis (right sided).

6

Malignant Neoplasms of the Larynx, Hypopharynx, and Trachea

■ **Lester D. R. Thompson**

■ PRECURSOR SQUAMOUS LESIONS

The definition of *precursor lesions* is difficult to quantify because they are lesions that have an increased likelihood of progressing to squamous cell carcinoma (SCC). A constellation of architectural and cytologic features comprises dysplasia or laryngeal intraepithelial neoplasia, but these features are not uniformly accepted or interpreted, thereby leading to differences in intraobserver and interobserver interpretation. It is wise to use "atypia" in the context of reactive, inflammatory, or regenerative changes, while reserving "dysplasia" for the premalignant group of lesions. Whichever classification system is adopted, consistent application of the criteria will allow clinicians to correctly manage their patients. Current terminology includes carcinoma in situ (CIS), keratosis with atypia, dysplasia (mild, moderate, severe), squamous intraepithelial lesion or neoplasia, laryngeal intraepithelial neoplasia, basal/parabasal hyperplasia, and atypical hyperplasia. For purposes of this book, keratinizing dysplasia and CIS are used. Keratinizing dysplasia is a potentially reversible alteration in epithelial cells that has an increased likelihood of progressing to SCC. CIS is a *noninvasive* malignant alteration of the full thickness of the surface epithelium.

CLINICAL FEATURES

Precursor lesions are mostly seen in the adult population (6th to 7th decades) with a male predilection that is especially pronounced after the 6th decade. There is a strong association with tobacco smoking and alcohol abuse, with a potentiating effect between the two—an increased risk directly proportional to duration of use. The etiologic role of human papillomavirus (HPV) infection remains unsettled, although it is detected in ~12% of cases. Symptoms depend on the location and severity of the disease and are usually present for at least a few months before clinical attention. Hoarseness, voice changes, throat irritation, sore throat, and/or chronic cough are frequently reported. Endoscopically, these lesions have a varied appearance: discrete to diffuse; leukoplakia to erythroplakia; and a small, flat patch to a large, warty plaque. Leukoplakia, in contrast to erythroplakia, tends to be well demarcated. Although inconsistent, leukoplakia alone seems to have a lower risk of malignant transformation than pure erythroplakia.

In general, it is accepted that there is an increased risk of progression to invasive SCC over time. Low-grade dysplasia is potentially reversible if the inciting factor is removed. However, as the grade of dysplasia increases, it becomes more difficult to predict which dysplasia may be reversible and which may progress to invasive tumor. Although quite variable, keratosis has only a 1% to 5% risk of the development of invasive SCC. This risk is increased in keratosis with mild dysplasia (6%), moderate dysplasia (23%), and severe dysplasia (28%). Due to variations in nomenclature, CIS has a 23% to 27% risk of progression (although probably it is the same as severe dysplasia). The progression is usually slow, with an average latency from simple keratosis to invasive SCC of just under 4 years. It is important to realize that multifocal disease is a major factor in disease development, since the entire epithelium is exposed to the same etiologic risk agents.

PATHOLOGIC FEATURES

GROSS FINDINGS

There is no characteristic appearance of precursor lesions, which may be circumscribed or diffuse; smooth, granular, or irregular; flat or exophytic; and leukoplakic or erythroplakic. The anterior true vocal cords are involved most commonly (usually not the commissure), although no region of the larynx is exempt. Bilateral

Definition

- Squamous lesions with an increased risk/likelihood of progressing to squamous cell carcinoma (dysplasia)

Incidence and Location

- From 6% to 28% of precursor lesions progress to carcinoma
- Supraglottic and glottic regions are most common

Gender and Age Distribution

- Males >> female
- 6th decade peak

Clinical Features

- Tobacco and alcohol abuse (with potentiating effect)
- Hoarseness, throat irritation, sore throat, chronic cough

Prognosis and Treatment

- Progression to carcinoma is slow, but there is a well-defined risk of malignant transformation
- Surgery and radiation, dependent on lesion

Gross Findings

- Leukoplakia, erythroplakia, mixed (speckled), variegated
- Diffuse or discrete
- Flat patch or large warty plaque
- Anterior true vocal cord most often, with frequent bilateral disease

Microscopic Findings

- A continuum of architectural and cytologic features required, separated into low, moderate, and severe dysplasia based on increasing thickness of the mucosa involved by the cells
- Increased cellularity, nuclear crowding, irregular maturation, lack of polarity, dyskeratosis, keratin pearl formation, parakeratosis, increased mitotic figures
- Increased nuclear:cytoplasmic ratio, increased nuclear size, anisocytosis, poikilocytosis, anisonucleosis, nuclear pleomorphism, nuclear hyperchromasia, nuclear chromatin condensation, increased nucleolar size and number, atypical mitotic figures
- No evidence of basement membrane invasion

Pathologic Differential Diagnosis

- Hyperplasia, regeneration, repair, inflammation, reactive and radiation changes, necrotizing sialometaplasia, squamous cell carcinoma

disease is common (30% to 60%). Invasive carcinoma may be concurrently present adjacent to or remote from the precursor lesion.

MICROSCOPIC FINDINGS

Dysplasia is an alteration of surface epithelium that is *more* than hyperplasia but *less* than carcinoma. Needless to say, to identify the earliest forms of dysplasia and to arbitrarily separate and rigidly divide the dysplasias into different categories is fraught with tremendous intraobserver and interobserver variability and an overall lack of reproducibility.

Many architectural (maturation abnormalities) and cytologic features can be seen in dysplasia although none in isolation is pathognomonic for dysplasia. In fact, many of these same features are more fully developed in carcinoma, and so a rigid segregation between lesions is nearly impossible. In general, all of the various layers begin to cytologically resemble the basal layer cells (immature or uncommitted) as the lesion progresses from low-grade dysplasia toward CIS. Moreover, on a continuous spectrum, there is a quantitative increase in architectural and cytologic features for the diagnosis of dysplasia, with low-grade dysplasia usually limited to the lower third of the epithelium (Figure 6-1), moderate dysplasia involving the lower two-thirds (Figure 6-2), and severe dysplasia/CIS involving the full thickness (Figure 6-3). Architectural features of dysplasia include increased cellularity, nuclear crowding, irregular maturation toward the surface, lack of polarity, dyskeratosis (Figure 6-4), keratin pearl formation within rete, parakeratosis

(Figure 6-5), and pseudoepitheliomatous hyperplasia (PEH) or acanthosis with irregular rete extending into the submucosa (Figure 6-6). In general, dysplasia starts in the basal/parabasal zone and moves toward the surface. Cytologic features of dysplasia include increased nuclear:cytoplasmic ratio, increased nuclear size, anisocytosis, poikilocytosis, anisonucleosis, nuclear pleomorphism, nuclear hyperchromasia, nuclear chromatin condensation and contour irregularities, and increased number and size of nucleoli. Mitoses are increased, identified above the basal zone, and may include atypical mitotic figures (misalignment of chromosomes, unbalanced distribution of chromosomes, and multipolar figures). While axiomatic, invasion of the basement is not present.

CIS is essentially synonymous with severe dysplasia, although keratinizing dysplasias seldom involve the full thickness, and CIS tends to affect nonkeratinizing epithelia. Nearly all laryngeal lesions are keratinizing dysplasia, with only isolated cases of nonkeratinizing dysplasia. An inflammatory infiltrate, occasionally intense, is common. A commonly asked question is: How many features are necessary for the diagnosis? Here the art of pathology comes into scope, with the clinical, gross, and histologic features interpreted collectively. Other considerations include the fact that a synchronous invasive SCC is frequently present. Furthermore, invasive carcinoma may develop from a nondysplastic surface epithelium. Finally, regarding dysplasia, glandular/duct extension must not be interpreted as invasive disease.

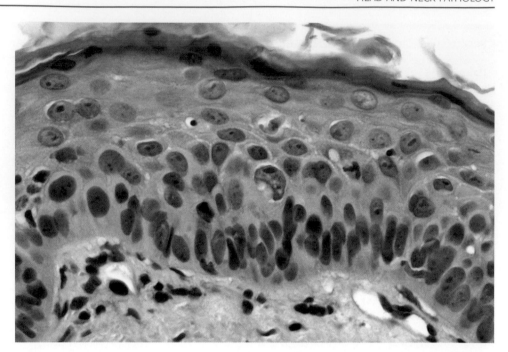

FIGURE 6-1

A mild dysplasia demonstrates focal disruption of the architecture and mild pleomorphism limited to the lower third of the mucosa. Parakeratosis is noted.

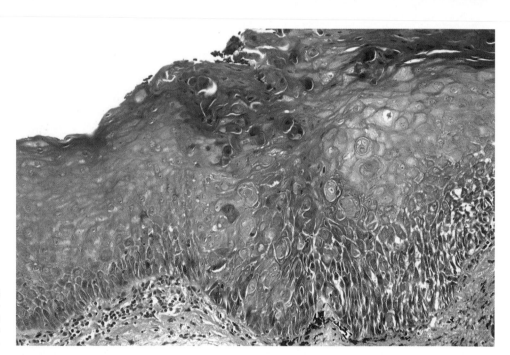

FIGURE 6-2

Moderate dysplasia has atypical features extending to the middle third of the epithelium. The thickened epithelium in the area of dysplasia sometimes makes determination of grade of dysplasia difficult.

Technical factors are important to accurate diagnosis. Multiple biopsy samples of sufficient size from within the diseased area are necessary to assess the full extent of the lesion. Avoiding tangential sections is paramount, which usually precludes frozen section diagnoses. Additional deeper sections may be needed to fully demonstrate diagnostic features of dysplasia. Glandular/duct extension must not be interpreted as invasive disease. Various immunohistochemical and molecular studies have been proposed to separate hyperplasia, dysplasia, and carcinoma, but in practical application they are currently too inconsistent and have too much overlap to be clinically meaningful.

DIFFERENTIAL DIAGNOSIS

Reactive, regenerative, reparative, or *hyperplastic* squamous proliferations (for example in response to trauma, inflammation, irradiation, or ulceration) may manifest architectural and cytologic atypia. However, morphologic

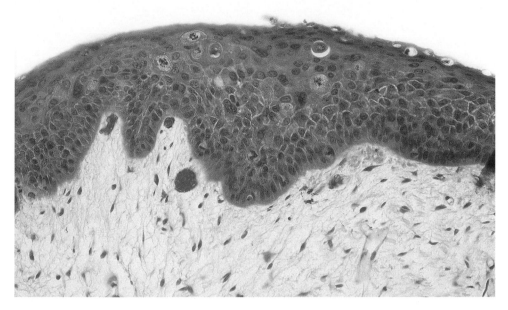

FIGURE 6-3

Severe dysplasia/carcinoma in situ. Full-thickness replacement of the epithelium by markedly atypical cells, with numerous atypical mitotic figures, but without basement membrane penetration.

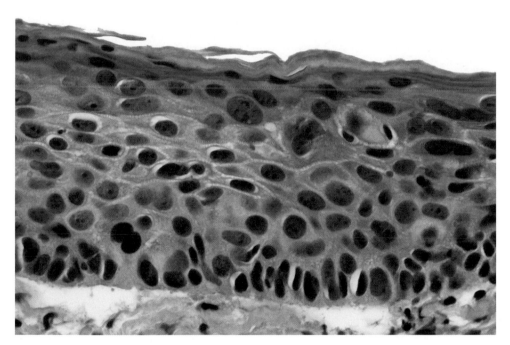

FIGURE 6-4

Increased nuclear:cytoplasmic ratio, nuclear pleomorphism, nuclear hyperchromasia, and binucleation in a dysplastic epithelium.

changes suggestive of the inciting event (e.g., ulceration, inflammation, hemorrhage, radiation-induced mesenchymal, and/or endothelial nuclear enlargement and hyperchromasia) may be present. Inflammatory infiltrates caused by infectious agents should be excluded with special stains or cultures. In addition, stratification and maturation are usually present and atypical mitotic figures are absent. The clinical history may also be helpful. *Transitional vocal cord epithelium* is sometimes confused with dysplasia, but knowledge of the normal histology will help make this separation. *Basal zone hyperplasia* has a columnar arrangement to the basal cells, which maintain a vertical polarity and hyperchromatic nuclei. There is an abrupt termination of the process at the upper edge of the prickle layer with a very sharp zone of transition horizontally oriented (see reactive lesions, Figure 4-22). *Granular cell tumor* can cause atypical epithelial changes, most importantly PEH, which often mimics invasion. However, the identification of large eosinophilic cells with abundant granular cytoplasm

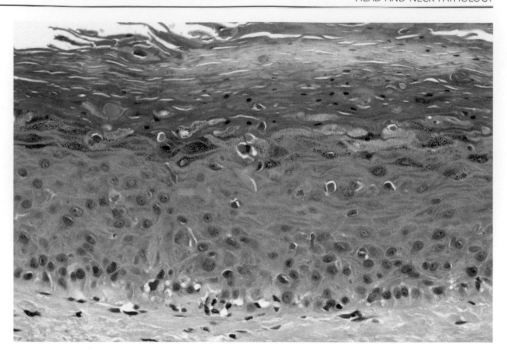

FIGURE 6-5

This atypical epithelium contains dyskeratosis, parakeratosis, keratosis, and loss of architecture, placing it in the mild dysplasia category.

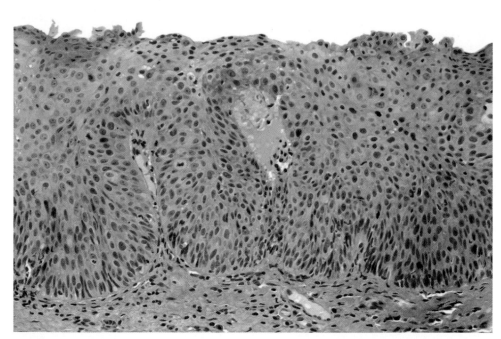

FIGURE 6-6

Severe dysplasia/carcinoma in situ. There is complete loss of maturation, loss of polarity, pleomorphism, dyskeratosis, and mitotic figures.

should confirm the diagnosis. Definitive evidence of dissociated squamous cells below the basement membrane confirms invasive SCC.

PROGNOSIS AND THERAPY

Some precursor lesions are self-limiting and reversible, others persist and some progress to SCC, with notable differences in incidence based on site of involvement

and the presence or absence of dysplasia. Lesions that arise in the anterior commissure nearly always convert to invasive SCC, while other topographic sites only convert about 15% of the time. Lesions classified as mild to moderate dysplasia have an ~10% rate of malignant transformation, implying the need for close clinical follow-up. Patients with CIS usually require more extensive management including close follow-up, although this is clinically dictated. Treatments are not standardized but include cessation of contributing factors, biopsy, vocal cord stripping, laser ablation, cordectomy, hemilaryngectomy, and radiation, used individually or in various combinations. Recurrence or persistence may develop from gland-duct extension left behind in a stripping or ablation.

■ SQUAMOUS CELL CARCINOMA

SCC is the most common malignancy of the head and neck and accounts for >90 % of all laryngeal carcinomas. However, it still accounts for only ~1 % of all carcinomas. About 1/10,000 men and 1/100,000 women are affected. The most important risk factors are, independently, tobacco and tobacco use, while susceptibility (immunologic factors and age), gastroesophageal reflux, environmental (including radiation), and occupational factors may also play a role. Smoking and alcohol use seem to have a multiplicative rather than additive effect in carcinoma development. Viruses (HPV, Epstein-Barr virus) are also linked to the development of SCC, although association versus direct effect remains unresolved. Associated genetic disorders include Lynch syndrome, Bloom syndrome, and Li-Fraumeni syndrome, among others. All of these factors probably interact in a multistep process.

As a malignant neoplasm characterized by squamous differentiation, SCC demonstrates infiltration into the stroma, abnormal keratinization, irregular nests of squamous epithelium, and cellular pleomorphism. Most laryngeal SCCs develop from a precursor lesion, with an arc of development, culminating in invasive SCC. Axiomatic, not all dysplasias progress to invasive carcinoma, but a multifactorial, multistep process is well characterized.

CLINICAL FEATURES

Men are affected much more frequently than women (6:1), although there is an increased incidence in women over recent years. All ages are affected, but patients usually present in the 6th to 7th decades of life. Patients present with symptoms referable to the anatomic site of the primary, including hoarseness, dysphagia, dysphonia, dyspnea, changes in phonation, foreign body sensation in the throat, difficulty swallowing, and stridor.

Radiographic imaging is usually done before endoscopy, as endoscopy may decrease the sensitivity of imaging. Imaging highlights the extent of the disease, shows submucosal invasive patterns, and helps with staging (extent of disease and lymph node status). Endoscopy is recommended to evaluate the extent of the disease, rule out other synchronous primaries (seen in up to 10 % of patients), and obtain a biopsy sample.

CONVENTIONAL SQUAMOUS CELL CARCINOMA—DISEASE FACT SHEET

Definition
- A malignant neoplasm characterized by squamous cell differentiation

Incidence and Location
- About 1% of all cancers, but >90% of head and neck cancers
- Supraglottic and glottic regions are most common

Morbidity and Mortality
- Loss of phonation
- Up to 25% mortality (site and stage dependent)

Gender and Age Distribution
- Males >> females (6:1)
- 6th to 7th decades

Clinical Features
- Tobacco and alcohol abuse
- Hoarseness, dysphagia, dysphonia, changes in phonation

Prognosis and Treatment
- Site, size, and stage specific, with ~90% 5-year survival for T1 versus <50% for T4 lesions
- Surgery and radiation

PATHOLOGIC FEATURES

CONVENTIONAL SQUAMOUS CELL CARCINOMA—PATHOLOGIC FEATURES

Gross Findings
- Glottic, supraglottic, subglottic, transglottic
- Flat, well-defined, raised edge, polypoid, exophytic
- Surface ulceration is seen

Microscopic Findings
- In situ, superficially or deeply invasive
- Well, moderately, or poorly differentiated
- Keratinizing, nonkeratinizing
- Disorganized growth, lack of maturation, dyskeratosis, keratin pearl formation, intercellular bridges, increased nuclear:cytoplasmic ratio, nuclear chromatin distribution irregularities, prominent nucleoli, increased mitotic figures, atypical mitotic figures
- Inflammatory infiltrate and tumor desmoplasia

Pathologic Differential Diagnosis
- Hyperplasia, radiation changes, necrotizing sialometaplasia, papilloma, variants of squamous cell carcinoma

GROSS FINDINGS

The anatomic sites—supraglottis, glottis, and subglottis—are embryologically distinct and separately compartmentalized (Figure 6-7), resulting in unique lymphatic drainage, and consequently have implications in the type of surgery and oncologic management. Glottic tumors for the most part are smaller (due to early clinical presentation), while supraglottic tumors are often clinically silent, resulting in a much larger tumor at the time of diagnosis. Interestingly, in Europe, supraglottic tumors predominate, while in the United States, glottic tumors are most common. SCCs can be ulcerative and endophytic, flat, polypoid, verrucous, or exophytic. They range from minute mucosa-thickened areas to large masses filling the luminal space, although they are usually <2 cm. The borders are rolled, raised to irregular and abrupt. Tumors can be erythematous to tan to white and firm to palpation.

MICROSCOPIC FINDINGS

SCC is generally divided into three histologic categories: (1) in situ (see earlier), (2) superficially invasive,

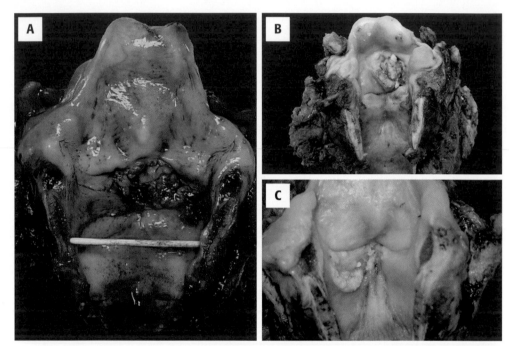

FIGURE 6-7

Laryngectomy specimens showing the various locations of tumor: transglottic (**A**), supraglottic (**B**), and subglottic (**C**). *(Courtesy of J. Fowler.)*

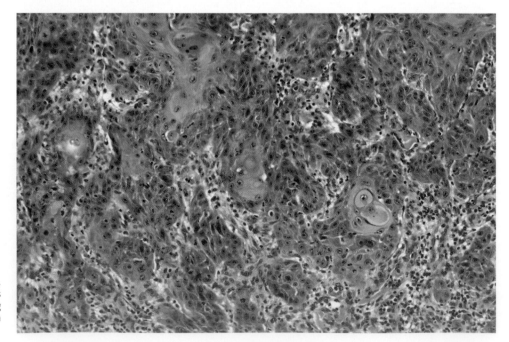

FIGURE 6-8

Squamous cell carcinoma with uneven, finger-like infiltration of the squamous cell carcinoma cells into the underlying stroma. Marked nuclear pleomorphism and cellular disarray are evident.

or (3) deeply invasive carcinomas, with additional modifiers based on histologic grade, including well-differentiated (closely resembles normal squamous mucosa), moderately differentiated (distinct nuclear pleomorphism and less keratinization), or poorly differentiated (immature cells with little maturation or keratinization), along with the presence or absence of keratinization (Figures 6-8 through 6-12). "Conventional" SCCs are composed of variable degrees of squamous differentiation, with the neoplastic cells invading through and disrupting the basement membrane (Figure 6-8). The overlying surface may not be atypical, and yet invasion may develop from the base (Figure 6-9). Broad infiltration or jagged, irregular cords, or individual cell infiltration can be seen, the latter correlating with a worse prognosis. SCC shows disorganized growth, a loss of polarity, dyskeratosis, keratin pearls (including paradoxical keratinization at the base), intercellular bridges, an increased nuclear:cytoplasmic ratio, nuclear chromatin irregularities, prominent eosinophilic nucleoli, and mitotic figures (including atypical forms). Keratinizing type is seen more frequently than nonkeratinizing or poorly differentiated types (Figure 6-10). Mitotic figures and necrosis tend to increase as the grade of the tumor becomes more poorly differentiated

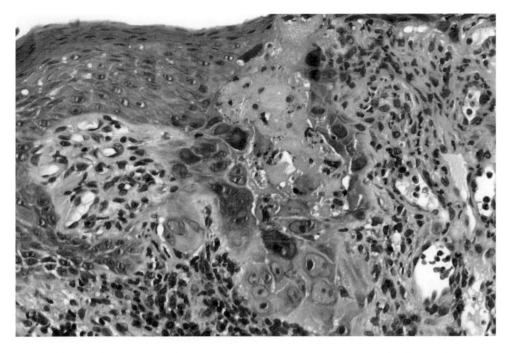

FIGURE 6-9

A moderately differentiated squamous cell carcinoma is noted arising from an unremarkable surface epithelium, underscoring the necessity for a biopsy of adequate size and depth.

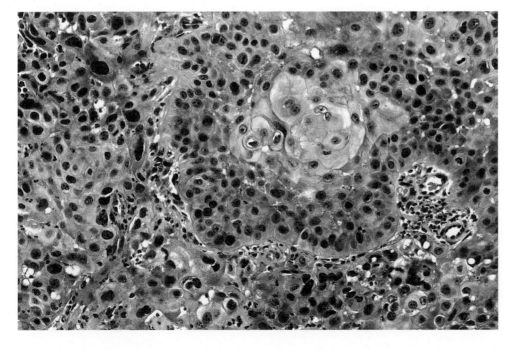

FIGURE 6-10

A moderately differentiated squamous cell carcinoma with loss of polarity, disorganization, increased nuclear:cytoplasmic ratio, and focal keratosis.

(Figure 6-11). A rich inflammatory infiltrate (usually of lymphocytes and plasma cells) is seen at the tumor to stroma junction, along with a dense, desmoplastic fibrous stroma. Perineural and vascular invasion can be seen, with a positive correlation to metastatic potential. Tumors may directly extend into cartilage (Figure 6-12), adjacent structures or organs. Margins are often difficult to assess, as shrinkage (up to 50%) may be seen after removal. There are also differences between frozen versus permanent sections. Special studies are rarely needed to document the epithelial nature of the tumor, although specific keratin subtypes may relate to histologic grade, degree

of keratinization and likelihood of metastases. *p53* mutations are an early event in carcinogenesis and so may help in separating benign from malignant lesions. Tumor site, size, histology (poorly differentiated), degree of invasion, positive surgical margins of resection, lymph node metastases (especially when there is extranodal capsular extension), and multifocal disease all correlate with a poorer prognosis. Separation of residual carcinoma from radiation changes in the postradiation sample may be difficult. While cellular enlargement is common, radiation usually does not change the nuclear:cytoplasmic ratio, as does carcinoma (Figure 6-13).

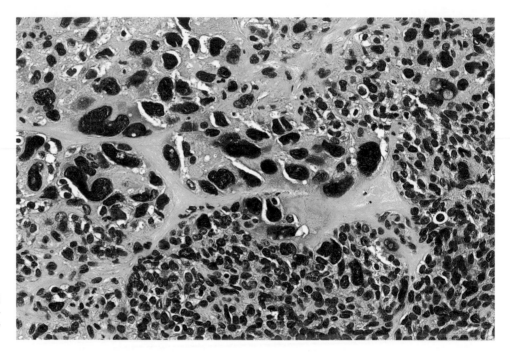

FIGURE 6-11

A poorly differentiated squamous cell carcinoma is arranged in a sheet-like distribution with only occasional cells suggesting squamous differentiation.

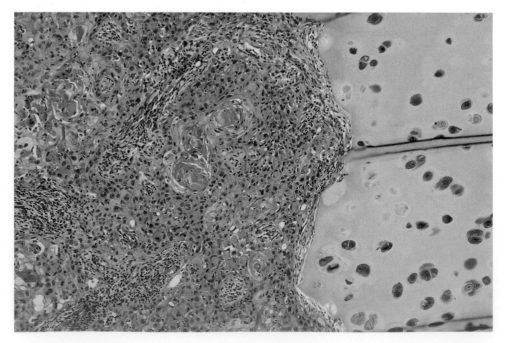

FIGURE 6-12

A moderately differentiated squamous cell carcinoma approaches but does not invade into the perichondrium of the laryngeal cartilage. Inflammation and fibrosis are noted.

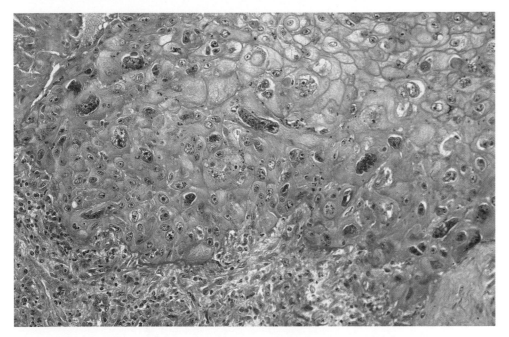

FIGURE 6-13

Radiation can induce changes in residual carcinoma, resulting in bizarre cells and nuclei, but the cells do not appear degenerated, nor do they have a low nuclear:cytoplasmic ratio. Nucleoli are frequently obvious in a squamous cell carcinoma after radiation therapy.

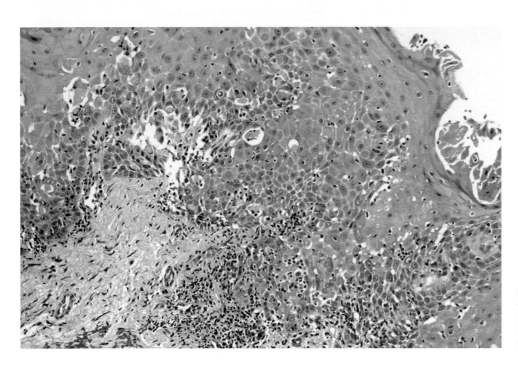

FIGURE 6-14

The difficulty of determining invasion is highlighted in this illustration of a jagged, hyperplastic squamous epithelium with inflammation. Note the parakeratosis.

DIFFERENTIAL DIAGNOSIS

The diagnosis of SCC is usually clear-cut, although occasionally other lesions are included in the differential diagnosis, such as hyperplasia (with atypia; Figure 6-14), radiation, necrotizing sialometaplasia, and papilloma. Marked PEH may be mistaken as SCC. However, the reactive nature of the proliferation, the lack of "finger-like" invasion, and the association with infectious agents and granular cell tumor will help to make this distinction. Radiation changes can affect epithelium, endothelial cells, and the stroma. Glands may become atrophic. There is often profound nuclear pleomorphism; however, these cells maintain a very low nuclear:cytoplasmic ratio. Necrotizing sialometaplasia has a preserved lobular architecture despite the degree of cytologic atypia (see Figures 4-30 to 4-32). A biopsy sample of sufficient size is necessary to secure this diagnosis. A papilloma does not have disorganized growth and unequivocal morphologic features of malignancy. SCC should be separated from SCC variants (discussed later), as there is often a difference in management and prognosis.

PROGNOSIS AND THERAPY

The TNM tumor classification, which incorporates site, size, and stage, correlates closely with both disease-free and overall survival (approximately 75%). Overall, 5-year survival rates approach 90% for T1 lesions, while being <50% for T4 tumors. Glottic tumors have an associated 80% to 85% survival rate, while the rate for subglottic tumors is ~40%. Regional lymph node metastases are relatively common, with extracapsular spread associated with a worse prognosis. A number of prognostic factors are available (EGFR, CCND1, CDK4, CDKN2A) although not yet commonly used. Larynx function–preserving treatment is the goal, with negative resection margins (3 to 5 mm). Laser excision, limited resection, and radical resection along with radiation therapy are variably used to achieve the best potentially curative voice-sparing outcome. There is a trend toward noninvasive management. Occasionally, neoadjuvant chemotherapy and radiation therapy are used to maintain laryngeal function. However, if these modalities fail, delayed salvage partial or total laryngectomy can still achieve a good patient outcome.

VARIANTS OF SQUAMOUS CELL CARCINOMA

Variants make up in aggregate <10% to 15% of all SCCs and include, among others, verrucous, exophytic or papillary, spindle cell (sarcomatoid) carcinoma, basaloid, and adenosquamous (Table 6-1). Rather than give an exhaustive review, only the unique features of each variant will be presented here.

VERRUCOUS SQUAMOUS CELL CARCINOMA

Verrucous SCC (VSCC) (Ackerman tumor) comprises ~3% of all SCCs, is pathogenetically related to HPV (specifically genotypes 16 and 18), and has specific loss of heterozygosity patterns not identified in hyperplasia. It usually affects the anterior true vocal cords and measures up to 10 cm.

VSCC is a highly differentiated type of SCC, composed of an exophytic, warty tumor (Figure 6-15) with multiple filiform projections, which are thickened and club-shaped, and lined by well-differentiated squamous epithelium (Figure 6-16). The advancing margins of the tumor are usually broad or bulbous rete ridges with a blunt, pushing rather than an infiltrative appearance, occasionally showing coalescing rete (Figure 6-17). The downward dipping epithelium may create a "cup" or "arms" around the periphery of the tumor. There is often a dense inflammatory response in the subjacent tissues. The epithelium is extraordinarily well differentiated without any of the normally associated malignant criteria identified in SCC. The cells are arranged in an

---

VERRUCOUS SQUAMOUS CELL CARCINOMA

Definition
- Well-differentiated exophytic/verrucous growth with pushing border of infiltration in a cytologically bland, amitotic squamous epithelium

Prognosis and Treatment
- 85% to 95% 5-year survival (20% recurrence/persistence)
- Surgery

Gross Findings
- Broad-based, warty, exophytic, fungating mass

Microscopic Findings
- Broad border of pushing infiltration
- Multiple projections of well-differentiated squamous epithelium with club-shaped to filiform projections
- Maturation toward surface
- Abundant keratosis (orthokeratosis and parakeratosis; church-spire), parakeratotic crypting
- Limited mitotic figures, if present at all

Pathologic Differential Diagnosis
- Verrucous hyperplasia and conventional squamous cell carcinoma

---

orderly maturation towards the surface, with abundant surface keratosis (parakeratosis and/or orthokeratosis (called "church-spire" keratosis; Figure 6-18). Parakeratotic crypting (collections of parakeratotic cells with debris) is a common feature. Mitotic figures are not easy to identify, and when found, they are not atypical (Figure 6-19). If dysplasia is present, it is focal and limited to the basal zone. A foreign body giant cell reaction may develop to extravasated keratin. p53 overexpression is seen in ~40% of cases. Both a benign keratinizing hyperplasia (or verruca vulgaris) and a very well differentiated SCC can share all of these features somewhere in the tumor, making separation of these lesions a most vexing problem. The relationship of the lesion to the stroma **must** be adequately assessed in a sample of sufficient size that has been accurately oriented (not tangential) before a definitive diagnosis is rendered.

The differential diagnosis rests between verrucous hyperplasia and conventional SCC. It is argued that the difference between verrucous hyperplasia and VSCC is only in stage and size, the lesions representing a developmental spectrum. The distinction on histologic features alone is often impossible. However, true verrucous hyperplasia does exist (hyperplastic squamous epithelium with regularly spaced, verrucous projections and hyperkeratosis, sharply defined at the epithelial–stromal interface; Figure 6-20). VSCC can include an invasive component of "ordinary" SCC at the base or demonstrate

TABLE 6-1

Clinical and Histologic Features of Squamous Cell Carcinoma Variants

| Feature | Variant | | | | |
	Verrucous	Papillary/ Exophytic	Spindle Cell (Sarcomatoid)	Basaloid	Adenosquamous
Gender	M > F, except oral	M >> F	M >>> F	M >> F	M slight > F
Location	Oral > larynx	Larynx > oral > nasal	Larynx > oral > nasal	Base of tongue > supraglottic larynx	Tongue > floor of mouth > nasal
Frequency (of all SCCs)	~3%	~1%	~3%	<1%	<1%
Etiologic agent?	HPV	? HPV	? Radiation	Unknown	Unknown
Macroscopic	Broad-based warty and fungating mass	Polypoid, exophytic, bulky, papillary, fungiform	Polypoid mass	Firm to hard with central necrosis	Indurated submucosal nodule
Size (cm)	Up to 10	1-1.5 (mean)	2 (mean)	Up to 6	1 (mean)
Microscopic	Pushing border of infiltration; abrupt transition with normal; large, blunt club-shaped rete pegs; no pleomorphism; no mitotic activity; abundant keratin, including parakeratin crypting and "church-spire" keratosis	>70% exophytic or papillary architecture; "cauliflower-like" versus "celery-like;" unequivocal cytomorphologic malignancy; surface keratinization; invasive, but difficult to demonstrate; koilocytic atypia	Biphasic; SCC present, but ulcerated; blended/ transition with atypical spindle cell population; hypercellular; variable patterns of spindle-cell growth; pleomorphism; opacified cytoplasm; increased mitotic figures	Biphasic; invasive; lobular; basaloid component most prominent; palisaded; high nuclear: cytoplasmic ratio; abrupt squamous differentiation (metaplasia, dysplasia, CIS or invasive); ↑ mitotic figures; comedonecrosis; hyaline material	Biphasic; SCC and adenocarcinoma; undifferentiated component; separate or intermixed with areas of transition; infiltrative; ↑ mitotic figures; sparse inflammatory infiltrate
Special studies	HPV identified	None	~70% positive with epithelial markers	Keratin, EMA, CK7, p63, and K903	Mucin positive
Differential diagnosis	Verrucous hyperplasia; SCC	In situ SCC; squamous papilloma; reactive hyperplasia	Benign and malignant mesenchymal process; melanoma; synovial sarcoma	Adenoid cystic carcinoma; neuroendocrine carcinoma (small cell carcinoma)	Basaloid SCC; mucoepidermoid carcinoma; adenocarcinoma with squamous metaplasia
Treatment	Surgery	Surgery ± radiation	Surgery with radiation	Surgery; radiation; chemotherapy	Surgery with neck dissection
Prognosis	75% 5-year survival	~ 70% 5-year survival	~ 80% 5-year survival	~ 40% 2-year survival	~ 55% 2-year survival
Pitfalls	Inadequate biopsy; tangential sectioning; radiation is acceptable	Orientation; adequacy of specimen	No surface; mesenchymal markers; needs "excisional" biopsy initially	Association with 2nd primary; high chance of nodal metastases	Separation on small biopsies from adenocarcinoma or SCC

CIS, carcinoma in situ; EMA, epithelial membrane antigen; HPV, human papillomavirus; SCC, squamous cell carcinoma.

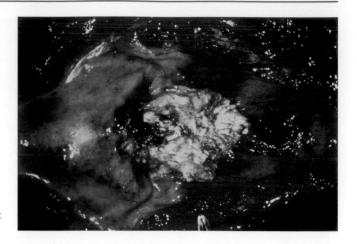

FIGURE 6-15

Multiple projections are seen in this macroscopic view of a large, transglottic verrucous squamous cell carcinoma.

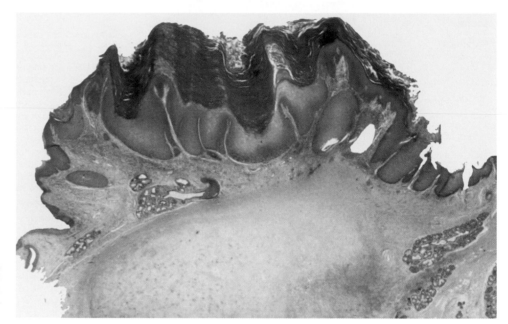

FIGURE 6-16

A broad, pushing border of infiltration is noted immediately above the laryngeal cartilage. Extensive keratosis is noted along with an increased number of layers of squamous epithelium.

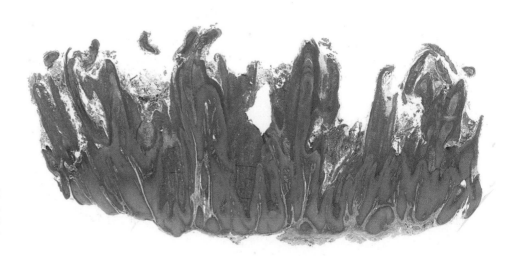

FIGURE 6-17

The size of the lesion is often a helpful indicator of the underlying diagnosis. Broad, pushing border of infiltration with extensive, "church-spire"–type keratosis, and parakeratotic crypting.

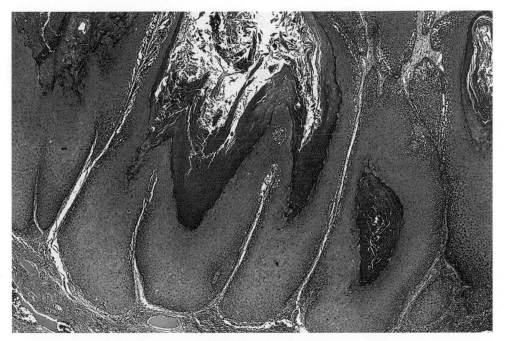

FIGURE 6-18

The proliferation in verrucous carcinoma is cytologically bland, shows maturation and appropriate polarity, demonstrating a broad, bulbous-type infiltration into the stroma with associated inflammation. There is "church-spire"–type keratosis at the surface.

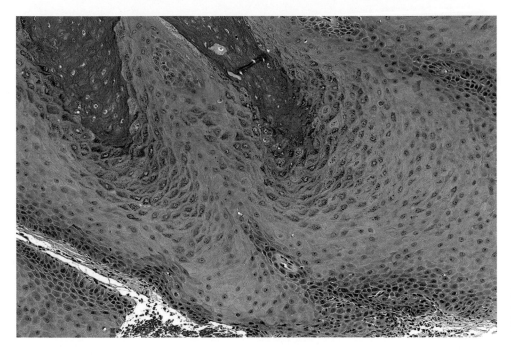

FIGURE 6-19

Keratosis is noted (*left*) in a cytologically bland, but "pushing" epithelium without mitotic figures.

atypical cytologic features; these tumors need to be managed as well-differentiated SCC. Squamous papilloma has thin, well-formed papillae, limited keratinization, and koilocytic atypia.

Biologically, VSCC behaves as an "extremely well differentiated squamous cell carcinoma," with an approximately 85% to 95% 5-year survival rate depending upon site and stage. Most tumors are pT1 at presentation without lymph node metastases. Persistence/recurrence is seen in up to 20% of patients, usually a function of the type of treatment. Voice preservation techniques are encouraged, with surgery alone the mainstay of therapy. Radiation is sometimes used for functional preservation in nonsurgical candidates.

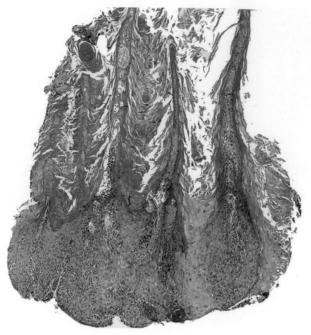

FIGURE 6-20

Verrucous hyperplasia with papillary fronds of squamous epithelium covered with keratin and lacking architectural and cytologic features of malignancy. The separation of verrucous hyperplasia from verrucous carcinoma is often difficult, demanding clinical correlation.

EXOPHYTIC AND PAPILLARY SQUAMOUS CELL CARCINOMA

Definition
- Exophytic or papillary architecture in squamous cell carcinoma

Prognosis and Treatment
- Recurrences in ~35%
- Better prognosis than conventional squamous cell carcinoma (site and stage dependent)

Gross Findings
- Mean of 1 to 1.5 cm
- Polypoid, exophytic, bulky, papillary or fungiform

Microscopic Findings
- >70% exophytic or papillary architecture
- **Exophytic:** broad-based, bulbous, rounded "cauliflower-like" growth
- **Papillary:** multiple, thin, delicate, filiform, finger-like projections
- Both types have malignant cytologic features
- Stromal invasion is difficult to identify

Pathologic Differential Diagnosis
- Squamous papilloma, verrucous squamous cell carcinoma

EXOPHYTIC AND PAPILLARY SQUAMOUS CELL CARCINOMA

Exophytic SCC (ESCC) and papillary SCC (PSCC) are uncommon but distinct variants of SCC, separable from verrucous SCC (as outlined earlier). By definition, ESCC and PSCC are de novo malignancies without a preexisting or coexisting benign lesion (i.e., squamous papilloma). However, since HPV is a suggested etiology in up to 20% of cases, malignant transformation of a preexisting squamous papilloma may be seen. The average size of exophytic and papillary tumors is between 1 and 1.5 cm. Most tumors present at a low tumor stage (T1 or T2),

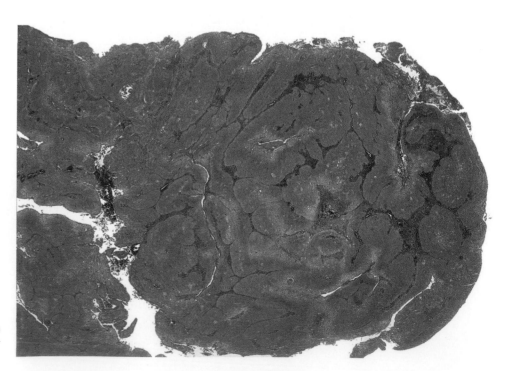

FIGURE 6-21

An exophytic squamous cell carcinoma has a rounded "cauliflower-like" projection to the projections.

although multifocality is described. Tumors are seen in the supraglottis much more commonly than the in glottis or subglottis. Macroscopically, ESCC and PSCC are polypoid, exophytic, bulky, papillary, or fungiform tumors, soft to firm, and arising from a broad base or from a narrow pedicle/stalk.

By definition, the neoplastic squamous epithelial proliferation must demonstrate a dominant (>70%) exophytic or papillary architectural growth pattern with unequivocal cytomorphologic evidence of malignancy. Cytologically, there is nuclear enlargement, pleomorphism, loss of polarity, limited surface keratosis, and an immature phenotype. The exophytic pattern consists

of a broad-based, bulbous to exophytic growth of the squamous epithelium (Figure 6-21). The projections are rounded and "cauliflower-like" in growth pattern. Tangential sectioning yields a number of central fibrovascular cores, but the superficial aspect is lobular, not papillary. The papillary pattern consists of multiple, thin, delicate filiform, finger-like papillary projections (Figure 6-22). The papillae contain a delicate fibrovascular core surrounded by the neoplastic epithelium (Figure 6-23) Tangential sectioning yields a number of central fibrovascular cores but appears more like a bunch of celery cut across the stalk. It is not uncommon to have extensive overlap between these patterns, and

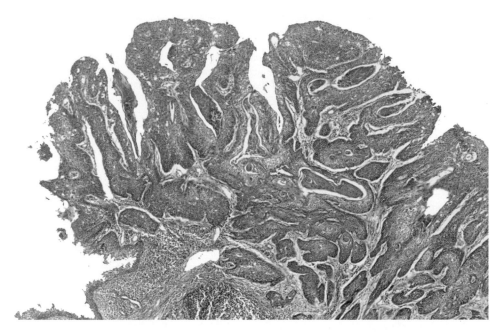

FIGURE 6-22

A papillary squamous cell carcinoma demonstrates multiple papillary projections above the surface, but an invasive component is also noted. Keratinization is prominent.

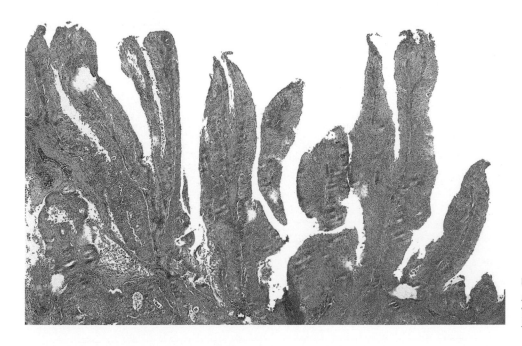

FIGURE 6-23

A papillary squamous cell carcinoma with individual, delicate finger-like projections with fibrovascular cores.

when that is the case, ESCC should be the default diagnosis. Both types have the features of SCC that have already been described (Figure 6-24). Necrosis may be seen. Invasion may be difficult to define, especially in superficial biopsy samples. However, the significant proliferation of this carcinomatous epithelium, often forming a large clinical lesion, is rather beyond the general concept of CIS. When in doubt, the significantly proliferated appearance of the lesion should be heavily weighted in the direction of carcinoma. The cytomorphologic features of malignancy would exclude the diagnosis of a papilloma, as well as the consideration of a verrucous carcinoma.

Approximately one-third of patients develop recurrence, frequently more than once. However, patients with these variants seem to have a better prognosis compared to site- and stage-matched conventional SCC patients. PSCC has a better prognosis than ESCC, both of which are better than that for conventional SCC. Lymph node metastases are uncommon, and most patients present at low stage. Radiation is used after surgery in most patients.

SPINDLE CELL "SARCOMATOID" CARCINOMA

Spindle cell "sarcomatoid" carcinoma (SCSC) (Lane tumor) is recognized as a morphologically biphasic neoplasm containing an epithelioid and spindle-shaped neoplastic proliferation. It comprises up to 3% of SCC. There is a profound male:female ratio (12:1). The

SPINDLE CELL "SARCOMATOID" CARCINOMA

Definition
- Morphologically biphasic tumor with squamous cell and malignant spindle cell component with a mesenchymal appearance but an epithelial origin

Prognosis and Treatment
- 80% 5-year survival, with most patients having a low stage
- Surgery and radiation

Gross Findings
- Polypoid mass arising from true vocal cord
- Ulcerated surface and firm cut surface

Microscopic Findings
- Surface ulceration with fibrinoid necrosis
- Dysplasia, carcinoma in situ, or infiltrating squamous cell carcinoma
- Imperceptible blending of carcinoma with spindle cell population
- Storiform, interlacing fascicles, or herringbone pattern
- Hypercellular, but hypocellular with collagen also
- Mitotic figures easily identified

Immunohistochemical Features
- Keratin, EMA, CK18, and p63 in epithelioid and spindle cell populations (~70% of cases)

Pathologic Differential Diagnosis
- Contact ulcer, myofibroblastic tumor, synovial sarcoma, spindle cell melanoma

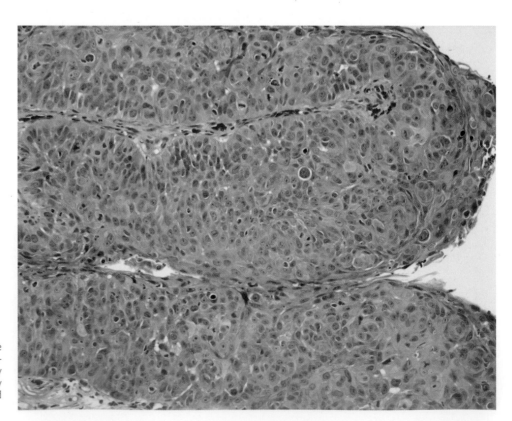

FIGURE 6-24
Papillary squamous cell carcinoma. The papillary projections have thin fibrovascular cores and remarkably cytologically atypical epithelium lining the papillary projections. Dyskeratosis and jumbled architecture is prominent.

majority (70%) are glottic tumors. Nearly all cases are described as ***polypoid*** masses with a mean size of ~2.0 cm (Figure 6-25). They are frequently ulcerated with a covering of fibrinoid necrosis. They have a firm and fibrous cut surface.

Considering the frequency of surface ulceration with fibrinoid necrosis (Figure 6-26), it may be difficult to discern the transition between the surface epithelium and the spindle cell element. In fact, the carcinomatous and sarcomatoid components will abut directly against one another with imperceptible blending and continuity

between them (Figure 6-27). However, if meticulously and diligently sought, dysplasia, CIS, or infiltrating SCC can be identified, although it is usually minor to inconspicuous with the sarcomatoid part dominating. Frank squamous differentiation can be found at the base of the polypoid lesion, the advancing margins, or within invaginations at the surface where the epithelium is not ulcerated or denuded. The sarcomatoid or fusiform fraction of the tumor can be arranged in a diverse array of appearances, including storiform, interlacing bundles or fascicles, and herringbone (Figure 6-28). Generally,

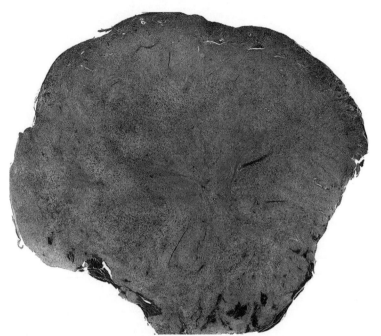

FIGURE 6-25

A macroscopic view of a spindle cell "sarcomatoid" carcinoma shows the polypoid projection attached to the underlying stroma by a narrow stalk. Surface ulceration has denuded most of the epithelium.

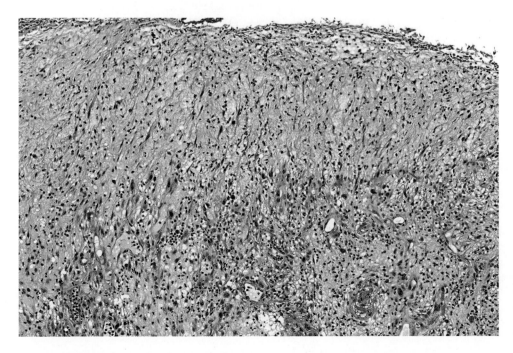

FIGURE 6-26

Complete loss of the surface epithelium with fibrinoid necrosis is characteristic for a spindle cell "sarcomatoid" carcinoma, with markedly atypical, hyperchromatic nuclei identified within the spindle cells of the "stroma."

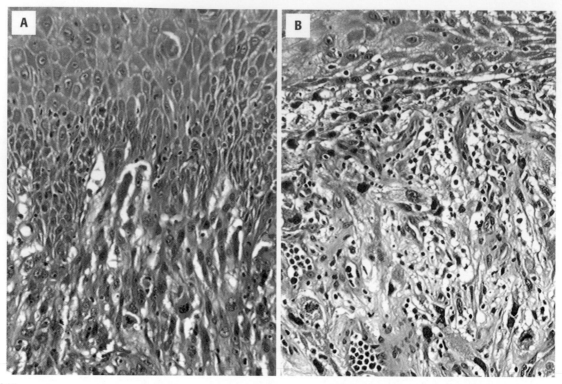

FIGURE 6-27
A and **B**, The surface epithelium blends imperceptibly with the spindled pattern of growth. Mitotic figures, pleomorphism, and inflammation are noted.

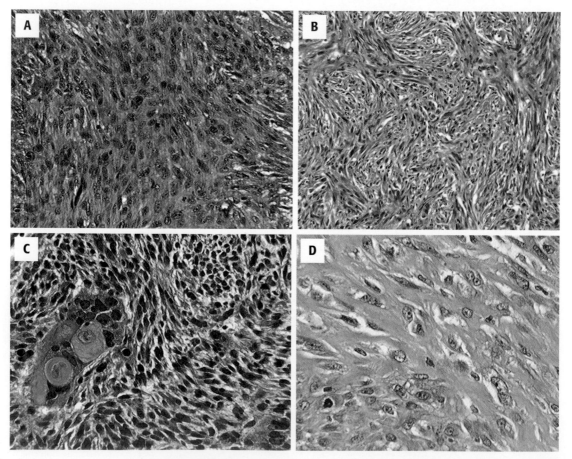

FIGURE 6-28
Variable patterns of growth, including solid-compact (**A**), fascicular and storiform (**B**), a focus of abrupt squamous differentiation (**C**), and a hypocellular atypical spindle cell population with mitotic figures (**D**).

hypercellular, hypocellular tumors with dense collagen deposition are also seen. A desmoplastic stroma is present in ~50% of cases. Pleomorphism is often mild to moderate, without a severe degree of anaplasia. The tumor cells are plump fusiform cells, although they can be rounded and epithelioid. Opacified, dense, eosinophilic cytoplasm gives a hint of squamous differentiation but is difficult to quantify or qualify accurately. Mitotic figures, including atypical forms, are easily counted in most tumors (Figure 6-29). Necrosis is usually absent. Rarely, metaplastic or frankly neoplastic cartilage or bone can be seen.

This is the one SCC variant in which immunohistochemistry may be of value. The individual spindle neoplastic cells react variably, although most sensitively and reliably with keratin (AE1/AE3), epithelial membrane antigen (EMA) (Figure 6-30), and CK18, although only ~70% of cases will yield any epithelial immunoreactivity. p63 is positive in many cases. Other mesenchymal markers can be identified focally,

although this phenotypic plasticity or lineage infidelity supports the sarcomatoid transformation seen in SCSC. Whereas a positive epithelial marker helps to confirm the diagnosis of SCSC, a nonreactive or negative result should not dissuade the pathologist from the diagnosis, especially in the correct clinical setting.

The differential diagnosis includes any spindle cell lesion, but suffice it to say that authentic primary mucosal sarcomas or benign mesenchymal tumors of the larynx are exceptional. *Contact ulcer* has a more vascular appearance and lacks cytologic atypia. A *myofibroblastic tumor* has a tissue culture–like growth of spindle to stellate cells with inflammatory cells throughout (Figure 6-31). *Synovial sarcoma* (especially monophasic) may cause the most diagnostic difficulty, but the age at presentation (young people), tumor location (usually hypopharynx and soft tissue rather than mucosal), and the presence of a specific chromosomal translocation t(X;18) (p11;q11) can aid in this distinction. *Spindle cell melanoma* would react with melanocytic markers.

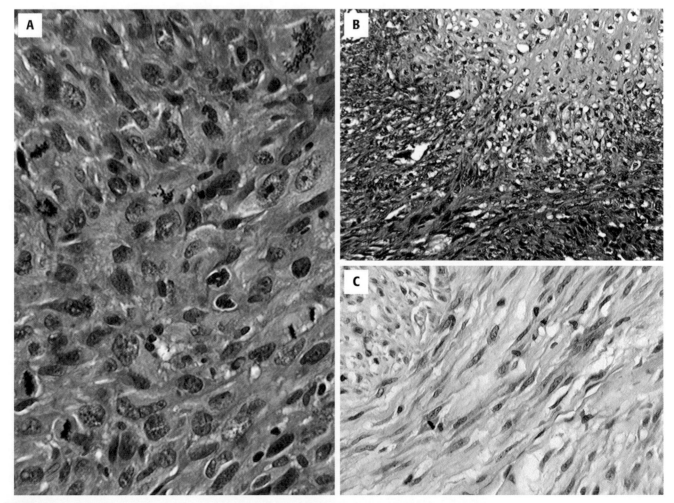

FIGURE 6-29

A, Spindle cell "sarcomatoid" carcinoma (SCSC) composed of haphazard atypical spindle cells with increased mitotic figures, including atypical forms. **B**, Metaplastic cartilage has undergone malignant transformation into a chondrosarcoma within this SCSC. **C**, Deceptively bland spindle cells may be the dominant finding.

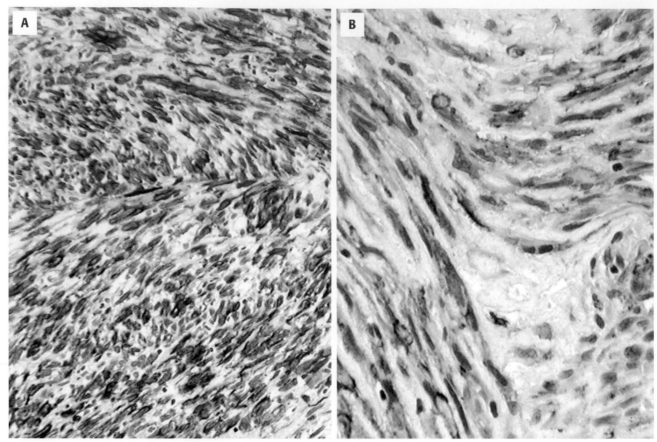

FIGURE 6-30

Spindle cell "sarcomatoid" carcinoma. It is unusual to find such a strongly immunopositive keratin reaction (**A**), while the more focal epithelial membrane antigen stain is more characteristic of the quality of the reaction (**B**).

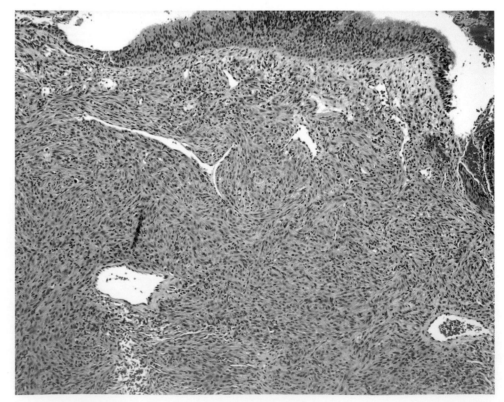

FIGURE 6-31

An inflammatory myofibroblastic tumor below an intact epithelium. Note the haphazard arrangement of this cellular tumor. But, there is a lack of atypia.

There is an overall 80% 5-year survival. Most patients (85%) present at a low stage (T1 and T2). When metastatic disease develops (~20%), cervical lymph nodes and pulmonary involvement is most frequent. There is a worse outcome for patients with a history of radiation, large tumors, fixed vocal cords, and the presence of epithelial markers immunohistochemically. Surgery, usually followed by radiation therapy, seems to yield the best long-term patient outcome, similar to conventional SCC, although site and stage specific. Polypectomy may be curative.

BASALOID SQUAMOUS CELL CARCINOMA

Basaloid SCC (BSCC) is a high-grade variant of SCC showing predominantly basaloid cells with associated squamous differentiation (keratinization, dysplasia, in situ, or invasive tumor). It affects primarily men in the 6th to 7th decades. As a high-grade lesion, it has a predi-

---

BASALOID SQUAMOUS CELL CARCINOMA

Definition
- High-grade squamous cell carcinoma variant with basaloid small cells arranged in a palisaded architecture; focal areas of squamous differentiation

Clinical Features
- Multifocal, older men, high cervical lymph node metastases

Prognosis and Treatment
- 40% survival
- Multimodality therapy (surgery, radiation, chemotherapy)

Gross Findings
- Firm tumors with central necrosis, up to 6 cm

Microscopic Findings
- Solid, lobular, **comedonecrosis**, cribriform, trabecular, glands, and cystic architecture
- Frequently ulcerated, easily identified lymphovascular invasion
- Basaloid cells with small closely opposed moderately pleomorphic cells with peripheral palisading
- Hyperchromatic to vesicular nuclei with coarse nuclear chromatin
- Abrupt keratinization, squamous pearl formation, individual cell keratinization
- High mitotic index
- Prominent, eosinophilic, hyaline, "cylindrical" matrix material

Immunohistochemical Features
- Keratin, K903 (34βE12), CAM5.2, EMA, CK7, CK5/6, p63, p53

Pathologic Differential Diagnosis
- Neuroendocrine carcinoma, adenoid cystic carcinoma, adenosquamous carcinoma, squamous cell carcinoma

---

lection for multifocal presentation and frequent cervical lymph node metastases at presentation. The piriform sinus and supraglottic areas are most frequently affected. Macroscopically, these tumors are usually firm to hard with associated central necrosis, occurring as exophytic to nodular masses, measuring up to 6 cm in greatest dimension.

Many patterns are seen in this infiltrating tumor, including solid, smooth-contoured lobules, comedonecrosis (Figure 6-32), cribriform, cords, trabeculae, nests, and glands or cysts. Surface ulceration may belie the deeply invasive nature of the tumor, which has frequent lymphovascular invasion, although neurotropism is less common. The basaloid component is the most diagnostic feature, incorporating small, closely opposed moderately pleomorphic cells with hyperchromatic to vesicular nuclei and scant cytoplasm into a lobular configuration with peripheral palisading (Figure 6-33). These basaloid regions are in intimate association with areas of squamous differentiation including abrupt keratinization in the form of squamous pearls (Figure 6-34), individual cell keratinization, dysplasia, or SCC (in situ or invasive). Marked mitotic activity, as well as comedonecrosis in the center of the neoplastic islands, is common. The tumor cells are separated by a prominent dense pink hyaline material, often cylinder shaped, with small cystic spaces containing mucoid-type material. Rosettes may be seen, with a spindled cell component in a few cases. In metastatic disease, both basaloid and squamous cell components can be seen, although the basaloid features predominate. The neoplastic cells are reactive with pan-keratin, K903 (34βE12), CAM5.2, EMA, CK7, CK5/6, p63, and p53.

A sample of sufficient depth to show the heterogeneous nature of the tumor will usually resolve the differential consideration of a neuroendocrine carcinoma, adenoid cystic carcinoma, adenosquamous carcinoma, and SCC. A lack of neuroendocrine nuclear features and immunoreactivity eliminates *neuroendocrine tumors* from consideration. *Adenoid cystic carcinoma* does not have squamous differentiation, prominent pleomorphism, mitoses, or necrosis. The nuclei are angulated with no nucleoli. S100 protein is frequently positive. *Adenosquamous carcinoma* (discussed later) shows a dual composition of true squamous carcinoma and adenocarcinoma. A poorly differentiated SCC will have a small basaloid population but without the characteristic lobular pattern with comedonecrosis. When the diagnosis of a basaloid squamous carcinoma is made, there is an increased possibility of a contemporaneous primary elsewhere.

Despite aggressive therapy, the overall mortality rate is high (60% die of disease). Regional and distant metastases are common. Patients present at a higher stage than conventional SCC. BSCC requires aggressive multimodality therapy, including radical surgery (including neck dissection), radiotherapy, and chemotherapy (especially for metastatic disease).

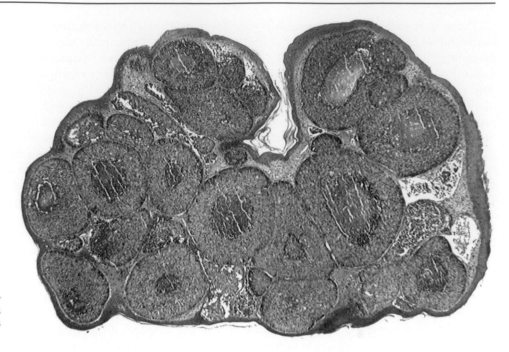

FIGURE 6-32

The neoplastic infiltrate is dominated by a lobular arrangement of basaloid cells with areas of comedonecrosis in this basaloid squamous cell carcinoma.

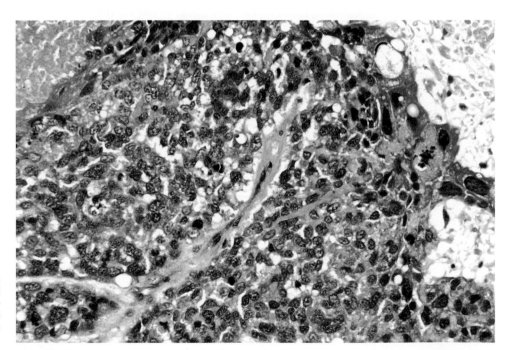

FIGURE 6-33

Frank squamous cell carcinoma is seen (*left*) with an area of necrosis, juxtaposed to the characteristic basaloid, small, peripherally palisaded nuclear architecture of a basaloid squamous cell carcinoma (*right*).

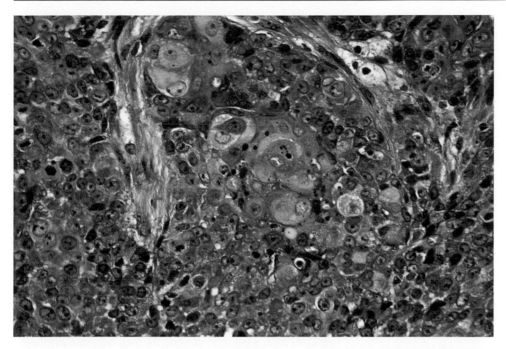

FIGURE 6-34

Abrupt keratinization intimately admixed with the basaloid cells, which are smaller in size and have a high nuclear:cytoplasmic ratio and hyperchromatic nuclei in this basaloid squamous cell carcinoma.

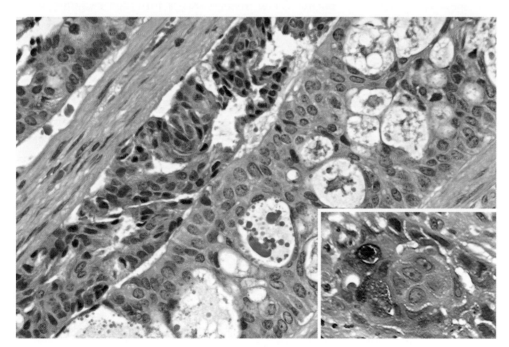

FIGURE 6-35

Adenosquamous carcinoma demonstrates blended adenocarcinoma and squamous cell carcinoma within a single tumor mass. *Inset* demonstrates a positive mucicarmine reaction.

ADENOSQUAMOUS CARCINOMA

Adenosquamous carcinoma (ASC) is a high-grade variant of SCC composed of an admixture of SCC and true adenocarcinoma. Most patients (up to 75%) present with lymph node metastases. ASC occurs throughout the upper aerodigestive tract, often as an indurated, ulcerated, submucosal to exophytic nodule, up to 5 cm in maximum dimension, although most are <1 cm. Any site of the larynx can be affected.

By definition the tumor demonstrates biphasic components of adenocarcinoma and SCC, with an undifferentiated cellular component in several tumors (Figure 6-35). The SCC can be in situ or invasive, ranging from well to poorly differentiated. Squamous differentiation is confirmed by pavemented growth with intercellular bridges, keratin pearl formation, dyskeratosis, or individual cell keratinization. The adenocarcinoma component tends to develop away from the surface (deep), appearing tubular, alveolar, and glandular. Mucous cell differentiation is not essential for the diagnosis, but mucin production is usually

ADENOSQUAMOUS CARCINOMA

Definition
- Composite of true adenocarcinoma and squamous cell carcinoma

Prognosis and Treatment
- Lymph node metastases in up to 75%
- Poor prognosis (~20% 5-year survival)
- Surgery

Gross Findings
- Indurated, submucosal nodule ~1 cm (mean)

Microscopic Findings
- Biphasic adenocarcinoma and squamous carcinoma
- Undifferentiated or transitional components between lesions
- Separate, intermixed, commingled, transitions
- Scant inflammatory infiltrate
- Squamous component: CK7, CK5/6, and p63 positive
- Glandular component: CEA, CK7

Pathologic Differential Diagnosis
- Basaloid squamous cell carcinoma, mucoepidermoid carcinoma, adenocarcinoma with squamous metaplasia, necrotizing sialometaplasia

easily identified. The cells in the adenocarcinoma can be basaloid, and separation from basaloid SCC can at times be arbitrary. The two carcinomas may be separate or intermixed, with areas of commingling and/or transition of the SCC to adenocarcinoma. The "undifferentiated" areas between the two distinct carcinomas are often composed of clear cells. Both carcinomas may demonstrate frequent mitoses, necrosis, and infiltration into the surrounding tissue with affiliated perineural invasion. There is typically a sparse inflammatory cell infiltrate at the tumor–stromal interface with minimal to absent desmoplastic fibrosis. The squamous component is CK7, CK5/6, and p63 immunoreactive, while the glandular component is carcinoembryonic antigen (CEA) and CK7 positive.

In contrast to *BSCC*, ASC shows a prominent squamous cell component, absence of basaloid cells with peripheral nuclear palisading, and the presence of glandular differentiation. Although separation of ASC from mucoepidermoid carcinoma may be impossible in some cases, mucoepidermoid carcinoma demonstrates intermediate-type cells, generally does not have true squamous cell differentiation, and does not have two distinctly separate carcinomas (adenocarcinoma and SCC). An *adenocarcinoma with squamous metaplasia* generally does not demonstrate the nuclear criteria of a malignant squamous cell component. Likewise, *necrotizing sialometaplasia* shows squamous epithelium lining the scaffolding of preserved duct-gland units that have been infarcted or destroyed. A contemporaneous SCC and adenocarcinoma may affect the upper aerodigestive tract, but these lesions are usually temporally separated. Aggressive surgery with neck dissection and follow-up radiation

yields an ~15% to 25% 5-year survival. Along with a high lymph node metastatic rate, distant metastases are seen in ~25% of patients (lung most commonly).

■ NEUROENDOCRINE CARCINOMA

The terminology for this family of neoplasms is fraught with a great deal of confusion. The terms "carcinoid," "atypical carcinoid," and "small cell carcinoma," similar to pulmonary nomenclature, have been suggested by the World Health Organization. Equivalent terminology includes well-differentiated (carcinoid), moderately differentiated (atypical carcinoma), and poorly differentiated (small cell carcinoma) neuroendocrine carcinoma, respectively. By definition, this is a heterogeneous group of neoplasms characterized by the presence of epithelial and neuroendocrine differentiation, the latter often limited to immunohistochemistry, as it is most uncommon to have systemic manifestations or paraneoplastic syndromes (Cushing, Lambert-Eaton, and Schwartz-Bartter). The histogenesis is unsettled but thought to be of epithelial origin.

CLINICAL FEATURES

NEUROENDOCRINE CARCINOMA (CARCINOID, ATYPICAL CARCINOID, SMALL CELL CARCINOMA)—DISEASE FACT SHEET

Definition
- Malignant epithelial neoplasm with neuroendocrine differentiation

Incidence and Location
- Most common non–squamous cell malignancy of the larynx
- Usually supraglottic

Morbidity and Mortality
- Variable based on histologic grade
- Metastatic disease rather than recurrence is cause of death
- Usually to lymph nodes, liver, lung, and bone

Gender and Age Distribution
- Men >> women (3:1)
- Peak in 7th decade

Clinical Features
- Strong tobacco association
- Dysphagia, hoarseness, sore throat, hemoptysis, lump in throat

Prognosis and Treatment
- Tumor dependent:
- **Carcinoid:** good long-term prognosis; surgery alone
- **Atypical carcinoid:** 45% metastatic disease; 48% 5-year survival; surgery and radiation
- **Small cell carcinoma:** rapidly fatal; 16% 2-year survival

Although there are slight differences between the various grades of neuroendocrine neoplasms, most patients are males (male:female is 3:1) between 45 and 80 years of age with a peak in the 7th decade and a strong tobacco use association. As with all laryngeal tumors, dysphagia, hoarseness, sore throat, hemoptysis, and the feeling of a lump are the most common presenting symptoms. Atypical carcinoid represents the most common nonsquamous malignancy of the larynx. Patients will small cell carcinoma frequently have lymph node metastases (50%).

PATHOLOGIC FEATURES

GROSS FINDINGS

Neuroendocrine neoplasms occur most frequently in the supraglottic region, presenting as a submucosal mass in the aryepiglottic fold or arytenoid. The gross appearance ranges from polypoid (Figure 6-36) and pedunculated to ulcerated, ranging in size up to 4 cm (average, 1.6 cm).

MICROSCOPIC FINDINGS

Neuroendocrine tumors are usually unencapsulated, although carcinoids and atypical carcinoids are circumscribed, covered by an uninvolved surface mucosa. The tumors present with a variety of different histologic patterns, including an organoid or a trabecular growth in carcinoid tumors (Figure 6-37); the addition of cords, solid, single-file and cribriform patterns in the atypical carcinoids; and all of these patterns along with sheets, ribbons, pseudoglands, and rosette formations in small cell carcinoma. Atypical carcinoid and small cell carcinoma may demonstrate surface ulceration. A fibrovascular

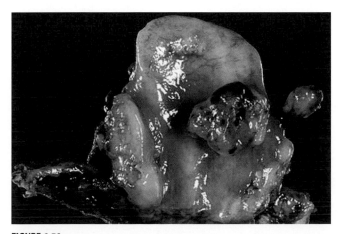

FIGURE 6-36

A supraglottic polypoid tumor is quite characteristic for a neuroendocrine carcinoma. *(Courtesy of J. Fowler.)*

NEUROENDOCRINE CARCINOMA (CARCINOID, ATYPICAL CARCINOID, SMALL CELL CARCINOMA)—PATHOLOGIC FEATURES

Gross Findings
- Supraglottic
- Submucosal mass, with ulceration in higher-grade tumors
- Polypoid, pedunculated
- Up to 4 cm (mean, 1.6 cm)

Microscopic Findings
- **Carcinoid:** organoid and trabecular with monotonous cells with round nuclei and low nuclear:cytoplasmic ratio and finely stippled chromatin
- **Atypical carcinoid:** cords, solid and single-file infiltration, vascular invasion, vesicular to hyperchromatic nuclei with a higher nuclear:cytoplasmic ratio, and nucleoli
- **Small cell carcinoma:** sheets, ribbons and pseudorosettes, invasive growth, pleomorphism, high nuclear:cytoplasmic ratio, nuclear molding, necrosis, mitoses, crush artifact

Immunohistochemical Features
- Keratin, EMA, and CEA
- Chromogranin, synaptophysin, CD56, CD57, calcitonin and other neuroendocrine markers and hormones

Pathologic Differential Diagnosis
- Poorly differentiated squamous cell carcinoma, medullary thyroid carcinoma, adenoid cystic carcinoma, melanoma, lymphoma, metastatic carcinoma

stroma is generally absent in small cell carcinoma, although it is seen in carcinoids and atypical carcinoids. Lymphovascular, perineural, and soft tissue invasion is seen in the atypical carcinoids or small cell carcinomas. Amyloid and tumor cell spindling is occasionally noted. Concurrent SCC may be present.

The cytologic appearance of the cells is determined by the subtype of neuroendocrine carcinoma. Glandular (with mucin production) or squamous differentiation can be seen in neuroendocrine neoplasms, along with occasional neural-type rosettes. The degree of cellular pleomorphism, mitotic activity, and necrosis increases as the tumor becomes more poorly differentiated (small cell carcinoma). There is virtual absence of pleomorphism, necrosis, and mitoses in a carcinoid, while there is prominent pleomorphism, necrosis, and mitoses in a small cell carcinoma, with atypical carcinoid exhibiting intermediate features (Figure 6-38). Due to the fragility of the cells, crush artifact is frequently prominent in small cell carcinoma.

Carcinoid tumors have small, monotonous cells with a low nuclear:cytoplasmic ratio and round vesicular nuclei with finely stippled chromatin. Atypical carcinoid tumors have vesicular to more hyperchromatic nuclei within polygonal cells that have an increased nuclear:cytoplasmic ratio (Figure 6-39). The location of

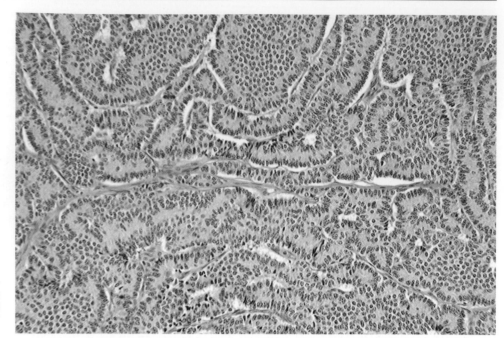

FIGURE 6-37

Well-differentiated cells arranged in ribbons and festoons in this carcinoid. The cells have pale cytoplasm surrounding round nuclei with granular, coarse nuclear chromatin.

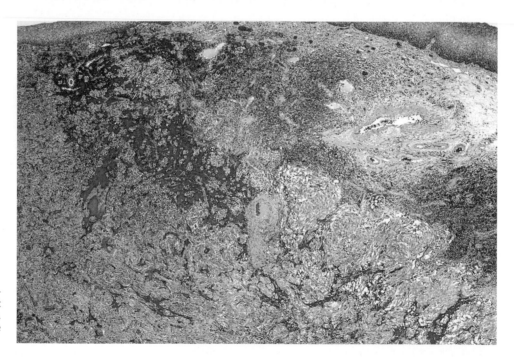

FIGURE 6-38

Atypical carcinoid. The surface epithelium is intact, with a number of different patterns of growth within the stroma. Note the tumor cell spindling and the inflammatory infiltrate.

the nucleus is variable (central, eccentric), surrounded by amphophilic to eosinophilic cytoplasm. Nucleoli are variable, from absent to prominent (Figure 6-40). Small cell carcinoma is hypercellular, composed of cells with a high nuclear:cytoplasmic ratio, indistinct cell borders, and intensely hyperchromatic oval to spindled nuclei without nucleoli (Figure 6-41). Nuclear molding is seen. Crush artifact, mitotic figures, necrosis, and occasional multinucleated neoplastic giant cells are present. There is usually limited stroma, which may be mucoid. Laryngeal neuroendocrine neoplasms are on a morphologically continuous spectrum, with an

aggregate of features distinguishing between the tumors. Concurrent squamous cell or adenocarcinoma may be present.

ANCILLARY STUDIES

ULTRASTRUCTURAL FEATURES

Electron microscopy will demonstrate membrane-bound, electron-dense neurosecretory granules, ranging

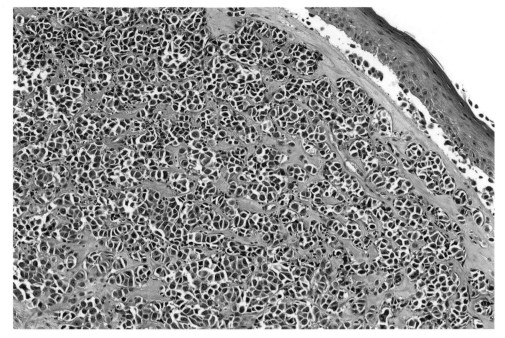

FIGURE 6-39

Atypical carcinoid. The surface epithelium is uninvolved by the neoplastic proliferation of moderately pleomorphic cells with coarse, hyperchromatic nuclei surrounded by ample, pale cytoplasm. There is a rich vascular stroma.

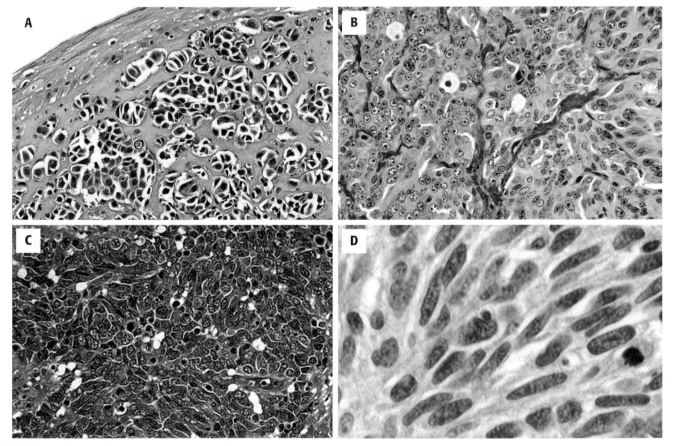

FIGURE 6-40

Atypical carcinoid. The cells can be arranged in nests and balls (**A**), glandular profiles with round nuclei and salt-and-pepper chromatin (**B**), to solid sheets of cells with a high nuclear:cytoplasmic ratio (**C**), to fascicles of spindle cells with stippled nuclear chromatin (**D**).

CHONDROSARCOMA—DISEASE FACT SHEET

Definition

- Chondrosarcoma is a malignant tumor arising within the laryngeal cartilages and forming neoplastic cartilage

Incidence and Location

- Up to 1% of all laryngeal malignancies
- 75% of all laryngeal sarcomas
- Cricoid cartilage most commonly

Morbidity and Mortality

- Recurrences in up to 40% of patients
- Infrequently, patients die from tumor

Gender, Race, and Age Distribution

- Male >> female (4:1)
- Mean, 60 to 65 years

Clinical Features

- Hoarseness, dyspnea, dysphagia, stridor
- Thyroid cartilage lesions present as a mass
- Long duration of symptoms
- Subglottic submucosal swelling on endoscopy

Radiologic Features

- Fine, punctate, stippled to coarse ("popcorn") calcifications
- Ill defined, destructive, hypodense mass

Prognosis and Treatment

- >95% 10-year survival
- Complete, but conservative, laryngeal function-preserving surgery

RADIOLOGIC FEATURES

Either plain films or computed tomography images will show an ill-defined, destructive, hypodense mass with fine, punctate stippled to coarse ("popcorn") calcification (Figure 6-43). After identification of the tumor as "cartilaginous," the remaining features are nonspecific.

PATHOLOGIC FEATURES

GROSS FINDINGS

The cricoid cartilage (specifically the inner posterior midline lamina) is affected far more frequently (about 75%) than other laryngeal cartilages, followed by the thyroid and arytenoid cartilages. The tumors range in size up to 12 cm, with a mean of 3.5 cm. Tumors are hard, "crunchy" or "gritty," lobular and glistening on cut surface, with a blue-gray, semitranslucent, myxoid-mucinous matrix material (Figure 6-44). Dedifferentiated chondrosarcoma has fleshy areas.

MICROSCOPIC FINDINGS

Chondrosarcomas are recognized by their increased cellularity, nuclear atypia including binucleation and multinucleation (Figure 6-45), and propensity to invade and destroy surrounding structures. Most chondrosarcomas seem to involve only a single cartilage with very

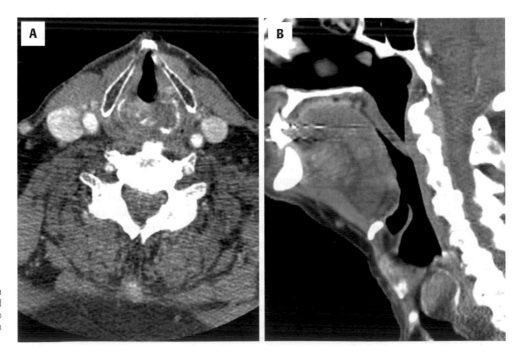

FIGURE 6-43

Computer tomography images of a chondrosarcoma destroying the cricoid cartilage and demonstrating stippled to coarse ("popcorn") calcifications within the tumor (axial and sagittal).

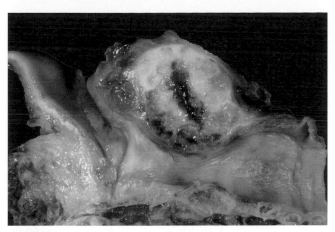

FIGURE 6-44

This macroscopic laryngectomy specimen shows a thin rim of bone invaded by the chondrosarcoma of the cricoid cartilage. A firm, lobular growth is noted, with central degenerative change.

CHONDROSARCOMA—PATHOLOGIC FEATURES

Gross Findings

- Cricoid cartilage (posterior plate) midline mass
- Mean, 3.5 cm
- Hard, crunchy, lobular, glistening blue-gray, semitranslucent, with myxoid-mucinous matrix

Microscopic Findings

- Bone invasion (ossification centers within cartilage)
- Increased cellularity
- Loss of normal architecture and distribution (cluster disarray)
- Nuclear atypia with binucleation and multinucleation
- Increased nuclear:cytoplasmic ratio
- Basophilic to metachromatic cartilaginous matrix
- Mitotic figures and necrosis only in high-grade tumors
- Separated into three grades

Pathologic Differential Diagnosis

- Chondroma, chondrometaplasia, spindle cell (sarcomatoid) carcinoma, pleomorphic adenoma

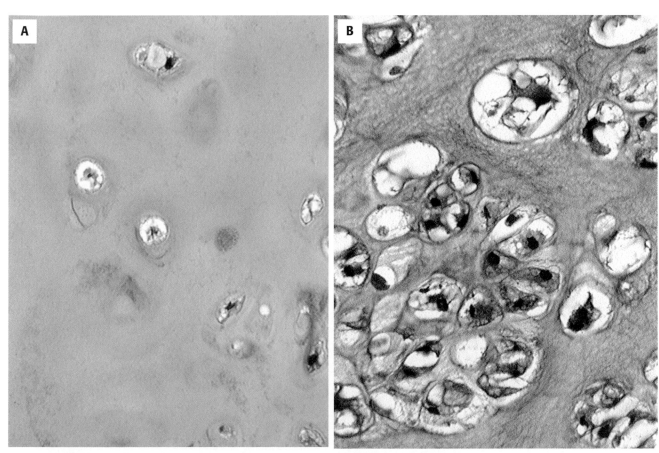

FIGURE 6-45

A, Normal cartilage cellularity and lacunar size. **B**, A chondrosarcoma has increased cellularity, pleomorphism, and increased nuclear size.

little tendency to infiltrate adjacent cartilages. When the native cartilage is included in the biopsy, the cartilage is frequently ossified and will show neoplastic chondrocytes invading into the ossified regions (Figure 6-46). The atypical, neoplastic chondrocytes are identified in a variable background of basophilic cartilaginous matrix material (Figure 6-47). There is an overall loss of normal architecture and distribution of the chondrocytes ("cluster disarray"). The tumor cytomorphology varies from slightly cellular tumors composed of small, hyperchromatic nuclei surrounded by abundant cytoplasm to hypercellular neoplasms consisting of enlarged, binucleated and multinucleated atypical cells with an increased nuclear:cytoplasmic ratio, nuclear chromatin distribution irregularities, and prominent nucleoli (Figure 6-48). There is less stroma between the lacunar spaces as the grade of tumor increases. Mitotic figures, including atypical forms, are only infrequently noted and only in high-grade tumors. Tumor necrosis, usually focal and of limited geographic distribution, is usually restricted to higher-grade tumors. Ischemic change (blue, granular cytoplasm) can be seen in the background.

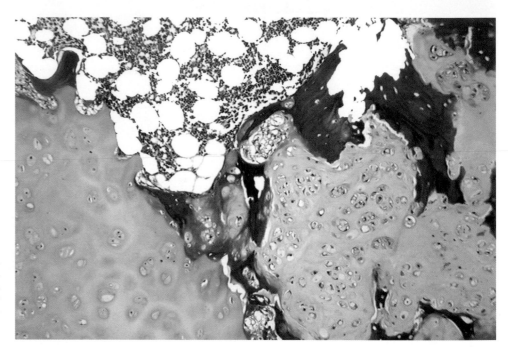

FIGURE 6-46

Hyaline cartilage with enchondral ossification is seen (*lower left*) immediately adjacent to the invasive component of a low-grade (grade 1) chondrosarcoma (*lower right*). Normal bone marrow elements are noted in the upper portion of the field.

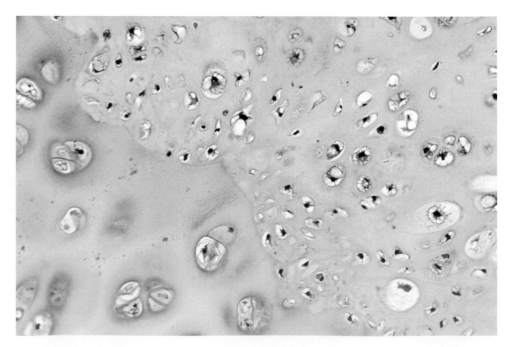

FIGURE 6-47

The lower left portion of the illustration demonstrates normal hyaline cartilage abutted by a grade 1 chondrosarcoma (*upper* and *right side*).

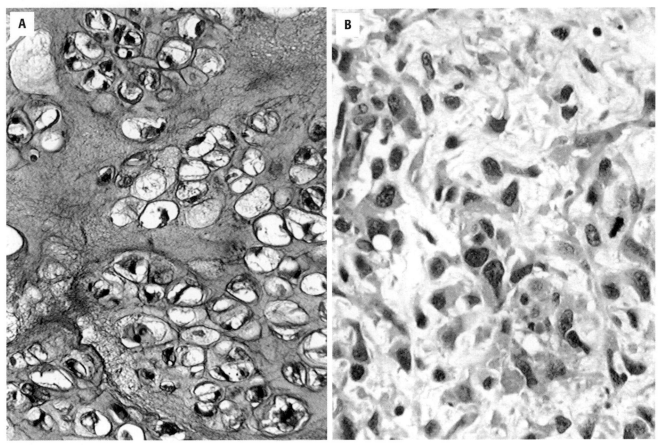

FIGURE 6-48

A, A grade 2 chondrosarcoma has moderate cellularity with binucleation, nuclear atypia, and nuclear hyperchromasia. **B,** A grade 3 chondrosarcoma has marked nuclear pleomorphism, multinucleation, and hyperchromatic nuclei. Mitotic figures are noted.

Chondrosarcomas are separated into grades based on increasing degrees of the aforementioned criteria. The vast majority (~65%) are well differentiated (low-grade, grade 1), followed by moderately differentiated (intermediate-grade, grade 2; 30%), and poorly differentiated (high-grade, grade 3; 5%; Figure 6-48) neoplasms. In the larynx, the grade does not seem to affect the overall patient outcome. The vast majority of tumors are chondrocytic chondrosarcomas, but myxoid, mesenchymal, and dedifferentiated chondrosarcoma are described. Immunohistochemistry is unnecessary, although the tumor cells will be S100 protein and vimentin immunoreactive.

DIFFERENTIAL DIAGNOSIS

The differential diagnosis is limited in practical terms to chondroma and chondrometaplasia. In general, true laryngeal *chondromas* are considered exceedingly rare, and a number of authors consider all laryngeal chondromas to be erroneous descriptions of low-grade chondrosarcomas. Given the frequent association of chondroma with chondrosarcoma, it is quite possible that "biopsy"

material does not sample the malignant component. Therefore, adequate tumor sampling (large biopsy) is critical to the accurate identification of tumor type and grade. While size alone is inaccurate in classification, tumors >3 cm are more likely to be chondrosarcomas. The microscopic separation of chondroma from chondrosarcoma can be a very difficult one, with chondromas containing slightly larger, albeit uniform nuclei with only slight architectural disorder. In practical terms, any *recurrent* cartilaginous tumor of the larynx should be considered a chondrosarcoma. A *spindle cell (sarcomatoid) carcinoma* may have metaplastic or malignant cartilage as part of the tumor, but they are polypoid, involve the glottis, and show keratin immunoreactivity in ~70% of cases. *Chondrometaplasia* of the larynx consists of multiple elastic-rich cartilage nodules usually located on the vocal cords and <1 cm, containing small, uniform chondrocytes without nuclear abnormalities. The margins of the lesions are indistinct with a peripheral zone of transition between the cartilage and the surrounding tissues. A cartilaginous-predominant *pleomorphic adenoma* may also enter the differential, although identification of epithelial and/or myoepithelial components will help resolve the matter.

PROGNOSIS AND THERAPY

Laryngeal chondrosarcomas are considered low-grade neoplasms. Overall, there is a >95% survival with a mean follow-up of >10 years. Death from disease is very uncommon and is usually the result of uncontrolled local growth into vital structures of the neck. The presence of the myxoid subtype (>10% of the tumor volume) and age >60 years at initial presentation has been reported to portend a worse patient outcome. A higher-grade tumor seems to suggest an increased chance of developing metastatic disease but not of dying from disease.

Conservative, laryngeal function-preserving surgery is the treatment of choice. When recurrences develop (in up to 40% of patients), wide excision can again be used, depending on the extent of the tumor, until functional compromise and the inability to reconstruct an adequate airway dictate the necessity for total laryngectomy. The voice-preserving surgeries allow for an improved quality of life and for a longer morbidity-free survival, which does not adversely impact the long-term patient survival.

■ METASTATIC/SECONDARY TUMORS

These are defined as tumors secondarily involving the larynx or hypopharynx that originate from, but are not in continuity with, primary malignancies of other sites.

CLINICAL FEATURES

Uncommon, these secondary lesions account for <0.2% of all laryngeal malignancies. Patients tend to be older men (male:female is 2:1), although sex predilection is tumor histology dependent. For mucosa-based metastases, the supraglottis is most commonly affected (40%), while metastases to the cartilages tend to affect those with ossification. Up to 35% of cases have multifocal involvement. Patients present with hoarseness, voice changes, and stridor.

PATHOLOGIC FEATURES

MICROSCOPIC FINDINGS

The tumors tend to be submucosal below an intact surface epithelium (Figure 6-49). The specific tumor type will dictate the histology, with melanoma and carcinoma the most common. Of the carcinomas, kidney

METASTATIC/SECONDARY TUMOR—DISEASE FACT SHEET

Definition
- Tumors secondarily involving larynx or hypopharynx that originate from, but are not in continuity with, primary malignancies of other sites

Incidence and Location
- Rare, <0.2% of all tumors
- Supraglottis (mucosa) and cricoid cartilage (cartilages)

Morbidity and Mortality
- Usually poor due to systemic nature of the underlying primary

Gender and Age Distribution
- Males > females (2:1)
- Older patients (due to nature of the underlying primary)

Clinical Features
- Multifocal disease
- Hoarseness, voice changes, and stridor

Prognosis and Treatment
- Matches underlying disease, but usually poor
- Excision for diagnosis and symptomatic relief

METASTATIC/SECONDARY TUMOR—PATHOLOGIC FEATURES

Microscopic Findings
- Submucosal mass with a tumor histology based on underlying primary site

Immunohistochemistry Studies
- Pertinent, selected immunohistochemistry to prove origin

Pathologic Differential Diagnosis
- Primary tumor; direct extension from adjacent organs

(Figure 6-49), breast, lung, prostate, and gastrointestinal tract account for the most common primary sites. Most tumors are adenocarcinomas. While rare, leiomyosarcoma is the most common mesenchymal tumor to metastasize to the larynx. Pertinent, selected immunohistochemistry can be used to confirm the site of origin (Figure 6-49).

DIFFERENTIAL DIAGNOSIS

Primary, poorly differentiated tumors may need to be separated from metastatic tumors. This is usually achieved by history, radiographic studies, and immunohistochemistry. Direct extension from adjacent organs

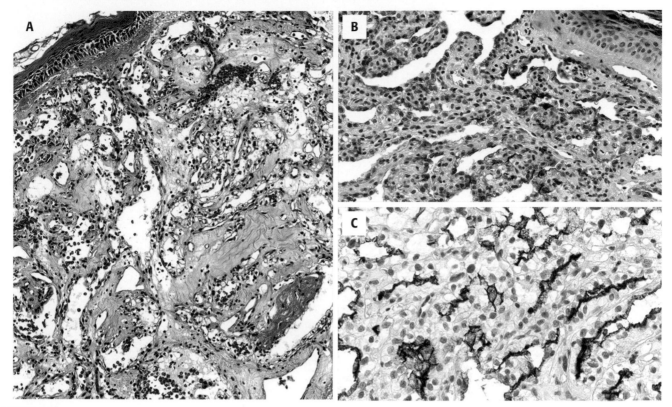

FIGURE 6-49

A, A metastatic renal cell carcinoma shows a pseudoalveolar pattern with extravasated erythrocytes. Note the cleared cytoplasm. The cells are immunoreactive with epithelial membrane antigen (**B**) and CD10 (**C**).

(thyroid and esophagus) and lymph nodes should also be considered.

PROGNOSIS AND TREATMENT

The prognosis is partly based on the tumor type but largely reflects the natural course of disseminated disease, which portends a grave outcome. Renal cell carcinoma is a possible exception, as isolated metastases, surgically removed, are associated with a good prognosis. Excision is advocated for diagnosis or symptomatic relief, and not for cure, since laryngeal metastases are seldom isolated.

SUGGESTED READINGS

The complete suggested readings list is available online at www.expertconsult.com.

7

Non-Neoplastic Lesions of the Oral Cavity and Oropharynx

■ Susan Müller

■ FORDYCE GRANULES

CLINICAL FEATURES

Fordyce granules are considered benign ectopic sebaceous glands (not associated with hair follicles) that occur on the oral mucosa. A normal variant, they are reported in up to 80% of adults, most commonly on the upper and lower lip and the buccal mucosa. They present as multiple, uniform-sized yellow or yellow-white papules (Figure 7-1), which may coalesce to form plaques. Usually asymptomatic, patients sometimes describe surface roughness.

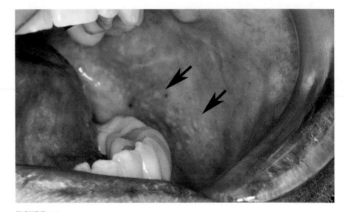

FIGURE 7-1

Clinical photograph of asymptomatic, multiple, small yellow papules on the buccal mucosa (*arrows*) in this example of Fordyce granules.

PATHOLOGIC FEATURES

Biopsy reveals normal sebaceous glands near the surface epithelium without hair follicles (Figure 7-2). Usually, multiple acinar lobules are present, although it may consist of one sebaceous lobule. A central duct sometimes connects the sebaceous lobules to the epithelial surface. Along the periphery, the sebaceous cells are basophilic and cuboidal, while the centrally located cells are polygonal in shape with abundant foamy cytoplasm and a centrally placed nucleus.

FORDYCE GRANULES—DISEASE FACT SHEET

Definition
- Benign ectopic sebaceous glands, considered to be a normal variant

Incidence and Location
- Reported in up to 80% of adults
- Present on the upper and lower lip and the buccal mucosa

Gender, Race, and Age Distribution
- Genders equally affected
- Less clinically evident in children and adolescents

Clinical Features
- Asymptomatic, multiple, small yellow papules

Prognosis and Treatment
- Considered a normal variant

FORDYCE GRANULES—PATHOLOGIC FEATURES

Microscopic Findings
- Normal sebaceous glands, below the surface, devoid of hair follicles

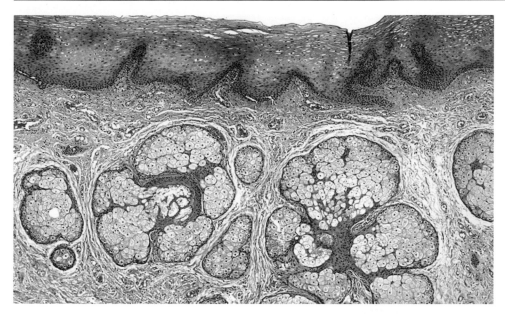

FIGURE 7-2
Multiple sebaceous glands in the superficial lamina propria.

DIFFERENTIAL DIAGNOSIS

Superficial mucoceles, which can present as 1- to 3-mm papules on the lower lip, generally are blue to clear in color and spontaneously resolve.

PROGNOSIS AND THERAPY

No treatment is indicated, although laser ablation can be offered to patients for cosmesis.

■ AMALGAM TATTOO

CLINICAL FEATURES

Amalgam tattoo is a common localized area of blue, gray, or black pigmentation caused by amalgam that has been embedded into the oral tissues during dental procedures. Amalgam is a common material used for dental fillings and contains silver, tin, mercury, and other metals. Amalgam tattoos are most commonly located on the buccal mucosa and gingiva (Figure 7-3), usually presenting as flat macules, anywhere from a few millimeters to larger, more diffuse areas of pigmentation.

RADIOLOGIC FEATURES

Generally, amalgam tattoos are not visible on dental radiographs. Larger tattoos may be visible on radiographs as densely radiopaque lesions.

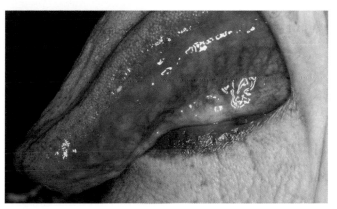

FIGURE 7-3
Clinical photograph of a blue-gray pigment present on the lateral border of the tongue. The pigmented area is flat with no ulceration or induration and is asymptomatic.

AMALGAM TATTOO—DISEASE FACT SHEET

Definition
- Localized pigmentation caused by amalgam which has been embedded in the oral tissues due to dental procedures

Incidence and Location
- Common
- Most common on the buccal mucosa and gingiva

Clinical Features
- Asymptomatic flat macules ranging from a few millimeters to more diffuse areas of blue, gray, or black pigmentation

Prognosis and Treatment
- No treatment necessary unless for cosmetic reasons or if clinical diagnosis is uncertain

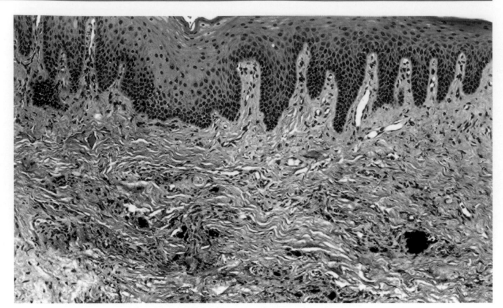

FIGURE 7-4

Black pigmented material is seen scattered in the lamina propria along collagen bundles and around blood vessels. The overlying epithelium is normal and scant inflammatory cells are present.

PATHOLOGIC FEATURES

An amalgam tattoo can demonstrate both discrete, fine black granules and scattered, irregular solid fragments (Figure 7-4). Pigment granules are often arranged along collagen fibers and around blood vessels and nerves. Most cases elicit no tissue reaction, although a foreign body giant cell reaction has been reported in up to 38% of cases.

DIFFERENTIAL DIAGNOSIS

Other exogenous pigmentations can mimic an amalgam tattoo. Melanin may be present in pigmented nevi, oral melanotic macule, oral melanoacanthoma, and melanoma. Further investigation is warranted if amalgam tattoos occur in sites distant from dental work or if the clinical diagnosis is uncertain.

AMALGAM TATTOO—PATHOLOGIC FEATURES

Microscopic Findings
- Discrete, black granules, and/or solid fragments findings of pigment arranged along collagen fibers, around blood vessels and nerves
- Foreign body reaction reported in up to 38% of cases

Pathologic Differential Diagnosis
- Other exogenous sources of pigmentation including pencil graphite, intentional tattoos, and coal dust

PROGNOSIS AND THERAPY

No treatment is generally required, unless for cosmetic reasons (surgery or laser treatment).

■ ECTOPIC THYROID

CLINICAL FEATURES

Ectopic thyroid is a result of the abnormal migration of the thyroglossal duct from the foramen cecum located at the junction of the anterior two-thirds and posterior third of the tongue to its normal prelaryngeal location. While uncommon, nearly 90% of all ectopic thyroids are located on the tongue between the foramen cecum and the epiglottis. In >75% of patients with lingual thyroid, this is the only functioning thyroid tissue. Females are affected 3 to 4 times as frequently as males. Symptoms, including dysphagia, dyspnea, globus sensation, and dysphonia, most often coincide with puberty onset, pregnancy, or menopause corresponding to elevated thyroid-stimulating hormone (TSH). Thyroid function tests should be evaluated as part of the workup. The endoscopic appearance at the base of the tongue is of a hyperemic mass (Figure 7-5).

RADIOLOGIC FEATURES

The iodine content of the thyroid tissue results in very high signal attenuation in relation to surrounding

ECTOPIC THYROID—DISEASE FACT SHEET

Definition

- Rare developmental anomaly due to the abnormal migration of the thyroid gland from the base of the tongue

Incidence and Location

- Uncommon, with reported incidence of 1/100,000
- 90% of ectopic thyroids are lingual thyroids

Morbidity and Mortality

- Larger lesions can cause airway obstruction
- Rare reports of carcinoma development

Gender, Race, and Age Distribution

- Female >> male (3 to 4:1)
- All ages (mean, 44 years)

Clinical Features

- Dysphagia, dyspnea, dysphonia, globus sensation
- One-third of patients are hypothyroid
- In >75%, ectopic tissue is only functional thyroid tissue

Prognosis and Treatment

- Suppression therapy with thyroxine to reduce size and symptoms
- Radioactive ^{131}I ablation
- Autotransplantation of lingual thyroid

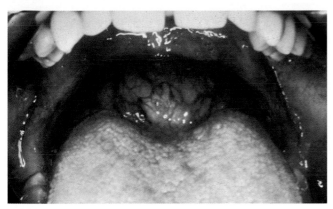

FIGURE 7-5
Clinical photograph of a lingual thyroid presenting as a midline nodular mass at the base of the tongue. The surface is smooth and hyperemic.

soft tissue using computed tomography. Radioisotopic studies (^{131}-Iodine and/or ^{99m}Tc: technetium-99m pertechnetate) may be needed to determine size, location, and activity of thyroid tissue.

PATHOLOGIC FEATURES

Immediately below the intact surface mucosa, unencapsulated ectopic thyroid follicles containing colloid and

ECTOPIC THYROID—PATHOLOGIC FEATURES

Microscopic Findings

- Nonencapsulated normal thyroid tissue insinuated through skeletal muscle
- Lymphocytic thyroiditis and adenomatoid nodules may develop

Pathologic Differential Diagnosis

- Metastatic thyroid carcinoma

lined by cuboidal epithelium are identified insinuating between the tongue musculature (Figure 7-6). Lymphocytic thyroiditis and adenomatoid nodules, as well as papillary carcinoma, have been reported.

ANCILLARY STUDIES

FINE NEEDLE ASPIRATION

Fine needle aspiration biopsy can be used to confirm the diagnosis of ectopic thyroid or to rule out neoplastic changes.

DIFFERENTIAL DIAGNOSIS

There are a number of clinical differential diagnostic considerations (hemangioma, lymphangioma, hypertrophic lingual tonsils, abscess, mucus retention cyst, squamous cell carcinoma), but the histologic features of ectopic thyroid are pathognomonic.

PROGNOSIS AND THERAPY

Thyroxine suppresses TSH with a subsequent reduction in size. Surgery is used if there is uncontrollable hemorrhage, airway obstruction, or inability to eat. Radioablation may be used in nonsurgical candidates. If no "normal" thyroid is identified in the anterior neck, autotransplantation can be performed. Malignancy is a rare complication (<1%), although it is more common in men.

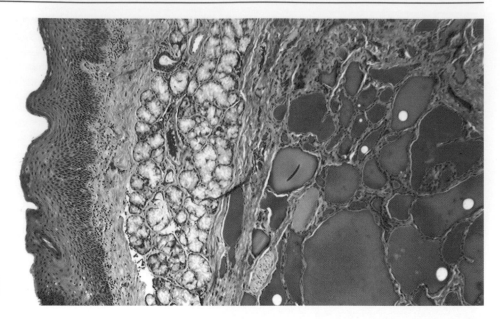

FIGURE 7-6
Normal stratified squamous epithelium overlying a nonencapsulated collection of thyroid follicles.

■ ORAL HAIRY LEUKOPLAKIA

CLINICAL FEATURES

Oral hairy leukoplakia (HL) is a benign epithelial disease associated with Epstein-Barr virus (EBV) and nearly always identified in HIV-infected and/or immunocompromised patients. The disease correlates with viral load and CD4 counts. HL usually presents on the

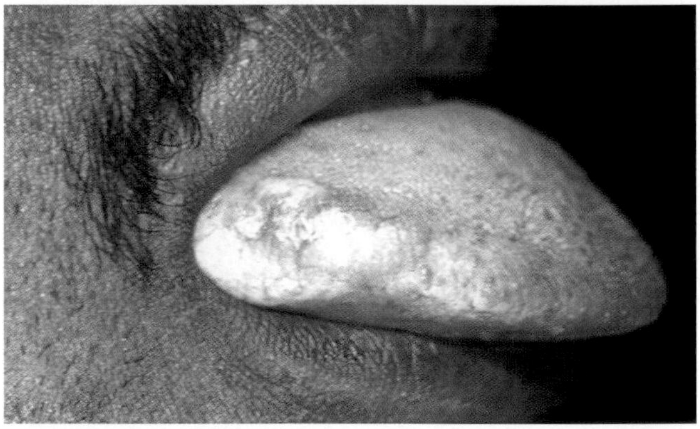

FIGURE 7-7
HIV-positive patient with a white patch on the lateral border of the tongue exhibiting a corrugated appearance in this example of oral hairy leukoplakia.

lateral border of the tongue as a white plaque, or vertical streaks, or with a corrugated surface (Figure 7-7). The lesions can become quite extensive, and in some cases cover the entire lateral and dorsal tongue. The lesion is asymptomatic and cannot be rubbed off.

ORAL HAIRY LEUKOPLAKIA—DISEASE FACT SHEET

Definition
- Benign, asymptomatic epithelial hyperplasia associated with Epstein-Barr virus nearly always in immunocompromised patients

Incidence and Location
- <10% of HIV-infected patients on highly active antiretroviral therapy
- Primarily occurs on the lateral tongue

Gender and Age Distribution
- Increased particularly in HIV-positive men
- No racial or age predilection

Clinical Features
- White patches that can have a corrugated or folded surface that cannot be rubbed off
- May be quite extensive and bilateral and involve dorsal tongue

Prognosis and Treatment
- 10% improve spontaneously
- No specific treatment, although secondary *Candida* may need to be treated

---

PATHOLOGIC FEATURES

HL is characterized by marked epithelial acanthosis with elongation of the rete ridges and prominent hyperkeratosis. In the superficial spinous layer, "balloon cells," characterized by intracellular ballooning degeneration, nuclear clearing, and margination of the chromatin indicative of a viral cytopathic effect, are present (Figure 7-8). These nonspecific findings require documentation of EBV within the lesion.

ORAL HAIRY LEUKOPLAKIA—PATHOLOGIC FEATURES

Microscopic Findings

- Epithelial hyperplasia, hyperparakeratosis, and acanthosis
- Balloon cells in the upper spinous layer
- Viral cytopathic effect can sometimes be seen
- Little or no inflammation
- Secondary candidal infection may be identified

Ancillary Studies

- Markers for Epstein-Barr virus antigens (EBER) show punctate nuclear staining in the balloon cells

Pathologic Differential Diagnosis

- Candidiasis, frictional keratosis, oral leukoplakia, lichen planus, and lichenoid reactions

ANCILLARY STUDIES

IMMUNOHISTOCHEMICAL FEATURES

Immunomarkers for EBV latent antigens (EBV nuclear antigen [EBNA], latent membrane protein [LMP]), replicative antigens (EA, VCA), or regulatory antigens (BLZF1) can be performed on both touch preps and biopsy specimens (Figure 7-9). Depending on the immunostain used, latent versus replicative EBV infection can be determined.

MOLECULAR STUDIES

Quantitative polymerase chain reaction (PCR) and in situ hybridization (ISH) assays (EBV-encoded RNA

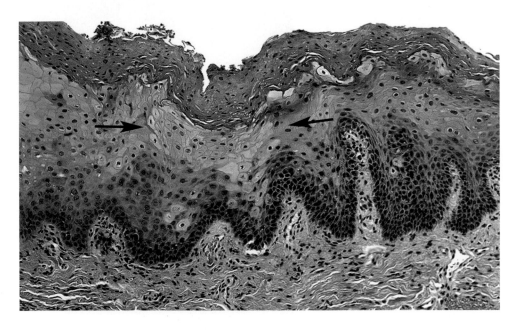

FIGURE 7-8

A corrugated hyperparakeratotic epithelium and a layer of balloon cells in the upper spinous layer (*arrows*).

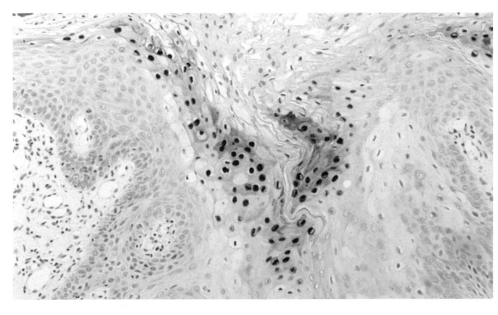

FIGURE 7-9

In situ hybridization for Epstein-Barr virus encoded RNA shows strong punctate nuclear positivity in the region of the balloon cells.

[EBER]) can be useful when immunohistochemical studies fail to detect EBV, and especially when investigating EBV latent genes.

DIFFERENTIAL DIAGNOSIS

Clinically, HL can mimic candidiasis, frictional keratosis (tongue biting), oral leukoplakia, lichen planus, and lichenoid reactions. Oral candidiasis can be rubbed off the mucosa, while HL cannot. However, HL is frequently colonized by *Candida* sp.

PROGNOSIS AND THERAPY

HL does not have any malignant potential. It reportedly improves spontaneously in 10% of cases. The incidence in HIV-infected patients has decreased to <10% with highly active antiretroviral therapy (HAART). Treatment for concurrent *Candida* may be necessary if "burning" is described by the patient.

■ INFECTIONS

CLINICAL FEATURES

There are numerous infectious conditions that can involve the oral cavity including bacterial, fungal, viral, and protozoal infections. These infections can present as an acute, rapidly progressive infection with constitutional symptoms, such as herpetic gingivostomatitis. Other infections can be chronic and slowly spreading, such as actinomycosis and leprosy. Sexually transmitted diseases, including syphilis and gonorrhea, can have oral manifestations. Deep fungal infections, including blastomycosis, coccidiomycosis, and histoplasmosis, can present as a nonspecific ulcer in the oral cavity. Since many infectious processes share clinical overlap, biopsy and/or culture is necessary to obtain a diagnosis. Three of the more common oral infections are caused by candidiasis, herpes simplex virus type 1 (HSV1), and actinomyces.

The most common fungal infection in the oral cavity and oropharynx is candidiasis. *Candida albicans* is the most common type, although other species have been isolated. Patients may complain of a burning sensation or a foul or salty taste or may be entirely asymptomatic. In many infections, other factors play a role: antibiotic therapy; immunosuppression, including the use of prednisone; diabetes; pregnancy; xerostomia; and anemia.

The clinical presentations are protean including the common acute pseudomembranous form (thrush) and erythematous (atrophic) variant. Median rhomboid

glossitis presents on the midline of the dorsal tongue as a red atrophic area (Figure 7-10), which may become nodular over time. Angular cheilitis presents as a red scaling, fissuring area at the corners of the mouth (Figure 7-11) and is predisposed by drooling, parafunctional lip habits, and ill-fitting dentures. Hyperplastic candidiasis presents as white plaques that are *not* removable by rubbing and occur most often on the hard palate and anterior buccal mucosa. Chronic mucocutaneous candidiasis presents as a chronic infection of the oral mucosa, nails, skin, and vagina, the familial form of which may

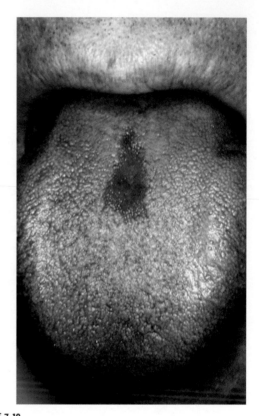

FIGURE 7-10

Clinical photograph of median rhomboid glossitis, with a red atrophic area on the midline of the dorsal tongue, corresponding to the loss of filiform papillae.

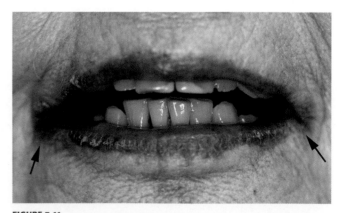

FIGURE 7-11

Clinical photograph of a patient with angular cheilitis; there is fissuring at the corners of the mouth, with painful red scaling areas (*arrows*).

INFECTIONS—DISEASE FACT SHEET

Definition
- **Candidiasis:** the most common oral fungal infection with a diverse clinical presentation and influenced by host immune status
- **HSV1:** a DNA virus transmitted via saliva or direct contact, with potential reactivation of latent disease
- **Actinomycosis:** acute or chronic infection by a normal saprophytic oral flora gram-positive anaerobic bacteria

Incidence
- **Candidiasis:** *Candida* species detected in up to 55% of healthy individuals
- **HSV1:** up to 90% of adults have antibodies to HSV1
- **Actinomycosis:** uncommon, exact incidence unknown

Morbidity and Mortality
- **Candidiasis:** usually a mild and self-limiting disease, although recurrent infections may signify an underlying disease
- **HSV1:** primary infection may be severely debilitating
- **Actinomycosis:** periostitis, osteomyelitis, and fistula formation

Gender, Race, and Age Distribution
- **Candidiasis:** there are no gender or ethnic differences, but particularly affects the very young and elderly
- **HSV1:** prevalence increases with age and correlates with socioeconomic status (inversely proportional)
- **Actinomycosis:** no gender, ethnic, or age predilection

Clinical Features
- **Candidiasis:** pseudomembranous, erythematous, median rhomboid glossitis, angular cheilitis, hyperplastic, and mucocutaneous types all have unique manifestations
- **HSV1:** primary HSV1 may have fever, malaise, lymphadenopathy, multiple mucosal ulcerations, and painful erythematous gingiva
- **Actinomycosis:** acute form presents with painful abscesses, while chronic form may be painless, hardened, and/or result in fistula formation with trismus

Prognosis and Treatment
- **Candidiasis:** topical and/or systemic antifungal medication
- **HSV1:** symptomatic or with topical/systemic antiviral drugs
- **Actinomycosis:** prolonged high doses of antibiotics, with abscess drainage and excision of the fistula, if present

PATHOLOGIC FEATURES

INFECTIONS—PATHOLOGIC FEATURES

Microscopic Findings
- **Candidiasis:** fungal hyphae or pseudohyphae and ovoid spores (PAS positive) associated with neutrophilic microabscesses
- **HSV1:** viral cytopathic effect includes acantholysis, ballooning degeneration, chromatin margination, and multinucleation
- **Actinomycosis:** colonies of club-shaped filaments arranged in a rosette pattern surrounded by neutrophils

Pathologic Differential Diagnosis
- **Candidiasis:** mucositis, leukoplakia, geographic tongue
- **HSV1:** erythema multiforme, herpes zoster, Epstein-Barr virus, HSV2, acute necrotizing ulcerative gingivitis, bacterial pharyngitis, traumatic ulcer
- **Actinomycosis:** abscess, other bacterial infections

border of the lip (herpes labialis), also called a "fever blister" or "cold sore" (Figure 7-12). There is often a prodrome of burning, tingling, or itching at the site of the eruption, up to 24 hours before the outbreak. A cluster of fluid-filled vesicles form, which rupture, crust, and heal within 7 to 10 days. Recurrent HSV1 can also occur intraorally on the hard palate and gingiva (Figure 7-13).

Actinomyces are saprophytic, gram-positive anaerobic bacteria that are part of normal oral flora. The primary pathogen is *A. israelii,* although other species can also cause infection. *Actinomyces* colonize tonsillar crypts, dental plaque, and gingival sulci. The presentation may be acute or chronic, with the bacteria entering through a site of trauma (tooth extraction site), infected tonsil, or soft tissue injury. In the acute suppurative phase, yellowish colonies of bacteria may be visible ("sulfur granules"), while the chronic form has extensive fibrosis, imparting a hard or "wooden" area of induration. A fistula may develop with extension to the surface, while periostitis and osteomyelitis may also develop.

present in early childhood and is associated with defects in cell-mediated immunity and endocrinopathies.

There are nearly ubiquitous antibodies (up to 90%) to the DNA of HSV1 virus, transmitted via direct contact or through saliva. Prevalence increases with age and correlates with socioeconomic status (lower status has increased prevalence). About 10% of patients when first exposed to HSV1 develop primary herpetic gingivostomatitis, while the remaining patients have subclinical symptoms. Symptoms include fever, lymphadenopathy, malaise, mucosal erythema, vesicles, and ulcers, which resolve in 7 to 14 days. The virus remains latent within sensory and autonomic ganglion, reactivated in the trigeminal ganglion to result in infection of the vermilion

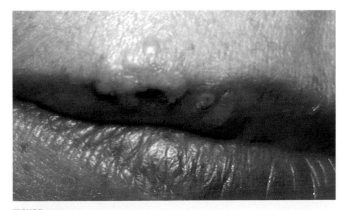

FIGURE 7-12

Clinical photograph of a cluster of fluid-filled vesicles of recurrent herpes simplex virus type 1 on the vermilion border.

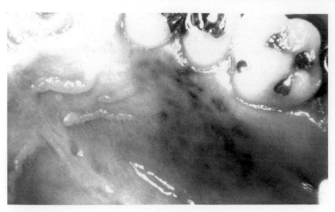

FIGURE 7-13

Clinical photograph of intraoral recurrent herpes simplex virus on the hard palate. Intraoral vesicles rupture immediately, leaving red, eroded mucosa.

CANDIDA (INCLUDING MEDIAN RHOMBOID GLOSSITIS)

Candida can be seen on an exfoliative cytologic examination using either a periodic acid–Schiff (PAS; magenta-stained hyphae) or KOH stain (normal cells are lysed, but hyphae remain). The 2-μm hyphae vary in length and can show branching along with ovoid spores or yeast forms (Figure 7-14). In tissue sections, the organisms are seen in the parakeratin layer (Figure 7-15), highlighted with a PAS stain, while neutrophilic microabscesses may be seen along with chronic inflammatory cells in the submucosa.

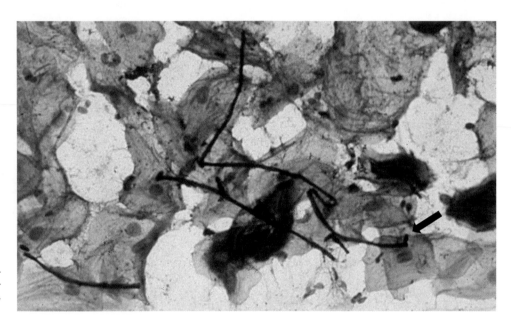

FIGURE 7-14

Exfoliative cytology with periodic acid–Schiff stain. The fungal hyphae, pseudohyphae and spores (at the terminal end, *arrow*) appear magenta.

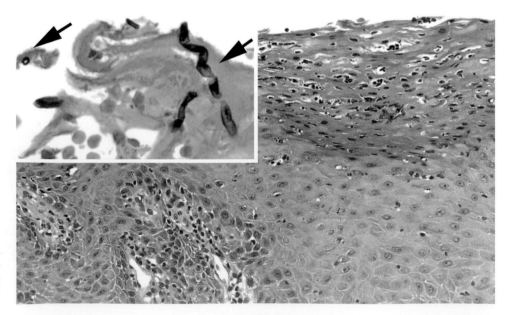

FIGURE 7-15

Marked parakeratosis with neutrophilic microabscesses present in hyperplastic candidiasis. *Inset:* Periodic acid–Schiff stain highlights yeast and hyphal forms noted within the parakeratin layer (*arrows*).

HERPES SIMPLEX VIRUS 1

Epithelial cells infected with HSV1 show marked acantholysis (Tzanck cells), nuclear enlargement (ballooning degeneration), and condensation of the chromatin around the periphery of the nucleus (Figure 7-16). Infected epithelial cells can fuse to form multinucleated cells. HSV1 ISH will demonstrate nuclear staining in virally infected cells (Figure 7-17). The adjacent mucosa is edematous with secondary inflammation.

ACTINOMYCOSIS

Biopsy results show granulation tissue, with a variable number of colonies of club-shaped, basophilic, filamentous organisms arranged in a radiating rosette pattern surrounded by neutrophils (Figure 7-18). The diagnosis of *Actinomyces* can be confirmed by culture; however, due to the overgrowth of other bacteria or lack of anaerobic conditions, recovery rates are <30%.

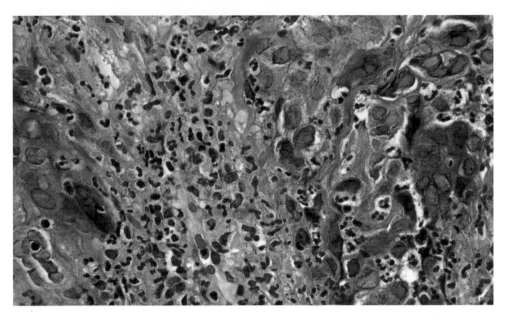

FIGURE 7-16

Acantholytic epithelial cells (Tzanck cells) and cells with nuclear enlargement. Numerous multinucleated cells also show chromatin condensation at the periphery.

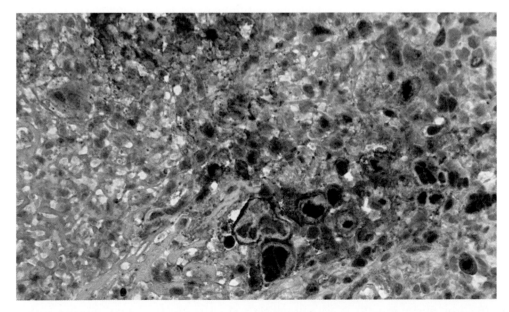

FIGURE 7-17

In situ hybridization for herpes simplex virus type 1 shows strong nuclear staining in the virally altered acantholytic and multinucleated cells.

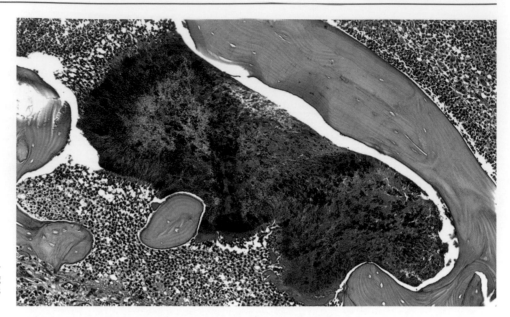

FIGURE 7-18

Colonies of club-shaped filamentous actinomycetes are arranged in a radiating rosette pattern surrounded by neutrophils and nonviable bone.

DIFFERENTIAL DIAGNOSIS

Careful clinical history and familiarity with the clinical signs can often be sufficient for arriving at a diagnosis. However, overlap in clinical presentation and lack of resolution after treatment may warrant a biopsy and/or culture. Mimics of candidiasis include severe mucositis, leukoplakia, geographic tongue, lichen planus, and squamous cell carcinoma.

Mimics of primary HSV1, especially in adults, include erythema multiforme, acute necrotizing ulcerative gingivitis (ANUG), pharyngotonsillitis of infectious mononucleosis, or streptococcal pharyngitis. Specific enzyme-linked immunosorbent assay (ELISA) testing of a culture from a vesicle can be performed in 24 hours and is definitive for diagnosis, while serologic tests for HSV1 antibodies document only past exposure. Changing social mores have increased the incidence of HSV2, but the infections are clinically and microscopically identical. Herpes zoster lesions can affect both keratinized and nonkeratinized mucosa, whereas HSV1 affects only keratinized mucosa.

Cervicofacial actinomycosis can masquerade as abscesses and benign or malignant neoplasms. *Nocardia* spp. are distinguished as acid-fast bacilli and stain well with a modified Ziehl-Neelsen stain, while *Actinomyces* spp. are not acid-fast.

PROGNOSIS AND THERAPY

Antimicrobial therapies represent an area of constant change and improvement, so specific drug therapies will not be included here. However, if a patient does not respond to antifungal therapy, culture is recommended to determine the definitive species of *Candida* and its drug sensitivity. If an otherwise healthy patient develops chronic oral candidiasis, then endocrine abnormalities and anemia studies should be evaluated. Any leukoplakic lesion that exhibits dysplasia with concomitant candidiasis should be treated with appropriate antifungals and then reevaluated.

Primary HSV1, especially in pediatric patients, requires management of fever, hydration, nutritional intake, and oral pain. Topical antiviral medications are most effective when initiated during the prodrome period or within the first few hours of vesicle formation.

Chronic actinomycosis is best managed by long-term, high-dose antibiotic therapy. Incision and drainage of any abscesses and excision of the sinus tracts are indicated.

ORAL LICHEN PLANUS

CLINICAL FEATURES

Lichen planus (LP) is a common mucocutaneous disease that can affect the skin, mucous membranes, nails, and eyes. Of patients with oral LP (OLP), only 15% to 35% develop cutaneous disease. LP is a self-limiting disease that affects mainly middle-aged adults, with women affected more often than men (2:1). OLP can manifest in various forms, most commonly the reticular and erosive types. The reticular variant is asymptomatic, presenting on the buccal mucosa with a lace-like network of fine white lines (Wickham striae) (Figure 7-19). On the dorsal tongue, it presents as a white plaque, rather than fine white striae. The erosive variant causes areas of erythema and superficial ulceration, often covered by a fibrinopurulent membrane, with symptoms of pain and burning that can interfere with speech and eating. At the periphery of the erythematous or eroded area, the more typical reticular form of OLP may be observed (Figure 7-20). Approximately 10% of OLP is confined to the gingiva, commonly presenting with marked erythema resulting in desquamative gingivitis. The gingiva bleeds readily and can lead to gingival recession and periodontal disease.

PATHOLOGIC FEATURES

While characteristic, the histology is not specific. OLP demonstrates hyperparakeratotic, acanthotic, and stratified squamous epithelium with either absent rete or hyperplastic rete descriptively called "sawtooth" rete. Basal cell liquefactive degeneration with an adjacent band-like lymphocytic infiltrate and occasional degenerating keratinocytes (colloid, cytoid, or Civatte bodies) are typical features (Figure 7-21). Biopsy samples from an erosive area may have epithelial separation or absence. No dysplasia should be present.

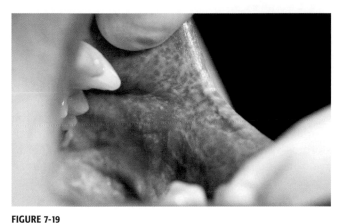

FIGURE 7-19
White lace-like striae (Wickham striae) affecting the buccal mucosa in a case of oral lichen planus.

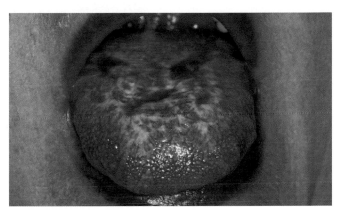

FIGURE 7-20
Clinical photograph of plaque-like erythema and erosions of the dorsal tongue in erosive lichen planus.

ORAL LICHEN PLANUS—DISEASE FACT SHEET

Definition
- Common chronic, self-limited inflammatory mucocutaneous disorder of unknown etiology that can affect the skin, mucous membranes, nails, and eyes

Incidence and Location
- 1% to 2% of world population

Gender, Race, and Age Distribution
- Female > male (2:1)
- Peak in middle-aged adults

Clinical Features
- Reticular variant: fine white lace-like striae
- Erosive variant: atrophic erythematous mucosa with ulceration

Prognosis and Treatment
- Symptomatic lesions controlled with topical corticosteroids

---

ORAL LICHEN PLANUS—PATHOLOGIC FEATURES

Microscopic Findings
- Hyperkeratosis, acanthosis, "saw-tooth" rete
- Destruction of epithelial basal cell layer
- Band-like lymphocytic infiltrate
- Degenerating keratinocytes (cytoid, Civatte bodies)
- Erosive form may have subepithelial separation from lamina propria

Immunofluorescence Features
- Direct immunofluorescence of *perilesional* tissue may show linear deposits of fibrin and fibrinogen at the basement membrane

Pathologic Differential Diagnosis
- Mucous membrane pemphigoid, lichenoid drug reaction, lichenoid reaction to amalgam, lupus, IgA disease, chronic graft-versus-host disease, chronic ulcerative stomatitis, dysplasia

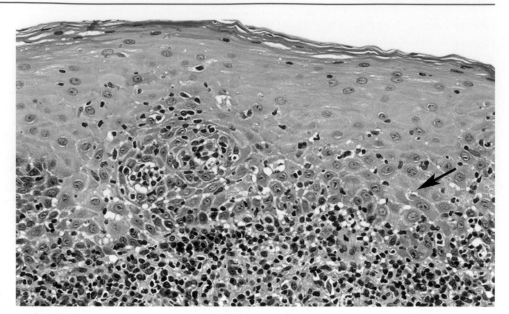

FIGURE 7-21

Lichen planus demonstrates parakeratotic, acanthotic stratified squamous epithelium with absent rete. Interface inflammation with basal cell liquefaction and band-like, lymphoplasmacytic infiltrate is seen. A cytoid body (*arrow*) is noted.

ANCILLARY STUDIES

Direct immunofluorescence (DIF) of *perilesional* mucosa often demonstrates linear deposits of fibrin and fibrinogen at the basement membrane zone. Although this finding is nonspecific, it is especially useful in excluding other vesiculoulcerative diseases.

DIFFERENTIAL DIAGNOSIS

The clinical appearance is most important, but with more complex patterns, including the erosive pattern, biopsy is often needed to rule out other vesiculoulcerative diseases. These include mucous membrane pemphigoid (MMP), lupus erythematosus, pemphigus vulgaris, chronic graft-versus-host disease, linear immunoglobulin (Ig)A disease, a lichenoid reaction to dental materials (e.g., amalgam), chronic ulcerative stomatitis, and lichenoid drug reactions. Both DIF and indirect immunofluorescence (IDIF) may help in delineating these disease processes. Furthermore, a solitary lesion should undergo biopsy to exclude a premalignant or malignant lesion, which would have cellular enlargement, nuclear pleomorphism, and increased or abnormal mitoses.

PROGNOSIS AND THERAPY

OLP is a chronic disease with symptoms that wax and wane over the lifetime of the patient. No treatment is necessary for asymptomatic patients, but corticosteroids are used for erosive or erythematous OLP. If extensive, a short course of systemic prednisone can reduce the symptomatic areas sufficiently so that topical corticosteroids can manage symptoms. Occasionally, topical cyclosporine and tacrolimus are employed. Extended topical corticosteroid use places the patient at increased risk for developing oral candidiasis. While controversial, malignant transformation may rarely develop in the atrophic, erosive pattern of OLP, suggesting the need for long-term clinical follow-up of patients with symptomatic OLP.

■ MUCOUS MEMBRANE PEMPHIGOID (CICATRICIAL PEMPHIGOID)

CLINICAL FEATURES

MMP is an autoimmune subepithelial blistering disease predominantly affecting the mucous membranes. The underlying pathogenesis is autoantibodies (at least 10 different types identified) that target the basement membrane zone. Serious sequelae include subglottic stenosis, airway obstruction, conjunctival scarring, and blindness. The scarring in MMP is referred to as cicatricial pemphigoid. Middle-aged to elderly patients (50 to 70 years) are most commonly affected, with women affected more often than men (1.5 to 2:1). Almost 100% of patients with MMP have oral involvement, with the gingiva affected most commonly (Figure 7-22). A positive Nikolsky sign, where clinically normal mucosa blisters on induced trauma, is seen in MMP.

MUCOUS MEMBRANE PEMPHIGOID—DISEASE FACT SHEET

Definition

- An autoimmune subepithelial blistering disease predominantly affecting the mucus membranes associated with autoantibodies that target the basement membrane zone

Incidence and Location

- Incidence is unknown

Morbidity and Mortality

- Erosions heal with scarring, which can result in blindness, airway obstruction, and epistaxis

Gender, Race, and Age Distribution

- Female > male (2:1)
- Mean, 50 to 70 years

Clinical Features

- Mucosal blisters, which collapse, resulting in red painful erosions
- Positive Nikolsky sign (blistering on induced trauma)

Prognosis and Treatment

- Waxing-waning, long-term course is usual
- Disease progression despite appropriate therapy
- Treatment includes topical and/or systemic corticosteroids, immunosuppressive therapy, and intravenous immunoglobulin

MUCOUS MEMBRANE PEMPHIGOID—PATHOLOGIC FEATURES

Microscopic Findings

- *Perilesional* tissue shows subepithelial cleft with intact basal cells with or without inflammatory cells

Immunofluorescence Features

- DIF demonstrates linear deposits along the basement membrane zone of IgG and/or C3, sometimes IgA, IgM

Pathologic Differential Diagnosis

- Lichen planus, erythema multiforme, lupus, linear IgA dermatoses, epidermolysis bullosa acquisita, pemphigoid-like drug reaction, pemphigus vulgaris, and paraneoplastic pemphigus

ANCILLARY STUDIES

DIF of perilesional mucosa demonstrates linear deposits along the basement membrane zone (BMZ) of IgG and/or C3 and sometimes IgA or IgM (Figure 7-24). These findings are not specific and require clinical correlation. Whereas IDIF of a patient's serum using salt-split skin can detect circulating antibodies to the BMZ, not all patients have detectable circulating antibodies; therefore, IDIF is not essential for the diagnosis. There is no correlation between circulating antibody titers and disease severity.

DIFFERENTIAL DIAGNOSIS

MMP must be separated from other blistering diseases of the oral cavity, including erosive lichen planus, erythema multiforme, pemphigus vulgaris, lupus erythematosus, linear IgA disease, epidermolysis bullosa acquisita, pemphigoid-like drug reactions, and paraneoplastic pemphigus. Both DIF and IDIF are essential to arriving at the correct diagnosis.

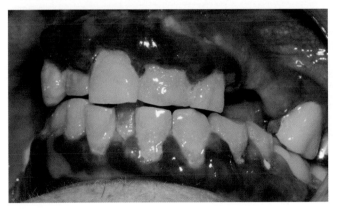

FIGURE 7-22
Mucous membrane pemphigoid presenting as desquamative gingivitis with large areas of red denuded mucosa resulting from sloughing of the epithelium of both the maxilla and mandible.

PATHOLOGIC FEATURES

Examination of *perilesional* mucosal tissue demonstrates a subepithelial cleft, with a sparse inflammatory cell infiltrate containing lymphocytes and plasma cells in the superficial lamina propria (Figure 7-23) with an intact basal cell layer. Occasionally, neutrophils and eosinophils are seen.

PROGNOSIS AND THERAPY

MMP confined to the oral cavity is more amenable to treatment and is rarely associated with scarring, in contrast to involvement of the eye, genital, laryngeal, and esophageal areas. There is often disease progression despite appropriate therapy, which includes topical corticosteroids, systemic corticosteroids, azathioprine, dapsone, and cyclophosphamide. Intravenous immunoglobulin has been used with success in patients resistant to other treatment regimens.

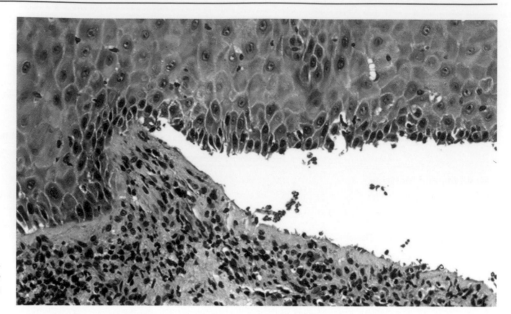

FIGURE 7-23

Perilesional tissue demonstrating subepithelial clefting and a sparse inflammatory cell infiltrate in the superficial lamina propria. No basal cell destruction.

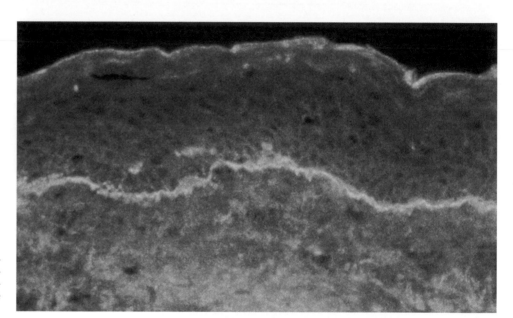

FIGURE 7-24

Direct immunofluorescence of perilesional mucosa from a patient with mucous membrane pemphigoid. A continuous linear band of IgG is seen at the basement membrane zone.

■ PEMPHIGUS VULGARIS

CLINICAL FEATURES

Pemphigus vulgaris (PV) is an autoimmune mucocutaneous blistering disease. Circulating IgG antibodies to desmoglein-1 and -3 (Dsg1, Dsg3) adhesion molecules of squamous epithelial cells are the underlying defects, causing loss of cell-to-cell adhesion. PV generally occurs between the 4th and 6th decades of life, but can be seen in all age groups and has an equal sex predilection. Although an uncommon disease, the incidence of PV is higher in patients of Mediterranean descent and among Ashkenazi Jews. Approximately 50% to 70% of cases first present in the oral cavity with blisters that rupture, leaving painful erosions that heal without scarring (Figure 7-25). Mucosal PV may precede cutaneous PV by an average of 5 months or may be the sole manifestation of the disease. PV can also affect other mucosal sites (esophagus, larynx, nasopharynx, conjunctiva, genitalia, anal mucosa). A flaccid blister on the upper trunk, head, neck, and/or intertriginous areas that readily ruptures is the clinical presentation. After rupture, large areas of painful, denuded epithelium remain. A positive Nikolsky sign and Asboe-Hansen sign (lateral pressure on a bullae extends it into uninvolved mucosa) are commonly seen.

PEMPHIGUS VULGARIS—DISEASE FACT SHEET

Definition
- Autoimmune mucocutaneous blistering disease associated with autoantibodies to adhesion molecules of squamous epithelium

Incidence and Location
- Incidence ranges 0.08 to 3.2/100,000 population
- 50% to 70% of cases first present with oral disease

Morbidity and Mortality
- Morbidity related to disease severity
- Mortality rate up to 10%, due to prolonged immunosuppression

Gender, Race, and Age Distribution
- Peak incidence between 4th to 6th decades
- Higher incidence in Ashkenazi Jews and people of Mediterranean descent

Clinical Features
- Bullae/blisters readily rupture leaving irregularly shaped, painful ulcerations and erosions, which may be quite extensive
- Skin lesions are flaccid, fluid-filled blisters, which rupture and leave painful ulcers

Prognosis and Treatment
- Steroid and immunosuppressive therapy
- Plasmapheresis or intravenous immunoglobulins
- Long-term therapy may achieve remission, especially if mild disease and rapid response to therapy

PEMPHIGUS VULGARIS—PATHOLOGIC FEATURES

Microscopic Findings
- Intraepithelial blister above the basal cell layer
- Intercellular edema, acantholysis, and loss of adhesion
- Basal cells remain attached to the basement membrane
- Mild inflammatory cell infiltrate

Immunofluorescence Features
- Direct immunofluorescence: intercellular deposits of IgG throughout the epithelium. C3 and IgA infrequent finding
- Indirect immunofluorescence: IgG autoantibodies detect on monkey esophagus substrate

Pathologic Differential Diagnosis
- Paraneoplastic pemphigus, pemphigus-like drug eruption, erythema multiforme, Grover disease, Hailey-Hailey disease

PATHOLOGIC FEATURES

A biopsy sample taken from the edge of a blister will show an intraepithelial clefting above the basal layer of the epithelium. Round, swollen, hyperchromatic acantholytic (Tzanck) cells are present in the cleft spaces (Figure 7-26). The basal cells remain attached to the basement membrane, giving a "tombstone" appearance. The superficial lamina propria may contain a mild inflammatory cell infiltrate.

ANCILLARY STUDIES

DIF of perilesional tissue demonstrates intercellular deposits of IgG throughout the epithelium (Figure 7-27). C3 and IgA can sometimes be noted, but less frequently than IgG. IDIF, using monkey esophagus as a substrate, detects circulating IgG autoantibodies in 80% to 90% of patients with PV. The titer of circulating antibody correlates with disease activity. ELISA can detect Dsg3 and Dsg1 autoantibodies, which correlate with disease severity.

DIFFERENTIAL DIAGNOSIS

The clinical differential includes many desquamative-blistering disorders (see the "Pemphigus Vulgaris—Pathologic Features" box), including, most importantly for discussion, paraneoplastic pemphigus (PNP). PNP affects both mucosal and cutaneous sites and is associated with malignancy (lymphoma, chronic lymphocytic leukemia, carcinoma, sarcoma). There is histologic and DIF overlap between PV and PNP, but more specific tests for PNP include IDIF, using the patient's serum and a substrate (monkey esophagus or transitional epithelium of rat bladder), as well as immunoprecipitation, immunoblotting, and ELISAs for the specific autoantibodies in the sera of patients with PNP.

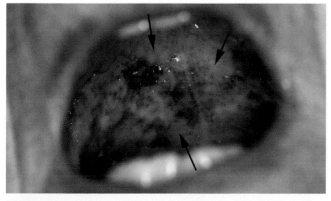

FIGURE 7-25

Large, irregularly shaped ulcer of the soft palate (*arrows*) from a patient with oral, oropharyngeal, and esophageal lesions.

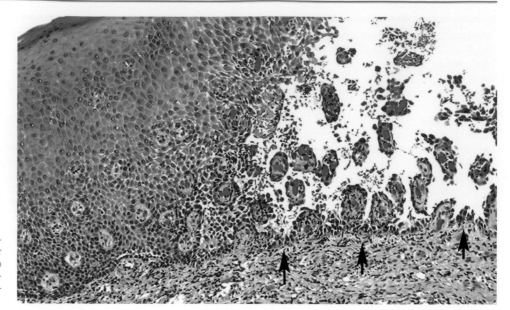

FIGURE 7-26

Perilesional mucosa showing acantholytic epithelial cells and a suprabasilar clefting, leaving the basal cell attached to the basement membrane ("tombstoning"; *arrows*). A mild chronic inflammatory infiltrate is noted.

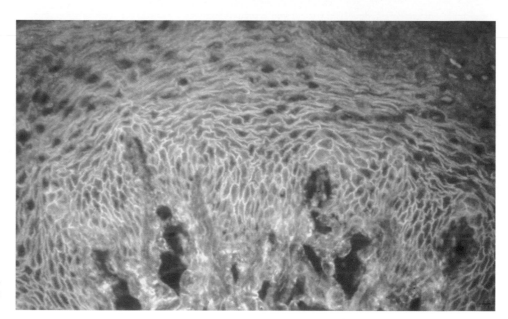

FIGURE 7-27

Perilesional mucosa depicting direct immunofluorescence with deposits of IgG in the intercellular areas of the epithelium.

PROGNOSIS AND THERAPY

Mortality from PV is up to 6%, mainly due today to complications from long-term immunosuppressive therapy, although mortality was much higher before the implementation of systemic corticosteroid therapy. Treatment consists of local or systemic therapy depending on the disease location and severity. Adjuvant immunosuppressants (methotrexate, azathioprine, cyclophosphamide, and cyclosporine) are used for their steroid-sparing effect. Drugs that also have an antiinflammatory effect, such as minocin, dapsone, or tetracycline, have also been used. Plasmapheresis or high-dose intravenous immunoglobulins are used in patients resistant to other therapies. The duration of treatment is variable, with the average time to achieve complete remission ranging from 2 to 10 years. Complete remission is highest in patients who present with mild disease and have a rapid response to treatment.

■ RECURRENT APHTHOUS STOMATITIS

CLINICAL FEATURES

Recurrent aphthous stomatitis (RAS), also known as canker sores, are common oral ulcers estimated to affect up to 30% to 35% of the population. These painful ulcers generally last from 10 to 30 days and range in size from a few millimeters to several centimeters. Minor aphthae, accounting for 80 % of all aphthae, are characterized as small (<1 cm) ulcers with a white, gray, or yellow fibrinopurulent membrane surrounded by an erythematous halo and present on nonkeratinized oral mucosa (buccal mucosa, labial mucosa, soft palate, floor of mouth, and lateral and ventral tongue; Figure 7-28). These ulcers typically heal within 10 to 14 days without scarring. Major aphthae (>1 cm) often take longer to heal and may heal with scarring. Herpetiform aphthous ulcers present as numerous pinpoint ulcers that can coalesce into a larger ulcer.

The etiology of RAS is thought to be multifactorial, including allergens, stress, anxiety, local mechanical trauma, and hormones. Reported food allergens include cinnamon, cereal products, tomatoes, nuts, citrus fruits, and chocolates. A familial association has been observed in ~40 % of cases. No known bacterial or viral infections are associated with RAS.

PATHOLOGIC FEATURES

The microscopic findings are of a nonspecific ulcer, covered by a fibrinopurulent membrane. The underlying connective tissue contains an acute and a chronic inflammatory cell infiltrate (Figure 7-29).

DIFFERENTIAL DIAGNOSIS

The clinical differential diagnosis is wide, although the microscopic differential of *nonspecific* inflammation is limited. The clinical differential includes HSV, herpangina, traumatic ulcer, pyostomatitis vegetans, and Behçet disease (ocular and orogenital ulcers). RAS typically develops on freely moveable mucosa, while herpes develops on "bound" or "taut" mucosa (hard palate, gingiva). Pyostomatitis vegetans is an uncommon pustular disorder that develops in patients with ulcerative colitis and is composed of microabscesses in the spinous layer. Lesions that fail to heal or respond to appropriate treatment, usually within 2 weeks, should undergo biopsy to exclude other diseases.

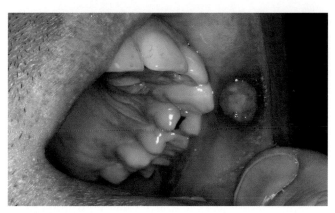

FIGURE 7-28
Clinical photograph of an aphthous ulcer present on the buccal mucosa. The ulcer is covered by a fibrinous membrane and surrounded by an erythematous halo.

PROGNOSIS AND THERAPY

The treatment of aphthous ulcer includes both over-the-counter products and prescription medications. Topical corticosteroids (triamcinolone, fluocinonide, and clobetasol) are effective in reducing the pain and decreasing healing time, while oral systemic corticosteroids can be administered to patients with severe disease. An important part of therapy is to detect and reduce local factors that trigger RAS. Elimination diets

---

RECURRENT APHTHOUS STOMATITIS—DISEASE FACT SHEET

Definition
- Common, noninfectious ulcers occurring on nonkeratinized oral mucosa of multifactorial etiology

Incidence and Location
- Up to 35% of the population

Gender and Age Distribution
- Ulcers usually start in childhood and persist through adulthood

Clinical Features
- Minor or major aphthae present as ulcers with a white-gray or yellow fibrinopurulent membrane and an erythematous halo on the nonkeratinized oral mucosa (buccal and labial mucosa, floor of mouth, soft palate, lateral and ventral tongue)

Prognosis and Treatment
- Treatment goals include reducing pain and promoting healing with the judicious use of topical/systemic corticosteroids, and identifying specific triggers to prevent future ulcer development

---

RECURRENT APHTHOUS STOMATITIS—PATHOLOGIC FEATURES

Microscopic Findings
- Nonspecific ulcer with a fibrinopurulent membrane overlying edematous granulation tissue that contains a mixed inflammatory cell infiltrate

Pathologic Differential Diagnosis
- Traumatic ulcer, pyostomatitis vegetans, herpes simplex virus

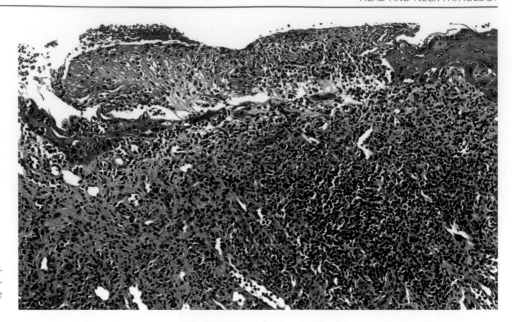

FIGURE 7-29

An aphthous ulcer exhibiting a fibrinopurulent membrane admixed with neutrophils. Granulation tissue beneath the ulcer bed contains inflammatory cells.

and patch testing may help in isolating the triggering agent. Patients who have more than four or five outbreaks a year should also be evaluated for systemic causes, including iron-deficiency anemia, pernicious anemia, celiac disease, and Crohn disease.

■ TRAUMATIC ULCERATIVE GRANULOMA

CLINICAL FEATURES

TRAUMATIC ULCERATIVE GRANULOMA—DISEASE FACT SHEET

Definition
- Chronic traumatic ulceration of the oral cavity with unique pathologic features

Incidence and Location
- Incidence unknown but most likely underreported
- Less frequent than recurrent aphthous ulcerations
- Can occur anywhere but most common on the lateral tongue

Gender and Age Distribution
- Can occur in all age groups including newborns (Riga-Fede disease)
- Males more commonly affected than females

Clinical Features
- 0.1 cm to >1 cm painful ulcer
- Zone of hyperkeratosis surrounding the ulcer
- Induration mimicking squamous cell carcinoma

Prognosis and Treatment
- Ulcers that do not resolve may need excision
- Intralesional steroids can induce ulcer resolution
- Source of trauma must be removed if possible or recurrence is likely

---

Traumatic ulcerative granuloma (traumatic granuloma, traumatic ulcerative granuloma with stromal eosinophilia [TUGSE], eosinophilic granuloma) is an oral ulcer of traumatic origin with unique histopathologic features. These ulcers most often occur on the lateral border of the tongue or buccal mucosa or in sites adjacent to an identifiable source of trauma, such as a fractured or malposed tooth. The ulcers are painful and range in size from 0.1 to 1 cm. A zone of hyperkeratosis surrounding the ulcer is noted along with induration, thus mimicking squamous cell carcinoma (Figure 7-30).

The true incidence of traumatic ulcerative granulomas is unknown but is less common than that of aphthous ulcers. These ulcers can occur in all ages. When present in an infant, it is termed Riga-Fede disease and presents as an ulceration on the ventral tongue caused by tongue thrusting against natal or neonatal teeth. Both electrical and thermal injury can induce a traumatic ulcerative granuloma as can factitious or self-induced injury, which

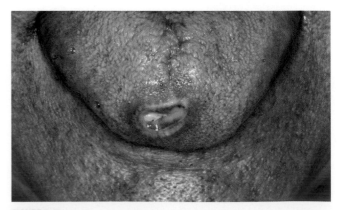

FIGURE 7-30

Clinical photograph of a traumatic ulcerative granuloma on the dorsal tongue. Note the zone of hyperkeratosis surrounding the ulcer.

can be observed in Lesch-Nyhan syndrome, Tourette syndrome, or obsessive-compulsive disorder.

PATHOLOGIC FEATURES

Traumatic ulcerative granulomas have a unique histologic appearance. A thickened fibrinopurulent membrane covers the ulcer and adjacent epithelium may exhibit pseudo-epitheliomatous hyperplasia (Figure 7-31). The ulcer bed is composed of granulation tissue with a mixed inflammatory cell infiltrate of lymphocytes, histiocytes, neutrophils, and occasionally plasma cells. The inflammation extends into the deeper tissue including skeletal muscle, and scattered eosinophils are observed (Figure 7-32). In a subset

TRAUMATIC ULCERATIVE GRANULOMA—PATHOLOGIC FEATURES

Microscopic Findings

- Ulcer bed composed of granulation tissue with mixed chronic inflammatory cell infiltrate
- May see pseudoepitheliomatous hyperplasia in adjacent epithelium
- Inflammation, including eosinophils, extends into skeletal muscle
- Atypical CD30+ histiocytes may be noted
- In thermal/electrical injury can see necrosis

Differential Diagnosis

- Recurrent aphthous ulcer, cutaneous CD30+ T-cell lymphoma

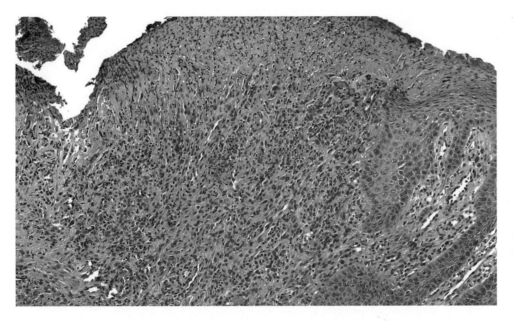

FIGURE 7-31

Traumatic ulcerative granuloma with characteristic thickened fibrinopurulent membrane with deep infiltrate of inflammatory cells. Marked epithelial hyperplasia is noted adjacent to the ulcer bed.

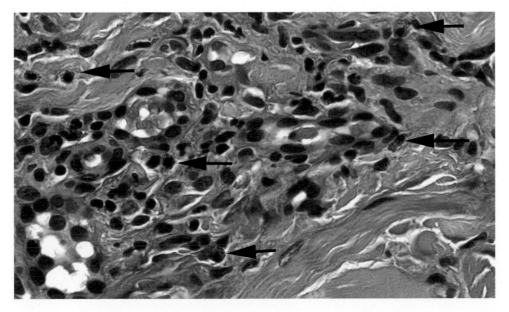

FIGURE 7-32

A mixed inflammatory cell infiltrate including histiocytes and numerous eosinophils (*arrows*) are noted within the striated muscle.

of traumatic ulcerative granulomas, atypical CD30$^+$ histiocytes are noted that may exhibit pleomorphism and mitotic figures. The significance of these findings is uncertain as most cases resolve after biopsy. Necrosis may be present when the ulcer is related to thermal or electrical injury.

DIFFERENTIAL DIAGNOSIS

Often, traumatic ulcerative granulomas undergo biopsy because, clinically, they mimic squamous cell carcinoma, presenting as a nonhealing ulcer with associated induration. Major aphthous ulcers may share clinical features, but on histologic examination these ulcers are superficial, not extending to the muscle. In the subset of traumatic ulcerative granulomas with atypical histiocytes, cutaneous CD30$^+$ T-cell lymphoma may be considered. Despite clonal T-cell receptor rearrangements

in some reported cases, no development of a T-cell lymphoproliferative disorder was noted and results should be cautiously interpreted.

PROGNOSIS AND THERAPY

Nonresolving ulcers may need total excision, although complete resolution has been reported in ulcers biopsied for diagnosis. Intralesional steroid injections are useful in resolving the ulcer. Recurrences of traumatic ulcerative granulomas are common, particularly if the source of the trauma persists.

SUGGESTED READINGS

The complete suggested readings list is available online at www.expertconsult.com.

8

Benign Neoplasms of the Oral Cavity and Oropharynx

■ Brenda L. Nelson

■ FIBROMA

The term *fibroma,* unless further qualified (e.g., ossifying fibroma, ameloblastic fibroma, etc.), refers to a localized proliferation of fibrous connective tissue in response to tissue irritation. As such, oral fibromas are reactive in nature, with some advocating the use of alternative designations, such as "localized fibrous hyperplasia" or "irritation fibroma." It is thought that these terms more accurately reflect the true reactive nature of this lesion, while the term "fibroma" may imply a neoplastic process.

Fibroma is the most common "tumor" encountered in the oral cavity. It occurs more often in women than in men by a 2:1 ratio. It usually presents during the 4th to 6th decades of life but can be found across a wide age range that includes children to the elderly. There is no racial predilection. Distribution within the oral cavity, not surprisingly, reflects those sites most prone to trauma. Consequently, fibromas favor the buccal mucosa, specifically along the bite line, and the lateral border of the tongue. They can, however, arise on the lips and gingiva as well. The classic clinical appearance is that of an elevated sessile nodule surfaced by smooth mucosa (Figure 8-1). Fibromas are painless; however, patients may find such lesions a nuisance.

CLINICAL FEATURES

FIBROMA—DISEASE FACT SHEET

Definition
- A localized proliferation of fibrous connective tissue in response to tissue irritation

Incidence and Location
- Most common "tumor" encountered in the oral cavity
- Most common in oral sites prone to irritation/injury (e.g., buccal mucosa along the bite line, lateral tongue)

Gender and Age Distribution
- Female > male (2:1)
- Most common between 30 and 50 years

Clinical Features
- Painless and asymptomatic
- Submucosal nodules with limited growth potential (usually a few millimeters in diameter)

Prognosis and Treatment
- Conservative surgical resection is curative
- Potential for recurrence if inciting trauma persists

PATHOLOGIC FEATURES

FIBROMA—PATHOLOGIC FEATURES

Gross Findings
- Dome-shaped nodule ranging from a few millimeters to 2 cm
- Smooth surface unless secondarily ulcerated

Microscopic Findings
- Histologic picture dominated by submucosal collagen
- Inconspicuous spindled fibroblasts sparsely dispersed among collagen bundles
- Squamous epithelium is usually unremarkable, but may demonstrate varying degrees of rete atrophy, hyperkeratosis, and/or superficial ulceration

Pathologic Differential Diagnosis
- Not easily confused with other oral submucosal nodules at the histologic level

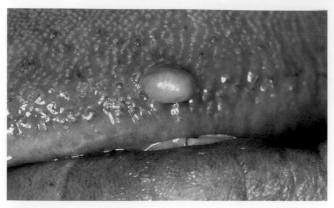

FIGURE 8-1

This fibroma arose along the lateral border of the tongue, and is seen as a raised sessile nodule with a smooth surface.

GROSS FINDINGS

Oral fibromas are generally seen as a round nodule with a smooth mucosal surface. The cut surface is solid and gray with a consistency that ranges from soft to firm. Most are only a few millimeters, and only the rare lesion reaches a diameter of 1 to 2 cm.

MICROSCOPIC FINDINGS

The histologic picture is dominated by the nodular deposition of submucosal collagen (Figure 8-2). Spindled fibroblasts and small blood vessels are dispersed among the pink, dense collagen bundles (Figure 8-3). The periphery of the nodule may be rounded and sharply

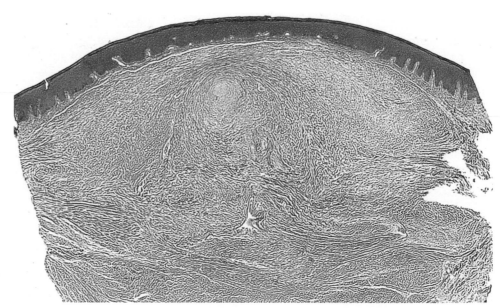

FIGURE 8-2

At low power, the deposition of connective tissue forms a discrete submucosal nodule.

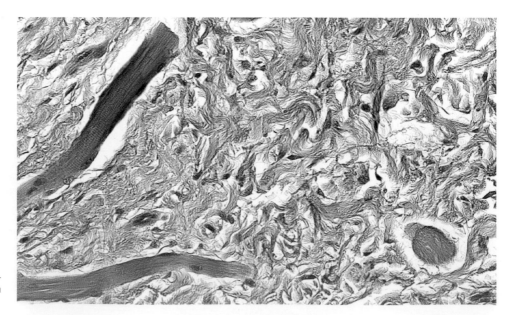

FIGURE 8-3

At higher power, the nodule is composed of inconspicuous fibroblasts in a collagen-rich stroma.

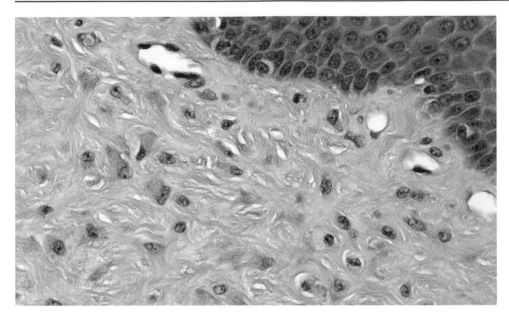

FIGURE 8-4

In contrast to the conventional (i.e., irritation) fibroma, the giant cell fibroma features stellate fibroblasts with large hyperchromatic nuclei.

demarcated or it may blend imperceptibly with the surrounding fibrous connective tissues. The overlying squamous epithelium may be attenuated with flattening of its rete ridges as if it were being tightly stretched over the nodular mass. Trauma to the nodule can incite secondary changes ranging from friction-induced hyperkeratosis to ulceration.

The fibroblasts of irritation fibromas are spindled and inconspicuous. The presence of larger stellate fibroblasts with large and multiple nuclei is characteristic of the *giant cell fibroma* (Figure 8-4). In contrast to the more common irritation fibroma, the giant cell fibroma is not associated with trauma, tends to occur in a younger age group, and favors the tongue and gingiva.

DIFFERENTIAL DIAGNOSIS

Although fibromas are common and clinically inconsequential, surgical removal with microscopic examination is prudent to rule out various benign and malignant neoplasms that can simulate the clinical appearance of fibromas, such as schwannomas, neurofibromas, granular cell tumors, and salivary gland neoplasms. This broad clinical differential diagnosis, however, is easily distinguished by microscopic examination.

PROGNOSIS AND THERAPY

As a reactive non-neoplastic process, fibromas have no malignant potential. Simple surgical resection is curative. If the source of inciting trauma has not been adequately addressed, the lesion may rarely recur.

■ SQUAMOUS PAPILLOMA (INCLUDING VERRUCA AND CONDYLOMA)

Squamous papilloma (SP) of the oral cavity is a localized benign exophytic proliferation of the squamous epithelium. Its classic microscopic presentation is that of a proliferation of keratinizing stratified squamous epithelium supported by fibrovascular connective tissue cores. It is one of several lesions of the oral cavity that has been associated with the human papillomavirus (HPV). Other HPV-associated lesions of the oral mucosa include verruca vulgaris (common wart) and condyloma acuminatum (venereal wart). The HPV serotypes 6 and 11 are most consistently detected in oral SPs and condyloma; while the HPV subtypes 2 and 4 are associated with verruca vulgaris.

CLINICAL FEATURES

SPs represent the most common benign neoplasm originating from the oral mucosa. They occur across a broad age range, affecting both children and adults. Most lesions, however, are diagnosed in individuals 30 to 50 years of age. Some large studies indicate that males are affected more commonly than females and whites more than blacks. They can arise from any intraoral mucosal location, but they show a definite predilection for the hard and soft palate and uvula.

SPs are clinically observed as soft, white pedunculated nodules that usually measure <1 cm (Figure 8-5). Their hallmark frond-like projections give rise to surface irregularities that range from granular, to spiny, to convoluted (i.e., "cauliflower-like"). Most papillomas of the oral cavity are solitary and may have a history of being present for years.

SQUAMOUS PAPILLOMA (INCLUDING VERRUCA AND CONDYLOMA)—DISEASE FACT SHEET

Definition

- A localized benign exophytic warty proliferation of the squamous epithelium driven in part by human papillomavirus, particularly by the nononcogenic serotypes 6 and 11

Incidence and Location

- Most common benign neoplasm originating from the surface epithelium
- May originate from any intraoral mucosal site, but with a preference for the hard and soft palate and uvula

Morbidity and Mortality

- Benign proliferations with little potential to undergo malignant transformation

Gender, Race, and Age Distribution

- May affect males slightly more often than females
- May affect whites slightly more often than blacks
- Occurs over a broad age range, but most commonly presents between 30 and 50 years

Clinical Features

- Painless and asymptomatic
- Warty exophytic growth
- Usually solitary and small (<1 cm)

Prognosis and Treatment

- Conservative surgical resection or laser ablation is curative

PATHOLOGIC FEATURES

GROSS FINDINGS

The SP tends to be exophytic, warty, friable, and white to gray. The degree of its surface irregularities reflects the length and complexity of the papillae.

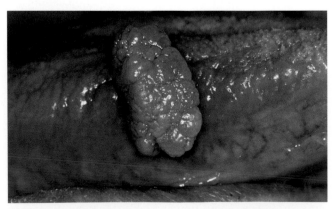

FIGURE 8-5

This squamous papilloma is located along the lateral aspect of the tongue and is seen as an exophytic cauliflower-like mass having a convoluted surface.

SQUAMOUS PAPILLOMA (INCLUDING VERRUCA AND CONDYLOMA)—PATHOLOGIC FEATURES

Gross Findings

- Exophytic, warty, friable, and white to gray
- Surface irregularities ranging from granular, to spiny, to convoluted

Microscopic Findings

- Fibrovascular cores lined by mature, stratified squamous epithelium
- The cells of the prickle layer may show koilocytic change: nuclear condensation and surrounding cytoplasmic clearing ("halos")
- Hyperplasia of the basal cell layer is common and should not be mistaken as a premalignant (i.e., dysplastic) change

Pathologic Differential Diagnosis

- Other human papillomavirus–induced squamous proliferations (verruca vulgaris, condyloma acuminatum), reactive papillary hyperplasia, proliferative verrucous leukoplakia, papillary squamous cell carcinoma

MICROSCOPIC FINDINGS

The trademark feature of SP, namely its papillary extensions, is histologically characterized by multilayered squamous epithelium supported by a central fibrovascular tissue core (Figure 8-6). The squamous layer is often thickened, but it demonstrates normal maturation (Figure 8-7). Hyperplasia of the basal cell layer with increased mitotic figures is not uncommon and should not be interpreted as a premalignant (i.e., dysplastic) change. HPV-induced cytopathic changes can sometimes be appreciated in cells within the prickle cell layer. These altered cells are referred to as koilocytes, and they are characterized by dark condensed nuclei with a surrounding zone of cytoplasmic clearing (Figure 8-8, *inset*).

ANCILLARY STUDIES

In situ hybridization analysis using type-specific HPV probes is a fairly reliable method of documenting the presence of HPV 6 or 11 in oral SPs, but this technique plays no practical role in diagnosing SP, determining treatment, or predicting clinical behavior.

DIFFERENTIAL DIAGNOSIS

SPs can be distinguished from other HPV-associated lesions of the oral cavity based on clinical and histopathologic characteristics. *Verruca vulgaris* usually occurs as

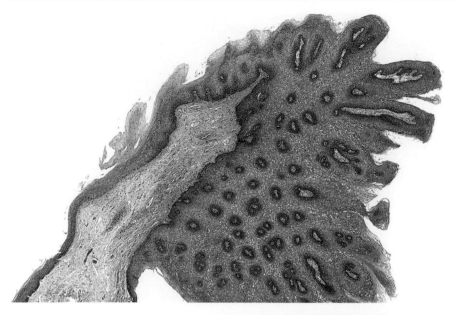

FIGURE 8-6

A low-power view demonstrates the complex branching papillary structures of a squamous papilloma.

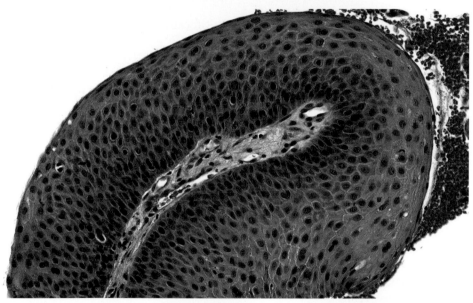

FIGURE 8-7

A higher-power view highlights the papillary frond composed of a fibrovascular core that supports a layer of squamous epithelium.

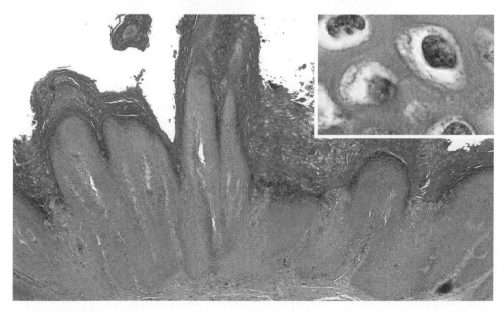

FIGURE 8-8

Low-power view of verruca vulgaris. In contrast to the squamous papilloma, verruca has a broad flat base, a prominent granular layer, and extensive hyperkeratosis. The inset demonstrates cells with dark condensed nuclei surrounded by a zone of cytoplasmic clearing. These koilocytic changes are viral-induced and are characteristic of human papillomavirus–related lesions of the oral cavity.

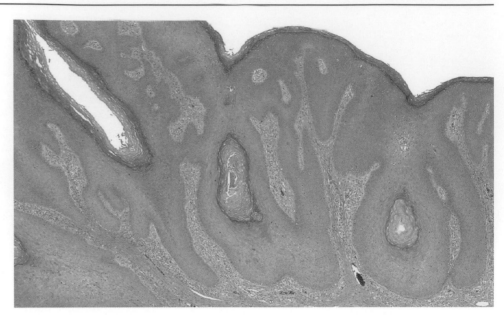

FIGURE 8-9

Oral condyloma exhibits papillary fronds that are broader and more blunted than the papillary projections of squamous papilloma.

warty excrescences located along the vermilion border, labial mucosa, and/or the anterior tongue of children. Histologically, verruca vulgaris will have projections of epithelium that appear to converge at the base. The epithelium demonstrates a prominent granular layer with spires of hyperkeratosis (Figure 8-8). *Oral condyloma* is considered a sexually transmitted disease. It is most commonly seen in young adults at sites of sexual contact (e.g., labial mucosa, soft palate). It is clinically seen as clusters of pink nodules that coalesce into broad-based exophytic masses. Microscopically, its papillary fronds are broader and more blunted than the papillary projections of squamous papilloma. Koilocytes are usually more prominent (Figure 8-9).

Other oral lesions that may be considered in the differential diagnosis include reactive *papillary hyperplasia, proliferative verrucous leukoplakia (PVL),* and *papillary squamous cell carcinoma.* The distinction between SP and papillary hyperplasia is usually determined clinically. Papillary hyperplasia is a reactive process that is generally seen in association with ill-fitting prostheses, usually dentures. PVL is characterized by multifocal lesions that may appear histologically similar to SPs. This condition represents a varied process that tends to spread and progress to malignancy. Papillary squamous cell carcinoma may share some of the architectural features of SP but will have malignant cytology.

PROGNOSIS AND THERAPY

As a benign neoplasm with a limited growth potential, the oral papilloma is cured by local excision or laser ablation. Local recurrence is uncommon and malignant transformation is exceedingly rare. Importantly, they do not share with juvenile laryngeal papillomas the penchant for multifocality, widespread growth, and rapid recurrence.

■ FOCAL EPITHELIAL HYPERPLASIA

Focal epithelial hyperplasia (FEH) (Heck disease) is a virus-induced benign proliferation of the oral squamous epithelium that arises primarily in children and adolescents. It has an ethnic predilection for those indigenous to North America, but it is not restricted to this population as was once thought. Cases involving populations from around the world are now well documented. HPV is the responsible agent, with HPV serotypes 13 and 32 being the most consistently identified.

CLINICAL FEATURES

FEH is not common, and incidence rates vary widely depending on age and ethnicity. Initially described in American Indians and Inuits, the ethnic incidence of FEH is broader than initially anticipated. It has been reported in populations from South and Central America, Africa, the Middle East, and elsewhere. Most initial diagnoses involve children and adolescents, and in certain ethnic groups, nearly 40% of children are affected. However, lesions can be seen throughout life. In some ethnic populations, females are affected more frequently than males by a 2:1 ratio. FEH has also been reported among those who are HIV positive and, interestingly, its frequency increases with the introduction of highly active antiretroviral therapy (HAART).

FEH has a distinct clinical appearance. It is seen as multiple clustered flat-topped papules and rounded

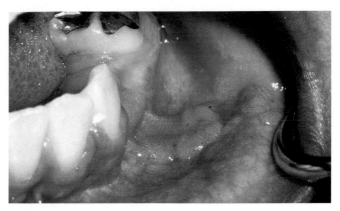

FIGURE 8-10

Focal epithelial hyperplasia involving the labial mucosa. Small, tightly packed papules merge to form larger confluent lesions.

GROSS FINDINGS

FEH is grossly seen as tan, soft nodules with a sessile base and a smooth surface.

MICROSCOPIC FINDINGS

The hallmark histologic feature is acanthosis of the squamous epithelium (Figure 8-11). The rete ridges are expanded and often fused. The keratinocytes show orderly maturation without atypia. Parakeratosis is a common finding. Virus-induced cellular alterations are sometimes present in the superficial keratinocytes. These alterations include koilocytic changes typical of HPV infection, and a more unique type of alteration characterized by fragmentation of the nuclei in a way that resembles a mitotic figure (the "mitosoid cell") (Figure 8-12).

ANCILLARY STUDIES

The presence of HPV can be documented using a variety of detection methods ranging from electron microscopy to type-specific DNA in situ hybridization. Viral detection, however, is a matter more of academic interest than of diagnostic relevance and methods of detection are generally not commercially available. Additionally, these techniques do not play any significant role in diagnosing FEH or predicting its clinical behavior.

nodules that have a predilection for the labial, lingual, and buccal mucosae (Figure 8-10). Individual papules are discrete and small (a few millimeters to 1 cm), but tightly clustered papules can coalesce to form large confluent lesions. Papules tend to be soft and painless.

PATHOLOGIC FEATURES

DIFFERENTIAL DIAGNOSIS

Careful correlation of the clinical and pathologic features should allow ready distinction of FEH from other papular eruptions of the oral cavity. *Condyloma acuminatum*, for example, can clinically present as multifocal

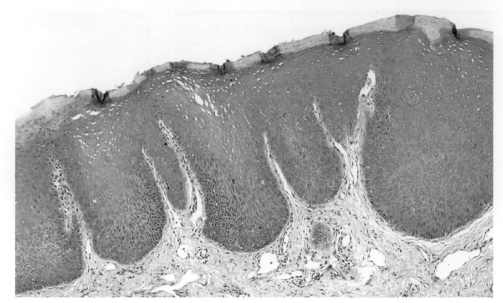

FIGURE 8-11

Low-power view showing acanthosis of the squamous epithelium with expansion and clubbing of rete ridges.

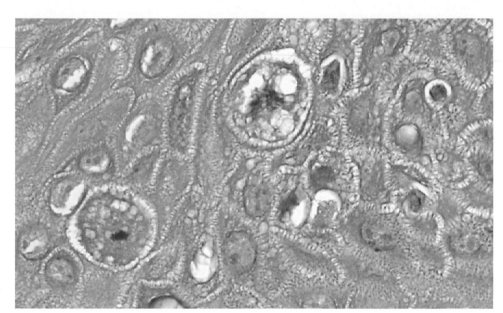

FIGURE 8-12

A high-power view of "mitosoid cells": The pattern of nuclear fragmentation in this keratinocyte has the appearance of a mitotic figure.

coalescent nodules of the oral mucosa. At the microscopic level, however, condyloma acuminatum and its family of HPV-related oral warts are characterized by a papillary growth as opposed to the simple squamous hyperplasia of FEH. The distinction is important as lesions may be submitted from children with the concern that they may be sexually transmitted and the result of abuse.

PROGNOSIS AND THERAPY

FEH is a benign epithelial proliferation that often undergoes spontaneous regression. Removal of individual lesions by surgical excision or laser ablation for cosmetic purposes is feasible when a few lesions are present but impractical when lesions are more numerous and widespread.

■ LOBULAR CAPILLARY HEMANGIOMA

Lobular capillary hemangioma (LCH), previously commonly referred to as "pyogenic granuloma," is a reactive soft tissue growth with a predilection for the oral cavity that is histologically characterized by a lobular arrangement of proliferating small blood vessels. The term "pyogenic granuloma," while entrenched in the culture and literature, is misleading as the lesion is neither infectious (related to pyogenic organisms) nor granulomatous. The later designation of "lobular capillary hemangioma" better reflects its true essence.

CLINICAL FEATURES

LCH occurs in all age groups. Although it occurs equally in both sexes overall, some have noted an unequal gender distribution across different age groups: Patients younger than 18 years are predominantly male, patients between 18 and 39 years are predominantly female, and patients older than 39 years are more evenly divided. The proportional increase in females during reproductive years reflects the contribution of hormonally driven lesions that occur during early stages of pregnancy. There is no race predominance.

The most frequently involved oral sites are the lips, gingiva, cheek, and tongue. Those lesions that arise during pregnancy almost exclusively involve the gingiva and are sometimes referred to as a *pregnancy tumor*. About one-third develop following minor trauma, while others are the result of a reaction to local irritation. Bleeding is the most common clinical complaint. Lesions of the oral cavity are almost always solitary. The

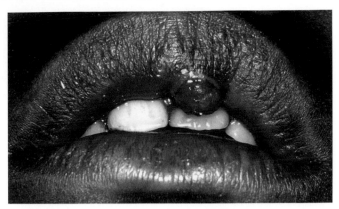

FIGURE 8-13
This pyogenic granuloma of the lip is seen as a purple polypoid nodule.

clinical presentation is that of a nonpainful, purple-red polypoid mass that is friable and bleeds easily; not surprisingly, bleeding is the most common clinical complaint (Figure 8-13). The surface is often ulcerated and sometimes covered with an exudate. Most lesions range in size from a few millimeters to a few centimeters.

PATHOLOGIC FEATURES

GROSS FINDINGS

LCH is grossly seen as a polypoid often pedunculated gray-tan mass. The surface is usually ulcerated, and the presence of an underlying exuberant granulation tissue often forms a prominent cap on a narrower stalk (Figure 8-14).

PYOGENIC GRANULOMA (LOBULAR CAPILLARY HEMANGIOMA)—DISEASE FACT SHEET

Definition
- An acquired polypoid form of capillary hemangioma that is histologically characterized by a lobular arrangement of proliferating vessels

Incidence and Location
- Common
- In the oral cavity the most frequently involved sites are the lips, gingiva, cheek, and tongue

Morbidity and Mortality
- Benign with no potential for invasive growth or malignant progression

Gender and Age Distribution
- Equal gender distribution
- A hormonally driven form affects a small percentage (1%) of pregnant women
- Occurs in all ages

Clinical Features
- Nonpainful, purple-red, polypoid mass that is friable and bleeds easily

Prognosis and Treatment
- Conservative local excision is usually curative, but a small percentage may locally recur if incompletely excised
- Pregnancy-associated lesions usually regress following parturition

---

PYOGENIC GRANULOMA (LOBULAR CAPILLARY HEMANGIOMA)—PATHOLOGIC FEATURES

Gross Findings
- Smooth, polypoid, pedunculated gray-tan mass

Microscopic Findings
- Lobular arrangement of compact capillaries around a central larger feeding vessel
- Surface ulceration with varying degrees of stromal edema, inflammation and fibrosis

Immunohistochemical Features
- Positive for endothelial markers including factor VIII–related antigen and CD31

Pathologic Differential Diagnosis
- Granulation tissue, nasopharyngeal angiofibroma, aggressive vascular neoplasms (e.g., Kaposi sarcoma, angiosarcoma, hemangiopericytoma)

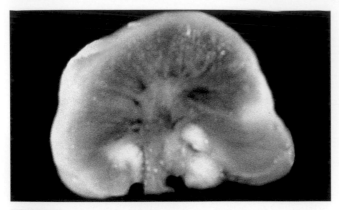

FIGURE 8-14

The cut surface of a pyogenic granuloma. An expanded cap of exuberant granulation tissue positioned on a stalk gives rise to a mushroom-like appearance.

MICROSCOPIC FINDINGS

At low magnification, LCH is an exophytic growth connected to the oral mucosa by a broad stalk that is often collared by hyperplastic squamous epithelium (Figure 8-15). The fundamental microscopic makeup is that of a lobulated capillary hemangioma. Each lobule consists of a compact proliferation of capillaries around a central larger feeding vessel (Figure 8-16). In the presence of ulceration, the stroma becomes inflamed and edematous, particularly in the superficial aspect of the lesion. When these secondary stromal changes are pronounced, the lobular pattern is lost and the distinction between a lobulated capillary hemangioma and an exuberant granulation tissue is obscured. The endothelial

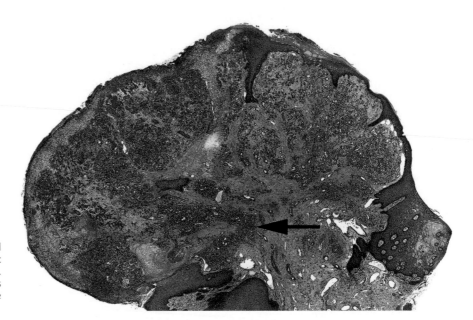

FIGURE 8-15

Low-power view showing the characteristic zonal pattern. The superficial aspect of this pyogenic granuloma is ulcerated, edematous, and inflamed. The lobular proliferation of small blood vessels is best appreciated in the deeper portion of the lesion (*arrow*).

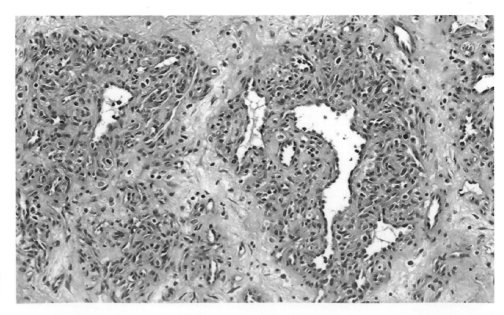

FIGURE 8-16

A high-power view of a lobule shows the compact proliferation of capillaries around a central larger feeding vessel.

cells lining the capillaries are often plump with an epithelioid appearance. Mitotic activity is variable and can be robust.

ANCILLARY STUDIES

The vascular component of LCH is immunoreactive with endothelial markers, including factor VIII–related antigen, CD34 and CD31; it is not immunoreactive for epithelial markers (e.g., cytokeratin) or melanocytic markers (e.g., S100 protein, HMB45, Melan-A/Mart-1). Immunohistochemical documentation of its vascular nature has diagnostic utility when the epithelioid appearance of some cellular LCH causes confusion with an epithelial or melanocytic neoplasm.

DIFFERENTIAL DIAGNOSIS

The differential diagnosis for an LCH is broad. Lesions with classic histology are not a diagnostic dilemma; however, lesions with prominent stromal edema can be dismissed as exuberant granulation tissue or as revolving mucoceles. In turn, LCHs that are in the process of resolving may share histologic features with fibromas. The possibility of malignancy is of bigger concern, as LCH with a predominant solid growth pattern and brisk mitotic activity can be mistaken for more aggressive vascular lesions, such as *angiosarcoma*, *Kaposi sarcoma*, and *hemangiopericytoma*. When the endothelial cells in these solid areas take on a more epithelioid appearance, the lesion can mimic *epithelioid hemangioma*, *angiolymphoid hyperplasia with eosinophilia*, and even carcinoma or melanoma. Brisk mitotic activity may lead to increased concerns of a possible malignancy. Unlike malignant vascular, epithelial, and melanocytic tumors, LCH is exophytic and circumscribed without infiltration of surrounding structures.

PROGNOSIS AND THERAPY

LCH is a benign vascular neoplasm with no potential for locally invasive tumor growth or metastatic spread. Conservative local excision is usually curative, but a small percentage may locally recur if incompletely excised. Gingival lesions should be excised down to periosteum and any local irritants should be addressed. Pregnancy-associated lesions usually regress following parturition.

■ PERIPHERAL OSSIFYING FIBROMA

Peripheral ossifying fibroma (POF) is a reactive non-neoplastic proliferation of fibrous tissue with focal mineralization forming a gingival mass (*peripheral* implies nonosseous, soft tissue involvement, while *central* implies within bone). The central ossifying fibroma is not, however, considered to be an intraosseous counterpart to the POF, as the former is a true neoplasm.

CLINICAL FEATURES

POF is a common lesion that occurs exclusively on the gingiva or alveolar ridge. It more commonly affects the maxilla than the mandible, and it favors the interdental papilla of the incisor/canine region. In some cases, a source of chronic irritation (e.g., ill-fitting dentures, orthodontics) or trauma is identified. It occurs over a broad age range with a concentration among teenagers and young adults. Females are affected more commonly than males at a ratio of 1.7:1. POF appears clinically as a sessile or pedunculated nodule that ranges in size from a few millimeters to 2 cm (Figure 8-17). The surface is often ulcerated.

PATHOLOGIC FEATURES

GROSS FINDINGS

POF is grossly seen as a polypoid sometimes pedunculated nodule. The surface may be intact or ulcerated.

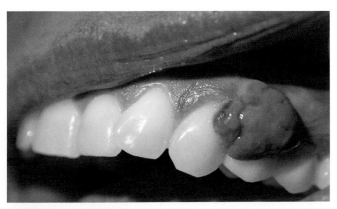

FIGURE 8-17
This peripheral ossifying fibroma is arising from the interdental papilla as a lobulated smooth, sessile nodule.

MICROSCOPIC FINDINGS

The fundamental makeup of the POF is fibroblastic tissue with randomly distributed deposits of mineralized material (Figure 8-18). However, there is some inconstancy in its histologic appearance due to variations in the cellularity and the extent and type of mineralization, as a result of lesion maturation. The fibroblastic proliferation is covered by a stratified squamous epithelium, but this epithelium is often ulcerated and replaced by an inflammatory exudate. The overall cellularity of the fibroblastic component varies according to the relative proportion of plump fibroblasts and stromal collagen. The nature of the mineralized material varies from dystrophic calcification to cementum-like material to well-formed bone (Figure 8-19). Mineralization may be scant and may require the review of multiple levels. Multinucleated giant cells may be present, but they are never numerous.

DIFFERENTIAL DIAGNOSIS

POFs can be confused with other fibrous lesions of the gingiva. Ulcerated lesions without conspicuous mineralization may be confused with *lobular capillary hemangioma*. A thorough microscopic examination, however, is usually sufficient in establishing a diagnosis of POF by demonstrating the presence of focal mineralized deposits and the absence of a lobular proliferation of capillaries. Although individual or clustered multinucleated giant cells are present in a subset of POFs, they are not nearly as numerous as in *peripheral giant cell granuloma*.

PROGNOSIS AND THERAPY

Even though a reactive, non-neoplastic process, ~16% of POFs recur following local surgical excision. Therefore,

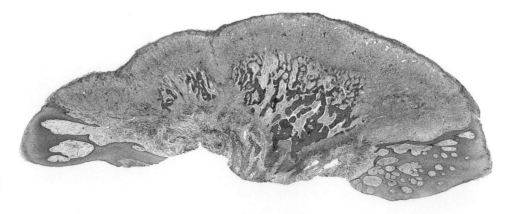

FIGURE 8-18

A low-power view demonstrates an exophytic mass of exuberant fibroconnective tissue emanating from a central nidus of mineralization. There is ulceration of the overlying epithelium.

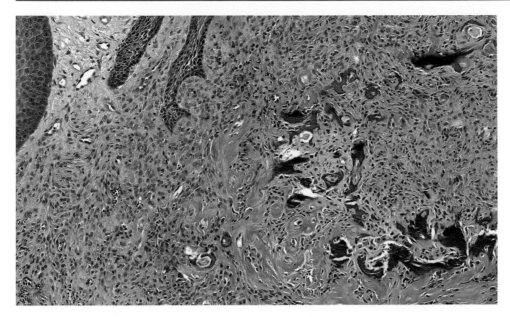

FIGURE 8-19
A higher-power view shows the mineralized component to be comprised of reactive, newly formed bone.

aggressive excision, down to the periosteum, along with the removal of the underlying inciting irritant, is recommended as a means of minimizing the long-term risk of local recurrence.

■ PERIPHERAL GIANT CELL GRANULOMA

Peripheral giant cell granuloma (PGCG) is a reactive proliferation caused by chronic irritation of the gingival mucosa. It is microscopically seen as an exuberant proliferation of multinucleated giant cells. The traditional term *peripheral giant cell reparative granuloma* is inaccurate as the multinucleated giant cells have little if any capacity for local tissue reparation. *Peripheral* implies soft tissue involvement, while *central* implies an intraosseous location.

CLINICAL FEATURES

PGCG is a relatively common exophytic lesion of the oral cavity. It occurs over a broad age range, but most patients are between 40 to 60 years. Females are affected slightly more often than males. The PGCG presumably arises from the periodontal ligament and thus occurs exclusively on the gingiva, usually between the permanent molars and incisors. The mandible and maxilla are involved at an almost equal frequency. PGCG classically presents as a solitary broad-based reddish-blue polypoid nodule (Figure 8-20). The surface epithelium is frequently ulcerated.

RADIOLOGIC FEATURES

Unlike central giant cell granuloma, the PGCG does not arise within the craniofacial bones. Nonetheless, it can occasionally induce focal resorption of underlying alveolar bone, thus giving rise to a superficial cup-shaped radiolucency on imaging.

PERIPHERAL GIANT CELL GRANULOMA—DISEASE FACT SHEET

Definition
- An exuberant reactive proliferation of multinucleated giant cells forming a gingival mass

Incidence and Location
- Relatively common
- Almost exclusively involves the gingiva

Morbidity and Mortality
- Reactive process with no malignant potential

Gender and Age Distribution
- More common in females
- Most patients 40 to 60 years old

Clinical Features
- Reddish-blue rubbery nodules that range in size from a few millimeters to 3 cm
- Surface ulceration is common

Prognosis and Treatment
- Local surgical excision down to bone
- Can recur locally

PATHOLOGIC FEATURES

PERIPHERAL GIANT CELL GRANULOMA—PATHOLOGIC FEATURES

Gross Findings
- Broad-based rubbery polypoid nodule with smooth surface

Microscopic Findings
- Histologic picture dominated by multinucleated giant cells admixed with mononuclear stromal cells
- Background features include hemorrhage, hemosiderin deposition, chronic inflammation, and islands of metaplastic bone

Pathologic Differential Diagnosis
- Other giant cell–rich tumors include central giant cell tumor, brown tumor of hyperparathyroidism, and cherubism

GROSS FINDINGS

PGCG grossly appears as a soft to rubbery, broad-based polypoid nodule that measures a few millimeters up to 3 cm. Its surface tends to be smooth.

MICROSCOPIC FINDINGS

The microscopic appearance is characterized by an exuberance of multinucleated giant cells (Figures 8-21 and 8-22). They are abundantly present and dominate the microscopic picture. The relationship of these cells to true osteoclasts is unclear, but they are certainly osteoclast-like in their appearance having abundant cytoplasm containing up to 100 nuclei (Figure 8-23). These multinucleated giant cells are interspersed among spindled to oval mononuclear cells. Secondary background features include hemorrhage, hemosiderin deposition, chronic inflammation, and islands of metaplastic bone.

DIFFERENTIAL DIAGNOSIS

There are a handful of lesions that closely resemble the PGCG in their histologic appearance. These include central *giant cell granuloma*, *brown tumor of hyperparathyroidism*, and *cherubism*. However, all of these occur within the craniofacial bones, in contrast to PGCG. Thus, the clinical features and radiographic findings are essential when it comes to distinguishing between the various giant cell–rich lesions of the oral cavity. Additionally, such correlation may assist in ruling out a central lesion that has perforated the bone, resulting in a gingival mass. Of course, giant cells may be found in other lesions, so the defining features of

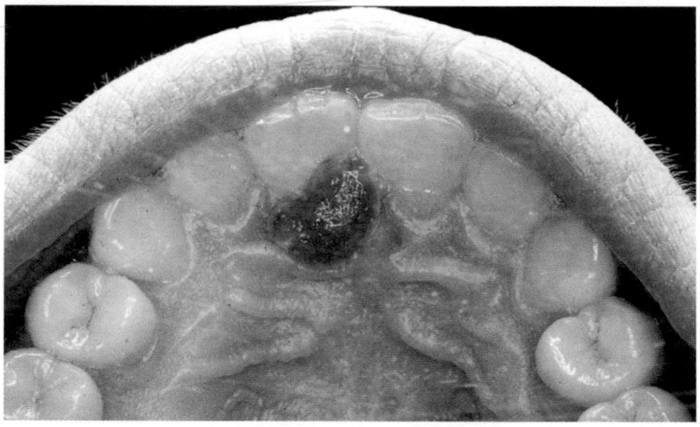

FIGURE 8-20

This peripheral giant cell granuloma is arising from the gingiva as a broad-based reddish-blue polypoid nodule.

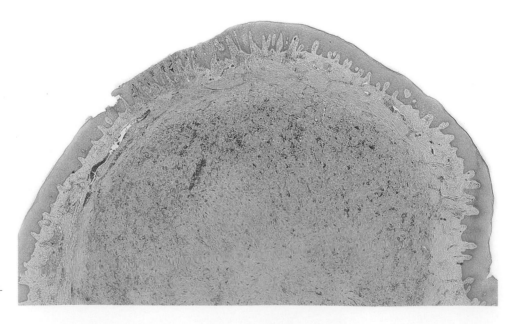

FIGURE 8-21

Proliferation of giant cells forms a submucosal nodule.

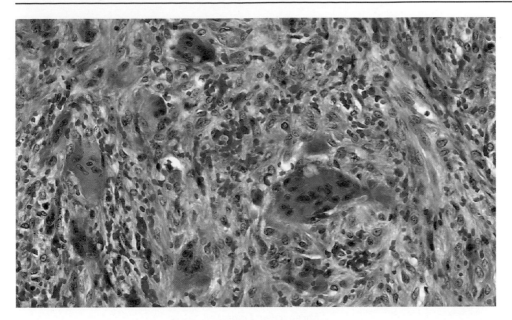

FIGURE 8-22

Giant cells are interspersed among stromal mononuclear cells in a hemorrhagic background.

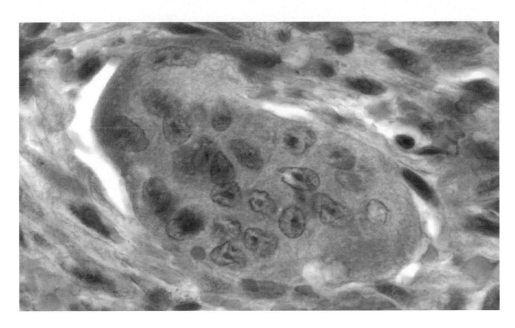

FIGURE 8-23

Giant cells have an abundant cytoplasm that contains numerous nuclei.

those entities must be considered before the diagnosis of PGCG is rendered.

PROGNOSIS AND THERAPY

The standard treatment of PGCG is surgical excision down to the bone. Failure to include the periosteum or periodontal ligament may result in an increased risk of local recurrence, which occurs in ∼10 % of lesions. In addition, efforts should be taken to identify and remove any inciting source(s) of chronic irritation.

■ CONGENITAL GRANULAR CELL EPULIS

Congenital granular cell epulis (CGCE) is a rare benign mesenchymal tumor composed of large cells with coarse granular cytoplasm. It is also known as *congenital epulis*, or as *congenital epulis of the newborn*, although the latter is redundant. It classically arises from the anterior alveolar ridge of the newborn. Its cell of origin remains elusive, and it is not to be regarded as the congenital counterpart of the Schwann cell–derived adult granular cell tumor.

CONGENITAL GRANULAR CELL EPULIS—DISEASE FACT SHEET

Definition
- A benign mesenchymal tumor arising from the anterior alveolar ridge of the newborn and composed of large cells with coarse granular cytoplasm

Incidence and Location
- Rare
- Almost exclusively involves the alveolar ridge with a distinct preference for gingiva overlying the future canine and lateral incisor teeth
- The maxilla is involved more commonly than the mandible

Morbidity and Mortality
- Obstructive masses may cause difficulty with respiration and feeding

Gender and Age Distribution
- Female >>> male (9:1)
- Newborns

Clinical Features
- Smooth nonulcerated polypoid masses with a broad-based attachment to the alveolar ridge

Prognosis and Treatment
- Stops growing at birth and often regresses over time
- Local conservative resection is curative
- Does not recur (even after incomplete excision)

CONGENITAL GRANULAR CELL EPULIS—PATHOLOGIC FEATURES

Gross Findings
- Tan-pink polypoid mass with a smooth nonulcerated surface

Microscopic Findings
- Submucosal proliferation of cells with abundant eosinophilic granular cytoplasm.

Immunohistochemical Features
- Absence of S100 protein staining, in contrast to adult granular cell tumors

Pathologic Differential Diagnosis
- Adult granular cell tumor, alveolar soft part sarcoma, rhabdomyoma

CLINICAL FEATURES

CGCE is a rare tumor that occurs almost exclusively in newborns. Females are affected much more commonly than males at a ratio of ~9:1. CGCE is a lesion of the alveolar ridge with a particular predilection for the gingiva overlying the future canine and lateral incisor teeth. The maxilla is involved more commonly than the mandible. They tend to be seen as smooth nonulcerated polypoid masses with a broad-based attachment to the alveolar ridge. The bone and teeth are uninvolved. Most lesions measure about 1 cm, but they can achieve sizes of >5 cm. Affected newborns often present with a mass protruding from the oral cavity (Figure 8-24). Mechanical obstruction can cause problems with feeding and respiration.

PATHOLOGIC FEATURES

GROSS FINDINGS

CGCE typically presents as a tan-pink polypoid mass with a smooth nonulcerated surface (Figure 8-25). The cut surface is homogeneous, firm, and tan to yellow.

MICROSCOPIC FINDINGS

The CGCE is composed of large, polygonal granular cells, characterized by an abundance of eosinophilic granular cytoplasm and round or oval basophilic nuclei. These distinctive cells grow in a sheet-like pattern supported by delicate fibrovascular septa (Figure 8-26). Incorporation of odontogenic epithelium is occasionally seen. The overlying surface epithelium is usually intact and atrophic.

ANCILLARY STUDIES

Immunohistochemical studies have focused on questions related to histogenesis, as the cell of origin remains elusive. The absence of staining for muscle markers, epithelial markers, and neural markers suggests an origin from an uncommitted mesenchymal cell. Notably, the lack of S100 protein staining has supported the argument that, histologic similarities aside, the CGCE and the Schwann cell–derived granular cell tumor (strongly

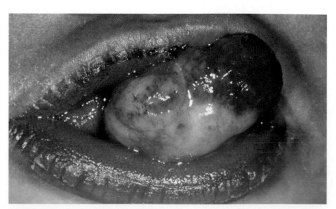

FIGURE 8-24
This congenital granular cell epulis arises from the alveolar ridge of the maxilla and emanates from the oral cavity as a large polypoid mass.

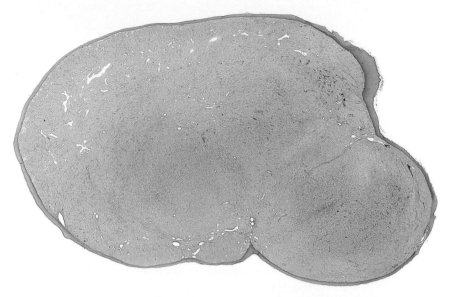

FIGURE 8-25
Low-power view showing sheets of granular cells filling the submucosa.

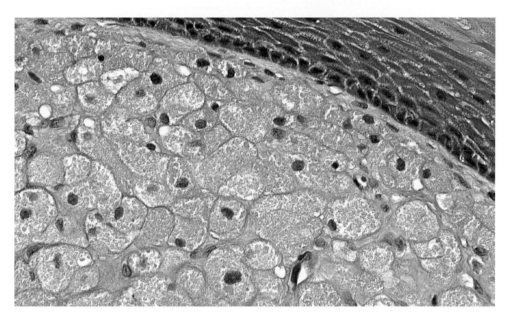

FIGURE 8-26
Higher-power view demonstrating the abundant pink granular cytoplasm of the granular cells.

S100 protein positive) are distinct, unrelated lesions. Moreover, electron microscopy fails to reveal any evidence of schwannian differentiation.

DIFFERENTIAL DIAGNOSIS

The granular cells in CGCE and *granular cell tumor* are microscopically identical, but they should not be regarded as equivalent tumors. In contrast to CGCE, granular cell tumors usually affect adults, have a site predilection for the tongue, are immunoreactive for S100 protein, and are associated with hyperplasia of the overlying epithelium (i.e., pseudoepitheliomatous hyperplasia). Other pink cell tumors that can involve the oral cavity include *alveolar soft part sarcoma* and *rhabdomyoma*, but these rarely cause diagnostic confusion when the histologic picture is considered together with the age of the patient and location of the mass.

PROGNOSIS AND THERAPY

The tumor stops growing at birth and regresses over time. In fact, complete regression without therapy has been reported. Most tumors are surgically excised. As they do not recur, even following incomplete removal, surgical excision should be conservative, to ensure the preservation of underlying developing teeth.

SUGGESTED READINGS

The complete suggested readings list is available online at www.expertconsult.com.

9

Malignant Neoplasms of the Oral Cavity and Oropharynx

■ **James S. Lewis, Jr.**

■ SQUAMOUS CELL CARCINOMA

Squamous cell carcinoma (SCC) arises from the epithelium lining the oral cavity and oropharyngeal tonsillar crypts. Although oral cavity and oropharyngeal SCC share many common carcinogenic factors, there are significant differences to justify considering them to be biologically and clinically distinct entities.

CLINICAL FEATURES

SCC is the most common cancer of the oral cavity and oropharynx, accounting for 90% of cases. Most develop in men (male:female, 3:1) over the age of 50. While the incidence of oral cavity SCC is higher among African Americans than whites, the opposite is true for the oropharynx. The rate of oropharyngeal SCC is increasing dramatically while that for oral cavity is declining slightly.

Carcinogen exposure, diet, and preexisting medical conditions may all play a role in tumor development. Tobacco is the most important risk factor for oral cavity SCC, while it is less important for oropharyngeal SCC. Depending on the number of cigarettes smoked ("pack years"), the risk of oral cavity or oropharyngeal SCC is 5 to 17 times higher. Although less substantial, other risk factors include snuff and chewing tobacco and, in some parts of the world, the chronic use of intraoral betel quid. Alcohol consumption is particularly significant for the way in which it *potentiates* the carcinogenicity of tobacco. Another risk factor is chronic sun exposure, which is a major cause of carcinoma of the lip vermilion.

In the oropharynx, human papillomavirus (HPV), particularly serotype 16, plays a causative role in the majority of cases (>70%). In the oral cavity, HPV DNA can be found in as many as 50% of tumors, but, unlike in the oropharynx, its biological and clinical significance is not well defined.

SQUAMOUS CELL CARCINOMA—DISEASE FACT SHEET

Definition

- A malignant neoplasm arising from the squamous epithelium of the oral cavity and oropharynx

Incidence and Location

- Most common malignancy of the oral cavity and oropharynx
- Over 25,000 cases diagnosed in the United States each year
- **Oral cavity:** most commonly arises from the lip, then tongue, floor of mouth, gingiva, palate, and buccal mucosa
- **Oropharynx:** most common in palatine tonsils followed by the tongue base

Gender, Race, and Age Distribution

- Male > female (~3:1)
- Most patients >50 years
- **Oral cavity:** higher incidence among blacks than whites
- **Oropharynx:** higher incidence among whites than blacks

Clinical Features

- Premalignant changes present as white (leukoplakia) or red (erythroplakia) mucosal patches
- Invasive carcinomas range from depressed ulcerated lesions to fungating masses
- Many patients have cervical lymph node metastases at presentation

Prognosis and Treatment

- Tumor stage has a dramatic impact on outcome and therapy
- Surgery with or without radiation and chemotherapy standard treatment for all oral cavity carcinomas; survival ~50% at 5 years
- Primary surgery and primary chemoradiation therapy are both effective treatment types for oropharyngeal carcinomas; survival at 5 years is ~50% for HPV negative and ~80% for HPV positive

Oral cavity carcinomas most commonly arise from the lip, followed by the tongue, floor of mouth, gingiva, palate, and buccal mucosa, in decreasing order. SCCs of the oral cavity are generally preceded by clinically visible, premalignant (dysplastic) mucosal lesions that clinically appear as leukoplakia or erythroplakia. "Leukoplakia" is a clinical term that refers to a white patch in the oral cavity (Figure 9-1) and corresponds to the presence of surface keratin. Leukoplakia varies in thickness, and its surface ranges from granular to nodular to fissured. "Erythroplakia" is a clinical term that refers to a thin, red patch of the oral mucosa (Figure 9-2). These white and red lesions frequently, but not always, have histologic evidence of dysplasia. Erythroplakia is much more likely than leukoplakia to be associated with dysplasia or carcinoma. During cancer progression, these lesions may evolve into expanding, nonhealing ulcers. Tumor invasion is heralded by bleeding, loosening of teeth, dysphagia, dysarthria, odynophagia, or a palpable neck mass.

Oropharyngeal carcinomas classically present as small primary tumors usually arising from the palatine tonsils (tonsillar pillar) followed by the base of the tongue. These sites harbor a large amount of lymphoid tissue associated with invaginated "crypt" epithelium, for which HPV is tropic. For most oropharyngeal SCCs, no obvious precursor lesions have been identified.

The clinical appearance of invasive carcinomas is highly variable, ranging from depressed, ulcerated lesions to fungating masses (Figure 9-3). Approximately 30% of patients with oral SCC and 80% with oropharyngeal SCC present with spread to regional/cervical lymph nodes. In fact, oropharyngeal SCC is sometimes clinically undetectable or presents as an "unknown primary" with bulky cervical metastases.

RADIOLOGIC FEATURES

Radiologic evaluation is primarily used for staging purposes. Computed tomography, magnetic resonance imaging, and occasionally positron emission tomography are used to determine the extent of local invasion and presence of metastatic spread to regional lymph nodes or distantly.

PATHOLOGIC FEATURES

SQUAMOUS CELL CARCINOMA—PATHOLOGIC FEATURES

Gross Findings
- Subtle grayish white thickening of the mucosa to large ulcerative, flat, or fungating masses

Microscopic Findings

Premalignant (Noninvasive) Stage (Dysplasia)
- Dysplastic cells limited to the surface squamous epithelium with abnormal cellular organization and maturation, increased mitotic activity, and nuclear enlargement with pleomorphism

Malignant (Invasive) Stage
- **Keratinizing-type SCC:** infiltrating nests and cords of cells showing varying degrees of squamous differentiation (pink cytoplasm, intercellular bridges and keratin pearl formation)
- Desmoplastic stromal reaction including stromal fibrosis and chronic inflammation
- **Nonkeratinizing-type SCC (oropharynx):** large, rounded nests of blue cells with little cytoplasm and hyperchromatic, ovoid nuclei; brisk mitotic activity and little keratinizing maturation.
- Specific variants characterized by verrucous, papillary (papillary variant), spindled or pleomorphic, or basaloid (basaloid variant) appearances of the tumor cells

Fine Needle Aspiration
- Atypical squamous cells in a background of keratinous and necrotic cystic debris

Immunohistochemical Features
- Immunoreactivity for epithelial markers (e.g., p63 and cytokeratins 5/6 and 34βE12)
- p16 positive: strong and diffuse nuclear and cytoplasmic expression in oropharyngeal carcinoma (HPV associated)

Pathologic Differential Diagnosis
- Pseudoepitheliomatous hyperplasia, verrucous hyperplasia, necrotizing sialometaplasia, squamous papilloma, sarcoma, malignant melanoma, solid variant of adenoid cystic carcinoma, high-grade neuroendocrine carcinoma

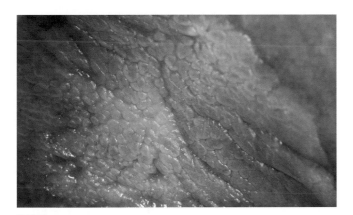

FIGURE 9-1

This patch of leukoplakia is seen as a white thickening of the buccal mucosa. *(Courtesy of Dr. J. Sciubba.)*

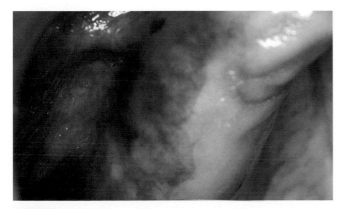

FIGURE 9-2

This patch of erythroplakia is seen as a subtle, red lesion of the buccal mucosa and alveolar ridge. *(Courtesy of Dr. J. Sciubba.)*

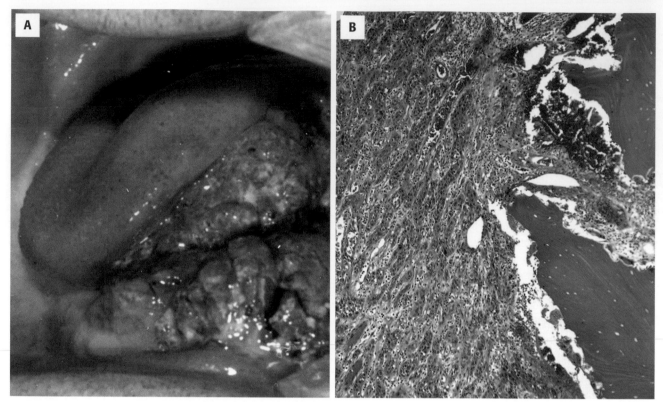

FIGURE 9-3

A, A large fungating squamous cell carcinoma involving the floor of mouth, tongue, and alveolar ridge. **B**, Histologic findings of squamous cell carcinoma, keratinizing type, showing a tumor with irregular nests of cells that have abundant, eosinophilic cytoplasm. The tumor invades the adjacent bone.

GROSS FINDINGS

The gross appearance of squamous lesions varies from subtle grayish-white thickening of the mucosa to large ulcerated, flat, or fungating masses with invasion of local structures. Depending on the degree of desmoplasia and tumor necrosis, the cut surface of invasive tumors ranges from solid and firm to cystic and friable.

MICROSCOPIC FINDINGS

Dysplasia refers to neoplastic alterations of the surface epithelium prior to invasion of the submucosa. These changes include abnormal cellular organization, increased mitotic activity, and nuclear enlargement with pleomorphism. Although terminology varies, pleomorphism limited to the lower third of the epithelium is generally referred to as mild dysplasia (Figure 9-4), pleomorphism limited to the lower two-thirds as moderate dysplasia (Figure 9-5), and pleomorphism involving the full thickness as severe dysplasia/carcinoma in situ (Figure 9-6). However, forms of severe dysplasia certainly can have less than full-thickness atypia.

With progression, cells invade through the basement membrane. With advanced tumor growth, tumor nests invade skeletal muscle and craniofacial bones (Figure 9-3) and frequently develop perineural and lymphovascular space invasion. Tumor grade in oral SCC varies from well to poorly differentiated. Well-differentiated carcinomas show robust squamous differentiation with interconnecting nests of cells with pink cytoplasm, intercellular bridges, and keratin pearl formation. At the other extreme, poorly differentiated tumors show little mature squamous differentiation. Regardless of tumor grade, nests of infiltrating SCC tend to elicit a prominent host fibrotic stromal reaction (desmoplasia) (Figure 9-3).

In contrast, HPV-related oropharyngeal SCC frequently adopts a "blue cell" morphology, characterized by scant cytoplasm and hyperchromatic nuclei, referred to as "nonkeratinizing" SCC. This type usually lacks surface involvement and has large nests with smooth edges, little or no stromal reaction, and no (or limited) squamous maturation (Figure 9-7). Mitotic activity is brisk. Lymphoepithelium-like oropharyngeal carcinoma and hybrid types having both keratinizing and nonkeratinizing features are also seen. Non-HPV-associated keratinizing SCC may also be seen in the oropharynx but are uncommon.

Certain variants of SCC depart from the typical appearance of conventional SCC. Except for the first variant, all of these can occur in the oropharynx as the result of HPV.

1. *Verrucous squamous cell carcinoma* (VSCC) is common in the oral cavity and presents as an exophytic

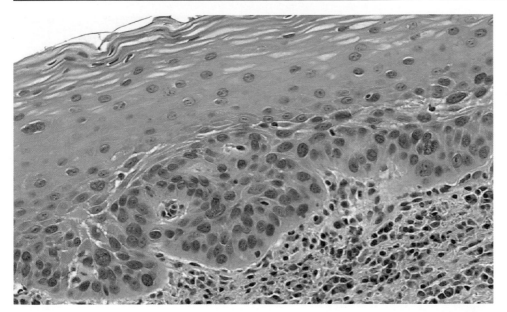

FIGURE 9-4

Mild dysplasia of the oral cavity with the atypical changes limited to the lower third of the epithelium.

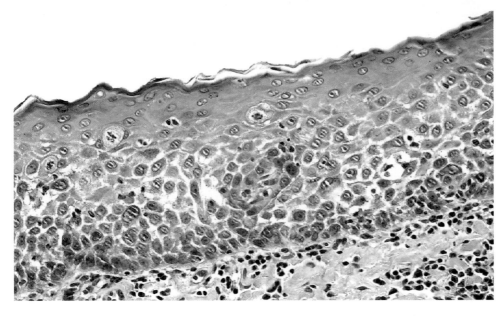

FIGURE 9-5

Moderate dysplasia of the oral cavity with the atypical cells present in up to two-thirds of the epithelium.

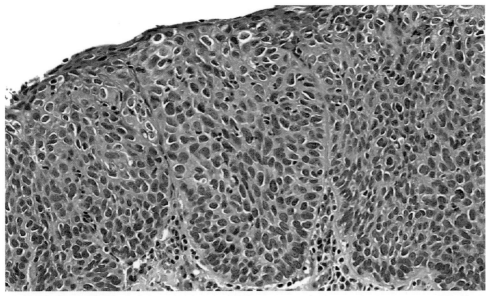

FIGURE 9-6

Severe dysplasia/carcinoma in situ with the atypical cells involving the full thickness of the epithelium, giving it a basophilic appearance and undulating contour.

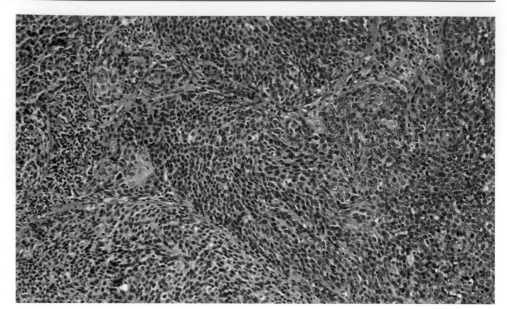

FIGURE 9-7

Nonkeratinizing squamous cell carcinoma of the oropharynx consisting of large sheets of tumor cells with oval nuclei, little cytoplasm, and no obvious maturing squamous differentiation. These findings are typical of human papillomavirus–related oropharyngeal carcinomas

mass with a warty, hyperkeratotic surface. Histologically, it has markedly thickened squamous epithelium with abundant hyperkeratosis and parakeratosis, with parakeratotic crypting (Figure 9-8). The tumor cells do not breach the basement membrane, so the tumor only invades as a pushing border. It lacks any significant atypia, shows limited mitoses (basal zone), and has no metastatic potential.

2. The *papillary variant* is common in the oropharynx and is characterized by a prominent exophytic component of papillae (Figure 9-9). In contrast to the benign squamous papilloma, these papillary fronds are diffusely lined by overtly malignant squamous cells.

3. The *spindle cell variant* is common in the oral cavity, classically presents as an exophytic, bosselated mass (Figure 9-10), and is characterized by sheets of spindled and/or pleomorphic cells, usually admixed with a component of typical invasive squamous carcinoma (Figure 9-11).

4. The *basaloid variant* is common in the oropharynx. It is characterized by expanding lobules of hyperchromatic, round, basaloid cells that have a "jigsaw puzzle" pattern, hyalinized, nodular stroma, and only focal areas of mature squamous differentiation (Figure 9-12).

5. The *adenosquamous variant* is seen rarely in both oral cavity and oropharynx and is defined by the presence of an SCC component admixed with true, rounded glands that are almost, but not always, associated with mucin production.

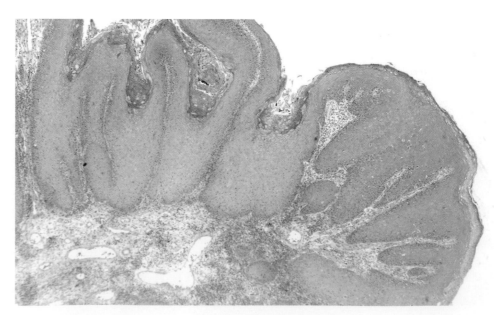

FIGURE 9-8

Verrucous carcinoma consists of masses of hyperkeratotic, thick, eosinophilic ("glassy") epithelium crowding into itself, while maintaining an intact basement membrane, such that it projects outward and develops a pushing downward stromal invasion.

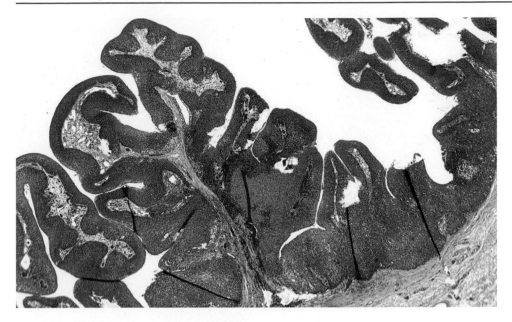

FIGURE 9-9

The papillary variant has delicate, papillary fronds diffusely lined by a cytologically malignant squamous epithelium.

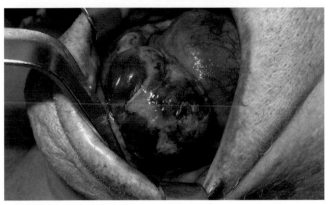

FIGURE 9-10

In spindle cell carcinoma, the gross appearance is usually of an exophytic, smooth, and partially ulcerated, polypoid mass—in this case, in the oral cavity. (*Courtesy of Dr. B. Nussenbaum.*)

ANCILLARY STUDIES

FINE NEEDLE ASPIRATION

Many patients present with cervical metastases, and some do not have an obvious primary lesion. Fine needle aspiration is effective in establishing a diagnosis of metastatic SCC. Cytologic smears are often cellular with both syncytial fragments of large pleomorphic cells as well as singly dispersed cells. These cells characteristically have large nuclei, prominent nucleoli, and dense, pink ("squamoid"-appearing) cytoplasm on Papanicolaou staining. If cell block material is obtained, staining for p16 may help to suggest an oropharyngeal primary site.

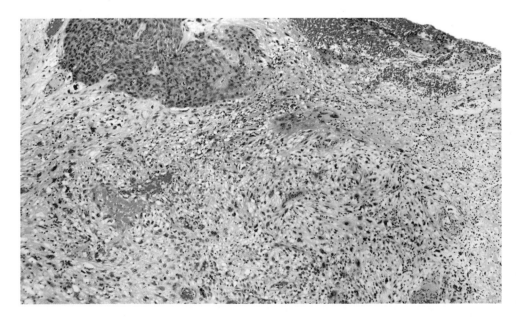

FIGURE 9-11

In spindle cell carcinoma, the spindled cells can be mistaken for a sarcoma. In this example, a component of severe dysplasia/carcinoma in situ is visible (*upper left*) with a sheet of malignant pleomorphic and spindled cells beneath it (*middle* and *lower right*).

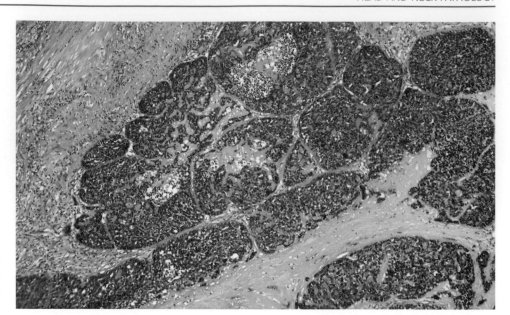

FIGURE 9-12

Basaloid squamous cell carcinoma infiltrates as rounded lobules of tumor cells having high nuclear:cytoplasmic ratios. The nests of tumor cells characteristically mold to one another, leaving only thin lines of intervening stroma.

IMMUNOHISTOCHEMICAL FEATURES

Immunohistochemistry is only rarely necessary for the diagnosis of poorly differentiated SCC. Most SCCs express a wide spectrum of cytokeratins (pan-keratin, CK5/6, 34βE12) and p63 and lack expression of lymphoid, melanocytic, and mesenchymal markers. In the oropharynx, p16, a tumor suppressor gene that is aberrantly overexpressed in HPV-infected cells, is strongly and diffusely expressed in HPV-related SCC (Figure 9-13).

DIFFERENTIAL DIAGNOSIS

SCCs can be mistaken for reactive non-neoplastic squamous proliferations of the oral cavity such as pseudo-epitheliomatous hyperplasia, radiation-induced atypia, and necrotizing sialometaplasia—a proliferation of metaplastic squamous cells within the ducts and acini of minor salivary glands. These reactive processes are generally preceded by an inciting event (e.g., ulceration,

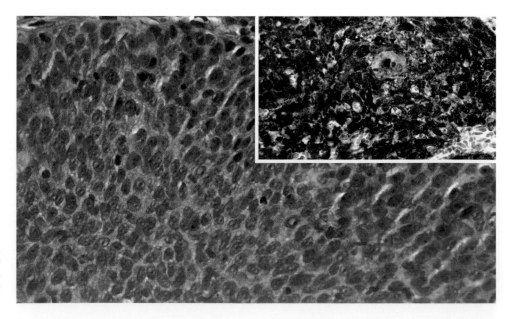

FIGURE 9-13

A nonkeratinizing squamous cell carcinoma with a sheet-like distribution of basaloid cells. *Inset:* Strong, diffuse, nuclear and cytoplasmic reactivity with p16 immunohistochemistry.

radiation) and, in contrast to SCC, do not display infiltrative growth, stromal desmoplasia, or overtly malignant cytology. At the other extreme, poorly differentiated and nonkeratinizing SCCs can be confused with various nonepithelial malignancies such as melanoma, sarcoma, or lymphoma. In this setting, immunohistochemistry may play a useful role in establishing the diagnosis of carcinoma by demonstrating positive staining for keratins and p63 and no staining for melanocytic, mesenchymal, or lymphoid markers. In addition, occasional tumors may resemble the solid variant of adenoid cystic carcinoma or a high-grade neuroendocrine tumor.

PROGNOSIS AND THERAPY

The overall 5-year survival rate for oral cavity SCC is ~50%. However, the tumor stage greatly determines outcome: stage I SCCs of the oral cavity are associated with survival rates of 80% to 90%, but this drops to 30% for locally or regionally advanced disease (stage III or IV). In contrast, oropharyngeal SCC has two distinct prognostic types—those related to high-risk HPV and those that are not. The p16 antibody is an effective surrogate marker for HPV infection. Overall 5-year survival for p16-positive cases is ~80% compared to 40% to 50% for those that are negative.

Treatment options are highly variable and depend on many factors, including size and location of the primary tumor, spread to regional lymph nodes or distant sites, and the patient's ability to tolerate treatment. For oral cavity SCC, primary surgery is the standard treatment. Adjuvant radiation and chemotherapy are often used for more advanced stage disease. For oropharyngeal SCC, all treatment approaches are effective, including primary radiation, primary chemoradiation, and primary surgery with or without adjuvant chemoradiation. Treatment type depends largely on the institution, but intensity-modulated radiation therapy seems to yield a better prognosis with HPV-associated tumors.

■ KAPOSI SARCOMA

Kaposi sarcoma (KS) is a malignant neoplasm of endothelial cells. Although historically rarely encountered in the oral cavity, an AIDS-related form of KS has resulted in a dramatic increase in the number of cases.

CLINICAL FEATURES

Four distinct clinical subtypes of KS are recognized: (1) *classic* form occurring primarily in older men of

---

KAPOSI SARCOMA—DISEASE FACT SHEET

Definition
- A vascular neoplasm unique to certain patient populations, most notably in individuals with AIDS

Incidence and Location
- Non–AIDS-related forms of KS are rare and mostly confined to older men of eastern European or Mediterranean descent, individuals in certain regions of Africa, and transplant recipients
- KS is common in patients with AIDS (~15% to 20%)
- Palate is the most common oral site, followed by the gingiva and dorsal tongue

Gender, Race, and Age Distribution
- In HIV-infected population, oral KS most commonly encountered in homosexual men with peak incidence in 4th decade

Clinical Features
- Oral lesions commonly multifocal
- Early lesions: flat, red, and asymptomatic
- Older lesions: larger, darker, nodular, and ulcerated

Prognosis and Treatment
- Mortality dependent on patient's immunologic status, presence of opportunistic infections, disease stage, and other factors
- General treatment: active antiretroviral therapy, radiation, chemotherapy
- Local treatment of problematic oral lesions: surgery, cryotherapy, laser ablation, intralesional injections of chemotherapeutic or sclerosing agents

---

eastern European (especially Ashkenazi Jew) or Mediterranean descent; (2) *endemic* form common to regions of Africa and particularly prevalent among young Bantu children of South Africa; (3) *transplant-associated* form occurring after high doses of immunosuppressive therapy; and (4) *AIDS-associated* form that is particularly prevalent among HIV-infected homosexual males. KS develops in 15% to 20% of patients with AIDS and is considered an AIDS-defining illness. Regardless of the form, all KS lesions are infected with human herpesvirus 8 (HHV-8). Immunosuppression is a critical cofactor in the pathogenesis and clinical expression of disease.

The AIDS-associated form is the most likely subtype to be encountered in the oral cavity. KS represents the most frequent HIV-associated oral cancer (followed by non-Hodgkin lymphoma). In the HIV-infected population, oral KS is most common in homosexual men with a peak incidence in the 4th decade. The palate is the most common subsite, often showing multiple lesions; moreover, concurrent cutaneous and visceral organ lesions are frequently present. The clinical appearance changes with lesion progression. Early lesions are flat, red, and asymptomatic, and later lesions become larger, darker, and raised (Figure 9-14). With continued growth,

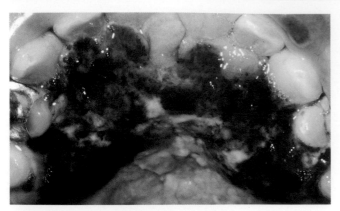

FIGURE 9-14

Clinical image of an advanced stage of oral Kaposi sarcoma seen as diffuse, reddish-purple nodules of the hard palate.

these large nodular lesions may become ulcerated and painful.

PATHOLOGIC FEATURES

GROSS FINDINGS

Early lesions are small, flat, and red. Advanced lesions are larger, deep-red to purple, and nodular.

MICROSCOPIC FINDINGS

KS is a nonencapsulated, infiltrative lesion. The histomorphology varies with stage of progression. The histologic findings in early stages of KS (patch stage) are

---

KAPOSI SARCOMA—PATHOLOGIC FEATURES

Gross Findings
- Early lesions: small, red, and flat
- Advanced lesions: large, deep-red to purple, and nodular

Microscopic Findings
- Early lesions (patch stage): proliferation of dilated, irregular blood vessels
- Maturing lesions (plaque stage): dilated vascular channels surrounded by aggregates of spindle cells
- Advanced lesions (nodular stage): cellular proliferation of spindle cells, slit-like vascular spaces, extravasated blood cells, hemosiderin deposits, and hyaline globules

Immunohistochemical Features
- Human herpesvirus 8 and variable expression for endothelial markers (CD31, CD34)

Pathologic Differential Diagnosis
- Reactive vascular ectasia, bacillary angiomatosis, lobular capillary hemangioma, well-differentiated angiosarcoma

---

subtle. The submucosa may show nothing more than an ill-defined proliferation of dilated, irregular, angulated blood vessels with associated chronic inflammatory cells (Figure 9-15). As the lesions progress (plaque stage), the dilated vascular channels become surrounded by aggregates of spindle cells. In advanced lesions, the histology is dominated by a highly cellular proliferation of spindle cells separated by slit-like vascular spaces containing red blood cells (Figure 9-16). The spindle cells are elongated with minimal atypia, and mitotic figures are not abundant. The presence of pleomorphism and high mitotic activity is unusual, and these generally portend a more aggressive behavior. The background shows an admixture of extravasated erythrocytes, hemosiderin, and small eosinophilic hyaline bodies (Figure 9-16, *inset*). Dilated vessels and chronic inflammatory cells are noted at the periphery of the lesion.

ANCILLARY STUDIES

KS tumor cells are immunoreactive for CD34, CD31, and other endothelial markers. However, as the differential diagnosis is virtually limited to other vascular proliferations, immunohistochemical confirmation of endothelial differentiation is not helpful. In contrast, the HHV-8-specific immunohistochemical stain is often helpful in separating KS from other vascular lesions.

DIFFERENTIAL DIAGNOSIS

The differential diagnosis is largely contingent on the histologic stage. Early lesions, due to their subtle changes, may be dismissed as reactive vascular ectasia. As the lesion progresses, the proliferation of vessels becomes more apparent, and may cause confusion with lobular capillary hemangioma (pyogenic granuloma), bacillary angiomatosis, and even well-differentiated angiosarcoma. Lobular capillary hemangioma classically shows a collarette of epithelium and lacks the hyaline globules of KS and HHV-8 positivity. In bacillary angiomatosis, a Warthin-Starry stain will reveal the slender bacilli of *Bartonella henselae* among the granular material in the interstitium. Angiosarcoma, with its classic endothelial "hobnailing," may show greater pleomorphism, mitoses, and necrosis and is also not HHV-8 associated.

PROGNOSIS AND THERAPY

The improved management and survival in HIV due to antiretroviral therapy, especially highly active

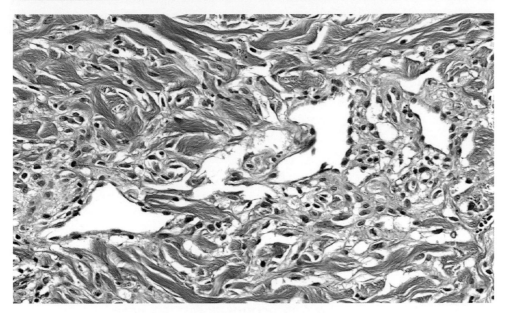

FIGURE 9-15

In the early (patch) phase, histologically, Kaposi sarcoma appears only as irregular, dilated blood vessels dissecting between collagen bundles.

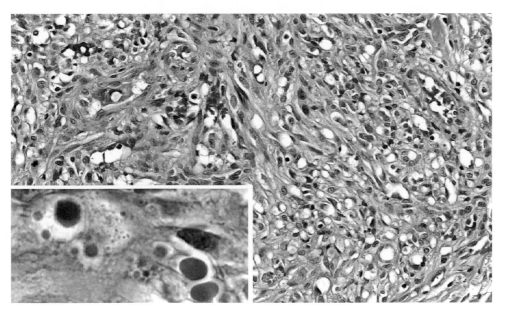

FIGURE 9-16

In the advanced (nodular) phase, the submucosa is infiltrated by cellular, nodular aggregates of spindled cells forming slit-like spaces. The background has abundant extravasated red blood cells and hyaline globules (*inset*).

antiretroviral therapy (HAART), has dramatically decreased the incidence of oral KS. Moreover, without correction of the underlying immunodeficiency, survival is poor—hence, the institution (or reinstitution) of HAART in combination with radiation and/or chemotherapy, which are the more general standard treatments of KS. Local symptoms can be controlled by intralesional injection of chemotherapeutic or sclerosing agents or by removal via surgery, cryotherapy, or laser therapy.

Nevertheless, the disease course and overall behavior depend greatly on the clinical subtype, amount of dissemination, disease stage, and presence of systemic symptoms and related comorbidities.

SUGGESTED READINGS

The complete suggested readings list is available online at
   www.expertconsult.com.

10

Non-Neoplastic Lesions of the Salivary Glands

■ **Mary S. Richardson**

■ DEVELOPMENTAL, INCLUDING HETEROTOPIA AND ONCOCYTOSIS

Salivary glands are composed of three paired major glands—the parotid, the submandibular, and the sublingual—and roughly a thousand minor seromucous glands that are distributed throughout the sinonasal tract, oral cavity, pharynx, larynx, and lower respiratory tract. The minor salivary glands secrete continuously, while the major glands secrete mainly in response to parasympathetic activity induced by stimuli. All the glands develop from ingrowths of surface epithelium and have a common architecture with varying acinar compositions of serous and mucus cell types: The parotid glands are almost entirely serous, the sublingual glands are predominantly mucous, and the submandibular glands contain both serous and mucous cells. These secretory units empty into excretory ducts lined by cuboidal to columnar epithelium. All salivary glands are vulnerable to the same disorders.

Not only are lesions of salivary gland uncommon, but they encompass a heterogeneous group of disorders. Enlargement of salivary glands is most often due to non-neoplastic or inflammatory conditions, including developmental abnormalities, hyperplasia, metaplasia, cysts, and inflammatory diseases. Of these, heterotopia and oncocytosis will be discussed.

CLINICAL FEATURES

Heterotopia of salivary gland is the existence of salivary gland tissue in locations external to the major and minor salivary glands. (In contrast, accessory salivary glands are defined as isolated lobules of glands situated along a major salivary duct.) Heterotopic or ectopic salivary gland tissue has been reported in a myriad of anatomic locations (Table 10-1) and is usually found incidentally, although it may be

DEVELOPMENTAL, INCLUDING HETEROTOPIA AND ONCOCYTOSIS—DISEASE FACT SHEET

Definition
- Heterotopia: salivary gland tissue in a location external to the major and minor salivary glands
- Oncocytes are transformed acinar or ductal cells with finely granular eosinophilic cytoplasm, categorized as oncocytic metaplasia, oncocytosis (nodular or diffuse), and oncocytoma

Incidence and Location
- Heterotopia most commonly involves the parotid and cervical lymph nodes
- Oncocytic tumors of salivary gland are rare (<1%)

Gender and Age Distribution
- Salivary gland heterotopia has no known age or gender predilection
- Oncocytic lesions are uncommon in patients <50 years, with a peak incidence in the 7th to 9th decades

Clinical Features
- Heterotopia is usually found incidentally or as a mass secondary to an inflammatory or neoplastic process
- Oncocytic lesions (oncocytosis/oncocytoma) may be multifocal within the gland, unilateral, or bilateral

Prognosis and Treatment
- Simple excision if clinically indicated for heterotopia
- Oncocytic lesions are usually not recurrent; however, oncocytoma has a 0% to 30% recurrence rate

discovered due to signs and symptoms associated with inflammation or neoplasia. The more common sites for heterotopic salivary gland are the middle ear, neck, mandible, and pituitary gland. Sites outside the head and neck include the mediastinum, stomach, prostate gland, rectum, and vulva. Removal of these salivary gland tissue deposits may occur for cosmetic reasons, as intervention for a congenital abnormality

TABLE 10-1

Reported Sites of Heterotopic Salivary Tissues

Middle ear	Mediastinum
External auditory canal	Pituitary gland
Neck	Cerebellopontine angle
Thyroglossal duct cyst	Stomach
Mandible (intraosseous)	Rectum
Cervical and paraparotid lymph nodes	Prostate gland

(oncocytosis), or due to neoplasia. In the case of malignancy, confusion may arise, particularly if the remaining normal gland architecture has been destroyed, as to whether the tumor is primary in heterotopic salivary gland tissue versus a metastatic deposit from a nearby salivary gland.

Oncocytes are characterized by the presence of abundant finely granular, bright eosinophilic cytoplasm surrounding a round nucleus that contains a single nucleolus. The granular cytoplasm is due to an overabundance of mitochondria. The number and distribution of oncocytic cells in salivary gland vary, as does the growth pattern. The occurrence of oncocytic cells in salivary gland can be categorized as oncocytic metaplasia within a duct or isolated aggregate, focal and diffuse oncocytosis, multifocal oncocytic hyperplasia, and oncocytoma. *Oncocytic metaplasia* involves the abnormal change or transformation (metaplasia) of acinar cells (serous, mucous, and seromucous) and/or striated ducts to oncocytes. Oncocytic metaplasia is uncommon before the age of 50 and increases with advancing age. The metaplasia is usually seen focally within a duct and

may be found in conjunction with salivary gland neoplasms (pleomorphic adenoma, mucoepidermoid carcinoma). *Oncocytosis* is an unencapsulated (mass-forming) collection of oncocytes, which may occur in minor or major salivary glands. This alteration may involve either ducts, predominantly, or acini and may be associated with fatty infiltration and acinar atrophy. The rare condition *multifocal nodular oncocytic hyperplasia (MNOH)* is characterized by multiple nodules of oncocytic cells in a lobular distribution within a salivary gland (Figure 10-1). MNOH has been reported associated with oncocytoma and benign or malignant salivary gland neoplasms. These nodules or islands may be large, but they lack the encapsulation of an oncocytoma. The oncocytic islands of MNOH may involve the intraparotid lymph nodes, which often contain salivary gland ducts, or the hilum of the lymph node. It is worth highlighting that these oncocytic islands within the lymph nodes can be incorrectly confused with a metastatic deposit.

PATHOLOGIC FEATURES

GROSS FINDINGS

On gross examination, the heterotopic salivary gland tissue has the characteristic features of normal salivary gland tissue, which usually has a yellow-tan firm and lobulated appearance. There is no definitive gross for oncocytosis, but larger lesions (which may measure up to 7 cm) may reveal tan to light brown nodules.

MICROSCOPIC FINDINGS

Like any salivary gland, histologic sections of heterotopia reveal a variably mixed population of large pale

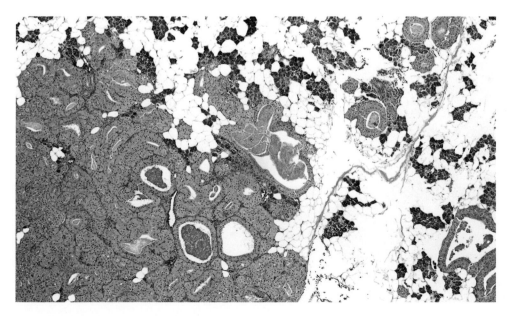

FIGURE 10-1

At medium power, notice the distribution of oncocytic proliferation within the salivary gland tissue. This proliferation can be seen diffusely throughout the salivary gland tissue.

DEVELOPMENTAL, INCLUDING HETEROTOPIA AND ONCOCYTOSIS—PATHOLOGIC FEATURES

Gross Findings

- Oncocytic nodules may measure up to 7 cm, with small, cystic areas

Microscopic Findings

- Oncocytic cells are characterized by finely granular, eosinophilic cytoplasm
- There is a single round nucleus with conspicuous nucleolus
- Architectural growth patterns are usually organoid with variable areas showing cording and prominent capillaries
- Oncocytes may undergo "clear cell" change

Ancillary Studies

- PTAH stain accentuates granules

Pathologic Differential Diagnosis

- When clear cell oncocytes are present, differential includes metastasis from clear cell mucoepidermoid carcinoma, clear cell acinic cell, and renal cell carcinoma

mucous cells with poorly staining mucigen granules and condensed peripheral nuclei and the more basophilic serous cells with strongly staining zymogen granules and central nuclei. Intermixed are the intercalated ducts with a lining of cuboidal secretory cells.

Histologic examination of an oncocytic lesion shows the characteristic polygonal cells with abundant finely granular eosinophilic cytoplasm. This oncocytic transformation can involve acinar and ductal cells and the cytologic distinction can be striking (Figure 10-2). The nuclei are usually uniformly round with granular chromatin and contain a single nucleolus. Mitotic figures are absent or rare. The presence of a complete or partial fibrous capsule surrounding an oncocytoma will aid in the distinction between an oncocytoma and nodular oncocytic hyperplasia. Oncocytes may grow as a solid nodule of cells or within ducts. There may be unencapsulated focal cystic areas with papillary proliferations within ducts or as an isolated parenchymal aggregate. The architectural growth pattern of the cells within a solid nodule is often organoid or forming cords in a hepatoid pattern. The individual cells show a variable eosinophilic staining quality (Figure 10-3) and, on a rare occasion, may contain focal or diffuse clear cells.

ANCILLARY STUDIES

Although not necessary for the diagnosis, the following may be useful in demonstrating the presence of mitochondria within oncocytic lesions.

ULTRASTRUCTURAL FEATURES

On ultrastructural evaluation, abundant mitochondria may completely fill the cytoplasmic compartment. The mitochondria show some variability in their shape, ranging from round to irregular and elongate. Desmosomal cell attachments are identified.

HISTOCHEMICAL FEATURES

A phosphotungstic acid–hematoxylin stain (PTAH) will stain mitochondria varying intensities of blue. The results of this stain, however, are not always consistent.

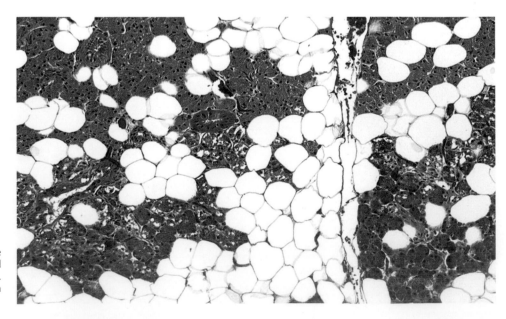

FIGURE 10-2

At medium power, the tinctorial difference between the basophilic acinar cells and the eosinophilic oncocytes is easily noted. Oncocytic metaplasia may be seen in acinar and ductal cells.

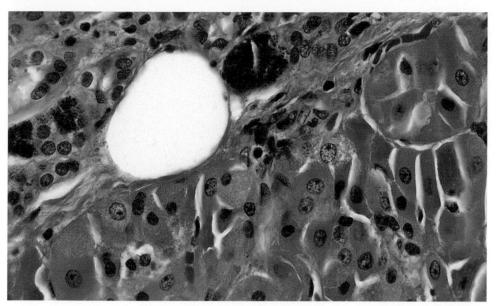

FIGURE 10-3
At high power, the finely granular eosinophilic cytoplasm and round nuclei with a single nucleolus are seen. Note the variability in eosinophilic staining of the oncocytic cytoplasm.

FINE NEEDLE ASPIRATION

On fine needle aspiration, oncocytes are easily identified with abundant, well-defined, finely granular cytoplasm and large round nuclei with prominent nucleoli. Distinguishing oncocytic metaplasia from oncocytomas, however, is done on excised lesions.

DIFFERENTIAL DIAGNOSIS

Distinguishing between nodular hyperplasia, nodular oncocytosis, and oncocytoma may be problematic and sometimes impossible. Some authorities define an oncocytoma as a *single* nodule, while others require the presence of at least a partial *capsule*. The distinction between oncocytic hyperplasia and neoplasia is still not well defined. Oncocytic metaplasia and a variety of clear cell neoplasms are included in the differential diagnosis with oncocytoma. Areas of oncocytic metaplasia have been reported in pleomorphic adenomas and within mucoepidermoid carcinomas; however, these areas are usually isolated. Furthermore, oncocytomas lack the architectural patterns of these two neoplasms: Focal mucus cell differentiation and squamous metaplasia are exceedingly rare within oncocytomas and help distinguish oncocytoma from mucoepidermoid carcinoma; and oncocytomas do not have myoepithelial cell proliferation with ductal structures, or myxoid or chondroid differentiation, which is characteristic of pleomorphic adenoma.

Acinic cell carcinoma may be difficult to distinguish from a multinodular oncocytic hyperplasia. However, the presence of zymogen granules combined with the microcystic and papillary follicular growth patterns of acinic cell carcinoma is not seen in oncocytic hyperplasia.

PROGNOSIS AND THERAPY

Oncocytic metaplasia and oncocytosis are usually identified in a gland removed for another reason. No therapy is necessary for these benign reactions. Heterotopias are excised for symptomatic relief in some cases, with an excellent prognosis.

■ MUCUS RETENTION CYST, MUCOCELE, AND SIALOLITHIASIS

CLINICAL FEATURES

The most common non-neoplastic lesion of salivary gland tissue is the mucocele. The mucocele is defined as the pooling of mucin in a cystic cavity. Two types of mucoceles are described: (1) the retention type (Figure 10-4), characterized by mucin pooling confined within a dilated excretory duct (Figures 10-5 and 10-6), and (2) the extravasation type (Figure 10-7), showing escape of salivary-secreted mucin from the duct system into connective tissue (Figures 10-8 and 10-9). The extravasated type is the most common mucocele, and its peak incidence is in the 3rd decade. The lower lip is the most common site, followed by the tongue, floor of mouth, palate, and buccal mucosa. These often appear as blue-tinged, dome-shaped swellings. A large mucocele that may arise in the floor of the mouth from the sublingual or minor salivary gland and descend into the soft tissues of the floor of the mouth is called a ranula. The mucus retention cyst is more common in the parotid and submandibular glands, and the peak incidence is in the 7th to 8th decades.

MUCUS RETENTION CYST, MUCOCELE, AND SIALOLITHIASIS—DISEASE FACT SHEET

Definition
- The pooling of salivary mucus within a cystic cavity resulting from blockage/rupture of a salivary gland duct

Incidence and Location
- Most common non-neoplastic lesion of salivary glands
- Lower lip is the most common site, followed by tongue, floor of mouth, palate, and buccal mucosa
- Mucoceles in the floor of mouth are called "ranula"

Gender and Age Distribution
- Equal gender distribution
- Peak incidence in 3rd decade
- Most common intraoral lesion in the first two decades of life

Clinical Features
- Soft, fluctuant, semitranslucent, painless swelling that may be noted to occur after a traumatic event
- The lesion may fluctuate with meals or when ruptured secondary to trauma
- Lesion may be recurrent to the same site

Prognosis and Treatment
- Complete excision, including minor salivary gland, usually is adequate
- Recurrence is usually seen with inadequate excision

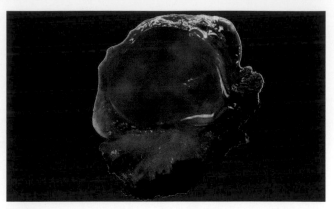

FIGURE 10-4

A macroscopic view of a mucocele showing a well-defined border filled with mucin.

RADIOLOGIC FEATURES

Sialoliths are always visible on radiographic examination. The Wharton duct of the submandibular gland is the most common site for a sialolith, which can be visualized easily on a radiograph (Figure 10-10).

PATHOLOGIC FEATURES

Histologically, the retention cyst captures the mucus within an epithelium-lined lumen. The cyst shows an attenuated epithelium. There is usually scant to no inflammatory infiltrate within the wall (Figure 10-5) unless there is adjacent rupture. In contrast, the lesions of extravasated mucin (mucocele) show compression of the adjacent connective tissue with a brisk inflammatory reaction circumscribing the mucin pool (Figure 10-8). Often within the infiltrate of the mucocele wall, there are

A sialolith is a collection of often laminated concretions that form a stone within the salivary gland excretory duct system. Sialolithiasis most frequently involves the submandibular gland and may cause a chronic sclerosing sialadenitis distal to the stone (Figure 10-10). The stone will cause distention of the duct system and retention of secreted fluids, resulting in glandular swelling and pain.

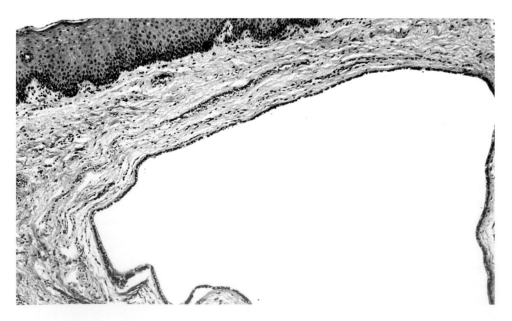

FIGURE 10-5

At low power, the dilated, epithelial lined cavity of a mucus cyst is apparent. The mucus has not extravasated into the tissues.

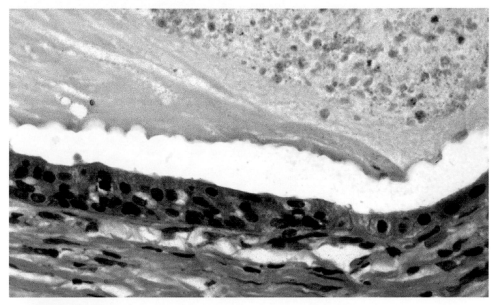

FIGURE 10-6

At high power, the low cuboidal lining of the cyst is seen. There is very little inflammatory response in the subjacent connective tissue.

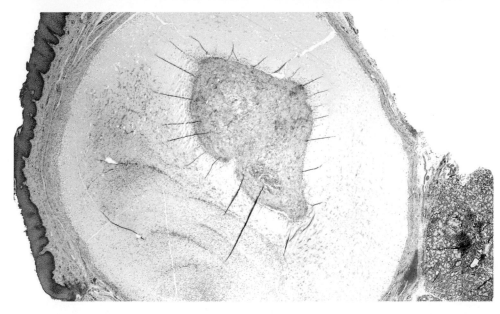

FIGURE 10-7

At low power, the circumscribed extravasated mucus is identified.

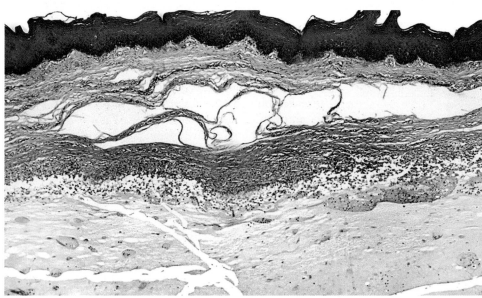

FIGURE 10-8

At medium power, the absence of an epithelial lining and mixed inflammatory infiltrate is noted at the mucus and connective tissue interface.

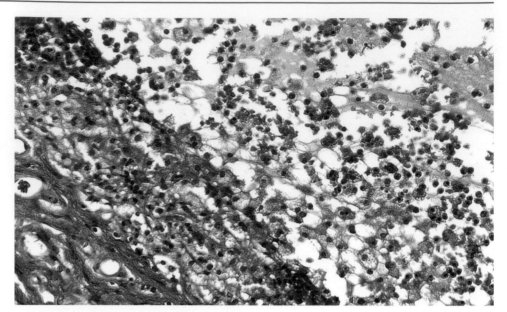

FIGURE 10-9

At high power, a prominent inflammatory infiltrate and foamy, mucin-laden macrophages are noted within the connective tissue and within the mucin. No epithelium is identified.

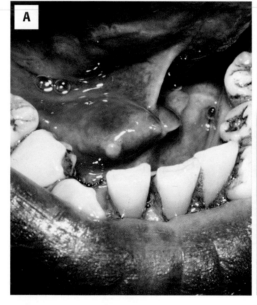

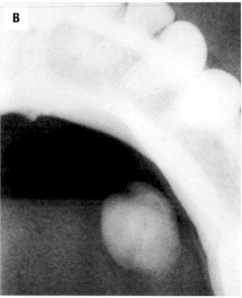

FIGURE 10-10

A, A sialolith (stone) present at the orifice of Wharton duct is just beginning to protrude from the lumen of the duct. **B**, Sialoliths are common in Wharton duct of the submandibular gland. The lamination of the sialolith can be appreciated on this radiograph.

MUCUS RETENTION CYST, MUCOCELE, AND SIALOLITHIASIS—PATHOLOGIC FEATURES

Gross Findings

- Cystic cavity within connective tissue containing glistening fluid

Microscopic Findings

- Circumscribed mucin with inflammation within the wall
- Retention cyst has epithelial lining of the lumen

Ancillary Studies

- PAS and mucicarmine stain mucin

Pathologic Differential Diagnosis

- Organizing hematoma

---

numerous foamy macrophages containing phagocytized mucin (Figure 10-9). As the lesion progresses, granulation tissue from the wall becomes more prominent and organizes to obliterate the lumen of the mucocele. In a primarily granulation tissue–laden lesion, a mucicarmine stain will highlight the residual mucin-containing macrophages.

A sialolith will frequently demonstrate a nidus of cellular debris found in the center of the concentric laminated calcium deposits (Figure 10-11).

DIFFERENTIAL DIAGNOSIS

Few entities enter into the differential diagnosis of an extravasated-type mucocele. Certainly, a resolving

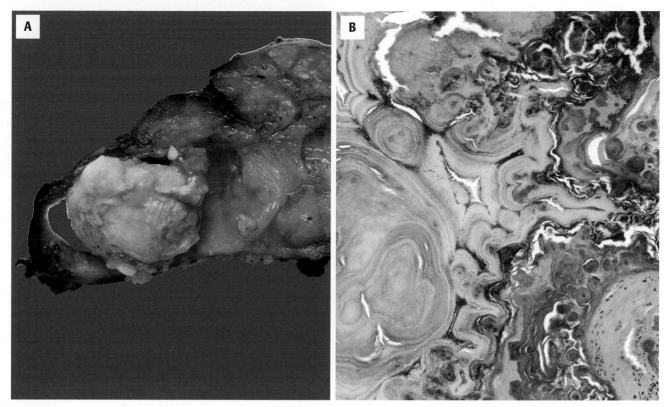

FIGURE 10-11
A, Macroscopically, there is a sialolith within the duct of the submandibular gland. **B**, At low power, the laminated concretions around nidi of cellular debris are seen in this section of a sialolith.

extravasated mucocele with only remaining granulation tissue may be misinterpreted as a small hematoma or a thrombus. The use of mucicarmine, however, would illustrate the presence of mucin-laden macrophages and aid in this distinction. The mucus retention cyst is lined by a thin layer of cuboidal epithelium with little to no inflammatory cell infiltrate. Mucoepidermoid carcinoma could enter the differential diagnosis of a mucus retention cyst. Mucoepidermoid carcinoma, however, contains three cell types: mucus goblet cells, intermediate cells, and squamous cells. Moreover, within mucus retention cysts, the epithelium is attenuated and lacks papillary projections that protrude into the lumen.

Prognosis and Therapy

Surgical excision to include the minor mucoserous gland is suggested, as clinically indicated by the patient's condition. Alginate has been used by some with varying results. Recurrence is seen in patients with inadequate excision. Lithotripsy, sialoendoscopy, and other supportive measures are used for symptomatic sialoliths.

■ NECROTIZING SIALOMETAPLASIA

CLINICAL FEATURES

NECROTIZING SIALOMETAPLASIA—DISEASE FACT SHEET

Definition
- Ischemic necrosis of salivary gland tissue that maintains a lobular distribution

Incidence and Location
- Palate is most frequent site of involvement

Gender and Age Distribution
- Male predominance
- All ages affected

Clinical Features
- Rapid swelling of the mucosa with ulceration in a few days
- Lesion slowly heals over several weeks
- Patients complain of pain or numbness which simulates malignancy

Prognosis and Treatment
- No therapy is necessary for this self-healing process

Necrotizing sialometaplasia is an uncommon destructive reactive inflammatory process of the salivary gland. The clinical and histologic characteristics resemble those of malignant neoplasms and can lead to misdiagnosis and inappropriate therapy. The age range of reported patients with necrotizing sialometaplasia is from 1.5 to 83 years, with the average age of approximately 46 years. The lesion has a 2:1 predominance in men. Its etiology is somewhat speculative, although strong evidence suggests the cause may be vascular compromise leading to ischemic necrosis. The vast majority of these lesions affect the minor salivary glands in the hard palate or at the junction of the hard and soft palate (Figure 10-12). Lesions are most commonly unilateral; however, occasional bilateral or midline lesions develop. Other common sites for this lesion are oral cavity, lower lip, retromolar trigone, tongue, and buccal mucosa, although the entire upper aerodigestive tract can be affected. Occurrence of this lesion in major salivary glands, primarily the parotid gland, is uncommon, representing 8.5% of necrotizing sialometaplasia cases.

Clinically, the lesion appears in the palate as a deep, sharply defined, up to 3 cm crater-like ulcer that develops rapidly over a few days and fails to heal for an extended period of time. Duration of healing of this lesion can range up to 6 months, although most heal within 1 month. All such lesions that fail to resolve usually undergo a biopsy. Other symptoms associated with this lesion (pain or numbness) may simulate malignancy.

PATHOLOGIC FEATURES

GROSS FINDINGS

On gross examination, there is only a slight suggestion of softening of these submucosal tissues with a glistening cut surface. Usually there is no distinguishing mass.

NECROTIZING SIALOMETAPLASIA—PATHOLOGIC FEATURES

Gross Findings
- Usually the overlying mucosa shows ulceration
- Ulcer may be up to 3 cm

Microscopic Findings
- Lobular coagulative necrosis of glandular acini
- Prominent squamous metaplasia of salivary gland ducts
- Inflammation is present
- Pseudoepitheliomatous hyperplasia of the overlying mucosal epithelium may be seen

Pathologic Differential Diagnosis
- Squamous cell carcinoma, mucoepidermoid carcinoma

MICROSCOPIC FINDINGS

Microscopically, the characteristic feature of necrotizing sialometaplasia is ischemic necrosis or infarction, which is thought to be the primary pathogenetic mechanism of this lesion, with preservation of the lobular architecture. The key histologic features in identifying this lesion are (1) lobular coagulative necrosis of the salivary gland acini (Figures 10-13 and 10-14), (2) prominent and proliferative squamous metaplasia of the excretory ducts, (3) pseudoepitheliomatous hyperplasia of the overlying mucosa, and (4) prominent inflammatory infiltrate. The most prominent and useful features histologically are the coagulative necrosis and ductal metaplasia (Figure 10-15). In addition, the overall acinar architecture is preserved, despite necrotic mucinous acini showing the "ghosted" outline of coagulative necrosis, and with associated salivary ducts showing metaplastic squamous mucosa (Figure 10-16).

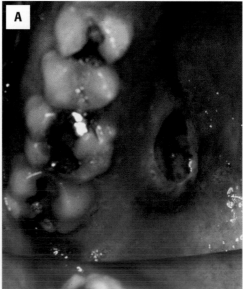
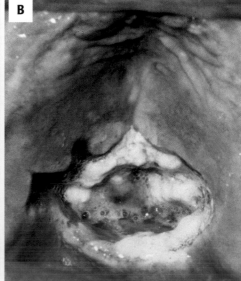

FIGURE 10-12

Two cases of necrotizing sialometaplasia as seen in the palate. **A**, A unilateral ulcer, showing a raised border and center crater. **B**, A large, crater-like ulceration in the midline. It is sharply defined, filled with exudate.

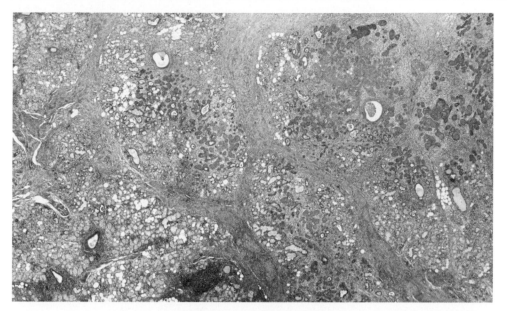

FIGURE 10-13

The lobules of salivary gland show multiple areas of squamous metaplasia as it replaces the areas of coagulative necrosis. Fibrosis is noted between the lobules.

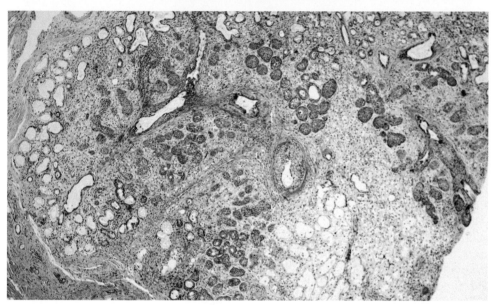

FIGURE 10-14

At low power, acinar alteration is noted; however, fibrous septa and ducts define the retained lobular architecture.

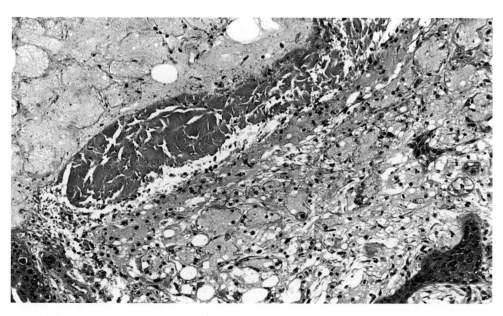

FIGURE 10-15

At medium power, there is extensive degeneration and necrosis with islands of squamous metaplasia (*lower*).

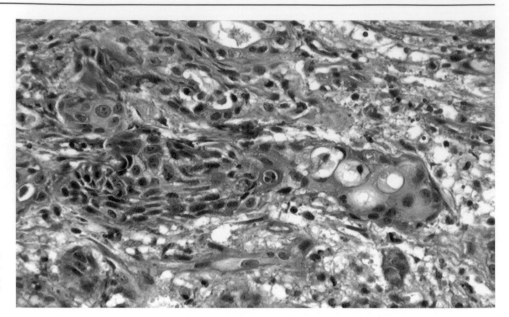

FIGURE 10-16

At high power, islands of squamous metaplasia are cytologically bland, not to be confused with malignancy. There is inflammation surrounding the outlines of the acini and ducts.

DIFFERENTIAL DIAGNOSIS

The diagnosis of necrotizing sialometaplasia can be problematic if the biopsy is not adequate or oriented properly. The chief differential diagnoses for this lesion are mucosal squamous cell carcinoma and mucoepidermoid carcinoma. In an adequately oriented biopsy, it is easy to distinguish these lesions based on the maintenance of the salivary gland lobular architecture. Also, the cytologic features of necrotizing sialometaplasia are bland. In addition, the inflammatory infiltrate characterizing necrotizing sialometaplasia is more prominent than that frequently associated with squamous cell carcinoma and mucoepidermoid carcinoma. Moreover, these two malignancies infiltrate the salivary gland parenchyma.

PROGNOSIS AND THERAPY

No specific therapy is required for necrotizing sialometaplasia. These lesions are self-healing.

■ BENIGN LYMPHOEPITHELIAL LESION

Benign lymphoepithelial lesion (BLEL) is used to describe a characteristic effacement of salivary parenchyma by a dense lymphocytic infiltrate. The term does not commit to an etiologic cause but refers to histologic findings.

CLINICAL FEATURES

Clinically, the lesions present as unilateral, bilateral, or diffuse enlargement of salivary glands (usually parotid) or lacrimal glands. This lesion may occur in children and adults of either gender; however, most cases present in women in the 4th and 5th decades.

BENIGN LYMPHOEPITHELIAL LESION—DISEASE FACT SHEET

Definition
- Salivary gland tissue with an intense lymphocytic infiltrate with associated epimyoepithelial islands

Incidence and Location
- Uncommon lesion

Morbidity and Mortality
- Increased risk of lymphoma

Gender and Age Distribution
- Female predominance
- Mean age, 50 years

Clinical Features
- 85% of cases occur in the parotid gland
- Diffuse swelling of the affected gland

Prognosis and Treatment
- Prognosis relates to development of lymphoma, which is usually a low-grade extranodal marginal zone B-cell lymphoma (MALT lymphoma)
- Surgery

BLEL is associated with, or a precursor to, Sjögren syndrome, a systemic autoimmune disease characterized by chronic inflammation in exocrine organs. In some cases, it is a precursor lesion to salivary mucosa-associated lymphoid tissue (MALT) lymphoma. Patients experience facial swelling with or without pain, dry mouth, and keratoconjunctivitis.

PATHOLOGIC FEATURES

GROSS FINDINGS

On gross examination, BLEL may be seen as diffuse enlargement of the gland or present as discrete tan micronodules. The gross appearance can be mistaken for a neoplastic process due to the multinodularity; however, the capsule in major salivary glands is intact.

BENIGN LYMPHOEPITHELIAL LESION—PATHOLOGIC FEATURES

Gross Findings
- Small tan nodules to diffuse replacement of gland by creamy tan tissue

Microscopic Findings
- Heavy lymphocytic infiltrate associated with destruction of salivary acini
- Proliferating epimyoepithelial islands

Pathologic Differential Diagnosis
- Lymphoma

MICROSCOPIC FINDINGS

BLEL is characterized histologically by irregular, multifocal islands of epithelial proliferations surrounded by a dense lymphocytic infiltrate (Figure 10-17). The extent of the lymphocytic infiltrate can vary within a lobule and ultimately progresses to total acinar atrophy with only remaining ducts (Figure 10-18). The remaining excretory ducts are usually infiltrated by intermediate-sized lymphocytes. Similar changes to those seen in the major salivary glands in BLEL can occur in the minor salivary glands of patients with Sjögren syndrome. The changes in minor glands include a chronic lymphocytic sialadenitis usually without epithelial hyperplasia. The changes seen in a labial minor salivary gland biopsy are supportive but not pathognomonic evidence for the diagnosis of Sjögren syndrome (Figure 10-19). Numeric grading systems are used based on the number of lymphocytic aggregates present in salivary gland lobules, but clinical and serologic confirmation is required for a definitive diagnosis. An aggregate (50 lymphocytes) is referred to as a "focus," resulting in a "focus score." It is important that the sample be obtained from normal tissue (i.e., not infected, inflamed, ulcerated, etc.) and that lymphocytes must be within the parenchyma, not in a periductal (sialodochitis) location or in association with heavy fibrosis (chronic sialadenitis).

ANCILLARY STUDIES

The lymphoid infiltrate that is present in these lesions is a mixture of T and B lymphocytes similar to those seen in hyperplastic lymph nodes. Plasma cells, eosinophils, and

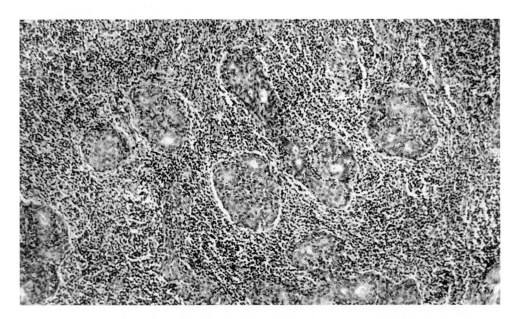

FIGURE 10-17

At intermediate power, the proliferative ductal epithelium is evident. The epimyoepithelial islands show infiltration by the lymphocytic infiltrate.

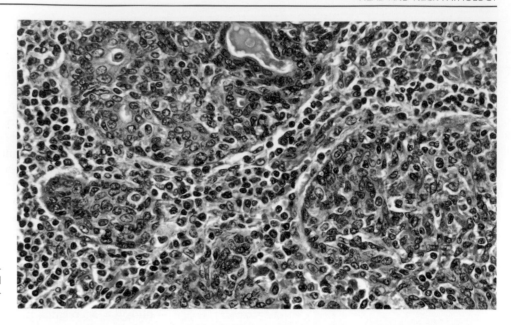

FIGURE 10-18

A well-developed lymphoepithelial lesion (BLEL) shows an epimyoepithelial cell proliferation. There are many infiltrating lymphocytes.

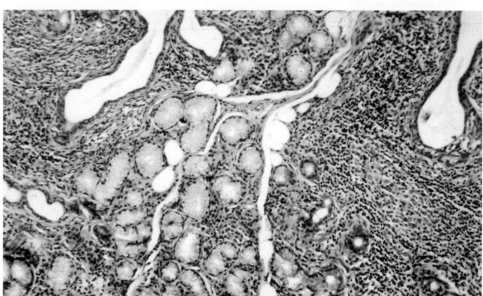

FIGURE 10-19

Focal lymphocytic sialadenitis is adjacent to normal-appearing acini. Germinal center formation in the lymphocytic infiltrate is noted. This biopsy specimen is from a patient with Sjögren syndrome.

polymorphonuclear leukocytes are not usually present. Use of immunohistochemistry for CD3 (T-cell marker) or CD20 (B-cell marker) can reveal a mixed population of T and B lymphocytes. Fresh tissue at the time of biopsy may be submitted for flow cytometry analysis and gene rearrangement studies to exclude a lymphoma.

DIFFERENTIAL DIAGNOSIS

The differential diagnosis includes malignant lymphoma, metastatic carcinoma, chronic sialadenitis, and sarcoidosis. The following are helpful in distinguishing lymphoma from a BLEL: the infiltrate remaining within the normal lobular architecture of the gland, lack of invasion of capsule and periglandular tissue, lack of infiltrated epithelial islands, and lack of the atypical nuclear features of malignant lymphocytes. Metastatic carcinoma can be excluded by the benign appearance of the cells within the myoepithelial islands. The distinction between chronic sialadenitis and sarcoidosis is often not quite as clear. Chronic sialadenitis is composed of a mixed chronic inflammatory infiltrate containing plasma cells and neutrophils with prominent fibrosis. Sarcoidosis is characterized by noncaseating granulomas.

PROGNOSIS AND THERAPY

Lymphomas arising in benign lymphoepithelial lesions are most frequently characterized as low-grade B-cell lymphomas similar to lymphomas of other MALT. Any salivary gland undergoing biopsy for Sjögren syndrome or for a persistent mass should have material submitted for flow cytometry analysis, immunohistochemical techniques, and gene arrangements to exclude the possibility of lymphoma. Malignant lymphoepithelial lesions, though rare, may arise in a setting of BLEL. These lesions have only been reported in major salivary glands, usually the parotid gland, and women seem to be affected more often than men. There are, however, two subgroups who are particularly affected: Inuits (Eskimos) and Chinese. These carcinomas may present with regional lymph node metastasis. Within Inuits this lesion has more commonly been reported in parotid, while within the Chinese, it is more common in the submandibular gland with less frequent regional lymph node disease.

■ LYMPHOEPITHELIAL CYST

CLINICAL FEATURES

The benign cystic salivary gland lesions known as lymphoepithelial cysts occur most commonly in the parotid glands and oral cavity. The name reflects the two histologic components that constitute the lesions: lymphoid tissue and epithelium-lined cysts. The male-to-female

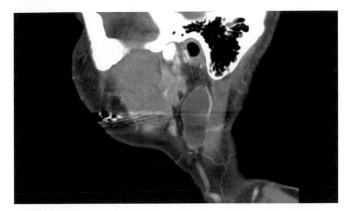

FIGURE 10-20
A sagittal computed tomography scan showing a large cyst within the parotid gland. This was part of a bilateral presentation in this HIV-positive patient.

ratio is 3:1, with a peak incidence in the 4th decade. These lesions are seen in a small minority of HIV-positive individuals, among whom it is more common in children. Although they may be present at birth, they may not become clinically obvious until later in adult life (Figure 10-20). They frequently present as a unilateral painful swelling. Pain may occur, however, due to secondary infection or nerve compression.

PATHOLOGIC FEATURES

GROSS FINDINGS

On gross examination, the cysts measure 0.1 to 8 cm. The cyst contents are usually a straw-colored serous fluid.

LYMPHOEPITHELIAL CYST—DISEASE FACT SHEET

Definition
- A cyst lined by epithelium that is surrounded by a dense lymphoid infiltrate

Incidence and Location
- Uncommon lesion
- Parotid gland most commonly affected

Morbidity and Mortality
- There may be facial nerve dysfunction with compression when involving the parotid gland

Gender, Race, and Age Distribution
- Male > female (3:1)
- Peak incidence in 4th decade
- HIV-associated lymphoepithelial cysts are more common in children

Clinical Features
- Lesions are usually asymptomatic with occasional associated pain or tenderness and rarely facial nerve dysfunction
- Unilateral or bilateral (HIV-related) parotid enlargement
- Small nodules may be located in minor salivary glands (floor of mouth, lateral tongue) or tonsillar tissues

Prognosis and Treatment
- Usually treated by surgical excision and is not known to recur

---

LYMPHOEPITHELIAL CYST—PATHOLOGIC FEATURES

Gross Findings
- Well-demarcated nodule or mass that varies in size by location from 0.1 cm (intraoral sites) to 8 cm (parotid)

Microscopic Findings
- Epithelium-lined cysts composed of stratified squamous, cuboidal, columnar, or pseudostratified-ciliated type
- Lymphoid tissue within the cyst wall, which may show follicular hyperplasia
- The lumen may be filled with desquamated cells
- In HIV-associated cysts, proliferating epimyoepithelial islands may be seen

Fine Needle Aspiration
- Composed of lymphocytes and desquamated squamous cells

Pathologic Differential Diagnosis
- Warthin tumor, cystic metastatic squamous carcinoma, metastatic nasopharyngeal carcinoma

MICROSCOPIC FINDINGS

Microscopically, the cyst lining is composed of squamous, columnar, or cuboidal epithelium (Figure 10-21). Occasionally, there may be goblet cells or oncocytic metaplasia identified within the cyst lining. The cyst wall is composed of lymphoid tissue that will contain germinal centers. Depending on the location of the cyst, it may be within an intraparotid lymph node or cervical lymph node.

ANCILLARY STUDIES

Due to the accessibility of lymphoepithelial cysts, they frequently undergo fine needle aspiration. However, findings on aspiration are fairly nonspecific. There can be a predominance of lymphoid cells with interspersed squamous cells. The differential diagnosis of an aspirate from these lesions may include cystadenoma and Warthin tumor.

DIFFERENTIAL DIAGNOSIS

These cysts are frequently misdiagnosed as tumors. They may be mistaken histologically for cystic low-grade mucoepidermoid carcinomas or metastatic cystic squamous cell carcinoma. However, the lining of the lymphoepithelial cyst is a benign squamous lining with no pleomorphism (Figure 10-22). The lining epithelium will be immunoreactive with keratin but negative for p16. p16 may show focal reactivity in areas where inflammatory cells are within the epithelium. In addition, lymphoepithelial cysts generally lack mucin cells with microcystic and macrocystic structures, contain no papillary projections, and have no intermediate cells.

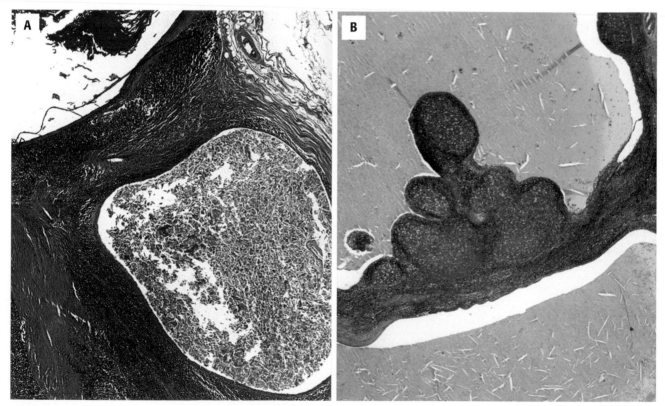

FIGURE 10-21

A and **B**, Two lymphoepithelial cysts. The dilated squamous-lined cysts are surrounded by a lymphocytic infiltrate within the parotid. Fine needle aspirate findings of squamous cells and lymphocytes are easily explained by the above tissue architecture.

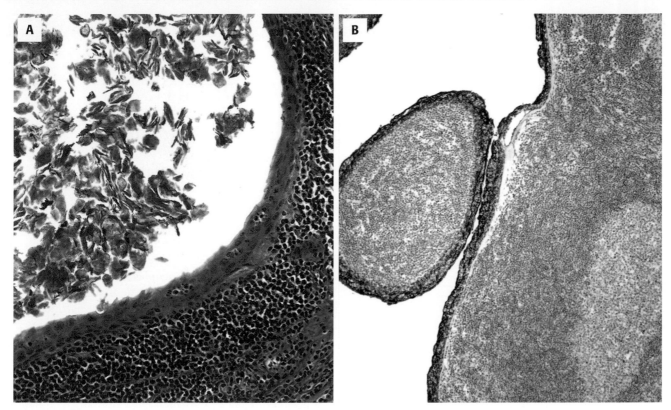

FIGURE 10-22

A, High power shows the attenuated benign squamous lining of a lymphoepithelial cyst. **B**, Although not required, the epithelium will be positive with keratin immunohistochemistry.

PROGNOSIS AND THERAPY

Surgical excision is curative. If a fistulous tract is present, then it is necessary to remove the sinus tract or fistula to prevent recurrence. There are alternative treatments to surgery for HIV-positive patients. Frequently, the only purpose for removing the cyst is for cosmetic reasons.

SUGGESTED READINGS

The complete suggested readings list is available online at
    www.expertconsult.com.

11

Benign Neoplasms of the Salivary Glands

■ **Kevin R. Torske**

■ PLEOMORPHIC ADENOMA

Pleomorphic adenoma (PA), also called benign mixed tumor or mixed tumor, is a benign salivary gland neoplasm composed of ductal epithelial and myoepithelial cell proliferations set within a mesenchymal stroma. This tumor displays remarkable histomorphologic diversity, including varying cellularity, cell morphology, matrix type, and encapsulation.

CLINICAL FEATURES

PA is the most common neoplasm within the salivary glands, accounting for 54% to 76% of all neoplasia. The vast majority of PAs are diagnosed in the parotid gland, followed by the minor salivary glands (especially the palate) and the submandibular gland. In adults, females are affected more often than males, with a wide age range peaking in the 4th to 5th decade. In children and adolescents, the incidence peaks between 5 and 15 years of age, and males are affected most frequently.

Presentation usually consists of a painless, slowly growing firm mass. Mucosal ulceration or paresthesia (due to nerve compression) is a rare finding. Nodules tend to be singular and mobile and may become very large if neglected.

PLEOMORPHIC ADENOMA—DISEASE FACT SHEET

Definition
- A benign neoplasm composed of ductal epithelial cells and myoepithelial cells set within a mesenchymal stroma

Incidence and Location
- Most common salivary gland neoplasm
- Comprises approximately 60% of parotid, submandibular, and minor salivary gland tumors

Gender, Race, and Age Distribution
- Female > male
- Male > female, in children and adolescents (peak 5 to 15 years)
- Peak incidence in 4th to 5th decades

Clinical Features
- Asymptomatic, slowly growing mass
- May become very large if neglected

Prognosis and Treatment
- 20% to 45% recurrence rate with enucleation
- Multinodular recurrences with potential for malignant transformation in up to 7% of patients
- Superficial or total parotidectomy, submandibular gland resection, or wide excision

---

PATHOLOGIC FEATURES

PLEOMORPHIC ADENOMA—PATHOLOGIC FEATURES

Gross Findings
- Well-circumscribed, round to oval, variably encapsulated mass
- White-tan, possibly shiny or translucent cut surface

Microscopic Findings
- Epithelial glandular ductal structures
- Myoepithelial cells in spindle, plasmacytoid, epithelioid, stellate, or basaloid morphologies
- Mesenchymal stroma either myxoid, mucochondroid, hyalinized, osseous, and/or fatty

Immunohistochemical Features
- Cytokeratin cocktail, S100 protein, SMA, p63, calponin, MSA, GFAP, and CD10 reactive

Pathologic Differential Diagnosis
- *Benign:* myoepithelioma, basal cell adenoma
- *Malignant:* adenoid cystic carcinoma, polymorphous low-grade adenocarcinoma

---

GROSS FINDINGS

The surgical specimen of a PA typically is a well-circumscribed, smooth to slightly lobular, round to oval mass. Encapsulation is highly variable, ranging from thick to nonexistent. The cut surface is white to tan and often shiny to translucent (Figure 11-1). Recurrent tumors are commonly multifocal, ranging in size from ~1 mm to several centimeters.

MICROSCOPIC FINDINGS

The histologic range of appearances of PAs is enormously varied; however, all mixed tumors display epithelial ductal structures, myoepithelial cells, and a mesenchymal stroma (Figure 11-2). Three main groups of tumor may be found: myxoid ("stroma-rich"; ~80% stroma), cellular ("cell-rich," "myoepithelial predominant"; ~80%

cellular), and mixed (classic), with the stroma-rich variant being more prone to recurrence.

Encapsulation is inconsistent in PAs, ranging from significant and well developed to nonexistent. Lack of encapsulation is particularly evident in tumors of the minor salivary glands (especially the palate) or those stroma-rich, with direct interface between the tumor and the surrounding gland or connective tissues (Figure 11-3).

Ductal epithelial cells comprise the minority of the cell population, forming variably sized ductal or cystic structures. The remainder of the cellularity is myoepithelial, with a wide range of cytomorphology, including spindled, plasmacytoid, squamoid, stellate, and basaloid. Neoplastic myoepithelial cells may be abluminal, individual and scattered, or in nests, solid sheets, or trabeculae (Figure 11-4). Oncocytic, sebaceous, and adipocytes may be present to a variable degree.

Mucochondroid stromal changes are most frequent. However, the amount of collagenation is variable, with stroma appearing from loose and myxoid to dense and hyalinized (Figure 11-4). Chondroid, osteoid, and adipose-like tissues may also occur.

Multinodular growth, although rare in primary mixed tumors, is common in recurrent disease. The nodules tend to be stroma-rich, widely scattered in the prior surgical area, and can number in excess of 100 (Figure 11-5).

PAs that display mild-to-moderate pleomorphism, prominent nucleoli, or numerous mitotic divisions may be termed *atypical*. If malignant features such as tumor necrosis, atypical mitoses, and profound nuclear pleomorphism are present but limited to the interior of the neoplasm (i.e., without capsular invasion), the diagnosis *carcinoma ex mixed tumor in situ* is appropriate. Other than indicating a stronger need for close clinical follow-up, these features do not appreciably alter the prognosis.

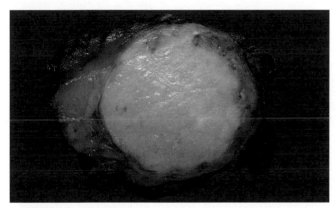

FIGURE 11-1

A very well-circumscribed and encapsulated neoplasm within the parotid gland. Note the shiny, translucent cut surface of this pleomorphic adenoma.

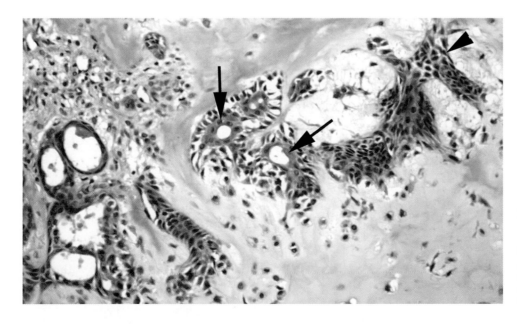

FIGURE 11-2

Pleomorphic adenoma, medium power. Ductal structures (*arrows*) are surrounded by abluminal myoepithelial cells, which are also present in sheets (*arrowhead*) and singly scattered. Hyalinized, myxoid, and chondromyxoid stroma types are evident.

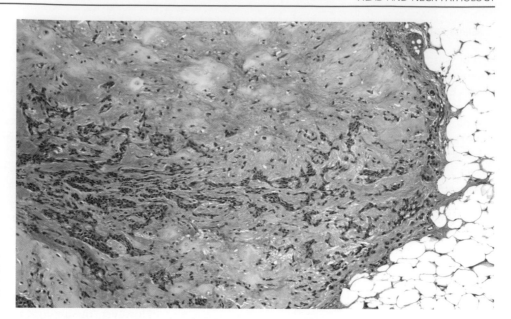

FIGURE 11-3

Pleomorphic adenoma, low power. Un-encapsulated myxoid (stroma-rich) variant showing direct apposition with the adjacent adipose tissue. Note the small tumor extensions into the fat.

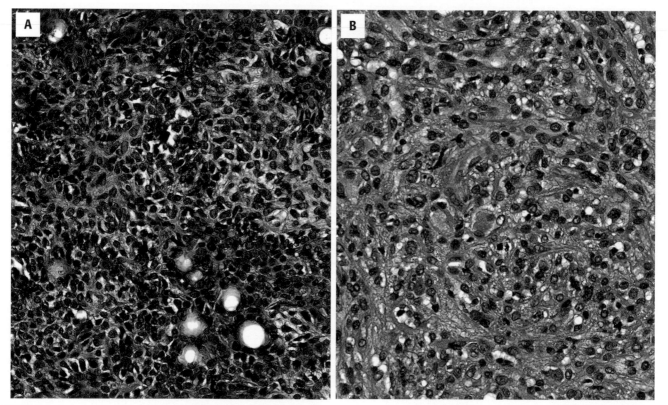

FIGURE 11-4

Pleomorphic adenoma may be quite cellular, showing focal small ductal lumen (**A**). Stromal hyalinization instead of a myxoid stroma may also be present (**B**), a feature that is seen more frequently in cases with malignant transformation.

ANCILLARY STUDIES

IMMUNOHISTOCHEMICAL FEATURES

Cytokeratin cocktail is strongly reactive in ductal epithelial and squamoid myoepithelial cells and variably reactive in other myoepithelial forms. Vimentin, S100 protein, p63, glial fibrillary acidic protein (GFAP), smooth muscle actin (SMA), calponin, smooth muscle myosin heavy chain, and CD10 decorate the myoepithelial component. CK7 highlights plasmacytoid cells. However, the staining patterns are irregular, with strongest reactivity for GFAP in the myxoid areas and SMA in the spindle cells.

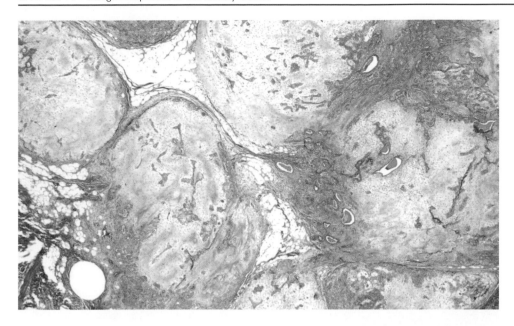

FIGURE 11-5

Recurrent pleomorphic adenoma, low power. Note the numerous, variably sized nodules that characterize recurrent disease.

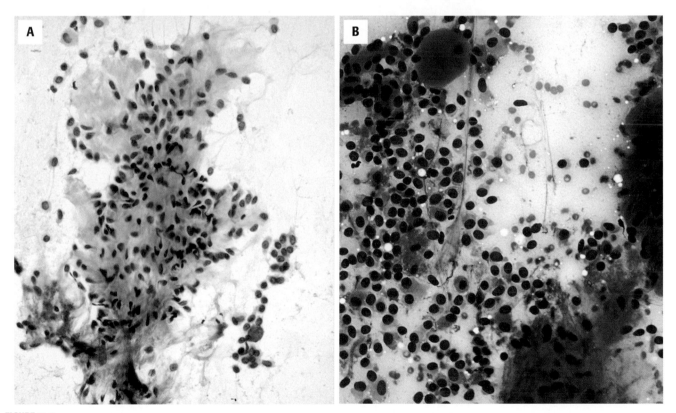

FIGURE 11-6

A, A Papanicolaou-stained fine needle aspiration (FNA) preparation shows small glands with a fibrillar matrix material intermixed with the epithelial component. **B**, A May-Grünwald-Giemsa stains the mucochondroid material bright magenta in this FNA preparation. The matrix material is intimately interspersed with the epithelial component.

FINE NEEDLE ASPIRATION

Aspirates are variably cellular, with a biphasic appearance of luminal (ductal) epithelial cells and abluminal myoepithelial cells. The ductal cells display ample cytoplasm with round to oval nuclei and small nucleoli. Myoepithelial cells may be single or clustered and plasmacytoid, spindle shaped, or stellate (Figure 11-6). Mucoid background material may also be present, taking on a bright, fibrillar, magenta quality with Wright- or Diff-Quik–stained material.

DIFFERENTIAL DIAGNOSIS

The differential includes myoepithelioma, a benign epithelial salivary gland neoplasm composed entirely of myoepithelial cells. This neoplasm may represent one end of the spectrum of mixed tumor in which ductal structures and myxoid matrix are absent. Plasmacytoid (Figure 11-7) or spindled (Figure 11-8) myoepithelial cells predominate, although any myoepithelial form may be present. Basal cell adenoma is also included in the differential. Unencapsulated tumors, especially those of the palate, may appear infiltrative, mimicking malignancies such as polymorphous low-grade adenocarcinoma or adenoid cystic carcinoma.

PROGNOSIS AND THERAPY

Recurrence rate after simple tumor enucleation approaches 45%. This is due to lack of encapsulation, which potentiates incomplete removal or tumor rupture with spillage. Therefore, superficial or total parotidectomy,

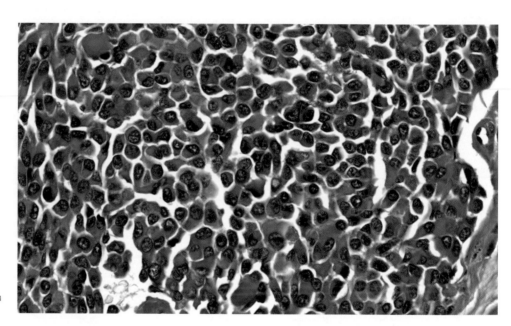

FIGURE 11-7
Myoepithelioma, plasmacytoid variant, high power.

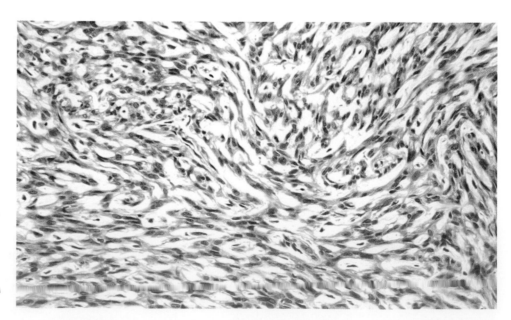

FIGURE 11-8
Myoepithelioma, spindle cell variant, medium power.

resection, or excision with a rim of uninvolved tissue is the treatment of choice for parotid, submandibular, or minor salivary gland tumors, respectively. Recurrence rate with such treatment is up to 2.5%, with most occurring in less than 10 years. Recurrent disease tends to include multiple nodules, with a resultant higher degree of surgical difficulty and risk of further recurrences. Malignant change develops in 2% to 7%. Influencing factors include multiple recurrences, age >40 years, male sex, nodule >2 cm in diameter, and deep lobe tumors.

■ BASAL CELL ADENOMA

Basal cell adenoma is a benign salivary gland epithelial neoplasm composed of a proliferation of small basaloid cells in solid, tubular, trabecular, or membranous patterns. Histogenesis is most likely from intercalated ducts or the basal cells of striated ducts.

CLINICAL FEATURES

Basal cell adenoma represents ~2% of salivary gland neoplasms, with a peak incidence in the 6th decade.

Usual presentation is of an asymptomatic, solitary, slowly growing mass, with almost 75% arising within the parotid gland. Females are affected slightly more commonly than males.

The membranous pattern of basal cell adenoma, however, has a different presentation. Males are affected more frequently and the tumor has a propensity for multicentricity. In addition, the membranous type (also known as *dermal anlage tumor*) may be part of the "skin/salivary gland tumor diathesis," a rare complex that includes concomitant skin neoplasms such as dermal cylindroma, trichoepithelioma, and eccrine spiradenoma.

PATHOLOGIC FEATURES

GROSS FINDINGS

Grossly, the tumor is well circumscribed, pink-brown, and smooth in texture, simulating an enlarged lymph node. It may be large but is generally <3 cm in diameter.

MICROSCOPIC FINDINGS

Basal cell adenoma is a well-circumscribed, usually encapsulated epithelial tumor that classically displays two cell morphologies. Peripheral cells line the outer surface of tumor nodules, often in a palisade-like fashion. These basaloid cells are small, with scant cytoplasm and dense basophilic nuclei. Central cells form the bulk of the nodules and solid sheets. Polygonal or angular in shape, they are larger with more abundant cytoplasm, and pale round nuclei (Figure 11-9). Small ductal structures or squamous metaplasia, including keratinization, may be observed.

BASAL CELL ADENOMA—DISEASE FACT SHEET

Definition
- Benign epithelial salivary gland neoplasm composed of small basaloid cells in solid, trabecular, tubular, or membranous growth patterns

Incidence and Location
- Represents 2% of salivary gland neoplasms
- 75% within parotid gland, remainder in submandibular and minor salivary glands

Gender, Race, and Age Distribution
- Female > male in solid and tubulotrabecular
- Male > female in membranous variant
- Peak incidence in 6th decade

Clinical Features
- Asymptomatic, slowly growing mass
- Membranous variant is associated with multifocality and skin adnexal tumors

Prognosis and Treatment
- 25% recurrence rate and small chance of malignant transformation for membranous type
- Low recurrence rate for other forms
- Surgical excision with possible parotidectomy

BASAL CELL ADENOMA—PATHOLOGIC FEATURES

Gross Findings
- Well-circumscribed, encapsulated, pink-brown mass

Microscopic Findings
- Solid, trabecular, tubular, and membranous patterns
- Small basaloid cells with peripheral palisading around sheets and islands
- Focal squamous metaplasia with keratinization

Immunohistochemical Features
- *Inner luminal cells:* cytokeratin cocktail, CK7, and CD117
- *Peripheral basaloid cells:* S100 protein, p63, SMA, and MSA

Pathologic Differential Diagnosis
- *Benign:* canalicular adenoma
- *Malignant:* basal cell adenocarcinoma, adenoid cystic carcinoma

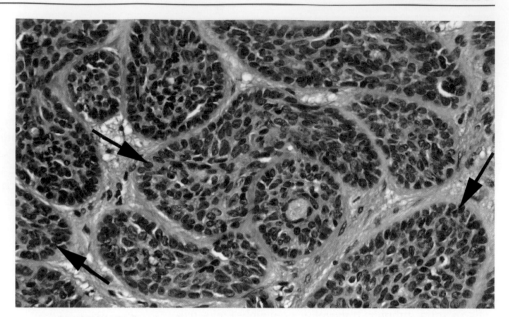

FIGURE 11-9

Basal cell adenoma, solid type, medium power. Nests of basaloid cells with peripheral palisading (*arrows*).

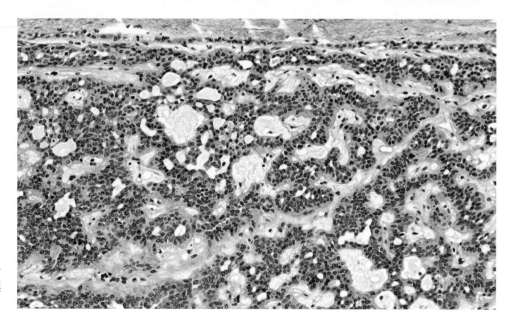

FIGURE 11-10

Basal cell adenoma, trabecular type, medium power. Encapsulated neoplasm composed of variably thick chains of basaloid cells in a loose fibrous stroma.

Four basic architectural patterns are seen: solid, tubular, trabecular (Figure 11-10), and membranous (Figure 11-11). A solitary tumor may display all patterns, but a specific configuration generally predominates. The membranous type is characterized by a "jigsaw" puzzle pattern, with nodules surrounded and separated by a dense, periodic acid–Schiff–positive hyaline band (Figure 11-12). The hyaline material may also form small round globules within the cellular islands. The membranous type may be multifocal or unencapsulated, with limited infiltration into the surrounding parenchyma.

ANCILLARY STUDIES

IMMUNOHISTOCHEMICAL FEATURES

Cytokeratin cocktail is reactive in all tumors, albeit with variable distribution and density. S100 protein, p63, SMA, and muscle-specific actin may display focal reactivity in the basal aspect of the peripheral epithelial cells (Figure 11-13), while CK7 and CD117 highlight the luminal cells.

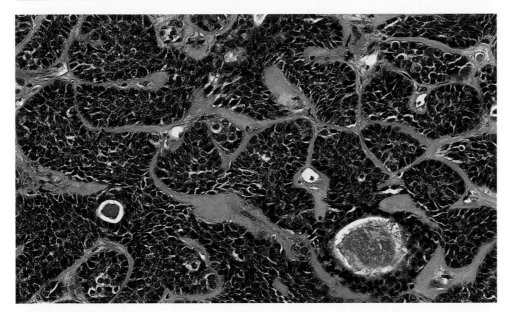

FIGURE 11-11

Basal cell adenoma, membranous type, medium power. Nests of basaloid cells are surrounded by a distinct hyaline band.

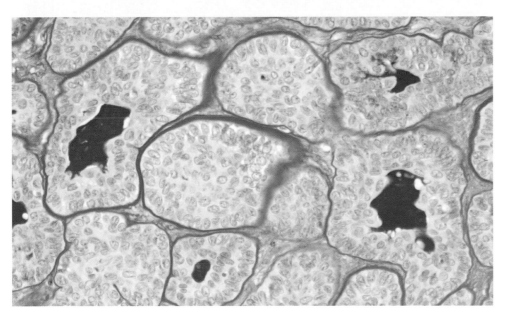

FIGURE 11-12

Basal cell adenoma, membranous type, medium power. The periodic acid–Schiff special stain accentuates the hyaline bands surrounding the basaloid cell nests.

FINE NEEDLE ASPIRATION

Aspirates consist of sheets or syncytial fragments of bland oval cells with scanty cytoplasm and round-to-oval nuclei. Nests or groups may be surrounded by a bright green (Papanicolaou) or pale magenta (Diff-Quik) hyaline band.

DIFFERENTIAL DIAGNOSIS

The differential diagnosis may include malignancies such as basal cell adenocarcinoma or adenoid cystic carcinoma. However, features of malignancy, such as cytologic pleomorphism, tumor necrosis, significant glandular infiltration, or perineural invasion, are seen in carcinoma but not in adenoma. Benign entities such as canalicular adenoma, PA, or myoepithelioma may also be considered, but they usually have different patterns of growth.

PROGNOSIS AND THERAPY

Surgical excision, to possibly include parotidectomy, is the treatment of choice. Although very low for most forms, the recurrence rate for membranous type is up to 25 %, possibly due to capsular infiltration or multifocality. In addition, malignant degeneration or concomitant skin lesions are possible with this variant.

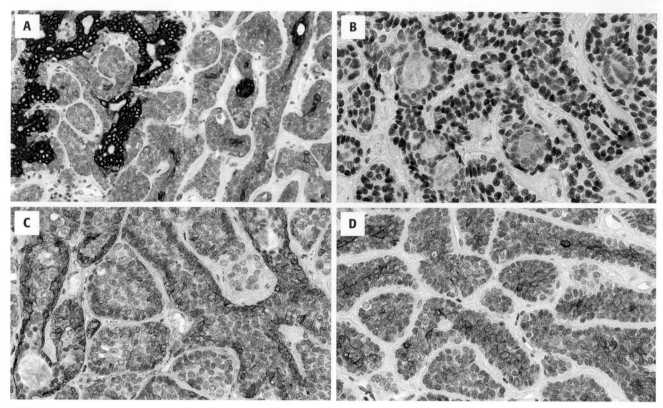

FIGURE 11-13
A variety of immunohistochemistry studies can be used to highlight the biphasic appearance of the neoplastic cells. **A**, Keratin highlights the inner luminal cells. **B**, p63 highlights the basal cells. **C**, Smooth muscle actin highlights the basal-myoepithelial zone. **D**, CD117 preferentially highlights the luminal cells.

■ CANALICULAR ADENOMA

Canalicular adenoma is a benign epithelial salivary gland neoplasm characterized by chains of columnar cells and preference for the minor salivary glands. An excretory duct origin is favored.

CLINICAL FEATURES

Canalicular adenoma is almost invariably associated with minor salivary glands, especially those of the upper lip, with occasional cases in the buccal mucosa or palate. Indeed, it is the second most common salivary gland neoplasm of the upper lip, just behind PA. It typically presents as an asymptomatic, firm to fluctuant, slowly growing, 1 to 2 cm submucosal nodule in the 7th decade of life. Although normally solitary, multifocal tumors may occur. Females are more commonly affected, as are blacks.

CANALICULAR ADENOMA—DISEASE FACT SHEET

Definition
- Benign epithelial salivary gland neoplasm characterized by chains of columnar cells and a loose connective tissue stroma

Incidence and Location
- 1% of all salivary gland neoplasms; 4% of all minor salivary gland neoplasms
- Minor salivary glands: especially upper lip

Gender, Race, and Age Distribution
- Female > male
- Black > white
- Peak incidence in 7th decade

Clinical Features
- Asymptomatic, potentially multinodular mass

Prognosis and Treatment
- Recurrence rare
- Simple excision with clear margins

PATHOLOGIC FEATURES

CANALICULAR ADENOMA—PATHOLOGIC FEATURES

Gross Findings
- Well-circumscribed, nonencapsulated, solid or cystic, pink-tan up to 2 cm mass

Microscopic Findings
- Long chains of columnar cells that may join and then separate
- Tubules, duct-like forms, and rare solid groups
- Loose, lightly collagenous stroma

Immunohistochemical Features
- Cytokeratin and S100 protein reactive
- GFAP reactive at tumor/connective tissue interface

Pathologic Differential Diagnosis
- *Benign:* pleomorphic adenoma, basal cell adenoma
- *Malignant:* adenoid cystic carcinoma, polymorphous low-grade adenocarcinoma

GROSS FINDINGS

Canalicular adenomas are well circumscribed yet nonencapsulated. Cut surface is pinkish-brown to tan, with a solid or cystic consistency.

MICROSCOPIC FINDINGS

Canalicular adenoma is commonly composed of long single-layered strands or tubules of cuboidal to short columnar epithelial cells within a loose, lightly collagenized stroma (Figure 11-14). The strands may run parallel to one another with a thin "canal-like" space in between and then attach to one another and separate, creating a "beaded" appearance (Figure 11-15). Cystic degeneration is common. The tumor may be multifocal, with possible small, unencapsulated "incipient" tumors evident within surrounding minor salivary glands.

The cuboidal or columnar cells have eosinophilic cytoplasm and basophilic, oval nuclei (Figure 11-16). Pleomorphism is minimal and mitotic figures are rare. Solid nests or sheets of smaller basaloid cells may also be evident, with the larger cuboidal to columnar cells present at the periphery.

ANCILLARY STUDIES

The cells are reactive for cytokeratin cocktail and S100 protein, while nonreactive for actin myofilaments and calponin. GFAP reactivity is focal, often at the tumor–connective tissue interface.

DIFFERENTIAL DIAGNOSIS

The differential includes benign neoplasms, including PA and basal cell adenoma. Malignancies commonly affecting the minor salivary glands, primarily adenoid cystic carcinoma and polymorphous low-grade adenocarcinoma, may also be considered.

PROGNOSIS AND THERAPY

Simple local excision to include a rim of normal surrounding tissue is the treatment of choice. Although true recurrence is rare, the presence of multiple lesions may set the stage for possible clinical persistence or recurrence.

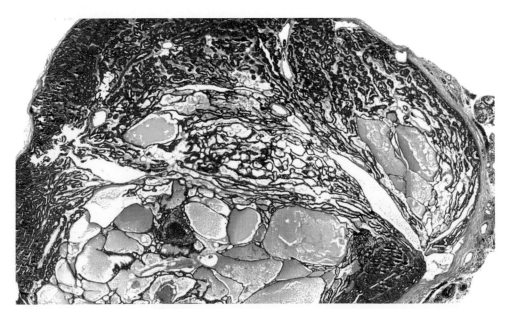

FIGURE 11-14

Canalicular adenoma, low power. Well-circumscribed neoplasm displaying chains of cells in a loose fibrous stroma. Note the numerous cystically dilated spaces.

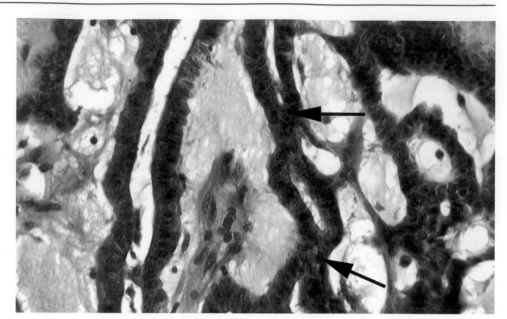

FIGURE 11-15

Canalicular adenoma, high power. Short columnar and smaller basaloid cells are arranged in a palisaded architecture with intervening loose stroma. "Beading" is noted where the cells come together and then separate (*arrows*).

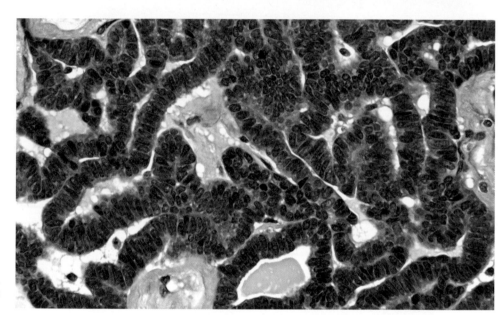

FIGURE 11-16

Canalicular adenoma, medium power. Single file chains of columnar cells with oval nuclei characterize this entity.

■ ONCOCYTOMA

Oncocytoma (oncocytic adenoma) is a putative neoplastic proliferation of oncocytically altered cells. Histogenesis may be associated with therapeutic radiation exposure.

CLINICAL FEATURES

Oncocytoma typically presents as an asymptomatic, slowly growing mass in the 7th to 8th decades of life. It affects the parotid gland in 80% to 90% of cases

and represents ~1% of all parotid gland neoplasms. A slight female predominance is noted. Approximately 7% of tumors have a bilateral presentation. White patients are affected much more commonly than other races.

PATHOLOGIC FEATURES

GROSS FINDINGS

Oncocytoma presents as a soft, well-circumscribed, tan-brown nodule. Usually solitary, the size may range from 1 to 7 cm.

ONCOCYTOMA—DISEASE FACT SHEET

Definition

- Neoplasm composed of large polygonal cells containing abundant, abnormal mitochondria

Incidence and Location

- Approximately 1% of all parotid gland neoplasms
- Parotid >> submandibular gland

Gender, Race, and Age Distribution

- Female > male
- Predominantly affects whites
- 7th to 8th decades

Clinical Features

- Asymptomatic, slowly growing mass

Prognosis and Treatment

- Minimal recurrence with adequate excision
- Parotidectomy

ONCOCYTOMA—PATHOLOGIC FEATURES

Gross Findings

- Single, soft, well-circumscribed tan-brown nodule

Microscopic Findings

- Large polygonal cells with abundant eosinophilic granular cytoplasm
- Solid, acinar, trabecular, or follicular patterns
- Clear cell change can be seen

Ancillary Studies

- Cytokeratin, p63, and PTAH reactive

Pathologic Differential Diagnosis

- *Benign:* Warthin tumor, nodular oncocytic hyperplasia
- *Malignant:* acinic cell adenocarcinoma, metastatic renal cell carcinoma, oncocytic carcinoma

MICROSCOPIC FINDINGS

Oncocytes are polygonal cells with abundant eosinophilic, finely granular cytoplasm and uniform, round, centrally placed nuclei, with or without nucleoli (Figure 11-17). Oncocytes may accumulate copious amounts of intracytoplasmic glycogen and, due to processing artifacts, appear "clear" and devoid of cytoplasmic staining (Figure 11-18).

Oncocytic metaplasia is identified as solitary or small groups of acinar cells (mucous or serous) that underwent cellular changes to become oncocytes, a process that increases with increasing age and becomes practically universal over 70 years of age. A distinct and immediate transformation of one cell type to another occurs, without alteration of the glandular architecture.

Oncocytosis (oncocytic hyperplasia) includes multiple areas of oncocytic change, ranging from isolated variably sized cellular groupings *(nodular form)* to a diffuse process affecting a majority of the gland *(diffuse form)*. An intimate, unencapsulated relationship between the glandular parenchyma and the oncocytic nodule is present and may include normal acini intermixed with oncocytes (Figure 11-19).

Oncocytoma is well circumscribed with variably thick encapsulation (Figure 11-20). Architectural patterns include monotonous solid sheets, acinar, trabecular, papillary-cystic, or follicular. Slight nuclear pleomorphism may be

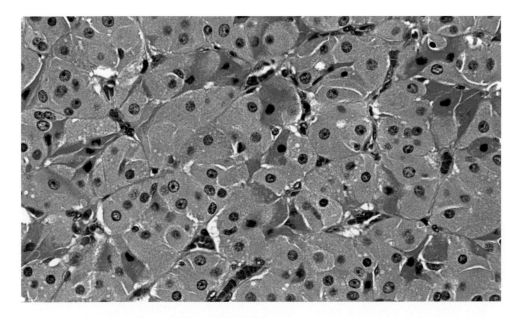

FIGURE 11-17

Oncocytoma, high power. Oncocytes are polygonal cells with abundant granular eosinophilic cytoplasm and round, centrally placed nuclei, with or without nucleoli.

256

HEAD AND NECK PATHOLOGY

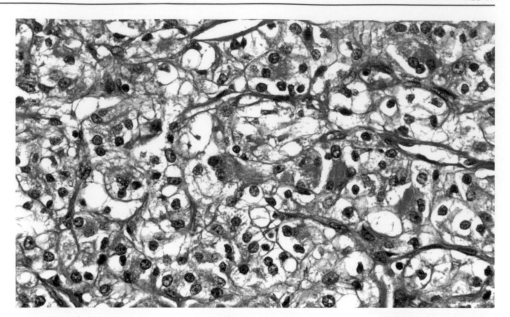

FIGURE 11-18

Oncocytoma, clear cell variant, high power. Note scattered cells still possessing eosinophilic granular cytoplasm.

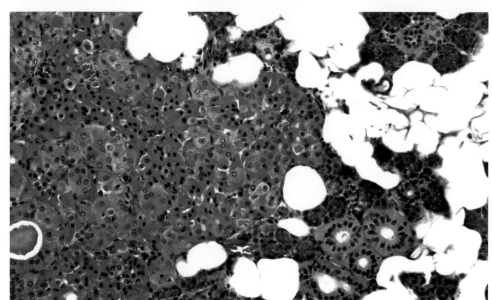

FIGURE 11-19

Oncocytosis, medium power. Sheets of oncocytes (*left*) showing an intimate association with the salivary gland parenchyma.

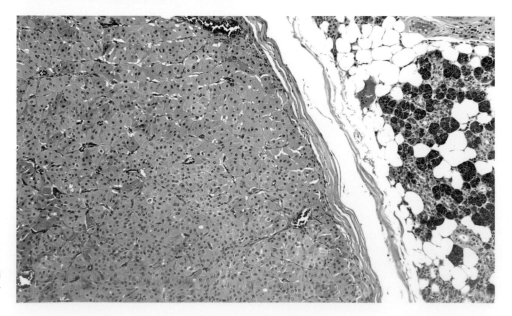

FIGURE 11-20

Oncocytoma, low power. Well-encapsulated neoplasm composed of sheets of oncocytically altered cells.

identified, including prominent nucleoli. Significant stromal hyalinization or vascularity is possible. It is common to appreciate focal areas of oncocytosis in conjunction with an oncocytoma. *Clear cell oncocytosis/ oncocytoma* may be applied if the majority of the oncocytes display cleared cytoplasm.

ANCILLARY STUDIES

HISTOCHEMICAL FEATURES

Phosphotungstic acid–hematoxylin (PTAH) highlights the abundant mitochondria, seen as deep blue cytoplasmic granularity, and ranging from focal or patchy to diffuse. Striated duct epithelial cells, with their basally oriented interdigitating cytoplasmic processes and associated columns of mitochondria, may act as a positive internal control.

ELECTRON MICROSCOPY

The organelles are shifted within the cytoplasm by an overwhelming number of surrounding mitochondria, many of which will show abnormal cristae (Figure 11-21).

FINE NEEDLE ASPIRATION

Aspirates contain polygonal epithelial cells in papillary fragments, sheets, acinar-like structures, or singly (Figure 11-22). Prominent nucleoli may be noted, but mitoses are rare to nonexistent. There is no background lymphoid component.

DIFFERENTIAL DIAGNOSIS

The benign differential includes Warthin tumor and a dominant nodule within oncocytic hyperplasia. Warthin tumor has prominent lymphoid elements and the oncocytic hyperplasia often blends with the surrounding parenchyma. Malignancies may include acinic cell adenocarcinoma or metastatic renal cell carcinoma, especially if clear cells predominate. Special studies usually help to resolve this differential. Oncocytic carcinoma is invasive with profound pleomorphism and necrosis. Oncocytoma and oncocytic carcinoma are reactive for p63 in a basal cell distribution, while metastatic renal cell carcinoma is nonreactive for this marker.

PROGNOSIS AND THERAPY

Superficial parotidectomy for lateral tumors, or total parotidectomy for deep lobe tumors, is the treatment of choice. Recurrence is minimal but may occur due to multifocality or incomplete removal. The rare tumors of the minor salivary glands require complete excision with a small margin of uninvolved tissue.

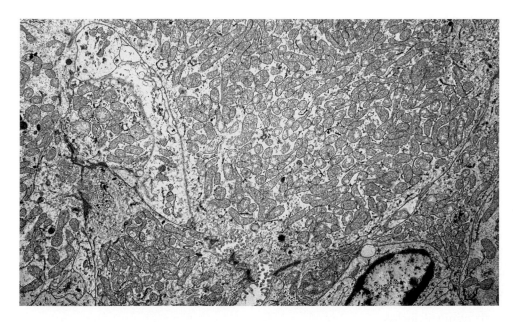

FIGURE 11-21

The cytoplasm is laden with mitochondria identified by this electron microscopic image of an oncocytoma. A small lumen is noted along with tight junctions and short microvilli. *(Courtesy of Dr. I. Dardick.)*

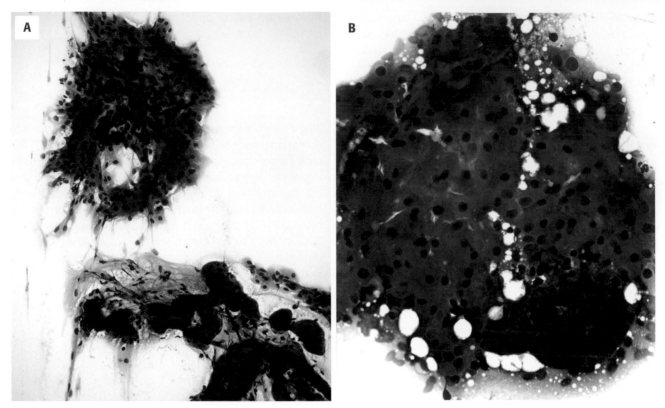

FIGURE 11-22
Fine needle aspiration shows sheets and nests of large cells with abundant granular-eosinophilic cytoplasm. **A**, Unremarkable acini are present in the lower field (Papanicolaou stain). **B**, Large, polygonal cells with small nuclei and abundant cytoplasm (Diff-Quik stained).

■ PAPILLARY CYSTADENOMA LYMPHOMATOSUM (WARTHIN TUMOR)

Warthin tumor is a relatively common lesion composed of a double layer of oncocytic epithelium, a papillary and cystic architectural pattern, and a dense lymphoid stroma. It is thought likely to arise from entrapped salivary tissue in intraparotid or periparotid lymph nodes.

CLINICAL FEATURES

Warthin tumor is the second most common benign salivary gland tumor and characteristically presents in the lower portion of the lateral lobe of the parotid gland. With slight caucasoid male predominance, presentation normally occurs in the 6th to 7th decades as an asymptomatic, slowly growing 1 to 4 cm mass. Bilaterality or multifocality occurs more frequently than with any other salivary gland tumor. Warthin tumor may also be synchronously identified with other salivary gland neoplasms. Cigarette smoking is a likely etiologic factor.

PAPILLARY CYSTADENOMA LYMPHOMATOSUM (WARTHIN TUMOR)—DISEASE FACT SHEET

Definition
- Biphasic tumor composed of bilayered oncocytic cells forming cysts and papillary fronds set within a dense lymph node–like stroma

Incidence and Location
- Second most common salivary gland tumor
- Parotid gland

Gender, Race, and Age Distribution
- Male > female
- White > black
- 6th to 7th decades

Clinical Features
- Asymptomatic, slowly growing mass
- Most common bilateral and "second" (synchronous) tumor

Prognosis and Treatment
- Recurrence rate 4% to 25%
- Lumpectomy to parotidectomy

PATHOLOGIC FEATURES

PAPILLARY CYSTADENOMA LYMPHOMATOSUM (WARTHIN TUMOR)—PATHOLOGIC FEATURES

Gross Findings
- Circumscribed, firm to cystic, brown, yellow, or red mass

Microscopic Findings
- Double layer of oncocytic epithelium with cuboidal basal cell and overlying columnar luminal cell
- Numerous cysts with papillary infoldings
- Dense lymph node–like stroma with possible reactive germinal centers

Immunohistochemical Features
- Epithelial component keratin reactive
- Lymphoid component reactive with B- and T-cell markers

Pathologic Differential Diagnosis
- Lymph node metastases; sebaceous lymphadenoma, cystadenoma

GROSS FINDINGS

Macroscopically, Warthin tumor is circumscribed, solid, papillary, or cystic, and brown, yellow, or red. Cysts may contain yellow-brown fluid.

MICROSCOPIC FINDINGS

The name "papillary cystadenoma lymphomatosum," while cumbersome, correctly describes the overall microscopic appearance (Figure 11-23). Papillary fronds and cystic spaces are lined by oncocytic epithelium, consisting of cuboidal basal cells supporting tall columnar cells with palisaded nuclei (Figure 11-24), often creating a "tram-tracking" nuclear appearance. The cystic spaces may be filled with fluid, desquamated epithelial cells, or lymphoid cells. Intimately associated with the epithelial component is a dense lymph node–like stroma, including reactive germinal centers. The proportion of the three elements is variable. Isolated mucocytes can be seen.

Trauma may lead to cyst rupture and subsequent foreign body giant cell reaction, fibrosis, squamous metaplasia, or necrosis. Such findings may occur after fine needle aspiration (FNA) biopsy.

ANCILLARY STUDIES

IMMUNOHISTOCHEMICAL FEATURES

The epithelial component is reactive for cytokeratin cocktail. The lymphoid portion is similar to a reactive lymph node, including κ and λ light-chain polyclonality.

FINE NEEDLE ASPIRATION

Aspirates display small collections of epithelial cells surrounded by lymphocytes. These epithelial islands demonstrate a "honeycomb" pattern, with well-defined cell borders and relatively large, centrally placed nuclei (Figure 11-25). Squamoid cells may also be evident. Background lymphoid elements are easily identified. The cytoplasm appears opacified and "blue" with air-dried preparations (Figure 11-25).

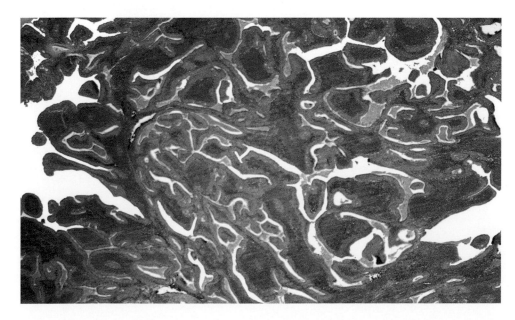

FIGURE 11-23

Warthin tumor, low power. Papillary-cystic tumor associated with a dense lymphoid stroma.

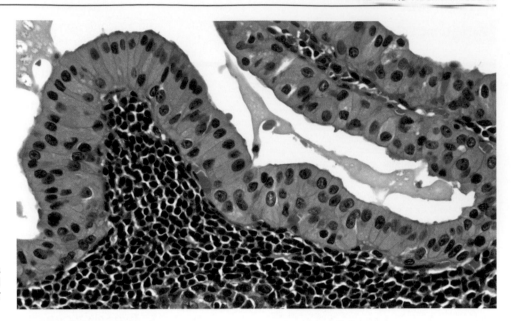

FIGURE 11-24

Warthin tumor, high power. Papillary fronds and cystic spaces lined by a double cell layer of oncocytes. A small germinal center is evident in the bottom center.

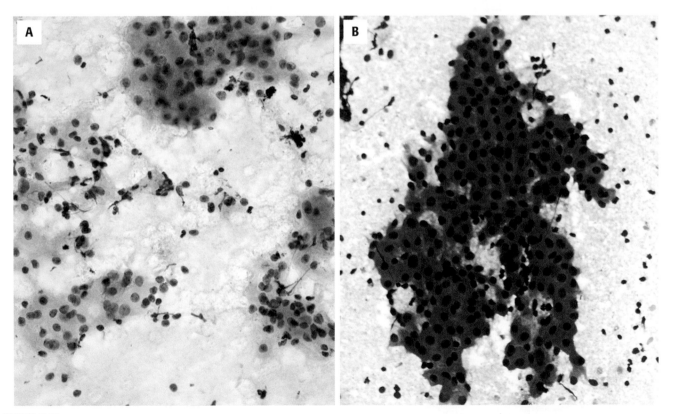

FIGURE 11-25

A, A Papanicolaou-stained smear demonstrates cohesive clusters of oncocytic epithelial cells in a honeycomb pattern with well-defined cell borders and background lymphocytes. **B**, A Diff-Quik preparation stains the papillary frond of epithelium a light blue. Lymphocytes and histiocytes are noted in the bloody background.

DIFFERENTIAL DIAGNOSIS

The differential diagnosis includes lymph node metastasis or sebaceous lymphadenoma. However, the cytologically bland, bilayered, oncocytic epithelial element mitigates against both. Cystadenomas may be oncocytic but do not have the lymphoid stroma and usually have small, multilocular cystic spaces.

PROGNOSIS AND THERAPY

The recurrence rate after excision is 4% to 25%, likely associated with multifocality or incomplete excision. Treatment may range from lumpectomy to total parotidectomy, depending on size and location. A low malignant transformation rate of 1% is recognized, interestingly, giving rise to squamous cell carcinoma (from epithelial component) or a low-grade B-cell lymphoma (from lymphoid component).

■ SEBACEOUS ADENOMA/LYMPHADENOMA

Sebaceous adenoma is a benign epithelial neoplasm composed of proliferating, incompletely differentiated sebaceous glands. Sebaceous lymphadenoma is a rare variant in which the epithelial proliferation is supported by a dense lymphoid stroma and possibly arises from entrapped salivary gland tissue within intraparotid or periparotid lymph nodes.

CLINICAL FEATURES

The clinical presentations of both neoplasms are similar and therefore discussed together. Both represent <1% of all salivary gland neoplasms and are rarely reported outside of the parotid gland. Males and females are affected equally, with most lesions presenting in the 6th to 7th decades of life as an asymptomatic, slowly growing mass.

PATHOLOGIC FEATURES

GROSS FINDINGS

Both sebaceous adenoma and lymphadenoma are firm, well-circumscribed masses. Cut section is pinkish-gray to white or yellow and may be solid or cystic (Figure 11-26).

SEBACEOUS ADENOMA/LYMPHADENOMA—DISEASE FACT SHEET

Definition
- Benign epithelial neoplasms composed of proliferating, incompletely differentiated sebaceous glands set within a fibrous (sebaceous adenoma) or dense lymphoid (sebaceous lymphadenoma) stroma

Incidence and Location
- Approximately 0.1% of all salivary gland neoplasms
- Parotid gland

Gender, Race, and Age Distribution
- Equal gender distribution
- 6th to 7th decades

Clinical Features
- Slowly growing, asymptomatic mass

Prognosis and Treatment
- Minimal recurrence rate
- Surgical excision with rim of normal tissue

SEBACEOUS ADENOMA/LYMPHADENOMA—PATHOLOGIC FEATURES

Gross Findings
- Well-circumscribed, solid or cystic, pink-gray mass

Microscopic Findings
- Solid nests or cystic structures
- Mature sebaceous differentiation in center of nodules or wall of cysts
- Fibrous stroma (sebaceous adenoma) or dense lymph node–like stroma (sebaceous lymphadenoma)

Immunohistochemical Features
- Epithelial component is cytokeratin and EMA reactive

Pathologic Differential Diagnosis
- Sebaceous adenoma: mucoepidermoid carcinoma and sebaceous adenocarcinoma
- Sebaceous lymphadenoma: Warthin tumor and metastatic carcinoma

---

MICROSCOPIC FINDINGS

Sebaceous adenoma is a well-circumscribed neoplasm composed of solid and cystic epithelial structures surrounded by a dense fibrous stroma (Figure 11-27). Epithelial nests are squamoid, displaying peripheral basaloid cells maturing inwardly into sebaceous cells (Figure 11-28). Sebaceous cells, either singly or in groups, may also be found within cyst walls.

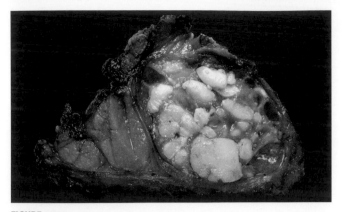

FIGURE 11-26

A sebaceous lymphadenoma showing a greasy cut surface, with multiple cystic spaces filled with sebaceous material. A background stroma is present.

Sebaceous lymphadenoma is composed of a similar epithelial component that is evenly distributed throughout the tumor. However, instead of a fibrous background, the stroma consists of a dense population of lymphocytes, to perhaps include reactive germinal centers (Figure 11-29). A histologically similar tumor, devoid of sebaceous differentiation, is termed *lymphadenoma*.

ANCILLARY STUDIES

IMMUNOHISTOCHEMICAL FEATURES

Cytokeratin cocktail and epithelial membrane antigen are reactive in the epithelial proliferation. S100 protein and SMA are nonreactive. As with Warthin

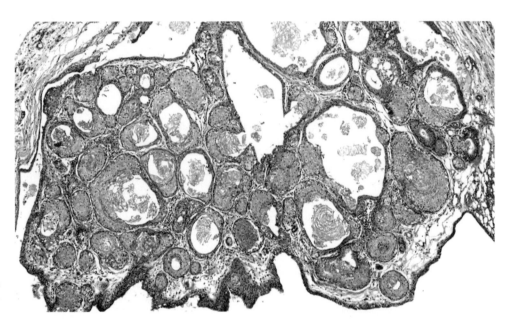

FIGURE 11-27

Sebaceous adenoma, low power. Numerous solid and cystically dilated nests of squamoid cells.

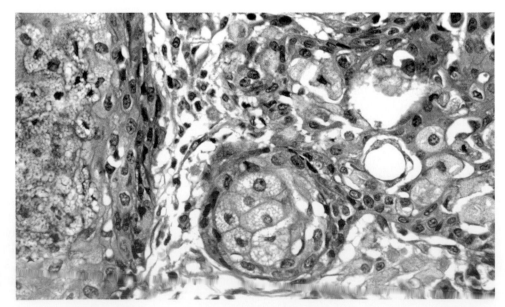

FIGURE 11-28

Sebaceous adenoma, medium power. Nests of squamoid cells displaying central sebaceous cell differentiation.

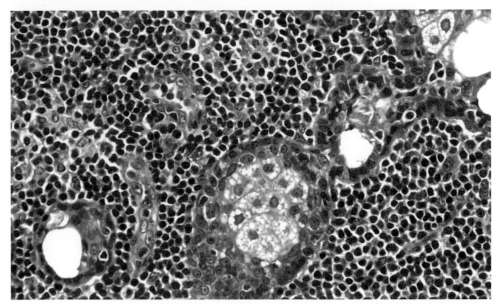

FIGURE 11-29
Sebaceous lymphadenoma, medium power. Solid and cystic nests of squamoid cells with sebaceous differentiation amid a dense lymphoid stroma.

tumor, the lymphoid component in sebaceous lymphadenoma is similar to a reactive lymph node.

FINE NEEDLE ASPIRATION

Aspirates of sebaceous adenoma demonstrate aggregates of large cells with foamy cytoplasm and central crenated nuclei, consistent with sebaceous cells. Less mature squamoid forms with dense cytoplasm and round to oval nuclei are also present. Sebaceous lymphadenoma is similar but also displays a background of small mature lymphocytes.

DIFFERENTIAL DIAGNOSIS

The sebaceous adenoma differential includes mucoepidermoid carcinoma and sebaceous adenocarcinoma. Sebaceous lymphadenoma may be confused with Warthin tumor and metastatic squamous cell carcinoma.

PROGNOSIS AND THERAPY

Treatment includes surgical excision to include a rim of normal surrounding tissue. The recurrence rate is minimal following complete removal.

■ HEMANGIOMA

Hemangioma is a soft tissue tumor composed of variably mature blood vessels and endothelial cells. All histologic variants of hemangioma occur in the salivary glands.

However, this discussion will be limited to the most common form, *juvenile (capillary) hemangioma (JH)*.

CLINICAL FEATURES

JH affects the very young, arising at birth or shortly thereafter, and is the most common salivary gland neoplasm to arise in this time frame. Females predominate, and the parotid gland is the affected site in a vast majority of cases. Bilaterality is found in ~25%. A rapid growth phase is followed by a very slow involutional phase. The tumor may become large,

---

HEMANGIOMA (JUVENILE)—DISEASE FACT SHEET

Definition
- Soft tissue tumor composed of variably mature blood vessels and endothelial cells

Incidence and Location
- Rare
- Parotid gland

Gender, Race, and Age Distribution
- Female > male
- Perinatal or neonatal

Clinical Features
- Rapid growth followed by slow involution
- Usually asymptomatic

Prognosis and Treatment
- Majority with spontaneous resolution over time
- Pharmacologic therapy if required

affecting more than half of the face, and extend into the ear, lip, subglottis, or nose. Usually asymptomatic, complications such as cutaneous ulceration, bleeding, airway compression, or, rarely, congestive heart failure may arise.

PATHOLOGIC FEATURES

GROSS FINDINGS

Macroscopically, parotid JH is hemorrhagic, lobular, and red to brown. As opposed to a discrete mass, the lesion diffusely affects the lobes of the gland.

MICROSCOPIC FINDINGS

JH appears as a diffuse replacement of the salivary gland parenchyma. The lobular architectural pattern and anatomic boundaries of the salivary gland are maintained, with replacement of the serous acini by sheets of small endothelial cells and immature capillaries (Figure 11-30). Striated ducts and peripheral nerves, however, seem unaffected.

The endothelial cells are small with indistinct cell borders. Nuclei are oval or irregular, with possible grooves and occasional inconspicuous nucleoli. Mitotic figures, normal in morphology, may be numerous. Dense cellularity may mask the vascular differentiation (Figure 11-31). Erythrocytes are noted within the lumens.

ANCILLARY STUDIES

IMMUNOHISTOCHEMICAL FEATURES

The endothelial cells are reactive with CD31, CD34, and factor VIII–related antigen (FVIII-RAg). Reticulin

---

HEMANGIOMA (JUVENILE)—PATHOLOGIC FEATURES

Gross Findings
- Hemorrhagic, lobular, red-brown

Microscopic Findings
- Interdigitation between salivary acini and intercalated ducts by immature endothelial cells and small capillaries
- Lobular architecture of gland intact

Immunohistochemical Features
- Endothelial cells are CD31, CD34, and FVIII-RAg reactive

Pathologic Differential Diagnosis
- Angiosarcoma

---

accentuates the vascularity. Cytokeratin cocktail highlights the residual ductal structures.

FINE NEEDLE ASPIRATION

Aspirates consist of a spindle cell proliferation, including cohesive groups of bland cells in a bloody background, or hypercellular groups arranged in compact, three-dimensional coils. The cells have scant to moderate cytoplasm and oval nuclei (Figure 11-32). Needless to say, FNA is not recommended if the clinical differential includes a vascular neoplasm.

DIFFERENTIAL DIAGNOSIS

Angiosarcoma is very rare in this age group, yet it is at the top of the differential. Bland cytomorphology and maintenance of glandular architecture favor JH.

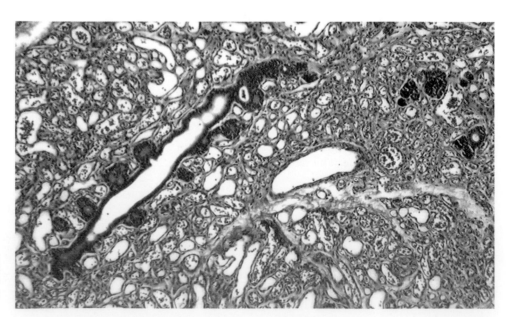

FIGURE 11-30
Juvenile capillary hemangioma, low power. Salivary gland lobules replaced by endothelial cells and small blood vessels. Note that the glandular architecture and excretory ducts are still intact.

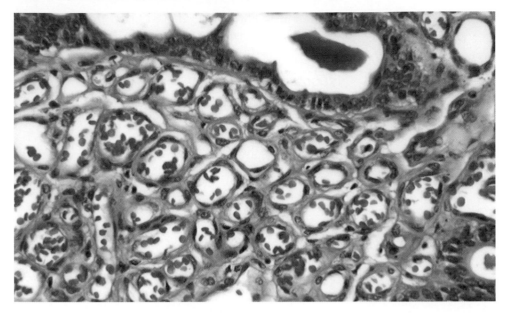

FIGURE 11-31
Juvenile capillary hemangioma, high power. Small uniform endothelial cells and small capillaries replace the glandular acini. Note the residual excretory ducts.

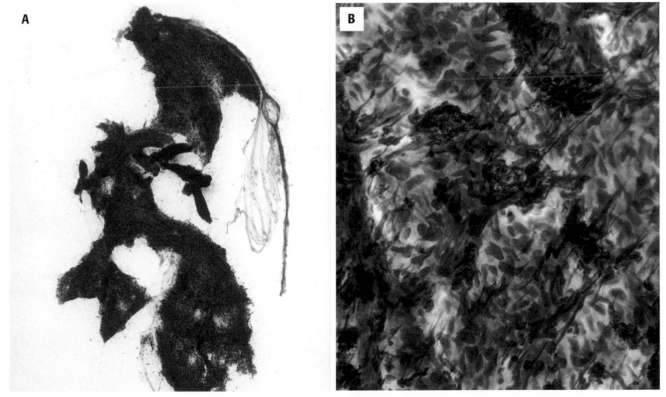

FIGURE 11-32

A, Papanicolaou-stained smear shows a hypercellular, compact three-dimensional cluster or coil. There is a relative lack of blood. **B**, Diff-Quik–stained material shows cohesive clusters of spindled cells without significant pleomorphism. This is a cellular smear of a hemangioma.

PROGNOSIS AND THERAPY

Most JHs involute over time, with 75% to 95% displaying spontaneous regression by 7 years. However, pharmacologic therapy, including corticosteroids and/or interferon (α-2a or α-2b), may be required if complications develop.

Resection is not advised due to blood loss or possible injury to the facial nerve.

SUGGESTED READINGS

The complete suggested readings list is available online at www.expertconsult.com.

12

Malignant Neoplasms of the Salivary Glands

■ John W. Eveson ■ Lester D. R. Thompson

■ ADENOCARCINOMA, NOT OTHERWISE SPECIFIED

CLINICAL FEATURES

ADENOCARCINOMA, NOT OTHERWISE SPECIFIED—DISEASE FACT SHEET

Definition

- Adenocarcinoma, not otherwise specified, is a malignant salivary gland tumor that shows ductal differentiation but lacks the histomorphologic features that characterize other specific types of salivary carcinoma

Incidence and Location

- Up to 17% of salivary gland carcinomas
- 60% of cases involve major glands, mostly the parotid
- 40% in minor glands: palate, buccal mucosa, and lips

Morbidity and Mortality

- 15-year survival rate of 54% to 3% depending on grade (low grade to high grade)

Gender, Race, and Age Distribution

- Slight female predominance
- Peak incidence in 6th decade
- Very rare in children

Clinical Features

- Usually forms a slow-growing mass
- Pain or facial nerve involvement in 20% of cases
- Tumors of minor glands may ulcerate and involve underlying bone

Prognosis and Treatment

- Prognostic factors include tumor grading, stage, and location
- Tumors in minor glands have better prognosis than major glands
- Surgery is treatment of choice, with radiotherapy and neck dissection in advanced or recurrent cases

---

Adenocarcinoma, not otherwise specified [AC (NOS)], is a diagnosis of exclusion and the variable reporting of these tumors makes the interpretation of published data difficult. It represents ~17% of all salivary gland carcinomas. There is a slight female preponderance, and the peak age incidence is in the 6th decade. It is rare in children. About 60% arise in the major glands, predominantly the parotid. Common intraoral sites are the junction of the hard and soft palates, buccal mucosa, and lips, accounting for the remaining 40%. Tumors usually present as a slowly growing, painless mass of 1 to 10 years' duration. About 20% of patients, however, have evidence of facial nerve involvement or pain. Tumors involving minor glands may ulcerate and extend into underlying bone.

PATHOLOGIC FEATURES

ADENOCARCINOMA, NOT OTHERWISE SPECIFIED—PATHOLOGIC FEATURES

Gross Findings

- Well defined or show irregular outline
- Hemorrhage and necrosis common in high-grade tumors

Microscopic Findings

- Duct-like structures with infiltrative growth
- Patterns include ducts, thèques, sheets, and trabeculae
- Cytologic variability used to grade the tumors into low-, intermediate-, and high-grade types
- Perineural and lymphovascular invasion may be seen

Fine Needle Aspiration

- Cellular smears with loose cohesion
- Features of malignancy include cytologic variability, nuclear pleomorphism, and occasional mucous cells

Pathologic Differential Diagnosis

- Diagnosis of exclusion, metastatic adenocarcinoma, undifferentiated carcinoma

---

GROSS FINDINGS

The tumor is well defined or has an irregular, infiltrative margin. There may be areas of intratumoral hemorrhage and necrosis.

MICROSCOPIC FINDINGS

AC (NOS) shows duct-like structures with evidence of an infiltrative growth pattern (Figure 12-1). By definition, they lack the characteristic features of more specific tumor types. There is wide variability in growth patterns, which can include ductal configurations, thèques, sheets, and trabeculae (Figure 12-2).

Cytologic variability can be used to grade these tumors into low-, intermediate-, and high-grade types. In most tumors, the cells are cuboidal or oval; and in low-grade AC (NOS), there is minimal cytologic atypia and infrequent mitotic figures. Ductal differentiation is typically a conspicuous feature of these tumors. Intermediate- and high-grade tumors show increasing cellular pleomorphism with hyperchromatism, high nuclear-to-cytoplasmic ratio, frequent and abnormal mitoses, and foci of hemorrhage and necrosis (Figure 12-3). The stroma is often fibrous and cellular in low-grade tumors but more scanty in higher-grade tumors, which often have a solid growth pattern with minimal ductal differentiation. There may be evidence of angiolymphatic and nerve involvement (Figure 12-4).

A previously poorly understood type of low-grade AC called cribriform AC of the tongue was thought to be a variant of polymorphous low-grade AC. However, it has recently been more fully characterized and renamed *cribriform AC of minor gland origin.*

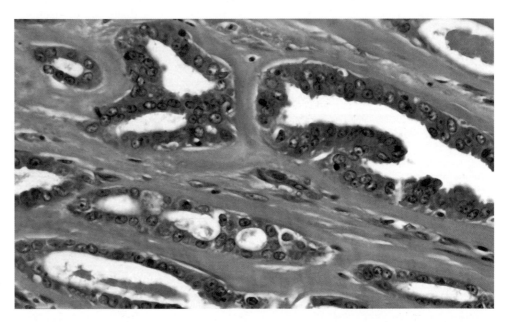

FIGURE 12-1

Heavy desmoplastic stroma separates these atypical epithelial cells arranged in glands in this adenocarcinoma, NOS.

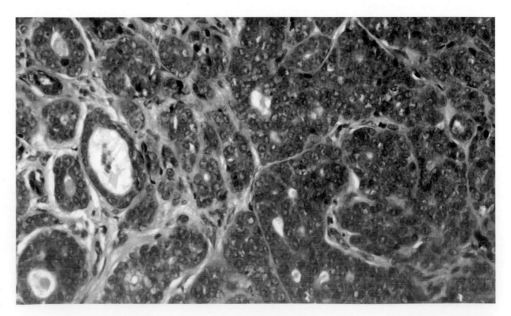

FIGURE 12-2

Trabeculae and tubules of atypical epithelial cells in this adenocarcinoma, NOS.

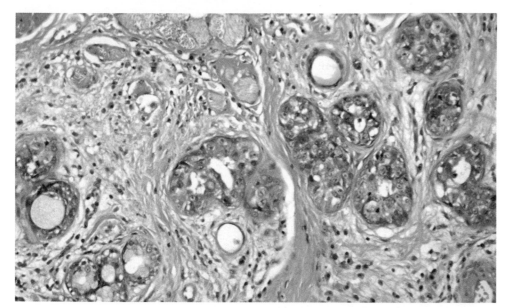

FIGURE 12-3

Glandular differentiation within a fibrous stroma. Mucin production and mitotic figures are seen in this intermediate-grade adenocarcinoma, NOS.

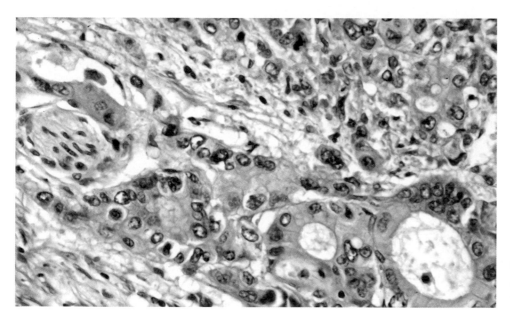

FIGURE 12-4

A high-grade adenocarcinoma, NOS shows glandular profiles with perineural invasion (*far left*). Mitotic figures are easily identified.

ANCILLARY STUDIES

IMMUNOHISTOCHEMICAL FEATURES

There are no characteristic immunohistochemical features.

FINE NEEDLE ASPIRATION

The aspirates of AC (NOS) are often diagnosed as "salivary gland neoplasm," covering a wide variety of tumors. Salivary gland tumors often have variable patterns within the same tumor, making fine needle aspiration (FNA) smears difficult to interpret. However, separation into benign and malignant tumors can usually be accomplished, with a low- versus high-grade designation. Cellular features of malignancy, remarkable cytologic variability, vague glandular differentiation, and rare mucin production may help in establishing a high-grade neoplasm, with definitive classification reserved for the surgical specimen (Figures 12-5 and 12-6).

DIFFERENTIAL DIAGNOSIS

The diagnosis of AC (NOS) is based on the exclusion of other specific tumor types. Metastatic disease must always be considered. Evidence of ductal differentiation aids in the distinction from undifferentiated carcinoma.

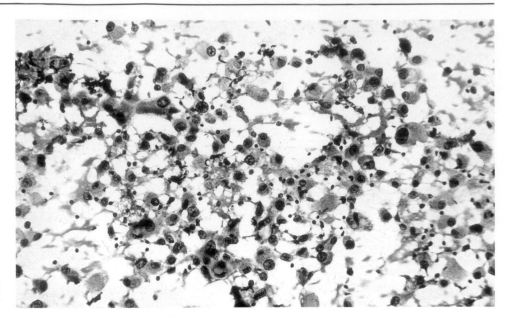

FIGURE 12-5

Highly cellular smear with slight dyscohesion of cells with a high nuclear-to-cytoplasmic ratio and focal mucin production (alcohol-fixed, Papanicolaou stain).

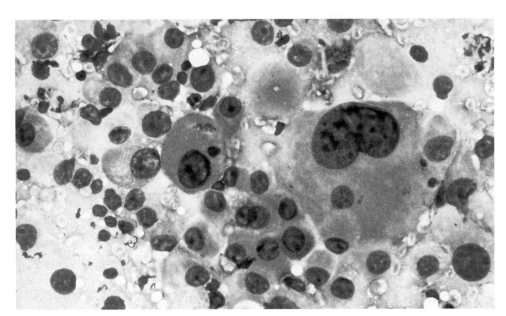

FIGURE 12-6

High power shows profound nuclear pleomorphism, confirming a high-grade malignancy, but no specific tumor type in this fine needle aspiration smear (air-dried, Diff-Quik stain).

PROGNOSIS AND THERAPY

Variability in the criteria used to define these tumors makes the determination of prognostic factors and assessment of outcome problematic. Prognostic factors include tumor grading, clinical stage, and location. Tumors in minor glands have a better prognosis than those in major glands. In the largest survey of this tumor, the 15-year survival rates for low-, intermediate-, and high-grade tumors were 54%, 31%, and 3%, respectively. Low-grade and -stage tumors are treated by complete surgical excision, and in higher-grade tumors, neck dissection and adjuvant radiotherapy need to be considered.

■ MUCOEPIDERMOID CARCINOMA

CLINICAL FEATURES

Mucoepidermoid carcinoma (MEC) is the most common malignant salivary gland tumor (12% to 29%). Over half of all cases involve major glands, particularly the parotid (Figure 12-7). Other sites include the mouth, particularly the palate (Figure 12-7), buccal mucosa, lips and retromolar trigone, and the upper and lower respiratory tracts. Rarely, intrabony tumors form in the mandible and maxilla.

Women are more commonly affected than men (3:2), with a mean age in the 5th decade. MEC is the most

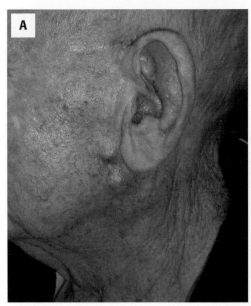
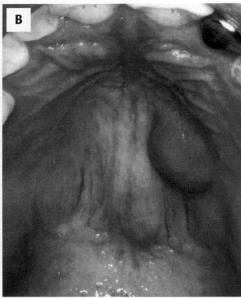

FIGURE 12-7

A, A multinodular mass is noted in the left parotid gland. There is erythema and focal ulceration. **B**, A mucosal covered slightly bluish mass in the left palate represents a mucoepidermoid carcinoma, although this finding is not specific.

MUCOEPIDERMOID CARCINOMA—DISEASE FACT SHEET

Definition

- A malignant glandular epithelial neoplasm characterized by mucus, intermediate, and epidermoid cells

Incidence and Location

- Most common malignant salivary gland tumor (12% to 29%)
- Nearly 60% in major salivary glands (parotid usually)
- Others develop in mouth, upper and lower respiratory tracts

Morbidity and Mortality

- About 40% of cases recur locally
- Spread to regional lymph nodes and distant sites in ~15% of cases
- 5-year survival rate of 80% overall

Gender, Race, and Age Distribution

- Female > male (3:2)
- Mean, 47 years (range, 8 to 92 years)
- Most common salivary malignancy in children

Clinical Features

- Usually forms a painless, fixed, slowly growing swelling
- Intraoral tumors often bluish red and may mimic mucoceles or vascular tumors
- Symptoms include pain, evidence of nerve involvement, otorrhea, dysphagia, and trismus

Prognosis and Treatment

- Prognosis depends on clinical stage, site, grading, and adequacy of surgical excision
- Most tumors are low grade with excellent prognosis
- Tumors of submandibular gland have poorer prognosis
- Tumors, particularly high grade, can show spread to regional lymph nodes and distant sites including lungs, bone, and brain
- Surgery, with or without neck dissection, is treatment of choice; palliative radiotherapy in some cases

common salivary gland malignancy in children. The tumor usually forms a painless, fixed, slowly growing swelling of widely varying duration; sometimes, it shows a recent accelerated growth phase. Symptoms include tenderness, pain, evidence of nerve involvement, otorrhea, dysphagia, and trismus. Intraoral tumors are often bluish-red and fluctuant and may resemble mucoceles or vascular lesions. The tumor occasionally invades the underlying bone.

PATHOLOGIC FEATURES

GROSS FINDINGS

MEC may be circumscribed and variably encapsulated or infiltrative and fixed, particularly in the higher grade tumors. Most tumors are less than 4 cm in diameter. Areas of scarring are relatively common. Cysts of variable sizes are often present and usually contain brownish, glairy fluid (Figure 12-8). Occasionally, tumors appear to be unicystic.

MICROSCOPIC FINDINGS

The cells of MEC form sheets, islands, duct-like structures, and cysts of varying sizes (Figure 12-9). Cysts may be lined by intermediate, mucous, or epidermoid cells (further described later) and are filled with mucus (Figure 12-10). Larger cysts often rupture, spreading tumor cells into the adjacent tissue and evoking an inflammatory reaction with hemorrhage, hemosiderin deposition, cholesterol cleft formation, and fibrosis. Some tumors show extensive mucinous lakes (mucin-rich variant). Papillary processes may extend into cyst lumen, and occasionally this is conspicuous.

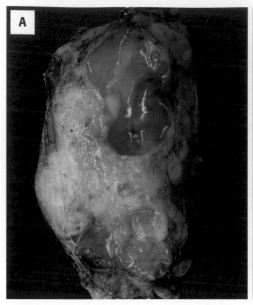
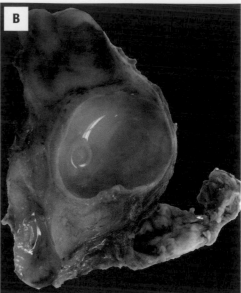

FIGURE 12-8

A, Gross photograph shows a tumor with a tan-yellow cut surface. Mucoid material glistens within the multiple cystic spaces. **B**, This gross photograph demonstrates a predominantly unilocular cyst of a mucoepidermoid carcinoma. The fluid is thick, mucoid, and tenacious. Note the lymph node (*upper*).

MUCOEPIDERMOID CARCINOMA—PATHOLOGIC FEATURES

Gross Findings

- May be circumscribed and variably encapsulated or infiltrative
- Cysts often present and contain brownish, viscid fluid

Microscopic Findings

- Consists of mucous, intermediate, and epidermoid cells
- Other cells include clear cells, columnar cells, and oncocytes
- Tumors show cystic and solid areas in varying proportions along with other patterns
- Inflammation and fibrosis are common
- Tumors separated into low, intermediate, and high grades

Immunohistochemical Features

- Intermediate and epidermoid cells are immunoreactive for cytokeratin and frequently EMA

Fine Needle Aspiration

- Cellular smears with background of mucinous material
- Cohesive epithelial clusters with sheets of cells and cells streaming in the mucus
- Mucocytes help to confirm diagnosis in presence of intermediate and epidermoid cells

Pathologic Differential Diagnosis

- Necrotizing sialometaplasia, mucocele, cystadenoma, cystadenocarcinoma, squamous cell carcinoma, adenosquamous carcinoma, clear cell neoplasms, metastasis

---

MEC consists predominantly of three cell types in widely varying proportions: epidermoid, mucous, and intermediate (Figure 12-11). Less common cell types seen include clear cells, columnar cells, and oncocytes. Intermediate cells frequently predominate and range in size from small, basal cells with scanty basophilic cytoplasm ("maternal" cells) to larger and more oval cells with more abundant pale, eosinophilic cytoplasm that appears to merge into epidermoid or mucous cells (Figure 12-12). The intermediate cells form islands or sheets and may form the basally located cells of intratumoral cysts. Mucous cells (mucocytes) can occur singly or in clusters and have pale and sometimes foamy cytoplasm, a distinct cell boundary, and peripherally placed, small and compressed nuclei. They often form the lining of cysts or duct-like structures (Figure 12-12). Occasionally, mucocytes are so scanty they can only be identified with confidence by using stains such as mucicarmine (Figure 12-13) or Alcian blue. Epidermoid cells may be uncommon and focally distributed. They have abundant eosinophilic cytoplasm but rarely show keratin pearl formation or dyskeratosis unless there has been a biopsy or FNA. Focal areas of clear cells are common but occasionally form the bulk of the tumor. The cells have distinct outlines, water-clear cytoplasm and small, centrally located nuclei (Figure 12-14). They contain minimal sialomucin but usually have a plentiful glycogen content, as demonstrated with periodic acid–Schiff diastase (PAS/D) staining. Columnar cells are uncommon and typically form the lining of cysts. Focal or generalized oncocytic metaplasia (known as MEC oncocytic variant) is seen occasionally.

Higher-grade tumors may show cytologic atypia, a high mitotic frequency, areas of necrosis, and neural invasion (Figure 12-15). Rarely, low-grade MECs undergo dedifferentiation. Stromal hyalinization is common and sometimes extensive and there is a sclerosing variant with intense central scarring, which may be due to infarction or mucous extravasation. In addition, there is a sclerosing variant associated with a florid eosinophilic infiltration. Patchy lymphocytic infiltration of MEC is frequent and there may be extensive lymphocytic proliferation with

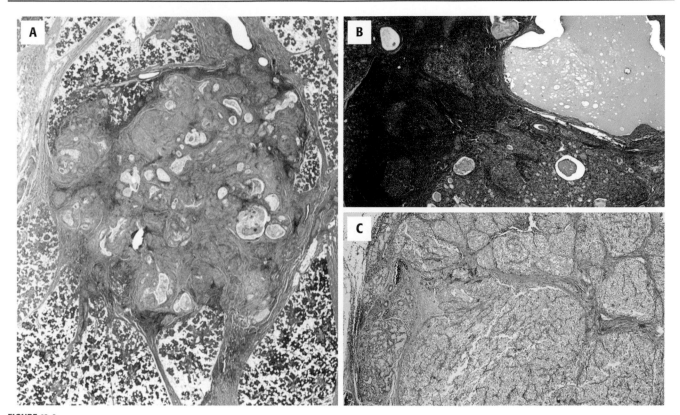

FIGURE 12-9

A, Mucoepidermoid carcinoma (MEC) often shows a variable growth pattern with cystic spaces and fibrosis. **B**, Tumor-associated lymphoid tissue is noted adjacent to the tumor. **C**, Predominantly mucinous epithelium is seen in this field of an MEC.

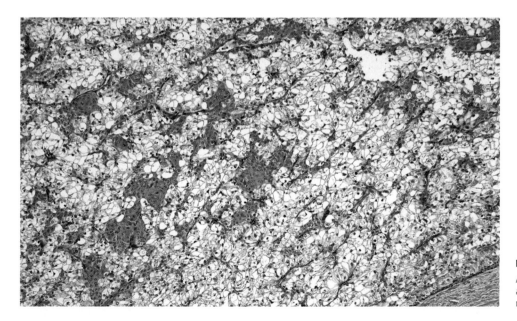

FIGURE 12-10

A sheet-like distribution of intermediate and mucous cells in this mucoepidermoid carcinoma.

germinal center formation, resembling lymph node infiltration (Figure 12-9).

TUMOR GRADING

MEC shows variability in clinical behavior and several microscopic grading systems have been advocated to predict outcome. Many rely on subjective evaluation of the relative proportions of the various cell types as well as (1) cystic component, (2) neural invasion (Figure 12-16), (3) necrosis, (4) increased mitoses, and (5) cellular pleomorphism (anaplasia). Low-grade tumors tend to be cystic, have abundant mucocytes, and show minimal atypia or mitotic activity. However, they usually show evidence of invasion. Higher grade tumors are more cellular with minimal cyst formation (Figure 12-17). They have few

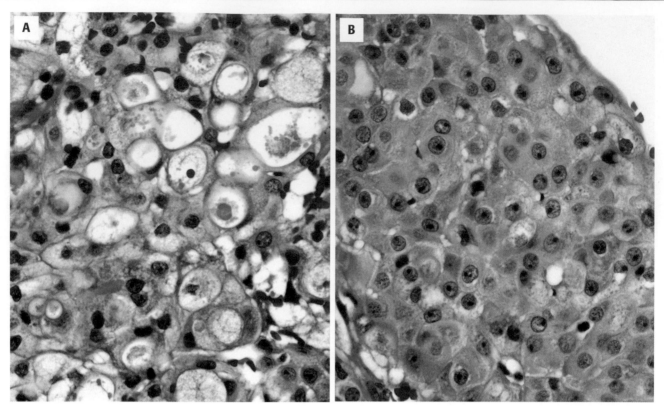

FIGURE 12-11

A, The intermediate cells are blending imperceptibly with the mucocytes in this mucoepidermoid carcinoma. **B**, A field of epidermoid cells. Note the lack of intercellular bridges and "hard" keratinization.

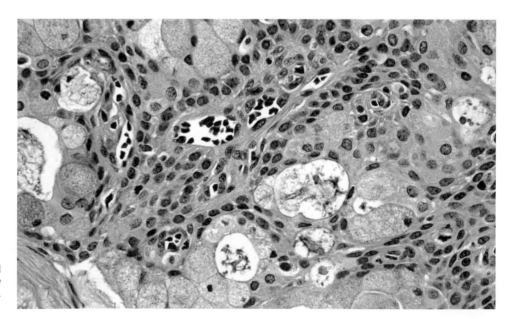

FIGURE 12-12

The intermediate cells are noted in small islands and form the "basal zone" below the cystic spaces lined by mucocytes. Mucocytes have fluffy cytoplasm.

mucocytes and consist mainly of cells similar to squamous cell carcinoma and may show necrosis and neural or vascular invasion. A numerical grading system using point scoring of five parameters appears to be useful in defining the tumors as low, intermediate, or high grade and predicting their behavior (Table 12-1). However, the grading of MEC of the submandibular gland using this system was less reliable. A seven-point grading system, including the additional parameters of the nature of the invasive front and bone invasion, has been proposed but requires additional validation. Lymphovascular invasion has not been included in grading scales to date.

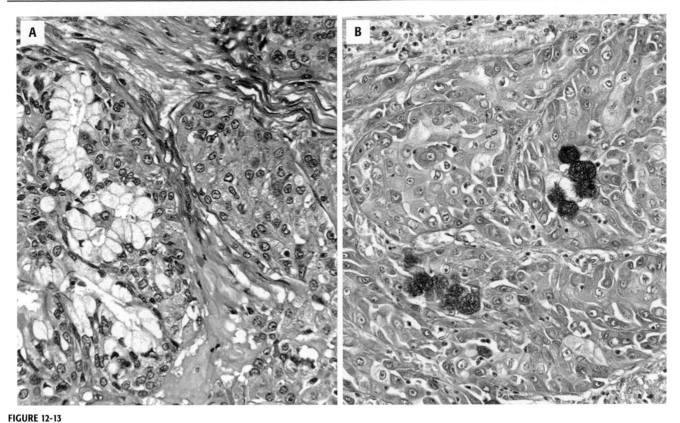

FIGURE 12-13

A, Mucocytes are identified in a cyst with intermediate cells at the base. **B**, Mucicarmine highlights intracytoplasmic mucin, especially in cells with eccentric, squashed nuclei.

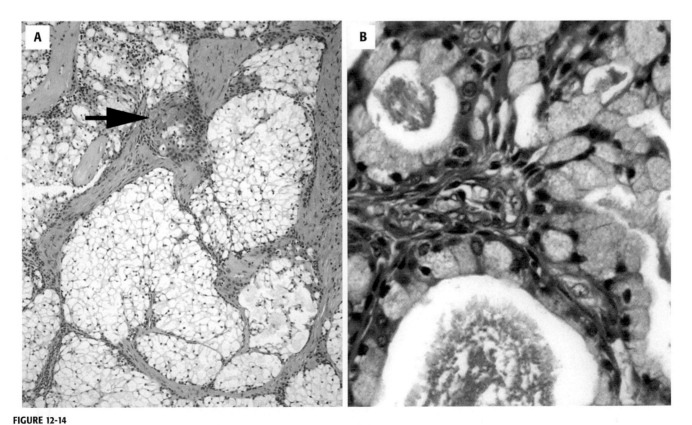

FIGURE 12-14

A, This mucoepidermoid carcinoma shows a predominantly clear cell pattern, although isolated mucocytes are noted (*arrow*). **B**, The mucocytes have fluffy cytoplasm and may surround secretions within the duct spaces.

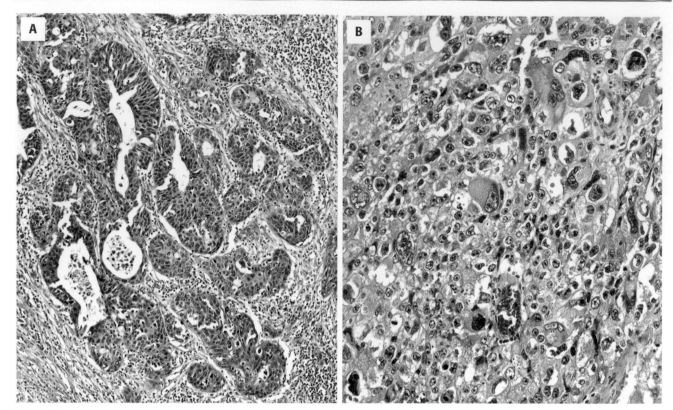

FIGURE 12-15

A, Intermediate-grade MEC showing limited cyst formation and nearly absent mucocytes. **B**, A high-grade tumor with increased mitoses and profound pleomorphism.

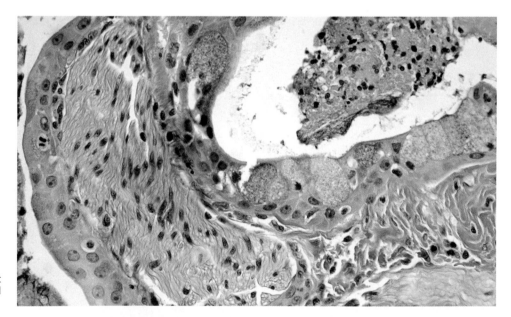

FIGURE 12-16

The degree of cytologic atypia is not profound, but there is well-developed perineural invasion in this tumor.

ANCILLARY STUDIES

IMMUNOHISTOCHEMICAL FEATURES

Intermediate, squamoid, and columnar cells are usually positive for cytokeratin but clear cells show inconsistent reactivity and mucocytes are negative. Epithelial membrane antigen (EMA) is positive in most tumor cells, but staining with this and other immunohistochemical markers (such as CK5/6 and p63) does not correlate with histologic grading and is rarely of diagnostic value (Figure 12-18).

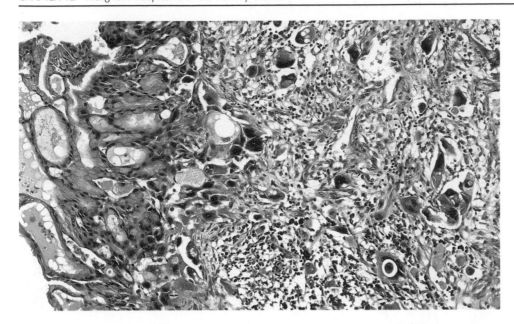

FIGURE 12-17

A low-grade tumor is noted to undergo dedifferentiation into a sarcomatoid carcinoma appearance (right-sided). This abrupt transition is usually the tip-off to sarcomatous transformation.

TABLE 12-1

Grading and Outcome for Mucoepidermoid Carcinomas

Parameter	Point Value	
Intracystic component <20%	2	
Neural invasion	2	
Necrosis	3	
Mitotic figures ≥4/10 HPFs	3	
Anaplasia	4	
Grade	**Total Score**	**Dead of Disease**
Low	0-4	3.3%
Intermediate	5-6	9.7%
High	≥7	46.3%

FINE NEEDLE ASPIRATION

Smears of an MEC may be difficult to separate from a mucocele or other benign cyst. However, MEC usually has cellular smears with abundant mucinous material and debris in the background (Figure 12-19). There are cohesive groups of epithelial cells arranged in sheets or streaming within the mucin (Figure 12-19). Cells are separated into mucocytes, intermediate, and epidermoid cells in variable proportions. Most of the cells have ample cytoplasm surrounding nuclei that are only mildly pleomorphic. Higher-grade tumors have less mucin and greater nuclear pleomorphism, which may be difficult to diagnose accurately on FNA. Occasionally, a diagnosis of "mucus-producing lesion" may be the only diagnosis that can be rendered with accuracy.

DIFFERENTIAL DIAGNOSIS

Both MEC and necrotizing sialometaplasia (NSM) can show squamous proliferation with foci of mucocytic differentiation in an inflamed, fibrous stroma. NSM, however, has a lobular distribution and usually shows areas of transition from the ducts to the solid islands of squamous cells formed by intraductal regenerative hyperplasia (Figure 12-20). There are no intermediate cells and cyst formation is not a feature. MEC can usually be distinguished from cystadenoma and cystadenocarcinoma by its much more variable cytologic and morphologic characteristics (Figure 12-21). High-grade tumors may resemble nonkeratinizing squamous cell carcinoma, but appropriate stains can demonstrate the presence of scattered mucocytes. In addition, it is exceedingly rare for MECs to show keratinization. Other mimics of high-grade MEC include adenosquamous carcinoma and salivary duct carcinoma. The sclerosing variant of MEC may be confused with chronic sialadenitis. Predominantly clear cell MEC must be distinguished from tumors such as epithelial-myoepithelial carcinoma (EMC), clear cell carcinoma (NOS), and metastatic tumors.

PROGNOSIS AND THERAPY

The prognosis is dependent on clinical stage, site, grading, and adequacy of surgery. Most MECs are low grade and the prognosis for these tumors is generally good (>95% survival with only rare regional metastases). The mortality rate, however, increases to about 45% in the much less common group of high-grade tumors. In addition, incompletely excised tumors have a very high recurrence rate, particularly high-grade tumors. Also,

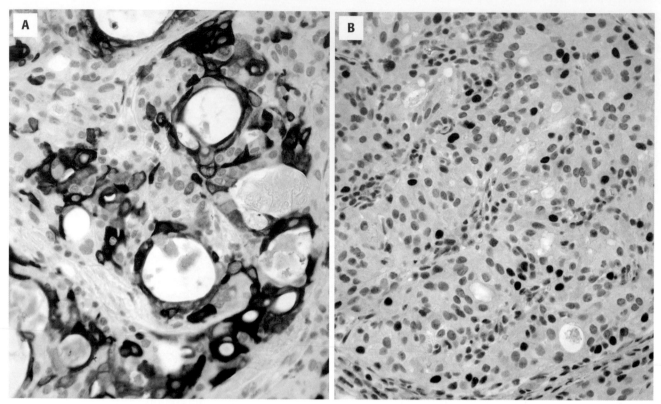

FIGURE 12-18

Immunohistochemistry can help to confirm the epithelial nature of the process and perhaps highlight the epidermoid cells (CK5/6, **A**), although basal markers (p63, **B**) are also positive.

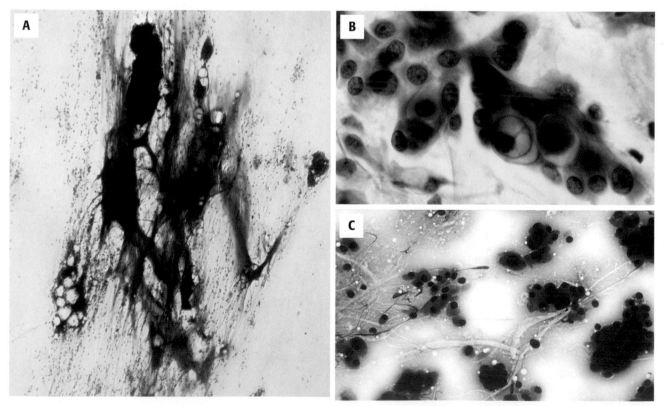

FIGURE 12-19

A, Epithelial cells are set in a sea of mucinous material. This type of mucinous material is the clue to the diagnosis. **B**, A cellular smear with intermediate-epidermoid cells arranged in sheets and streaming groups. Note the mucocyte in the center with mucin vacuoles (alcohol-fixed, Papanicolaou stain). **C**, A cellular smear with a background of mucinous material. Groups of epithelial cells with opaque cytoplasm comprise the intermediate component (air-dried, Diff-Quik stain).

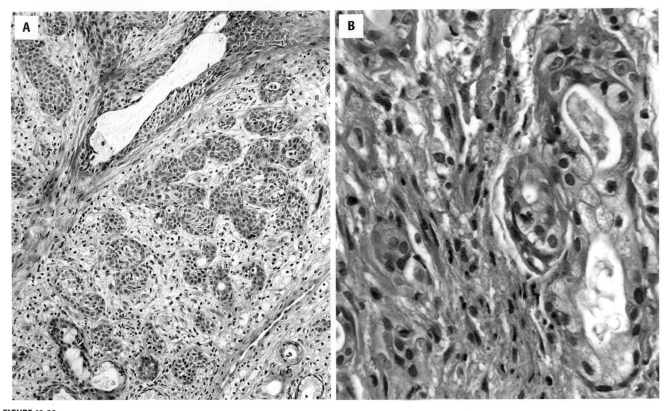

FIGURE 12-20
A, Necrotizing sialometaplasia has a lobular architecture with squamous metaplasia of the duct/lobular units. **B**, Residual mucocytes are replaced by metaplastic squamous epithelium. Inflammatory cells are noted in the background.

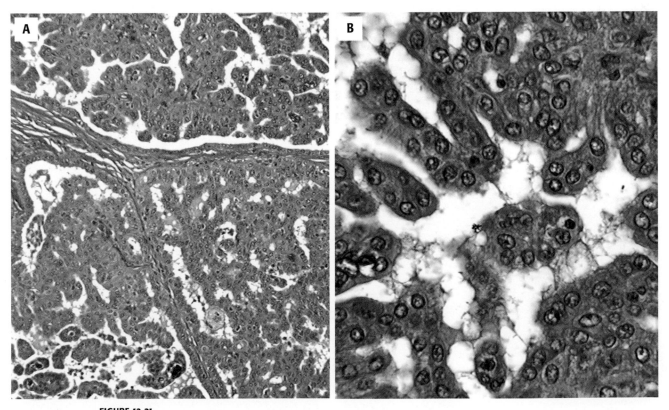

FIGURE 12-21
A papillary cystadenocarcinoma has complex, arborizing papillae (**A**) with nuclear atypia and mitotic figures (**B**).

MEC in the submandibular gland, floor of mouth, tongue, and maxillary antrum has a poorer prognosis. Death is usually due to uncontrolled locoregional disease and/or metastases to lung, bone, and brain. Treatment is by surgical excision, with or without neck dissection. Radiotherapy is generally palliative in advanced tumors but has little impact on outcome.

■ ACINIC CELL CARCINOMA

CLINICAL FEATURES

Acinic cell carcinoma (AcCC) accounts for about 6% of all salivary gland tumors and up to 17.5% of all salivary malignancies. About 80% form in the parotid gland, while the minor salivary glands are the second most common site (Figure 12-22). About 4% arise in the submandibular gland and 1% in the sublingual. Less common locations include the buccal mucosa, lips, and palate and, rarely, the lacrimal gland, mandible, and minor glands in the upper and lower respiratory tracts. There is a slight female predominance (3:2). Most cases are evenly distributed in the 2nd to 7th decades (mean, 44 years). It is the second most common malignant salivary gland tumor in children.

AcCC usually presents as a slowly growing mass with a duration ranging from a few weeks to 40 years. Pain or tenderness is present in up to half of patients. The tumor may be freely mobile or fixed to the skin or underlying tissues. Facial nerve involvement is seen in up to 10% of cases.

PATHOLOGIC FEATURES

GROSS FINDINGS

Most tumors are less than 3 cm in diameter and usually form a rubbery or firm, circumscribed, oval or round mass. Some have poorly defined margins or multifocal nodules and areas of hemorrhage or cystic change (Figure 12-22).

ACINIC CELL CARCINOMA—DISEASE FACT SHEET

Definition
- A malignant epithelial neoplasm demonstrating serous acinar cell differentiation with cytoplasmic zymogen secretory granules

Incidence and Location
- About 6% of salivary gland tumors
- 80% involve the parotid gland
- Minor salivary glands second most common site

Morbidity and Mortality
- 5-year and 10-year survival rates 82% and 68%, respectively

Gender, Race, and Age Distribution
- Female > male (3:2)
- 2nd to 7th decades (mean, 44 years)
- Second most common malignant salivary gland tumor in children

Clinical Features
- Slowly growing, mobile or fixed mass
- Duration varies from weeks to several decades
- Pain or tenderness in up to half of patients
- Facial nerve involvement in 5% to 10% of cases

Prognosis and Treatment
- About 35% develop recurrences
- Behavior does not correlate with patterns of growth
- Poor prognosis associated with large size, involvement of the deep lobe of the parotid, multinodularity, regional and distant metastases, cellular pleomorphism, increased mitotic frequency, areas of necrosis, and neural invasion
- Ki-67 staining may be an independent prognostic factor for survival
- Complete surgical excision treatment of choice

ACINIC CELL CARCINOMA—PATHOLOGIC FEATURES

Gross Findings
- Rubbery or firm tumors usually <3 cm
- Usually circumscribed (occasionally irregular)
- May show hemorrhage or cystic change

Microscopic Findings
- Characteristic cell is serous acinar type with granules in the cytoplasm (usually accentuated at the lumen)
- Other cell types include nonspecific glandular, intercalated ductal, vacuolated, and clear
- Wide variety of histomorphologic configurations including solid, microcystic, papillary-cystic, and follicular
- May have lymphoid infiltrate, occasionally prominent

Ancillary Studies
- PAS-positive, diastase-resistant zymogen granules
- Acinic cells may stain positively for amylase, transferrin, lactoferrin, CEA, VIP, and others
- About 10% show some positivity for S100 protein

Fine Needle Aspiration
- Cellular smears with clean background
- Cohesive, small, tight clusters
- Ample, granular to vacuolated cytoplasm surrounding round and regular nuclei with coarse chromatin (lymphocyte-like nuclei)

Pathologic Differential Diagnosis
- Normal salivary gland, sialadenitis, cystadenocarcinoma (especially papillary variants), mucoepidermoid carcinoma, thyroid carcinoma, clear cell tumors

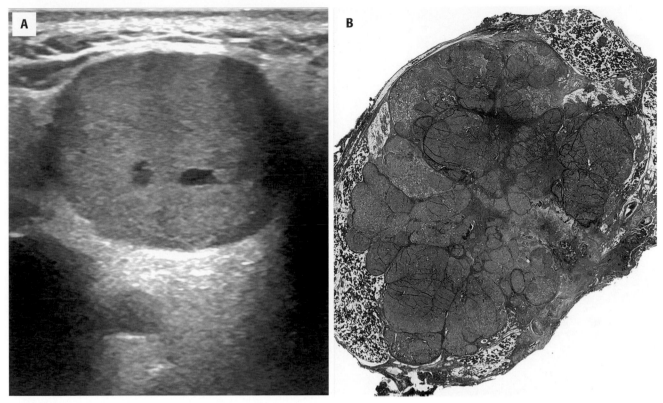

FIGURE 12-22

A, Ultrasound shows a well-circumscribed mass focally showing cystic change. **B**, There is an irregular and invasive periphery to this multinodular tumor. A capsule is not well developed, although internal tumor fibrosis is present.

MICROSCOPIC FINDINGS

AcCC is characterized by serous acinar cells, but several other cell types may be present. These include intercalated duct, nonspecific glandular, vacuolated, and clear cells. Individual tumors may show several cell types or one type may predominate. *Serous acinar* cells are the most common (Figure 12-23). They resemble serous cells of the normal salivary gland and have abundant pale, basophilic cytoplasm containing dense, grayish or blue zymogen granules. The granules may be fine or coarse and are variably PAS/D positive (Figure 12-24). Nuclei are round and basophilic or occasionally more vesicular and are usually located peripherally. *Intercalated duct-type* cells are smaller as they contain less cytoplasm, which is usually eosinophilic, and the nuclei tend to be central. These cells surround luminal spaces of varying sizes. *Vacuolated* cells may be a

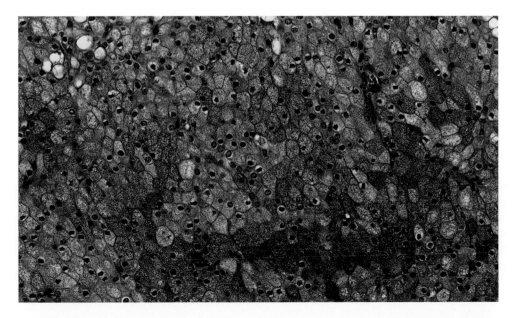

FIGURE 12-23

Serous acinar cells have abundant pale to basophilic, heavily granular cytoplasm in this low-grade acinic cell carcinoma.

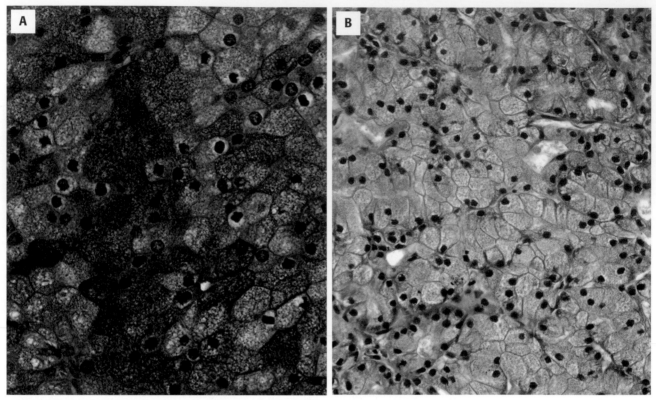

FIGURE 12-24

A, The granules, representing zymogen granules, are variable in size and often accentuated along the luminal border in acinic cell carcinoma. **B**, Sometimes the granules are less well developed, although the cell borders are usually quite prominent.

conspicuous feature. They have clear, PAS/D-negative, cytoplasmic vacuoles, and some cells also contain zymogen granules. Cells with *clear* cytoplasm and conspicuous cell boundaries are usually only seen focally. They do not contain glycogen and may be a fixation or processing artifact. *Nonspecific glandular* cells are polygonal or round and are usually smaller than acinar cells. The cytoplasm is eosinophilic or amphophilic, PAS/D negative, and lacks granules. There is greater variability in the size and staining characteristics of the nuclei. The nonspecific glandular cells often form sheets of cells with indistinct borders.

Growth patterns of AcCC include solid, papillary-cystic, microcystic, and follicular; individual tumors may show several configurations (Figure 12-25). In the *solid* type, the cells are closely aggregated in sheets or nodules. Acinic cells are the most common form, but nonspecific glandular and clear cells may also be seen. In the *papillary-cystic* variant, the cysts are usually prominent and show intraluminal papillary projections. The cells on the luminal layer may show a hobnail appearance. Intratumoral and intracystic hemorrhage is common in this variant, and sometimes the tumor cells phagocytose hemosiderin (Figure 12-26). The *microcystic* pattern, which is the most common, contains small spaces in the tumor that give it a lattice-like appearance (Figure 12-27). In addition to the acinic cells, vacuolated and intercalated type cells are common. The *follicular variant* consists of

multiple, variably sized cystic spaces. These are lined mostly by intercalated duct-type cells and contain homogeneous, eosinophilic, proteinaceous fluid, and the appearance closely mimics follicular thyroid carcinoma (Figure 12-27). Psammoma bodies are sometimes seen in a variety of AcCC types and may be a conspicuous feature.

Many tumors show focal areas of stromal infiltration by lymphocytes, but some have a very striking lymphocytic stroma in which germinal centers develop (Figure 12-28). These tumors are well circumscribed or encapsulated and usually of the solid or microcystic type. They may have a better prognosis than conventional types. Stromal fibrosis or sclerosis may be associated with a slightly worse prognosis (Figure 12-28). Rare dedifferentiated tumors showing high-grade malignant areas in an otherwise conventional AcCC have been described (Figure 12-29). Bilateral, multifocal, and hybrid tumors have also been reported.

ANCILLARY STUDIES

ULTRASTRUCTURAL FEATURES

While uncommonly used to identify tumors in modern practice, identification of secretory zymogen granules in the cytoplasm can help to confirm the diagnosis (Figure 12-30).

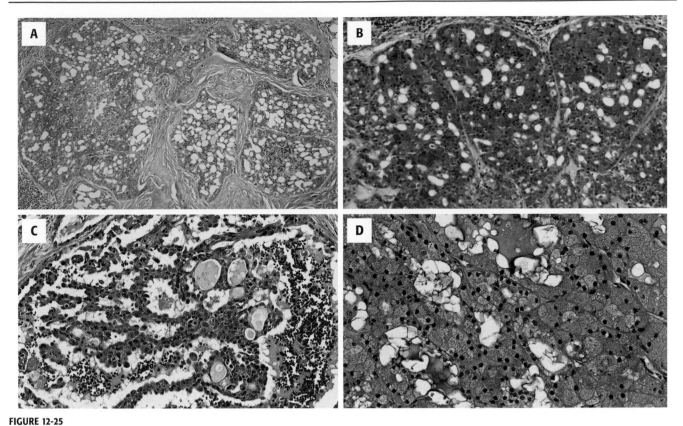

FIGURE 12-25

A, A microcystic or lattice-like pattern is created by multiple small cysts. **B**, A solid pattern still has small glandular spaces. **C**, A papillary-cystic variant has abundant papillary projections. Note the hobnail appearance with cystic spaces. **D**, This follicular pattern shows "colloid-like" material within some of the spaces.

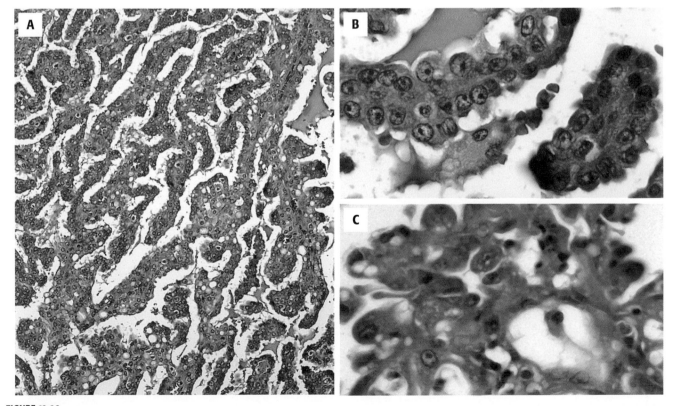

FIGURE 12-26

A, A microcystic pattern is seen in this acinic cell carcinoma. **B**, Note the hobnail-like appearance. **C**, Intracystic hemorrhage may show phagocytosed hemosiderin within the cytoplasm of some of the tumor cells.

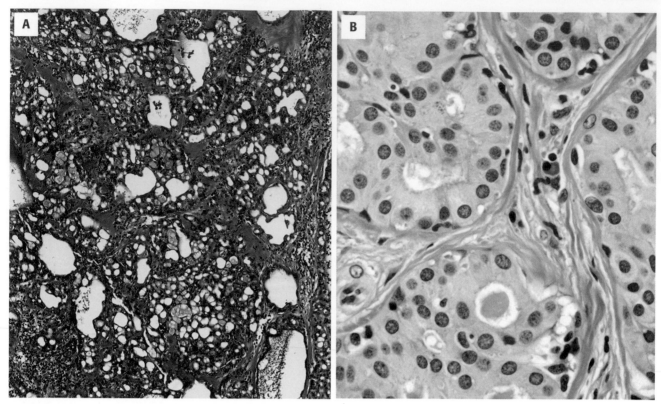

FIGURE 12-27

A, A lattice-like appearance is dominant in this case with fibrous bands noted. Secretions are frequently present. **B**, This tumor shows a follicular pattern with glandular-like spaces and concretions. Note the fine granules surrounding the lumen at the center of the image.

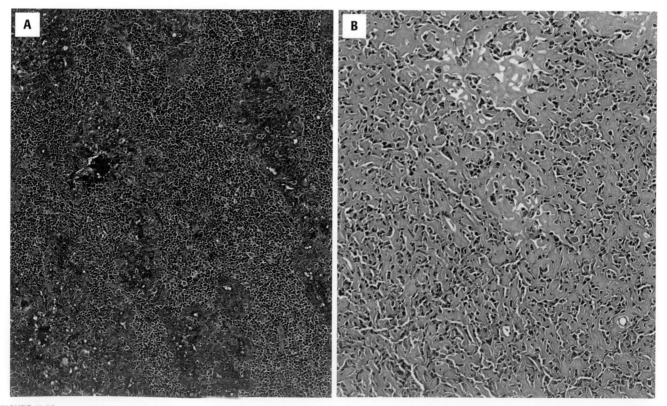

FIGURE 12-28

A, The stroma is infiltrated by lymphocytes (tumor-associated lymphoid proliferation) in this acinic cell carcinoma. **B**, Dense stromal fibrosis compressed the tumor cells into cords, making them difficult to accurately classify.

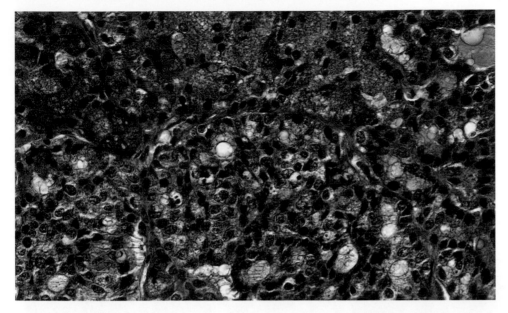

FIGURE 12-29

High-grade transformation (dedifferentiation) can be seen in acinic cell carcinoma. In this case, the lower half of the image shows the area of sheet-like to glandular appearance of the more pleomorphic cells (upper part shows classic tumor appearance).

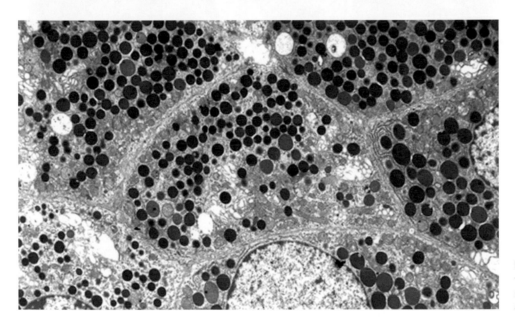

FIGURE 12-30

This ultrastructural examination demonstrates secretory zymogen granules. *(Courtesy of Dr. I. Dardick.)*

IMMUNOHISTOCHEMICAL FEATURES

AcCC shows reactivity with a variety of immunoagents, but staining tends to be unpredictable and of little value in diagnosis. Acinic cells may stain positively for amylase, transferrin, lactoferrin, carcinoembryonic antigen (CEA), vasoactive intestinal peptide (VIP), and others. However, staining for amylase is frequently weak or absent in routinely processed tissue. About 10% of tumors show some positivity for S100 protein.

FINE NEEDLE ASPIRATION

AcCC tends to yield cellular smears with a clean background. Tumor cells are cohesive, arranged in small, tight clusters, occasionally demonstrating a small central, fibrovascular core (Figures 12-31 and 12-32). The nuclei are usually round and regular with little pleomorphism surrounded by abundant, eosinophilic, finely granular to vacuolated cytoplasm (Figure 12-32). Separating other tumors from acinic cell on FNA preparations may be difficult.

DIFFERENTIAL DIAGNOSIS

The variants of AcCC may cause problems in diagnosis. The neoplasm needs to be distinguished from normal serous acini or *sialadenitis*, especially if there is limited material. Microcystic and papillary-cystic variants need

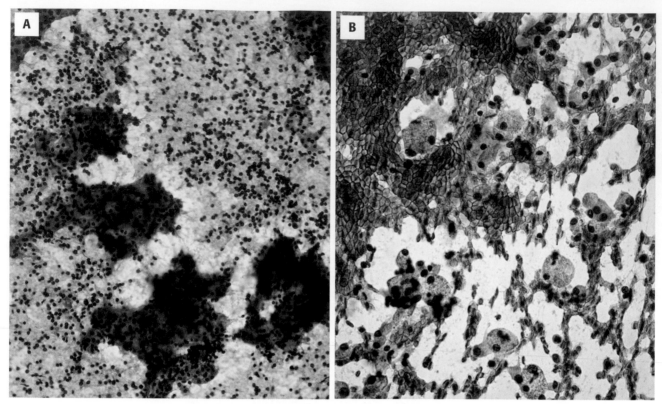

FIGURE 12-31

Acinic cell carcinoma. **A**, An acinar arrangement of cells with round, regular nuclei and granular cytoplasm along with numerous naked nuclei in the background (alcohol-fixed, hematoxylin and eosin stain) **B**, Isolated tumor cells with bubbly cytoplasm can suggest macrophages rather than epithelial cells (alcohol-fixed, Papanicolaou stain).

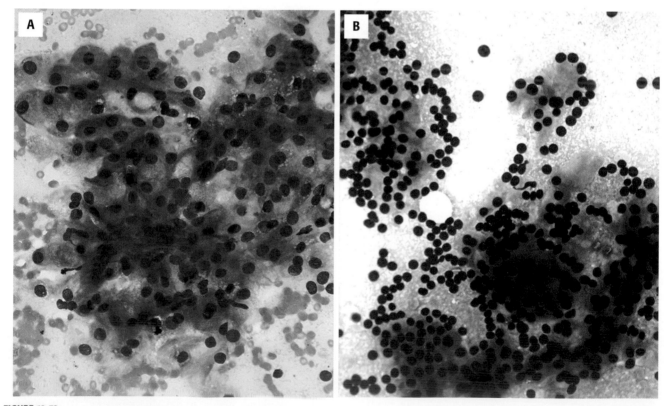

FIGURE 12-32

A and **B**, A cohesive cluster of cells is noted in a background of blood. There is only slight nuclear variability. Note the finely granular to vacuolated cytoplasm in these acinic cell carcinomas (air-dried, Diff-Quik stain).

to be differentiated from *cystadenocarcinoma*, particularly its papillary variant. Zymogen granules, vacuolated cells, and intercalated ductal differentiation support the diagnosis of AcCC. Microcystic variants may be misdiagnosed as *MECs* due to the strong mucicarmine positivity of the cystic spaces and the presence of small spaces being interpreted as mucocytes. Follicular variants can resemble *thyroid carcinomas* so closely that immunostaining for thyroglobulin is needed to separate the tumors. Although *clear cell tumors* are included in the differential diagnosis, this is rarely a practical problem as the clear cells in AcCC are usually focal.

PROGNOSIS AND THERAPY

Recurrences develop in ~35% of patients. There is an overall 5-year and 10-year survival rate of 82% and 68%, respectively. The tumor may involve regional lymph nodes and the most common sites for distant spread are lung and bones. Grading is not universally accepted and there is no correlation between prognosis and the four main histomorphologic patterns. Histologic features thought to be associated with poor prognosis include cellular pleomorphism, increased mitotic frequency, areas of necrosis, and neural invasion. Ki-67 staining may be an independent prognostic factor for survival. However, the clinical stage at presentation may be a better predictor of behavior than grading. Large size, involvement of the deep lobe of the parotid, multiple recurrences, multinodularity, and regional and distant metastases are indicators of poor prognosis. Tumors in minor glands have a much better prognosis than those in major glands. Complete surgical excision is the treatment of choice and failure to clear the tumor is associated with a poor outcome.

■ ADENOID CYSTIC CARCINOMA

CLINICAL FEATURES

Adenoid cystic carcinoma (AdCC) accounts for ~10% of all malignant salivary gland tumors. It affects a wide age range with a peak incidence in 40- to 60-year-olds. There is a slight female preponderance. Minor glands of the mouth, particularly the palate, and the upper aerodigestive tract, account for about half of all cases (Figure 12-33). Other common sites include the parotid (21%), submandibular gland (5%), and sinonasal tract (11%). Tumors usually present as a slowly growing mass of long duration. It may be tender or painful, and cranial nerve lesions, particularly facial nerve palsy, may be the presenting feature. Tumors of minor glands often show ulceration of the overlying mucosa.

PATHOLOGIC FEATURES

GROSS FINDINGS

The tumor is usually firm and may be well circumscribed, particularly when small. Most are unencapsulated. The gross appearance belies the true extent of the tumor, as neural infiltration is not discernible on macroscopic examination.

MICROSCOPIC FINDINGS

AdCC has three main morphologic patterns: cribriform or cylindromatous, tubular, and solid, in decreasing order of frequency. A mixture of these patterns may be seen (Figure 12-34). The *cribriform* variant consists of islands of modified myoepithelial cells containing rounded, pseudocystic areas forming a characteristic "Swiss cheese" appearance (Figure 12-35). The pseudocysts are basophilic and mucoid, or consist of hyaline, eosinophilic material. They are composed of glycosaminoglycans and reduplicated basement membrane material. Foci of ductal cells are present within

ADENOID CYSTIC CARCINOMA—PATHOLOGIC FEATURES

Gross Findings

- Usually firm, often well circumscribed, but unencapsulated

Microscopic Findings

- Composed of duct lining cells and abluminal modified myoepithelial cells
- Main patterns are cribriform, tubular, and solid in decreasing order of frequency; mixed patterns common
- Pseudocysts filled with basophilic mucoid ("blue-goo") or hyaline, eosinophilic material (reduplicated basement membrane material)
- Perineural invasion common and frequently extensive
- Cells are small with high nuclear-to-cytoplasmic ratio
- Nuclei are peg shaped ("carrot" shaped) to columnar with dense nuclear chromatin distribution
- Stroma is hyalinized

Ancillary Studies

- Pseudocysts positive for PAS, Alcian blue, laminin, and type IV collagen
- Epithelial cells positive for low-molecular-weight keratins, EMA, and CD117
- Myoepithelial cells positive with calponin, SMA, S100 protein, and p63

Fine Needle Aspiration

- Usually cellular smears with cohesive sheets of monotonous, only mildly atypical epithelial cells
- Cells surround spherical, hyaline globules (reduplicated basement membrane material resembling pink "gum balls"), best seen on air-dried preparations (bright magenta on Romanovsky stains)
- Nuclei are hyperchromatic and peg shaped/cuboidal within cells that have high nuclear-to-cytoplasmic ratios

Pathologic Differential Diagnosis

- Polymorphous low-grade adenocarcinoma, pleomorphic adenoma, basaloid squamous cell carcinoma, epithelial-myoepithelial carcinoma

the myoepithelial areas but may be inconspicuous. The *tubular* variant is double-layered and has more obvious ductal differentiation (Figure 12-36). There is an inner layer of eosinophilic, duct-lining cells, and the abluminal myoepithelial cells often show clear cytoplasm and irregular, angular nuclei (Figure 12-37). The uncommon *solid* variant consists of islands or sheets of basaloid cells with larger and less angular nuclei (Figure 12-38). Duct-lining cells may be sparse and indistinct, and comedonecrosis is common. Mitoses are sparse in the cribriform and tubular patterns but may be frequent in the solid type. Rarely, AdCC undergoes high-grade transformation (dedifferentiation) and shows pleomorphism, a high frequency of mitoses, and extensive necrosis.

AdCC is composed of luminal ductal cells and abluminal, modified myoepithelial cells. The latter predominate and have indistinct cell borders and frequently sparse, amphophilic or clear cytoplasm. The nuclei are uniform in size, with dense chromatin and may be round or angular (peg shaped). Ductal cells surround small and sometimes indistinct lumina (Figure 12-39). They are cuboidal and have more abundant, eosinophilic cytoplasm and round, uniform nuclei that may contain small nucleoli.

The stroma of ACC is usually hyalinized and in some cases is so abundant that tumor cells are attenuated into strands (Figure 12-40). It is continuous, even though appearing separated in histologic sections. Perineural or intraneural invasion is common and frequently conspicuous, and the tumor can extend along nerves over a wide area (Figure 12-38). It may invade bone extensively before there is any radiologic evidence of bone destruction. Lymph node involvement is often due to contiguous spread rather than lymphatic permeation or embolization.

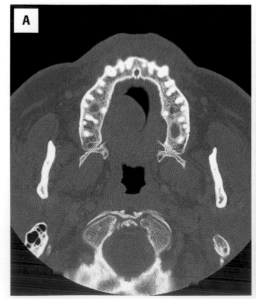 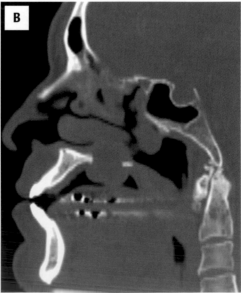

FIGURE 12-33

A tumor within the palate shows a projection into the oral cavity (**A**), while destroying the bony floor of the nasal cavity (**B**) in these computed tomography scans of adenoid cystic carcinoma.

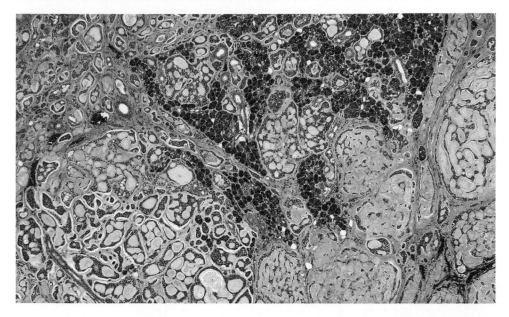

FIGURE 12-34

An adenoid cystic carcinoma showing multiple patterns of growth, although the cribriform and tubular areas predominate. Notice how the tumor is infiltrating between and around the parenchyma.

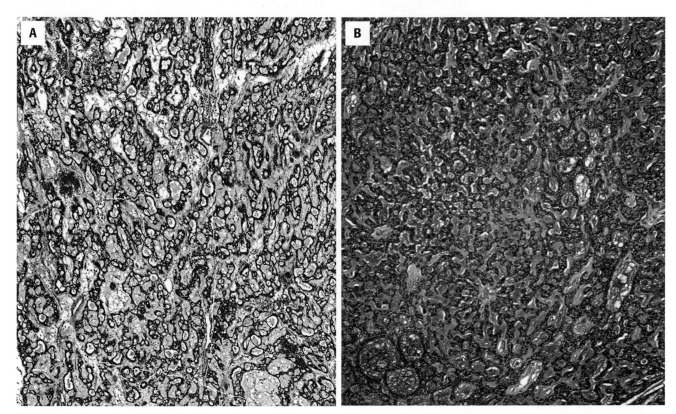

FIGURE 12-35

A, The characteristic cribriform or cylindromatous pattern is seen in this adenoid cystic carcinoma. **B**, Note a more trabecular appearance, although the glycosaminoglycan material is very prominent in this adenoid cystic carcinoma.

ANCILLARY STUDIES

HISTOCHEMICAL AND IMMUNOHISTOCHEMICAL FEATURES

The pseudocysts are positive for PAS and Alcian blue (Figure 12-39) and react with antibodies to basement membrane components such as laminin and type IV collagen. The epithelial cells are positive for low-molecular-weight keratins (including CK5/6) and EMA and CD117, and the myoepithelial cells are positive for markers such as calponin, smooth muscle actin (SMA), p63, and S100 protein (Figures 12-41 and 12-42).

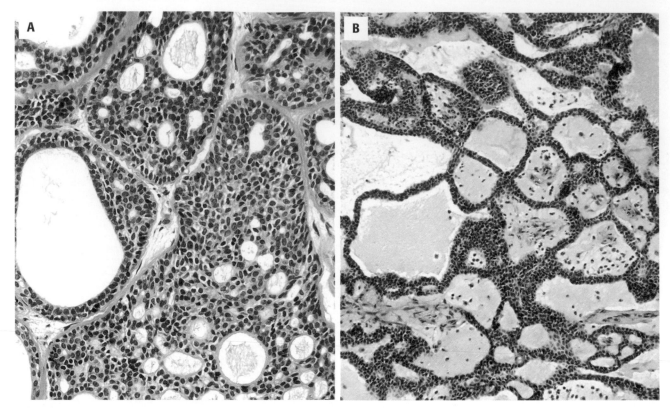

FIGURE 12-36

A, There is a mixture of patterns, but the peg-shaped nuclei are seen along with small duct-like spaces within the proliferation. **B**, This pattern suggests a canalicular adenoma pattern, although the matrix material is not similar.

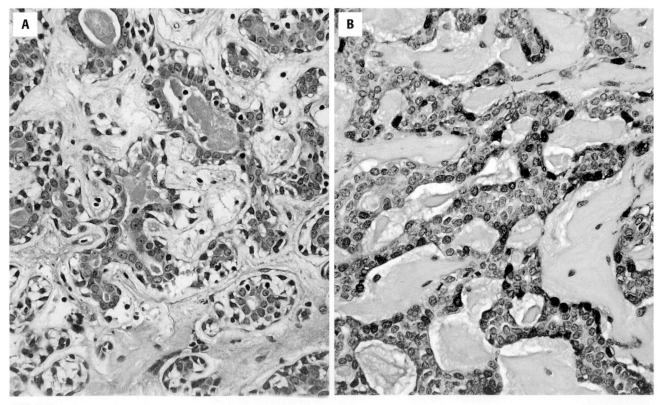

FIGURE 12-37

A, The epithelial-myoepithelial pattern is highlighted by the outer, clear cytoplasm of myoepithelial cells surrounding the ductal, luminal cells. **B**, The S100 protein stain highlights the basal-myoepithelial cell component.

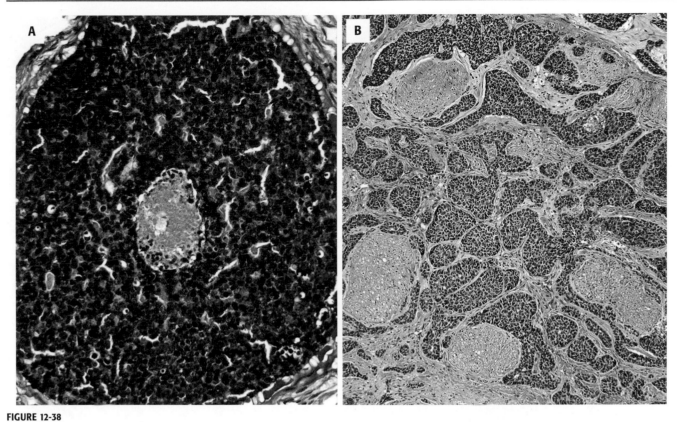

FIGURE 12-38
A, The solid variant of adenoid cystic carcinoma has large nests of cells with high nuclear-to-cytoplasmic ratio. Central comedonecrosis is noted. **B**, There is extensive perineural invasion in this tumor.

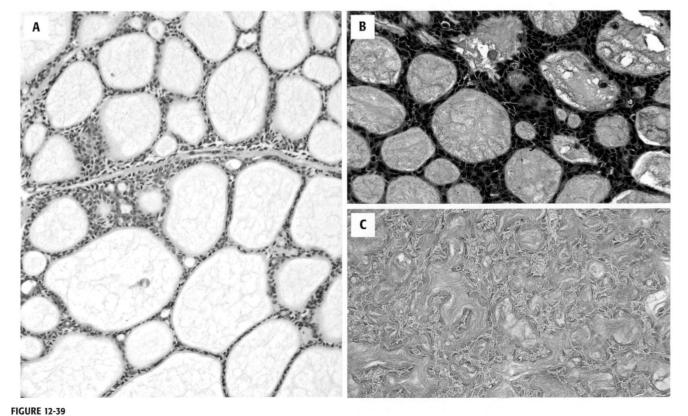

FIGURE 12-39
A, Pseudocystic spaces with mucoid and eosinophilic material. Note the peg-shaped nuclei, especially at the periphery of the cell groups as well as small duct-like spaces. **B**, A cylindrical appearance with mucoid, basophilic material in the center. **C**, Alcian blue highlights the pseudocystic glycosaminoglycan material.

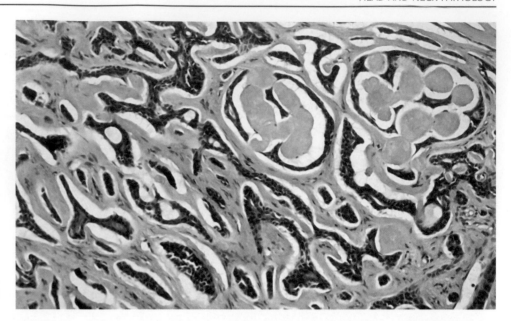

FIGURE 12-40

A heavily hyalinized stroma has compressed the neoplastic cells in this adenoid cystic carcinoma.

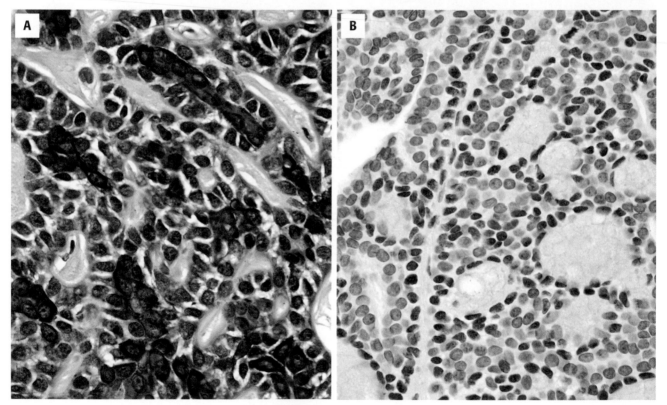

FIGURE 12-41

A, Keratin immunohistochemistry highlights the luminal epithelial cells. **B**, p63 immunohistochemistry highlights the basal-myoepithelial cells.

FINE NEEDLE ASPIRATION

AdCC contains intensely metachromatic spherical hyaline globules (resembling pink "gum balls"), which represent the reduplicated basement membrane material, intimately surrounded by the neoplastic cells (Figure 12-43), best seen on air-dried preparations (they stain pale blue or pink on Pap stain). The globules do not have a fibrillar or feathery edge as seen in pleomorphic adenoma (PA). There are often rounded stromal structures between the nests of tumor cells. The tumor cells are cohesive, often showing high cellularity and cellular overlap of cells that have little pleomorphism (Figure 12-44). The nuclei are often peg shaped, identified in cells with a high

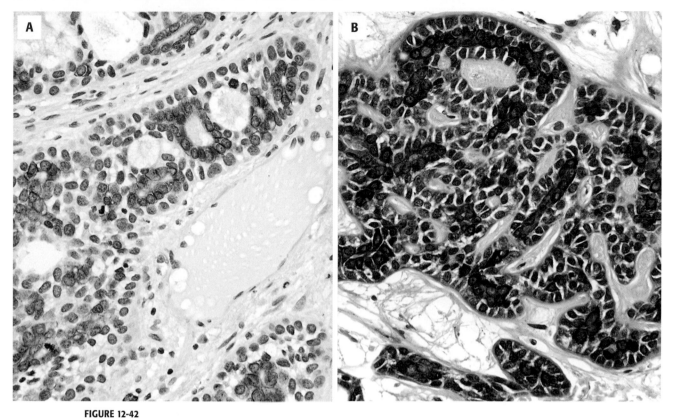

FIGURE 12-42

A, CD117 tends to highlight the luminal cells preferentially. **B**, Many times the luminal cells are highlighted with CK5/6.

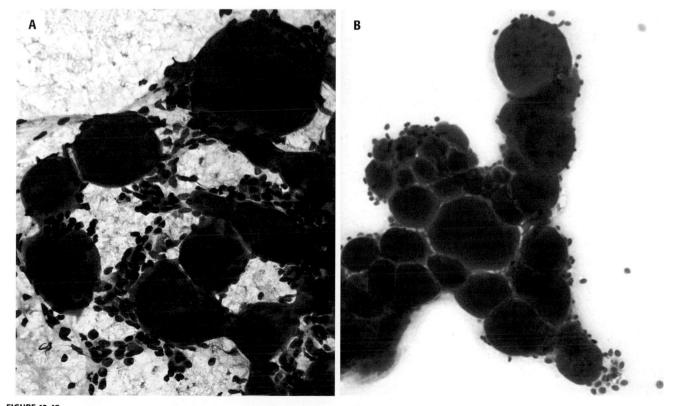

FIGURE 12-43

A and **B**, Air-dried, Romanovsky-stained fine needle aspiration material highlights the spherical hyaline globules with the intimately associated cells with small, hyperchromatic nuclei. Note the peripheral arrangement of the nuclei, rather than appearing within the matrix.

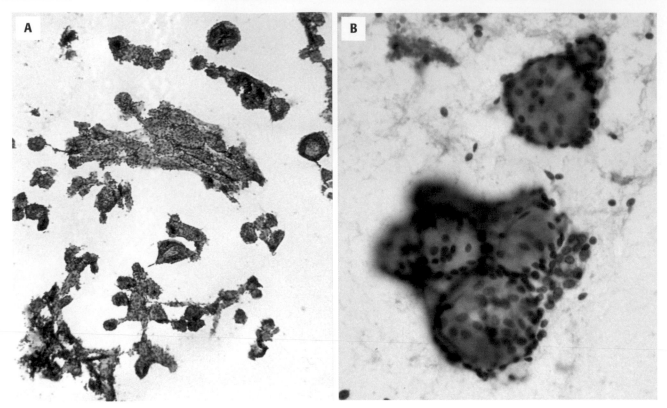

FIGURE 12-44

A and **B**, The epithelial cells form cohesive sheets that show rounded void areas, corresponding to the hyaline globules. These globules do not stain with Papanicolaou-stained preparations, but appear as voids.

nuclear-to-cytoplasmic ratio. The chromatin is heavy and coarse in distribution. FNA of AdCC may be difficult to separate from a PA.

DIFFERENTIAL DIAGNOSIS

It is important to distinguish AdCC from *polymorphous low-grade adenocarcinoma (PLGA)*. While both neoplasms have similar patterns of growth, PLGA consists of a uniform cell population with cytologically bland, round or oval and vesicular nuclei, and pale eosinophilic cytoplasm. PLGA has infiltrating single cords of cells and also has a striking targetoid arrangement, often centered on a nerve. Immunohistochemical separation still requires further validation. Although staining for CD117 and galectin-3 showed initial promise, more recent studies have questioned the value of these immunoagents. Occasional foci in *PA* can resemble AdCC but the presence of typical myxochondroid matrix and plasmacytoid or spindle-shaped cells helps to avoid confusion. *Basaloid squamous cell carcinoma* can resemble the solid variant of AdCC, but typically involves the hypopharynx and glottic region, shows squamous differentiation, and often involves the overlying mucosa. Both *EMC* and the tubular variant of AdCC

can show double-layered duct-like structures with an abluminal layer of clear cells. However, the other cytologic features allow for separation.

PROGNOSIS AND THERAPY

The 5- and 10-year survival rates are 62% and 40%, respectively, although most patients usually die of or with the tumor. Local recurrence is very common, especially in the first 5 years after surgery. The main prognostic factors are site, tumor size, clinical stage, and histologic pattern. Bone involvement and failure of primary surgery are associated with poor prognosis. Correlations between tumor morphology and outcome have yielded conflicting results due to the overall poor long-term prognosis. However, it appears that the tubular and cribriform variants have a better outcome than tumors with a solid component, especially if the solid component exceeds 30% of the tumor volume. Tumors in the submandibular gland have a poorer prognosis than those in the parotid. The relationship between nerve involvement and survival is contentious but invasion of larger nerves appears to correlate with more aggressive behavior. Lymph node involvement is relatively uncommon but distant metastases to lung, bone, brain, and liver are seen in up to 60 % of cases. Wide local excision, together with adjuvant radiotherapy, offers the best hope of local control.

■ POLYMORPHOUS LOW-GRADE ADENOCARCINOMA

CLINICAL FEATURES

PLGA is found almost exclusively in minor glands and accounts for about a quarter of the malignant tumors in these sites. Most present in patients aged 50 to 70 years, with a female predominance (2:1). The most common site is the palate (60 %), especially at the junction of the hard and soft palates (Figure 12-45). Other intraoral sites include the lip (particularly the upper), buccal mucosa, retromolar areas, and posterior third of the tongue. Rarely, tumors arise in the lacrimal gland, sinonasal tract, nasopharynx, and the upper and lower respiratory tracts. Tumors usually form a slow growing mass that may have been present

for many years. Ulceration, bleeding, and pain are uncommon presenting features.

PATHOLOGIC FEATURES

GROSS FINDINGS

The tumor usually forms a circumscribed, nonencapsulated, pale yellow or tan colored mass. Most measure up to 3 cm.

MICROSCOPIC FINDINGS

PLGA is an invasive tumor that is often circumscribed but not encapsulated, frequently identified immediately below an intact surface epithelium (Figure 12-46). There is typically a wide variety of morphologic patterns within individual tumors. The most common configurations include lobular, solid nests or thèques, cribriform areas, and duct-like structures of varying sizes (Figures 12-47 and 12-48). Concentric targeting or whorling, often by cells in a single file arrangement, producing an "eye of the storm" appearance, can often be seen around nerves and, less commonly, blood vessels and small ducts (Figures 12-49 and 12-50). The perineural infiltration is usually present within, or close to, the body of the tumor (Figure 12-50). Foci of oncocytic, mucous, and squamous metaplasia are occasionally present. Normal salivary gland acini are frequently incarcerated within the tumor (Figure 12-49).

POLYMORPHOUS LOW-GRADE ADENOCARCINOMA—DISEASE FACT SHEET

Definition
- A malignant epithelial tumor characterized by an infiltrative growth of cytologically uniform cells ("low-grade") arranged in architecturally diverse patterns ("polymorphous")

Incidence and Location
- Accounts for ~25% of intraoral malignant salivary gland tumors
- 60% of cases involve the palate; other sites include lip, buccal mucosa, retromolar areas, and tongue

Morbidity and Mortality
- Spread to regional lymph nodes in 9% to 15% of cases
- Death due to disease is uncommon

Gender, Race, and Age Distribution
- Female > male (2:1)
- Peak in 6th to 8th decades (wide age range)
- Rare in children

Clinical Features
- Usually forms a painless, slowly growing mass
- Tumors often present for many years
- Tumors may be mobile or fixed
- Ulceration, pain, and bleeding are uncommon

Prognosis and Treatment
- Prognosis usually excellent
- Local recurrences in 9% to 17% of cases
- Questionable aggressive behavior in younger patients
- Conservative surgery is the treatment of choice

POLYMORPHOUS LOW-GRADE ADENOCARCINOMA—PATHOLOGIC FEATURES

Gross Findings
- Circumscribed, but usually nonencapsulated mass
- Usually 1 to 3 cm

Microscopic Findings
- Cytologically uniform and architecturally diverse
- Wide variety of morphologic patterns in individual tumors
- Concentric targeting around nerves and blood vessels
- Encasement of benign residual salivary gland tissue
- Stromal hyalinization or mucinosis (slate-gray)
- Isomorphic, small to medium-sized cells with eosinophilic cytoplasm
- Cytologically bland, pale-staining (vesicular), round or oval nuclei
- Mitoses and necrosis uncommon

Immunohistochemical Features
- Cytokeratin, vimentin, and S100 protein positive
- Variable results with immunohistochemistry and rarely of diagnostic value

Pathologic Differential Diagnosis
- Limited biopsy specimens make diagnosis difficult; pleomorphic adenoma, adenoid cystic carcinoma, cystadenocarcinoma

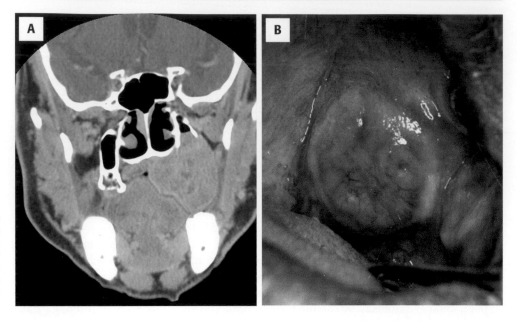

FIGURE 12-45

A, There is a large tumor growing into the base of the nasal cavity from the palate, resulting in bone destruction (computed tomography scan). **B**, An intact mucosa overlies a mass at the junction of the hard and soft palate. Note the vascular pattern. No surface ulceration is present.

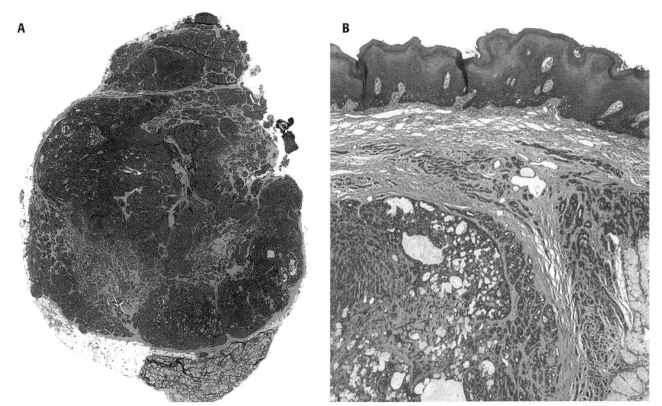

FIGURE 12-46

A, Low power shows an invasive tumor arranged in several patterns. **B**, A low-power magnification of polymorphous low-grade adenocarcinoma showing a well-circumscribed, although unencapsulated, mass with a variety of different growth patterns. The surface is intact and uninvolved. Note the encasement of the mucous glands (*far right*).

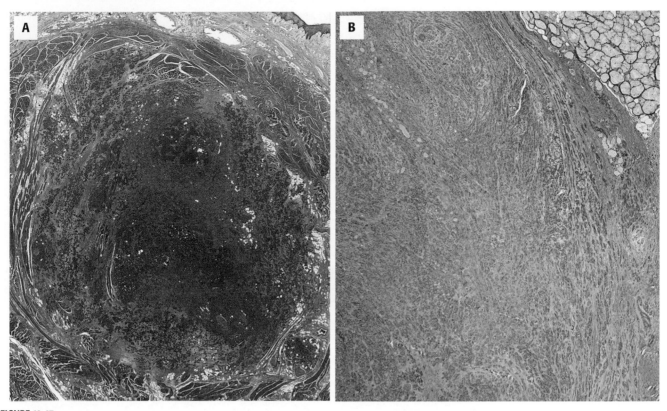

FIGURE 12-47
A, Low power shows a number of different patterns in this unencapsulated tumor. **B**, Note the single file infiltration at the periphery of this variably patterned tumor.

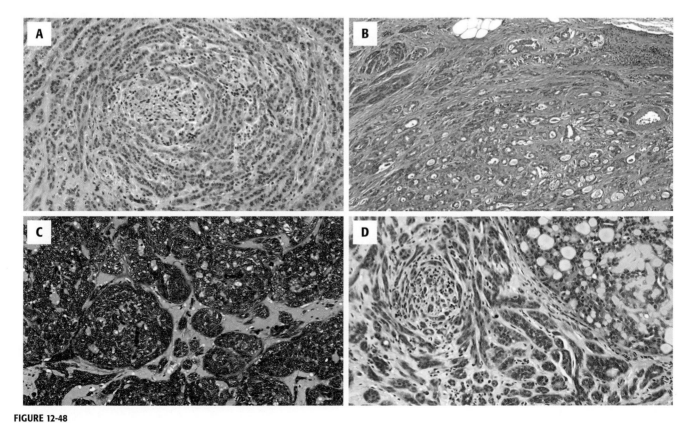

FIGURE 12-48
A–D, Variable architectures are seen within a single tumor, including cribriform, tubular, and trabecular. Note the stroma in the background, which can be mucinous, myxoid, slate gray-blue to eosinophilic and hyalinized.

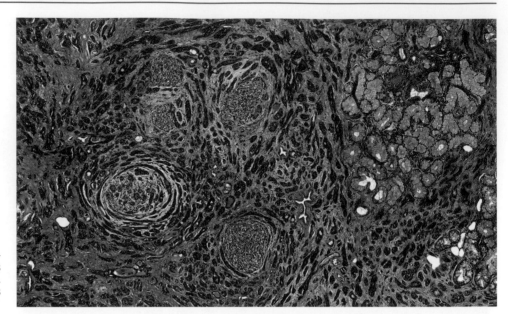

FIGURE 12-49

A targetoid pattern with single-file, concentric arrangement of the cells. Nerves are usually in the center of these targets. Note the entombed minor mucoserous glands (surrounded but not destroyed).

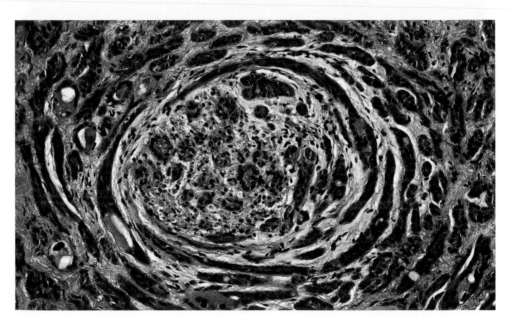

FIGURE 12-50

A targetoid arrangement around a nerve, with intraneural and perineural invasion easily identified in this polymorphous low-grade adenocarcinoma.

A characteristic stromal hyalinization with a slate-gray appearance is common (Figure 12-51), but chondroid or myxochondroid areas are not seen.

PLGA is characterized by cytologic uniformity ("low-grade") and architectural diversity ("polymorphous"). The cells are isomorphic, small to medium size, with pale eosinophilic cytoplasm. They have cytologically bland, pale-staining (vesicular), round or oval nuclei (Figures 12-51 and 12-52). It is uncommon to see mitotic figures or areas of necrosis.

ANCILLARY STUDIES

The immunohistochemical profile is variable and rarely of diagnostic value. Cytokeratin, vimentin, and S100 protein are the most consistent markers and will decorate some cells in the large majority of tumors, but the intensity and distribution are variable (Figure 12-53). Most cases of PLGA appear to overexpress bcl-2.

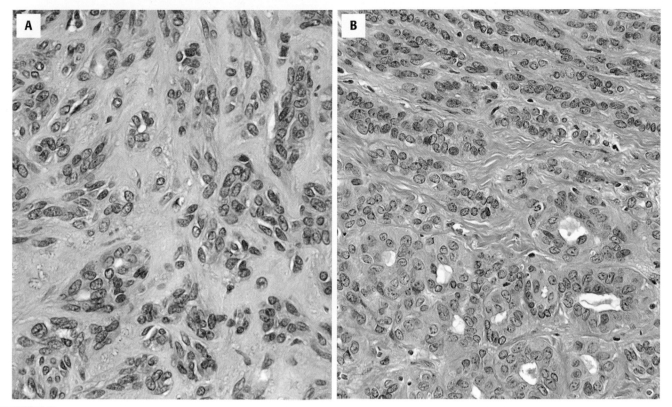

FIGURE 12-51
A and **B**, Stromal hyalinization and a slate-gray to blue mucinous material in the background is quite characteristic for a polymorphous low-grade adenocarcinoma. Note the open, vesicular nuclear chromatin and delicate, small nucleoli.

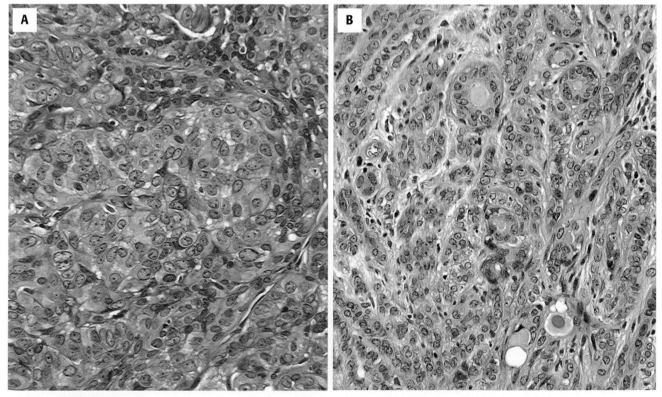

FIGURE 12-52
A and **B**, The nuclei are round to oval, with vesicular, pale nuclear chromatin, and small nucleoli. Mitotic figures are inconspicuous.

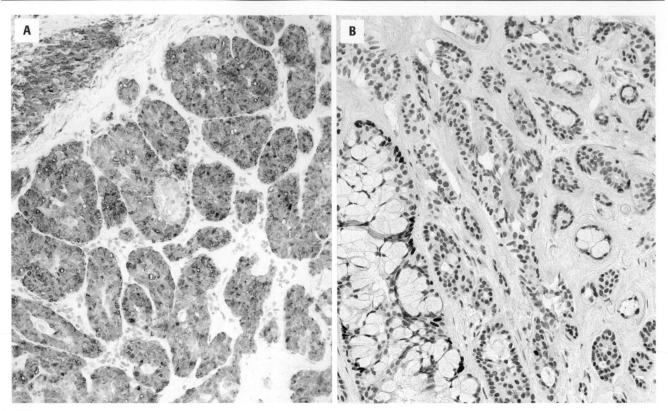

FIGURE 12-53

A polymorphous low-grade adenocarcinoma shows biphasic staining. **A**, S100 protein highlights the basaloid-myoepithelial cells (and a nerve in the *upper left*). **B**, p63 is noted within the basal zone of the tumor and in the minor mucoserous gland (*left*).

DIFFERENTIAL DIAGNOSIS

The differential diagnosis includes PA, AdCC, and papillary variants of cystadenocarcinoma. This separation is hampered if the biopsy is small. Typically, *PA* is circumscribed and often shows plasmacytoid differentiation in minor glands. Although both tumors can show stromal mucinosis and elastosis, myxochondroid or chondroid matrix is not seen in PLGA. It has been reported that staining for GFAP is very strong in PAs but weak or absent in PLGA. AdCC has hyperchromatic nuclei with a much higher nuclear-to-cytoplasmic ratio and tends to be more extensively infiltrative. *Cystadenocarcinoma* usually has a conspicuous papillary architecture and nuclear pleomorphism with mitotic figures.

PROGNOSIS AND THERAPY

The long-term prognosis is usually excellent. There is local recurrence in 9% to 17% of cases and spread to regional lymph nodes is seen in 9% to 15% of cases. Distant metastases are very rare and death due to disease is uncommon. Whether papillary PLGA exists is debatable, but papillary tumors have a much more aggressive behavior, suggesting they may not belong in this category. Complete but conservative surgery is the treatment of choice, together with neck dissection in cases with proven regional metastases.

■ EPITHELIAL-MYOEPITHELIAL CARCINOMA

CLINICAL FEATURES

EMC is a malignant neoplasm demonstrating a characteristic biphasic pattern of inner duct-like lining cells and an outer layer of myoepithelium-like cells. EMC accounts for ~1% of salivary gland tumors. It is usually seen in older age groups (50 to 60 years) and is rare in children. Women are affected twice as often as men. Most cases arise in the parotid gland where they typically form a slowly growing, painless mass, often of long duration. It can also arise from minor glands of the mouth and the upper and lower respiratory tracts where it has a tendency to ulcerate. Higher-grade tumors may undergo rapid growth and cause pain or facial nerve palsy.

EPITHELIAL-MYOEPITHELIAL CARCINOMA—DISEASE FACT SHEET

Definition

- A malignant neoplasm with biphasic duct-like structures composed of an inner layer of duct lining, epithelium-type cells and an outer layer of clear, myoepithelium-type cells

Incidence and Location

- About 1% of salivary gland tumors
- 60% of cases involve the parotid gland
- Also seen in the mouth, upper and lower respiratory tracts

Morbidity and Mortality

- Spread to regional lymph nodes and distant sites (~15%)
- 5-year survival rate of 80%

Gender, Race, and Age Distribution

- Female > male (2:1)
- Peak incidence in 6th to 7th decades
- Rare in children

Clinical Features

- Painless, slowly growing mass
- Tumors are often present for long periods
- Tumors involving mucosal sites often ulcerate
- Occasionally, tumors are rapidly growing and painful and may cause nerve palsies

Prognosis and Treatment

- Prognosis is usually good (5-year survival of 80%), although recurrences are common (40%)
- Clinical indicators of poor prognosis include incomplete surgical excision, large size, rapid growth, and involvement of minor salivary glands
- Microscopic features associated with a poor outcome include cellular atypia, high mitotic count, and aneuploidy
- Surgery is the treatment of choice, supplemented by radiotherapy in advanced or recurrent cases

EPITHELIAL-MYOEPITHELIAL CARCINOMA—PATHOLOGIC FEATURES

Gross Findings

- Well-defined, but usually nonencapsulated mass, 2 to 8 cm
- Often lobulated, cystic areas common
- Tumors in minor glands less well demarcated

Microscopic Findings

- Double-layered duct-like structures
- Inner cuboidal duct-lining cells and outer, single or multiple layers of myoepithelial cells with clear cytoplasm and eccentric, vesicular nuclei
- Wide variation in proportions of each cell type
- Duct-like structures may be widely separated by fibrous tissue or merge into cohesive sheets
- Papillary and cystic areas are present in 20% of cases
- Spindle cell areas and squamous metaplasia occasionally present
- Mitoses uncommon (2/10 HPFs)
- Perineural and vascular invasion commonly seen

Immunohistochemical Features

- Inner cells positive with keratins
- Outer myoepithelial cells calponin, SMA, p63, and, less reliably, S100 protein positive; CD117 and bcl-2 frequently positive

Pathologic Differential Diagnosis

- Pleomorphic adenoma, adenoid cystic carcinoma (tubular variant), myoepithelioma, clear cell oncocytoma, mucoepidermoid carcinoma, clear cell carcinoma (not otherwise specified), and metastases from the kidney and thyroid gland

PATHOLOGIC FEATURES

GROSS FINDINGS

The tumor typically forms a well-defined, but usually nonencapsulated, mass, 2 to 8 cm in diameter. The tumors are often lobulated with cystic areas common (Figure 12-54). Tumors in minor glands tend to be less well demarcated.

MICROSCOPIC FINDINGS

The characteristic feature of EMC is the formation of double-layered, duct-like structures (Figure 12-55). The luminal cells form a single, cuboidal, or columnar layer and have finely granular, eosinophilic cytoplasm, and a central round or oval nucleus. The outer cells may form single or multiple layers and have abundant, clear cytoplasm that is usually rich in glycogen, and they typically have eccentric and vesicular nuclei. However, in ~20% of cases, there is no evidence of clear cells; in contrast, occasionally both layers consist of clear cells (Figure 12-56). The proportion of each cell type and their architectural arrangements is extremely variable. The duct-like structures may be surrounded and separated by hyaline material or fibrous tissue (Figure 12-56). They can also form more cohesive sheets, and the ductal configuration may not be immediately apparent. Tumors may consist predominantly of clear cells with only scattered duct-lining cells that may form solid islands without canalization. Cystic or papillary areas are seen in about 20% of cases. Less commonly, areas show spindle cell or squamous differentiation, or oncocytic metaplasia, typically of the luminal cells (Figure 12-57). Mitoses are usually sparse and rarely exceed 2/10 high-power fields (HPFs). Perineural and vascular involvement is relatively common and bone invasion is occasionally seen (Figure 12-56). EMC can arise from a PA and a few cases of hybrid tumors have been described. Cases of EMC showing dedifferentiation have been reported. Recently described but rare variants include oncocytic-sebaceous EMC and apocrine EMC.

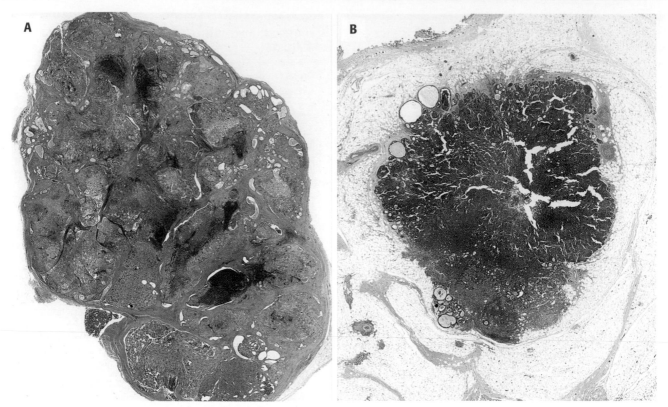

FIGURE 12-54

A, There is a well-defined but unencapsulated tumor showing invasion and irregular borders in this epithelial-myoepithelial carcinoma. **B**, An ill-defined tumor is noted in this minor salivary gland location.

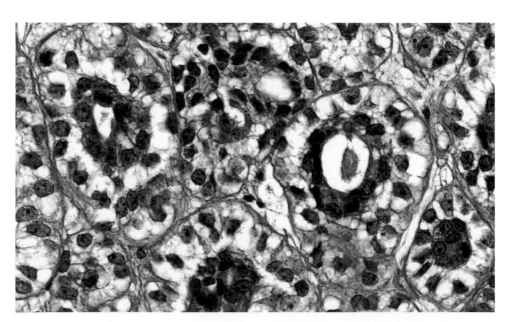

FIGURE 12-55

High power shows eosinophilic cytoplasm of the inner luminal duct-like cells. The myoepithelial cells have cleared cytoplasm with more vesicular nuclear chromatin.

ANCILLARY STUDIES

The inner duct-lining cells stain with low-molecular-weight cytokeratins, CAM5.2, and EMA (Figure 12-58). The outer clear cells stain with myoepithelial markers such as calponin, SMA, p63, and, less reliably, S100 protein (Figure 12-58). CD117 and bcl-2 are frequently positive (up to 70% of cases).

DIFFERENTIAL DIAGNOSIS

The differential diagnosis of EMC includes tumors showing double-layered duct-like structures and those consisting predominantly of clear cells. Double-layered duct-like structures can be seen in *PA* and the tubular variant of *AdCC*. The clear cells in these tumors tend to be focal, have less abundant cytoplasm, and have

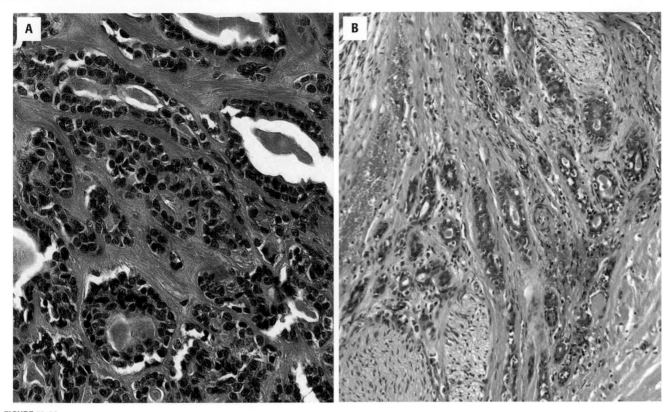

FIGURE 12-56

A, Duct-like structures separated by fibrous connective tissue. Note the double layer of inner cuboidal cells surrounded by myoepithelial cells. **B**, Perineural invasion is prominent.

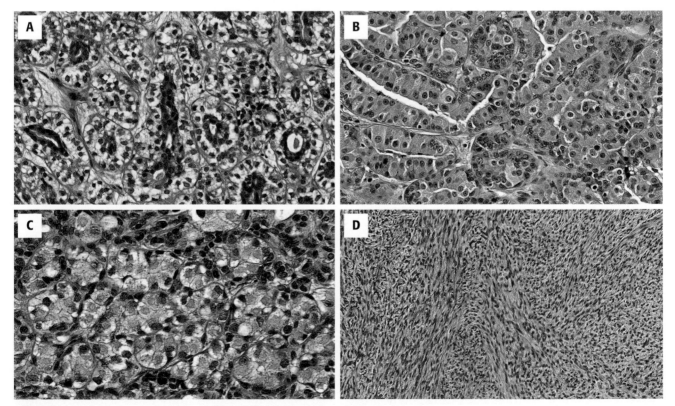

FIGURE 12-57

A variety of different cell types can be seen in an epithelial-myoepithelial carcinoma. **A**, The classic central duct-like structures surrounded by syncytial myoepithelial cells with cleared cytoplasm. **B**, The cells have an oncocytic appearance, although the biphasic appearance is still noted with the darker myoepithelial cells. **C**, A more solid area shows granular cytoplasm in the ductal cells and darker basaloid cells. **D**, The tumor cells are arranged in a spindled pattern without any easily identified epithelial component. Immunohistochemistry would be valuable in this setting.

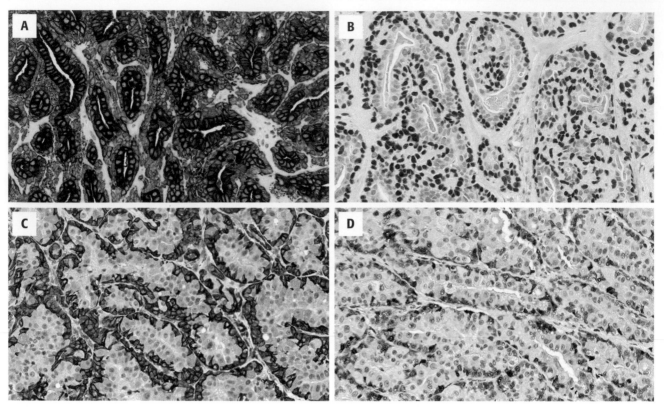

FIGURE 12-58

A, Keratin highlights the inner ductal type cells. **B**, p63 highlights the basal myoepithelial cells. **C**, A smooth muscle actin strongly stains the basal-myoepithelial cells. **D**, An S100 protein stain accentuates the outer myoepithelial cells.

hyperchromatic, angular nuclei. In addition, the clear cells of EMC are typically rich in glycogen. Nonetheless, in such circumstances, it may not be possible to distinguish between these tumors with confidence. Tumors showing focal or extensive areas of predominantly clear cells include clear cell variants of PA, myoepithelioma, oncocytoma, and MEC, as well as clear cell carcinoma (NOS). *Metastases* from the kidney and thyroid glands may need to be excluded by staining for p63, calponin, renal cell carcinoma (RCC) marker, PAX8, PAX2, thyroglobulin, and TTF-1.

PROGNOSIS AND THERAPY

EMC is a moderately aggressive salivary tumor with a high recurrence rate (40%) and metastases to regional lymph nodes and distant sites, such as the lung, liver, and kidney seen in nearly 15% of cases. The 5-year survival rate is 80% and the 10-year survival is 72%. Clinical features indicating poorer prognosis include incomplete surgical excision, large size, rapid growth, and involvement of minor salivary glands. Microscopic features associated with a poor outcome include cellular atypia, high mitotic count,

and aneuploidy. Surgery is the treatment of choice and neck dissection should be included in patients with evidence of regional lymph node spread. This can be supplemented by radiotherapy in advanced or recurrent cases.

■ SALIVARY DUCT CARCINOMA

CLINICAL FEATURES

Salivary duct carcinoma (SDC) can arise ab initio and is also a relatively common malignant element of carcinoma ex PA (Ca ex PA). It accounts for ~9% of malignant salivary gland tumors. The age at presentation ranges from 22 to 91 years but most patients are older than 50 years. There is a striking male predominance (4:1). The vast majority of cases arise in the major glands (96%), predominantly the parotid (Figure 12-59), and rarely in the sinonasal tract and larynx. They usually present as a rapidly growing mass, with ulceration and facial nerve palsy relatively common. In carcinomas arising ex PA, there may be a history of a long-standing mass with recent enlargement.

SALIVARY DUCT CARCINOMA—DISEASE FACT SHEET

Definition

- Salivary duct carcinoma is an aggressive adenocarcinoma that resembles high-grade breast ductal adenocarcinoma

Incidence and Location

- Represents ~ 9% of malignant salivary gland tumors
- Common type of malignancy arising ex pleomorphic adenoma
- Overwhelming majority affect major glands (usually parotid)

Morbidity and Mortality

- About a third of cases recur locally
- 65% of patients die from disease

Gender, Race, and Age Distribution

- Male >> female (4:1)
- Peak incidence in 6th to 7th decades

Clinical Features

- Presents as rapidly growing mass
- Ulceration and facial nerve palsy common
- If it is in a carcinoma ex pleomorphic adenoma, there is rapid enlargement in a long-standing mass

Prognosis and Treatment

- Most aggressive salivary gland tumor with regional metastasis in ~60% with distant spread in ~50% of cases
- Features associated with a poor outcome include large tumor size, distant metastases, and overexpression of HER-2/neu
- Radical surgery with adjuvant radiotherapy and chemotherapy (antiandrogen and trastuzumab)

SALIVARY DUCT CARCINOMA—PATHOLOGIC FEATURES

Gross Findings

- Predominantly solid white, gray, or tan
- Cysts, necrosis, and hemorrhage common
- Usually shows invasion into surrounding tissues
- Macroscopic features typical of a preexisting pleomorphic adenoma may be present

Microscopic Findings

- Resembles ductal adenocarcinoma of breast, both intraductal and infiltrative
- Vascular and neural invasion
- Large ducts with cribriform configurations, Roman-bridging, and comedonecrosis
- Solid, papillary areas, and squamous differentiation may be present
- Cytologically pleomorphic cells, often with granular or oncocytic cytoplasm
- Large, hyperchromatic nuclei with prominent nucleoli and high mitotic frequency

Immunohistochemical Features

- Positive for a wide range of cytokeratins, CEA, and EMA
- Strongly positive for androgen receptor (negative with estrogen/progesterone receptors)
- Most show overexpression of HER 2/neu protein

Pathologic Differential Diagnosis

- Metastatic breast carcinoma, squamous cell carcinoma, oncocytic carcinoma, cystadenocarcinoma, may be part of Ca ex PA

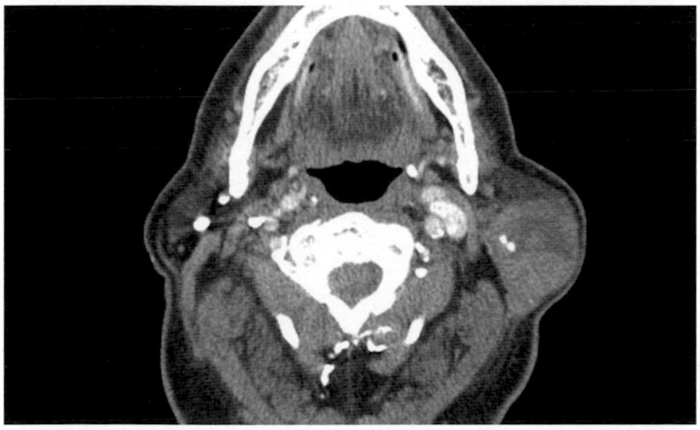

FIGURE 12-59

A computed tomography scan showing a right parotid gland tumor with cystic degeneration and small calcifications. The latter finding suggests a previous pleomorphic adenoma.

PATHOLOGIC FEATURES

GROSS FINDINGS

The cut surface is predominantly solid, white, gray or tan, with cysts, necrosis, and hemorrhage commonly seen. The tumor usually shows invasion into surrounding tissues but occasional cases appear to be relatively well circumscribed (Figure 12-60). Macroscopic features typical of a preexisting PA may be present.

MICROSCOPIC FINDINGS

SDC resembles in situ (intraductal) and infiltrative ductal AC of breast. The most characteristic feature is the formation of multiple large ducts with cribriform configurations, "Roman-bridging," and comedonecrosis (Figure 12-61). In addition, solid and papillary areas and evidence of squamous differentiation may be present. Stromal fibrosis or infarction and inflammatory infiltration are often conspicuous features (Figure 12-62). Vascular and neural invasions are common and frequently extensive (Figure 12-63). The tumor typically consists of cytologically pleomorphic cells with abundant pink, granular cytoplasm (Figure 12-64). Oncocytic metaplasia is a common and sometimes striking feature (Figure 12-65). The nuclei are large and hyperchromatic with prominent nucleoli, and there is usually a high mitotic frequency. Tumors are occasionally biphasic and have a malignant spindle cell, sarcomatoid stroma (Figure 12-66). Several other variants have been

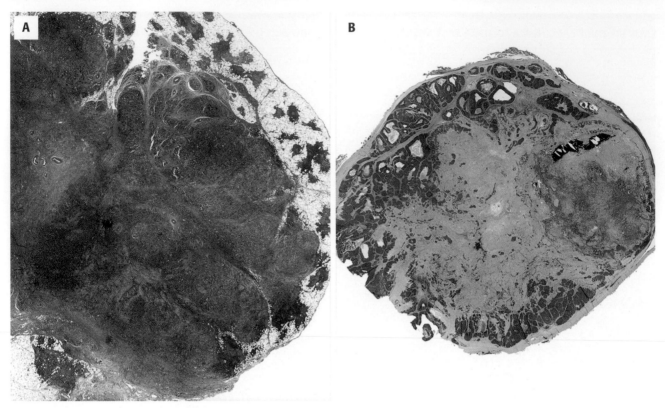

FIGURE 12-60

A and **B**, Low-power view of two tumors, showing an infiltrating pattern in both. The right-sided tumor shows extensive hyalinization and calcification with associated pleomorphic adenoma. The "carcinoma" of a carcinoma ex pleomorphic adenoma is frequently a salivary duct carcinoma.

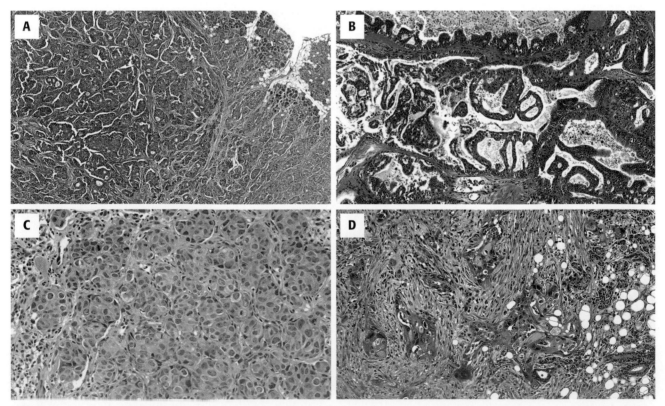

FIGURE 12-61

A number of different patterns of growth can be seen. **A**, A micropapillary architecture is noted in this tumor that infiltrates into the surrounding parenchyma. **B**, There is a well-developed papillary and "Roman-bridge" pattern in this tumor. **C**, A more solid pattern of growth is noted, composed of large, polygonal tumor cells. **D**, This area shows a sarcomatoid pattern to the cells that are infiltrating into the adjacent fat and parenchyma.

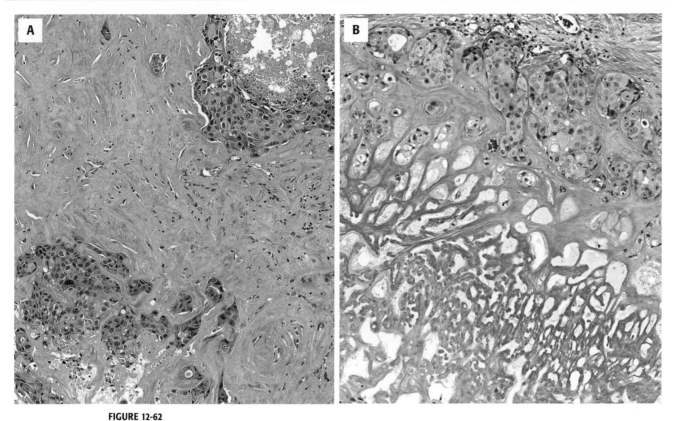

FIGURE 12-62

A, The pleomorphic cells are arranged as tumor nests, set in a heavy stromal fibrosis, showing infarction (**B**).

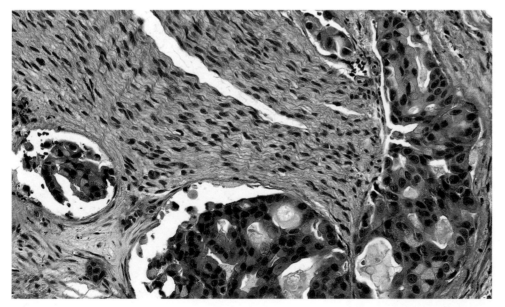

FIGURE 12-63

The characteristic cribriform pattern of tumor growth is identified within and adjacent to nerves.

described. The mucin-rich variant shows lakes of epithelial mucin containing malignant cells, in addition to more typical areas. Some tumors have an invasive, micropapillary component and a strong propensity for angiolymphatic and neural spread; these have a particularly poor prognosis. Recently, purely in situ variants of SDC have been reported.

ANCILLARY STUDIES

IMMUNOHISTOCHEMISTRY FINDINGS

SDC is usually positive for a wide range of cytokeratins, CEA, and EMA. It shows strong nuclear positivity for androgen receptors (Figure 12-67) and is usually negative for

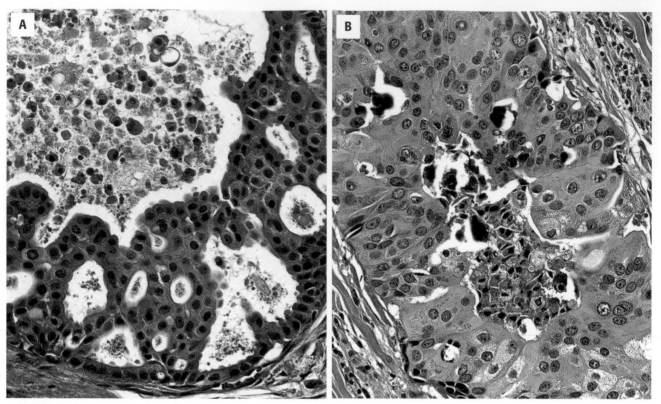

FIGURE 12-64

A, Cribriform areas with "Roman-bridge" formation and comedonecrosis are seen in this salivary duct carcinoma. Note the pleomorphism and mitotic figures. **B**, An area of comedonecrosis is noted in this mimic of breast ductal adenocarcinoma.

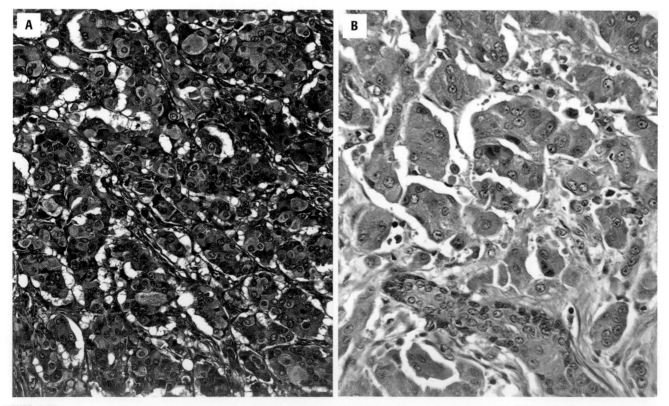

FIGURE 12-65

A, There are small packets of neoplastic cells showing a pseudoalveolar pattern with ample granular-eosinophilic cytoplasm. **B**, These cytologically pleomorphic cells have abundant granular, eosinophilic cytoplasm (normal duct in lower field).

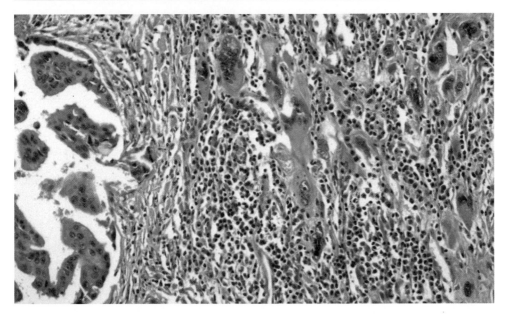

FIGURE 12-66

A papillary architecture blends into an area of spindle cell or "sarcomatoid" transformation in this salivary duct carcinoma.

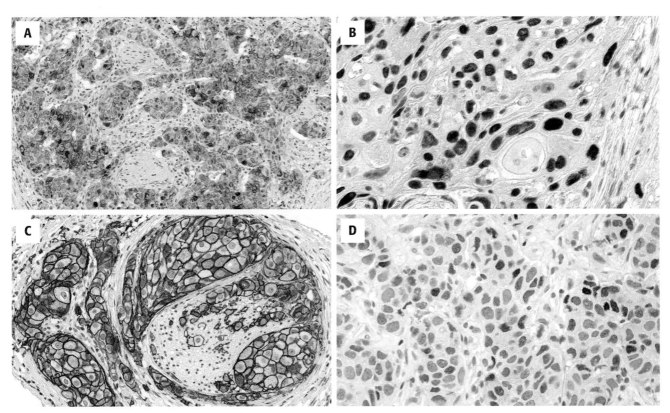

FIGURE 12-67

Immunohistochemistry highlights several different features. **A**, Epithelial membrane antigen highlights many of the neoplastic cells (nerve is negative). **B**, p63 strongly and diffusely highlights the atypical nuclei of this tumor. **C**, HER-2/neu usually gives a strong, diffuse, circumferential membrane reaction of >30% of the tumor cells. **D**, Androgen receptor gives a strong diffuse reaction in most of the tumor cell nuclei.

myoepithelial, estrogen, and progesterone markers. There is variable positivity for prostate-specific antigen and prostatic acid phosphatase. Peroxisome proliferator-activated receptor gamma is expressed in 80 % of SDC, often at high levels, and is topographically localized to the cytoplasm. Most tumors show overexpression of HER-2/neu protein with strong membrane staining (Figure 12-67).

Fine Needle Aspiration

The smears are usually very cellular with abundant background debris and necrotic material. The cells are arranged in cohesive and three-dimensional papillary clusters. A cribriform pattern can be seen. The cells range from round to polygonal, occasionally spindled, with abundant finely granular to vacuolated cytoplasm. Nuclei are large, pleomorphic, and often hyperchromatic. Nucleoli are frequently prominent. Mitotic figures can be easily identified. The background will frequently contain isolated highly atypical epithelial cells, frequently clustered at the periphery of the cell groups (Figure 12-68).

Differential Diagnosis

SDC must be distinguished from metastatic breast carcinoma. Although areas can resemble poorly differentiated squamous cell carcinoma, more typical cribriform areas and duct-like structures are typically present. Papillary areas can resemble cystadenocarcinoma, but these are usually focal and show more cellular pleomorphism in SDC. Some tumors are extensively oncocytic but their histomorphologic characteristics should aid differentiation from oncocytic carcinoma.

Prognosis and Therapy

SDC is the most aggressive salivary gland tumor, with an overall survival rate of ~35 %, most patients dying within 4 years. About a third of cases show local recurrence and ~60 % develop metastasis to regional lymph nodes. Systemic metastases to lung and bone are seen in up to 50 % of cases. A large primary tumor, evidence of metastases, and overexpression of HER-2/neu protein appear to be indicators of poorer prognosis. Aneuploidy, proliferation rate, and expression of p53 show no correlation with outcome. The treatment usually includes a total parotidectomy with a neck dissection and adjuvant radiotherapy. Antiandrogen and trastuzumab (Herceptin) have been used for systemic therapy for patients with advanced disease.

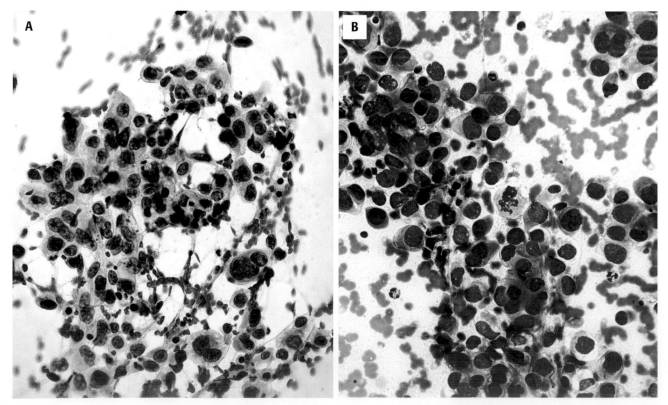

FIGURE 12-68
A, Cellular smears with loose clusters of atypical epithelial cells. The chromatin is coarse to open (alcohol fixed, Papanicolaou stain). B, Slightly cohesive cells with a high nuclear to cytoplasmic ratio. Note the mitotic figure in the center (air-dried, Diff-Quik stain).

■ CARCINOMA EX PLEOMORPHIC ADENOMA

CLINICAL FEATURES

Ca ex PA accounts for ~4% of all salivary tumors and ~12% of salivary malignancies. The sites of origin are usually the parotid (67%), minor glands (18%), submandibular (15%), and sublingual gland (<1%). Most cases are seen in 6th and 7th decades; it is rare in children. There is equal gender distribution. The typical history is that of a long-standing mass with recent rapid enlargement or previous surgery for a PA (Figure 12-69). They are often painless but some are painful, and ~40% of patients have nerve palsies.

PATHOLOGIC FEATURES

GROSS FINDINGS

Tumors range up to 25 cm. An area of circumscribed PA may be apparent, associated with an extensively infiltrative component, often showing areas of hemorrhage and necrosis. The preexisting PA may be represented by an area of scarring.

MICROSCOPIC FINDINGS

The relative proportions of preexisting PA and Ca ex PA vary widely. Some tumors show a carcinoma in direct juxtaposition to a typical PA (Figure 12-70); sometimes the benign remnant may be difficult to find, particularly in scarred tumors. The malignant component may overgrow the benign element, but the diagnosis can be implied on the basis of clinical history. The tumor frequently shows invasion, which may involve soft tissue, nerve, or vasculature (Figures 12-71 and 12-72). Ca ex PA has been subclassified into noninvasive, minimally invasive ($\leq$1.5 mm), and invasive ($\geq$1.5 mm) (Figures 12-73 and 12-74). Noninvasive carcinomas have also been referred to as intracapsular carcinomas, in situ Ca ex PA, or severely dysplastic PA. They show a PA with focal or diffuse areas of cytologically malignant cells but without evidence of invasion into the surrounding tissues. These areas are commonly associated with increased mitotic activity. The malignant component is frequently a poorly differentiated carcinoma, high-grade AC (NOS), or SDC (Figure 12-75). However, many other types of salivary gland carcinomas have been described in Ca ex PA, and some cases show diverse differentiation with several distinct types within the tumor mass (Figure 12-76). A carcinosarcoma is defined by the simultaneous presence of a carcinoma and a sarcoma (Figure 12-77), and this tumor may be associated with a residual PA; it is vanishingly rare.

CARCINOMA EX PLEOMORPHIC ADENOMA—DISEASE FACT SHEET

Definition
- A carcinoma arising in association with a PA

Incidence and Location
- 4% of all salivary tumors; 12% of salivary malignancies
- Parotid (67%), submandibular (15%), minor glands (18%)

Morbidity and Mortality
- Dependent on tumor size, type, and extent of invasion
- 25% to 65% at 5 years; 24% to 50% at 10 years; 10% to 35% at 15 years for tumors with >1.5 mm of invasion

Gender, Race, and Age Distribution
- Equal gender distribution
- Usually seen in 6th and 7th decades
- Rare in children

Clinical Features
- Typical history of long-standing mass with recent rapid enlargement
- Previous surgery for PA often reported
- Often painless, but some painful, and nearly 40% have nerve palsies

Prognosis and Treatment
- Noninvasive carcinomas have same prognosis as PA
- About 25% to 50% have local recurrence, usually within 5 years
- Minimally invasive tumors ($\leq$1.5 mm) relatively good prognosis
- Invasive tumors ($\geq$1.5 mm) poor prognosis
- Large and histologically high-grade tumors have poor prognosis
- Wide resection is the treatment of choice

CARCINOMA EX PLEOMORPHIC ADENOMA—PATHOLOGIC FEATURES

Gross Findings
- Range from to massive (25 cm)
- Area of circumscribed PA associated with infiltrative component

Microscopic Findings
- Proportions of preexisting PA and Ca ex PA widely variable
- Original PA may scar or be overgrown by malignant component
- Malignant element frequently a poorly differentiated carcinoma or a salivary duct carcinoma
- There may be several distinct carcinomatous components
- Sarcoma, carcinoma, and PA combinations are rare

Pathologic Differential Diagnosis
- Fine needle or infarction of PA, separation of noninvasive and invasive tumor, foci of carcinoma in hyalinized PA easily missed

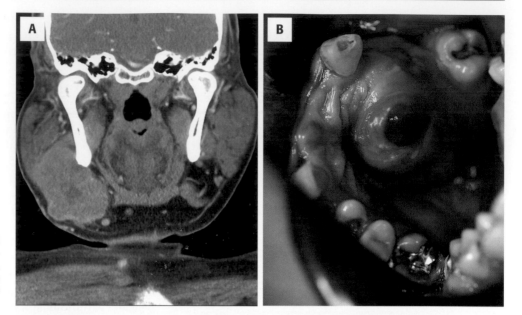

FIGURE 12-69

A, There is a mass in the parotid gland showing extensive necrosis and multinodularity. **B**, A tumor in the palate, showing ulceration and erythema. Both of these images are not specific for a carcinoma ex pleomorphic adenoma.

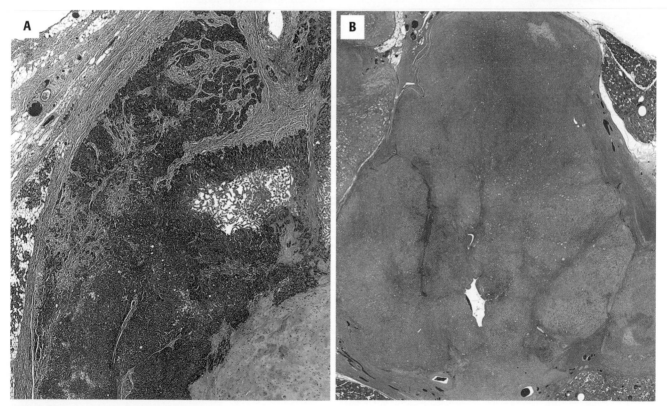

FIGURE 12-70

Two examples of carcinoma ex pleomorphic adenoma. **A**, The pleomorphic adenoma is noted in the lower right, with a malignant tumor expanding outward. **B**, There is extensive hyalinization in this tumor, which shows a multinodular-bosselated appearance.

DIFFERENTIAL DIAGNOSIS

FNA or spontaneous infarction of *PA* can cause secondary degenerative changes that may be confused with Ca ex PA. These include hemorrhage, necrosis, inflammation, reactive cellular atypia, and squamous or mucous metaplasia. It is important to distinguish between noninvasive, minimally invasive, and invasive tumors, as there are clear prognostic implications. Foci of carcinoma may develop in a hyalinized PA and be easily missed, particularly in large tumors. A *metastasizing PA* may be caused by surgical manipulation of a previous PA, with benign-appearing epithelial elements in the sites of metastasis (Figure 12-78).

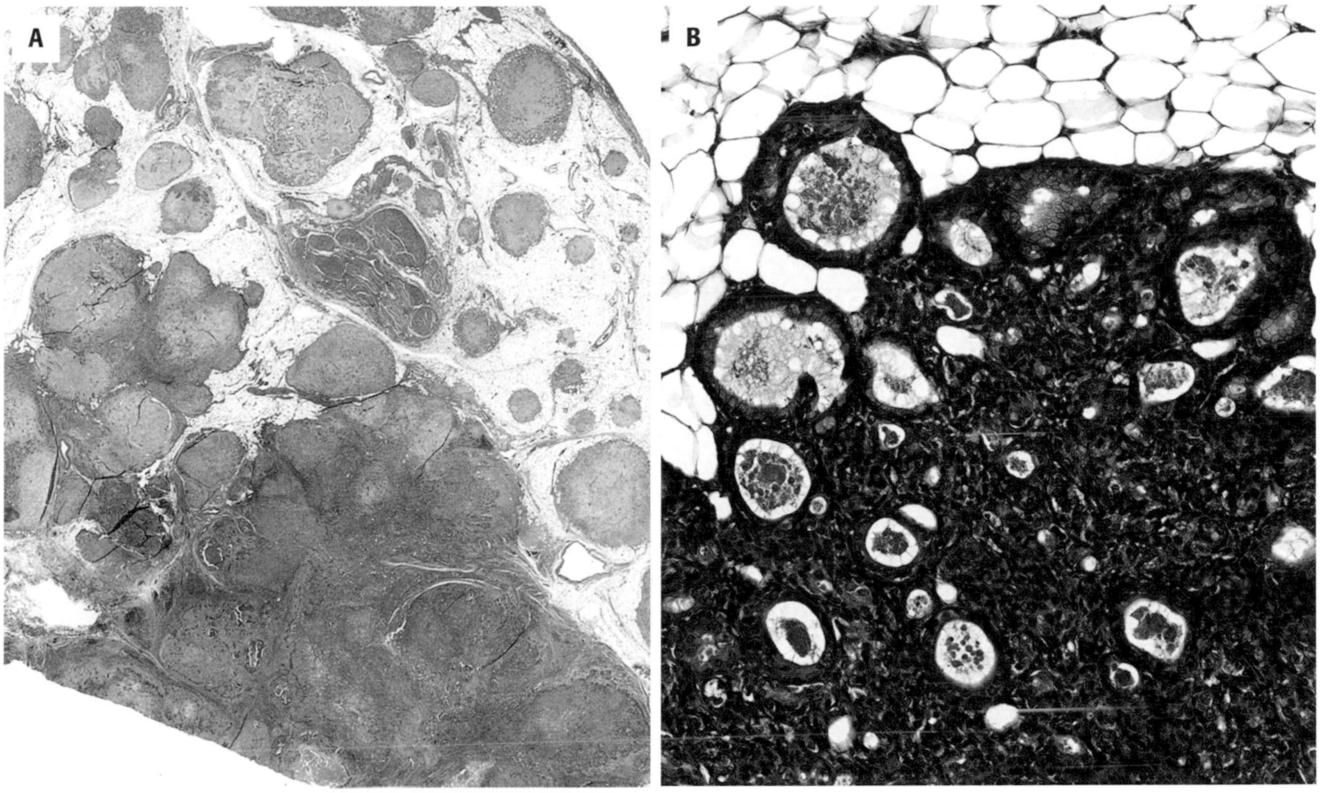

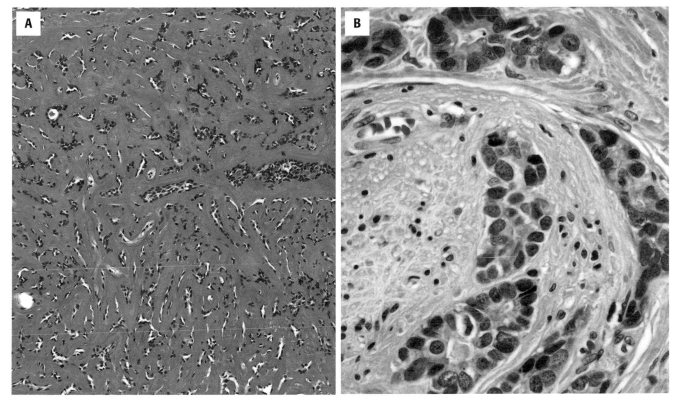

FIGURE 12-71

A, There are multiple nodules of tumor within the adipose tissue. These represent the recurrent pleomorphic adenoma. However, the area of carcinoma is noted in the lower part of the field. **B**, Note the infiltration of this carcinoma into the adjacent adipose tissue.

FIGURE 12-72

A, This tumor shows extremely heavy sclerosing or scarring, nearly completely obscuring the underlying tumor. **B**, Perineural invasion by the malignant epithelial cells.

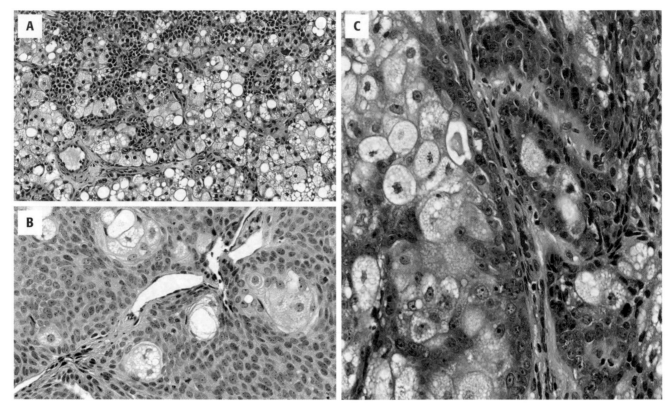

FIGURE 12-95

A–C, The variable degree of sebaceous differentiation is shown. It is important to note that the cells should show true microvesiculation and not degenerative change. Nucleoli are frequently quite prominent.

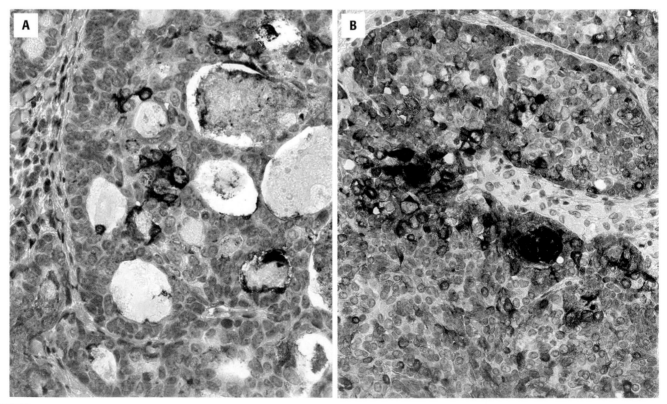

FIGURE 12-96

A, CD15 highlights the sebaceous cells in this sebaceous carcinoma. **B**, Epithelial membrane antigen preferentially highlights the sebocytes, although other cells are also positive.

The tumor is unencapsulated and consists of large, round, or polyhedral cells with abundant, granular, and eosinophilic cytoplasm and large, centrally placed nuclei with prominent nucleoli (Figure 12-97). The mitochondria-rich cytoplasm usually shows intensely blue, granular positivity with PTAH stain. There is variable pleomorphism and some tumors have cytologically bland areas, suggesting that they have arisen from a preexisting oncocytoma. Ki-67 staining may be of value in differentiating between benign and malignant oncocytic tumors. The cells are arranged in sheets, thèques, and cords, and sometimes duct-like structures are present. The tumor shows infiltration into surrounding tissue, and neural and vascular invasion are common (Figure 12-98). The diagnosis is usually made after oncocytic variants of other salivary gland

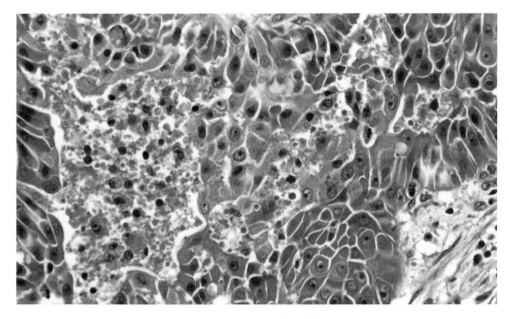

FIGURE 12-97

Large, polygonal cells with ample oncocytic-oxyphilic cytoplasm surround nuclei with prominent nucleoli. Note the necrosis.

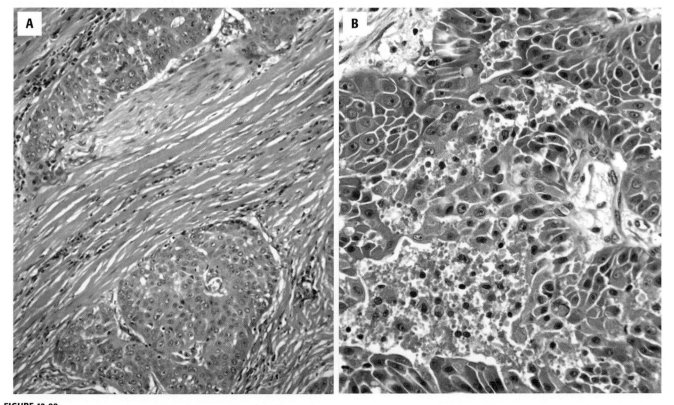

FIGURE 12-98

A and **B**, Oncocytic carcinoma cells are arranged in gland- or duct-like structures, seen surrounding a nerve in this infiltrative neoplasm. The cells have prominent nucleoli.

malignancies have been excluded. Oncocytic carcinoma is often high grade, showing frequent local recurrence and both regional and distant metastases.

UNDIFFERENTIATED CARCINOMAS

Undifferentiated carcinomas are rare high-grade malignant salivary tumors. They are too poorly differentiated to be placed in any other specific category of carcinoma but are now divided into three independent groups: small and large cell carcinomas and lymphoepithelial carcinoma (LEC).

SMALL CELL CARCINOMA

Small cell carcinoma is a type of undifferentiated carcinoma characterized by a proliferation of small anaplastic cells with scanty cytoplasm, fine nuclear chromatin, and inconspicuous nucleoli. Most show evidence of neuroendocrine differentiation. It is very rare in the salivary glands and most cases involve the parotid gland. There is a slight male predominance and the peak incidence is in the 5th to 7th decades. The tumor usually presents as a painless but rapidly growing mass, and facial nerve and regional lymph node involvement are common.

It typically forms a poorly circumscribed, infiltrative mass. It consists of sheets, cords, or nests of uniform, anaplastic cells that are usually less than 30 μm (Figure 12-99). Occasional larger or fusiform cells are present. The nuclear chromatin is finely granular and there are no nucleoli. The cytoplasm is scanty and cell borders are ill defined (Figure 12-100). Crush artifacts with nuclear smearing are usually present. Cells at the periphery of nests may show a suggestion of palisading, and occasionally cells are arranged in organoid or rosette-like patterns. Occasionally, there are small foci of ductal or squamous differentiation.

UNDIFFERENTIATED CARCINOMAS—FACT SHEET

Small Cell Carcinoma

Clinical

- A type of undifferentiated carcinoma characterized by a proliferation of small anaplastic cells. Most show evidence of neuroendocrine differentiation
- Represent <1% of salivary gland tumors
- Peak incidence in 5th to 7th decades
- Usually painless but rapidly growing mass with frequent facial nerve and cervical lymph node involvement
- Highly aggressive with 5-year survival of <50%

Pathology

- Poorly circumscribed infiltrative mass often with areas of hemorrhage and necrosis
- Sheets, cords, trabeculae of anaplastic small cells
- May show focal palisading or organoid patterns
- Numerous mitoses; stretch artifacts, necrosis, neural and vascular invasion
- Focal pan-cytokeratin paranuclear dot-like staining
- Must be separated from solid variant of adenoid cystic carcinoma, lymphoma, melanoma, Merkel cell carcinoma, metastases

Large Cell Carcinoma

Clinical

- A rare, high-grade, undifferentiated, malignant salivary tumor composed of pleomorphic, large cells with abundant cytoplasm
- Represents <1% of salivary gland tumors
- Most cases involve major glands, particularly the parotid gland
- Peak incidence 60 to 70 years
- Rapidly growing, firm, fixed mass, which is often tender or painful
- Facial nerve and regional lymph node involvement common
- Very aggressive with frequent local recurrence and distant metastases

Pathology

- Poorly circumscribed infiltrative mass often with areas of necrosis
- Characterized by lack of differentiation, with occasional foci of ductal or squamous differentiation
- Sheets, cords, or trabeculae of loosely cohesive cells in fibrous stroma
- Cells >30 μm with abundant, pale eosinophilic or clear cytoplasm
- Nuclei round or polygonal, and vesicular with prominent nucleoli and frequent mitoses
- Vascular and neural invasion frequent
- Must be separated from metastases, particularly nasopharyngeal; component of carcinoma ex pleomorphic adenoma; melanoma, anaplastic large cell lymphoma

Lymphoepithelial Carcinoma

Clinical

- A large cell undifferentiated carcinoma with prominent non-neoplastic lymphoplasmacytic infiltrate
- Represents <0.4% of salivary gland tumors
- 80% parotid, 20% submandibular
- Mean age 40 years (range: 2nd to 9th decades)
- Much higher incidence in Inuit and southern Chinese populations with a strong association with Epstein-Barr virus
- Often presents as long-standing mass with recent rapid growth, pain or nerve involvement
- 5-year survival rate 60% to 80%

Pathology

- Solid, firm mass that may be circumscribed and lobulated or extensively infiltrative
- Sheets, cords, nests of tumor cells in dense lymphoid stroma
- Carcinoma cells large and polyhedral with faintly eosinophilic, abundant cytoplasm and indistinct cell borders
- Nuclei round or oval with vesicular chromatin, conspicuous nucleoli, and frequent mitoses
- Must be separated from metastatic nasopharyngeal carcinoma, lymphoepithelial sialadenitis, large cell undifferentiated carcinoma, lymphoma

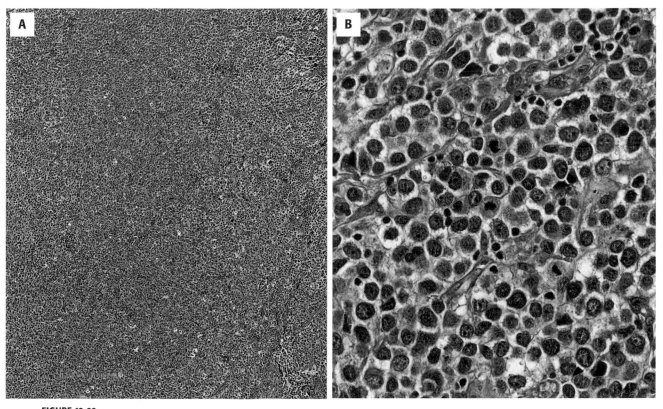

FIGURE 12-99
A and **B**, Small cell carcinoma showing sheets of small cells with densely hyperchromatic nuclei. Note the high nuclear-to-cytoplasmic ratio.

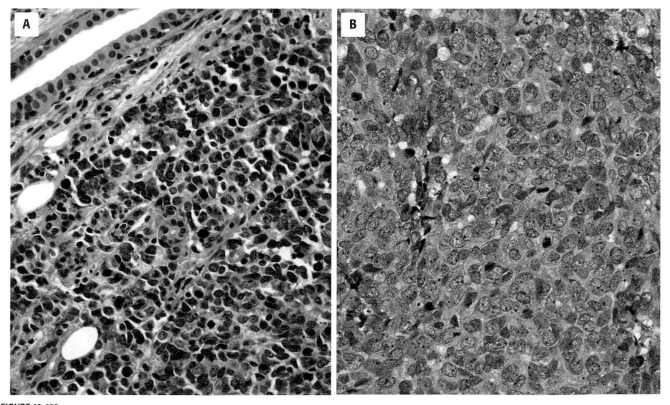

FIGURE 12-100
A, A streaming architecture of small cells with a high nuclear-to-cytoplasmic ratio. There is a normal duct in the upper left. **B**, A slightly larger cell appearance, with vesicular, open nuclear chromatin and small but easily identified nucleolus. Note the numerous mitoses.

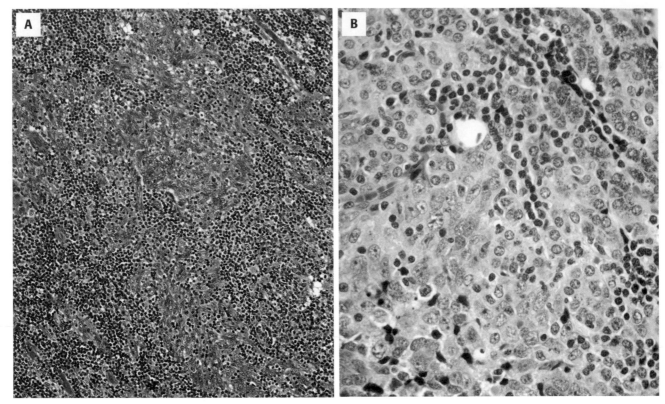

FIGURE 12-103

A, Lymphoepithelial carcinoma showing islands of epithelial cells surrounded and infiltrated by lymphocytes. **B**, The cells have a syncytial arrangement with prominent nucleoli identified in nuclei with vesicular nuclear chromatin. Note the heavy inflammatory infiltrate.

are usually large and polygonal with faintly eosinophilic, abundant cytoplasm and indistinct cell borders (Figure 12-103). This often produces a syncytial appearance. Occasionally, plumper or spindle-shaped cells are present. The nuclei are round or oval and have vesicular chromatin and conspicuous nucleoli. Extreme nuclear pleomorphism is rarely conspicuous. There is usually a high mitotic frequency and focal necrosis is common. Foci of squamous differentiation are infrequent. Some tumors show evidence of neural and angiolymphatic invasion. The stroma consists of a dense lymphoid infiltrate with smaller numbers of plasma cells. This infiltrate may be so dense that initially it can mask the underlying malignant component. Lymphocytes surround and permeate the tumor islands. Germinal centers are an inconsistent feature. Many tumors show pale, reactive histiocytes imparting a "starry sky" appearance. In some cases, the surrounding salivary parenchyma can show evidence of LESA. LEC cells are positive for pan-cytokeratin and EMA. There is increased expression of p53 and a high Ki-67 proliferative index. The lymphoid component is polyclonal and consists of B and T cells, with the latter predominating. CD4$^+$ T cells are prominent in the stroma and CD8$^+$ T cells predominate in the epithelial islands. EBV-encoded small RNA can usually be detected by in situ hybridization in the carcinoma cells of endemic cases.

The differential diagnosis includes metastatic *nasopharyngeal carcinoma, LESA, large cell undifferentiated carcinoma*, and *lymphoma*. In endemic populations, it may not be possible to exclude metastatic nasopharyngeal carcinoma of the lymphoepithelial type on the basis of morphology, immunocytochemistry, or virology.

Locoregional lymph node metastasis is common (40%), and ~20% of cases show distant metastases. Despite this, the 5-year survival rate is about 60% to 80%. Most cases are treated with a combination of local radical surgical excision and adjuvant radiotherapy to the surgical site and ipsilateral neck. Elective neck dissection is usually limited to patients with proven cervical metastases.

SUGGESTED READINGS

The complete suggested readings list is available online at
    www.expertconsult.com.

13

Non-Neoplastic Lesions of the Gnathic Bones

■ Uta Flucke ■ Pieter J. Slootweg

■ OSTEOMYELITIS

Osteomyelitis is an inflammatory process in the marrow cavities of the bone. It may be either acute or chronic.

CLINICAL FEATURES

Patients with acute osteomyelitis show all signs and symptoms of an acute inflammatory disease, such as fever, malaise, and regional lymphadenopathy. In chronic osteomyelitis, signs and symptoms usually are less prominent and may fluctuate in severity; they include swelling, pain, sinus formation, sequestration, and, in case of bone loss, pathologic fractures. The disease may occur at any age.

Sclerosing osteomyelitis and proliferative periostitis are specific subtypes. Sclerosing osteomyelitis causes recurrent pain, swelling of the cheek, and restricted jaw movement and may be either diffuse or focal. Proliferative periostitis is a periosteal reaction to inflammatory changes in the underlying jaw bone causing facial swelling and bony enlargement. All types of osteomyelitis predominantly affect the mandible.

RADIOLOGIC FEATURES

Radiographs show an irregular pattern of bone loss and increased density of bone. Cortical duplicating or "onion-skinning" is the radiologic hallmark of proliferative periostitis.

PATHOLOGIC FEATURES

OSTEOMYELITIS—DISEASE FACT SHEET

Definition
- Inflammatory changes in the mandibular bone causing both loss and increase of bone

Gender, Race, and Age Distribution
- Mandible most often involved in adults, maxilla in children

Clinical Features
- Fever, chills, regional lymphadenopathy in case of acute osteomyelitis
- Swelling, pain, and draining fistulae in both acute and chronic osteomyelitis
- Localized bony swelling in case of proliferative periostitis

Radiologic Features
- Mixed radiodense and radiolucent

Prognosis and Treatment
- Depends on eradication of the causative organisms and removal of necrotic bone

---

OSTEOMYELITIS—PATHOLOGIC FEATURES

Gross Findings
- Nonspecific

Microscopic Findings
- Necrotic bone that may be invested with microorganisms
- Sclerotic bone
- Infiltrate of polymorphonuclear granulocytes
- Granulation tissue
- Sinuses lined by squamous epithelium

Pathologic Differential Diagnosis
- Paget disease
- Fibrous dysplasia
- Osseous dysplasia

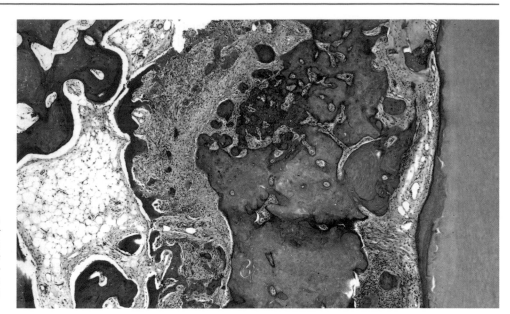

FIGURE 13-17

Osseous dysplasia is interposed between bone (*left side*) and tooth surface (*right side*). The lesional tissue may fuse with surrounding bone but the tooth surface is not touched. The variation in size, outline, and tinctorial qualities of bone in osseous dysplasia is also illustrated in this case.

fibroma is a single expansive predominantly radiolucent lesion. Separation by histology alone may be impossible, requiring radiographic and clinical features. Sclerosing lamellar bone and well-vascularized fibrous tissue with lymphocytes and plasma cells define *sclerosing osteomyelitis*. *Fibrous dysplasia* is composed of irregular woven bone without osteoblastic rimming, whereas osseous dysplasia shows woven and lamellar bone and mineralized particles resembling cementum.

PROGNOSIS AND THERAPY

Treatment for all forms of osseous dysplasia is needed when there is infection or sclerotic bone masses that result in cosmetic deformities.

SUGGESTED READINGS

The complete suggested readings list is available online at www.expertconsult.com.

14

Benign Neoplasms of the Gnathic Bones

■ **Brenda L. Nelson**

■ OSSIFYING FIBROMA

Benign fibro-osseous lesions are characterized by the replacement of native bone by fibrous and mineralized tissues. The ossifying fibroma is unique among these lesions as it is categorized as a neoplasm and requires more extensive treatment. The other benign fibro-osseous lesions, fibrous dysplasia and osseous dysplasia, can be difficult to differentiate, requiring radiographic and clinical correlation to make an accurate diagnosis. Bone and/or cementum may be present, and so *cementifying fibroma* and *cemento-ossifying fibroma* have also been used to describe these lesions. The World Health Organization (WHO) refers to this lesion as simply "ossifying fibroma."

CLINICAL FEATURES

Ossifying fibromas are found more commonly in the mandible (90%) than the maxilla, specifically affecting the molar-premolar area. Patients in the 3rd to 4th decades are most affected, with a high female-to-male ratio (5:1). Small lesions are usually asymptomatic, often incidental findings on routine dental radiographs, while larger lesions can result in significant cosmetic and functional morbidity, especially with resection and reconstruction.

RADIOLOGIC FEATURES

Radiographic images are essential to the diagnosis, and a diagnosis should not be rendered without radiographs or their reliable interpretation. Ossifying fibromas are characteristically well-demarcated unilocular or multilocular radiolucent lesions with varying degrees of radiopacity (Figure 14-1). The radiopacities

---

OSSIFYING FIBROMA—DISEASE FACT SHEET

Definition
- A well-demarcated neoplasm of gnathic bones composed of fibrocellular tissue and mineralized material of varying appearances

Incidence and Location
- Mandible >> maxilla (90%), premolar molar area specifically

Morbidity and Mortality
- Aggressive behavior is reported with functional morbidity and cosmetic disruption

Gender, Race, and Age Distribution
- Female >> male (5:1)
- Wide age range with a predilection for 3rd to 4th decade

Clinical Features
- Small lesions are asymptomatic, incidentally discovered
- Larger lesions may cause facial deformity, malocclusion, and pain

Prognosis and Treatment
- Clinical follow-up for recurrences
- Surgical curettage or enucleation

---

correlate with the mineralized component of the tumor. Large lesions may cause displacement of teeth, root divergence, or alterations of associated structures. Furthermore, a characteristic downward bowing of the mandible may be helpful in developing a radiographic differential diagnosis.

PATHOLOGIC FEATURES

GROSS FINDINGS

Lesions are well demarcated, frequently described as "shelling out" of the bone. The intact tumor is a smooth, glistening, white, firm-elastic mass.

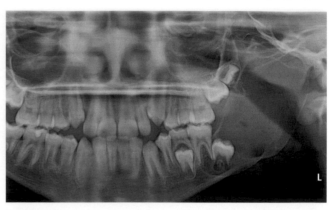

FIGURE 14-14

Panorex image features of an expansive, multiloculated cystic ameloblastoma of the left posterior mandible, inferiorly displacing the molar tooth and forming fine bony septa in the ramus.

bone; however, more frequently, thinning and expansion of the cortical plate are seen (Figure 14-15). Unicystic lesions are large solitary radiolucent cysts, associated with an impacted tooth (Figure 14-15). The cortical plate may be expanded and a dense sclerotic border is seen at the leading edge of the slowly expanding tumor. Maxillary tumors may show less distinct radiographic borders, often filling the maxillary sinus and appearing as a diffuse solid semiradiopaque mass within the sinus. Desmoplastic ameloblastoma usually presents as a mixed radiolucency/radiopacity. These lesions are often thought to represent a benign fibro-osseous lesion radiographically.

PATHOLOGIC FEATURES

as a subtype by the WHO, to stress its unique features. Unlike multicystic ameloblastomas, it favors the anterior mandible; however, treatment is essentially the same as a multicystic ameloblastoma. All forms of ameloblastomas are asymptomatic until later stages, when significant cosmetic deformity and pathologic fracture may occur.

RADIOLOGIC FEATURES

Multicystic lesions form large radiolucent loculations within the cortex of the bone with numerous distinct bony septa forming the walls of the compartments (Figure 14-14). Multicystic tumors progress anteriorly and posteriorly through the central medullary bone through the path of least resistance. The involved impacted tooth may be significantly displaced, with tooth resorption seen only in later stages of development. Large, long-standing lesions may perforate cortical

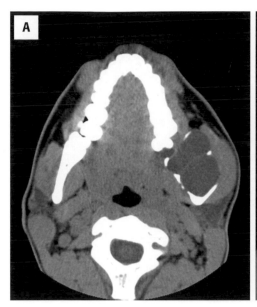
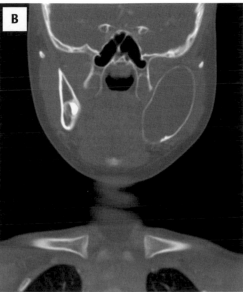

FIGURE 14-15

Computed tomography features an intraosseous ameloblastoma. **A**, Multilocular cyst with bone remodeling and tooth displacement. **B**, A unicystic ameloblastoma of the left mandible, showing a rim of bone around the periphery.

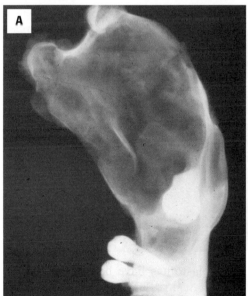
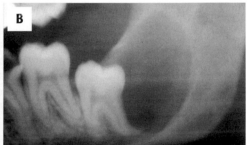
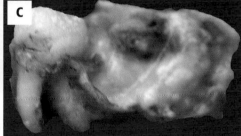

FIGURE 14-16

A, Specimen radiograph showing the remarkable extent of the tumor in this en bloc resection. **B**, Radiographic features of a solitary, unilocular radiolucent cystic ameloblastoma of right mandible with distinct sclerotic peripheral margin. **C**, Gross specimen with attached bisected cyst, showing intact cyst wall with hemorrhagic-appearing area representing a plexiform unicystic ameloblastoma.

GROSS FINDINGS

Early multicystic and unicystic ameloblastomas are typically cysts that have thick walls with rough luminal surface elevations. The cyst wall in early unicystic tumors is thin, uniform, and often filled by gray-brown gelatinous material representing tumor (Figure 14-16). Unicystic tumor with mural involvement shows mild thickening of the wall with corresponding variegated coloration of the luminal surface. Late-stage multicystic tumors are removed as en bloc resections of bone with tumor filling medullary spaces and appearing as dense fibrous tissue with cystic spaces.

MICROSCOPIC FINDINGS

The classic histologic (follicular) features, as described by Vickers and Gorlin, are seen in conventional tumors and characterized by islands of proliferating odontogenic epithelium reminiscent of the enamel organ (Figure 14-17). Epithelial tumor islands are enmeshed in hyperplastic fibrous connective tissue, displaying pale hyalinized areas at the epithelial connective tissue interface (Figure 14-18). The odontogenic elements are composed of basophilic columnar cells at the periphery, exhibiting reverse polarization of nuclei away from the connective tissue with vacuolization. The central

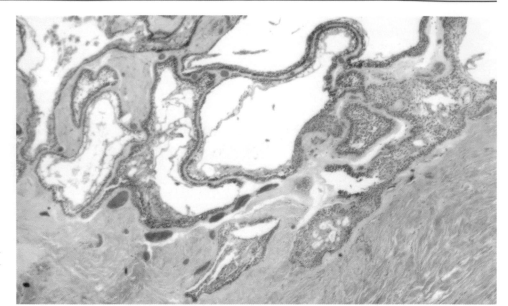

FIGURE 14-21

Low-power view of plexiform ameloblastoma with reticulated strands of epithelium proliferating into the cystic lumen and focal extension of a follicular pattern ameloblastoma into the fibrous wall.

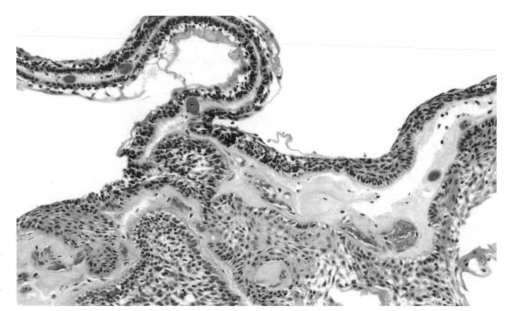

FIGURE 14-22

High-power view shows strands of plexiform ameloblastoma free floating in a cyst with little reverse polarization and a "basketweave" surface typical of unicystic ameloblastomas.

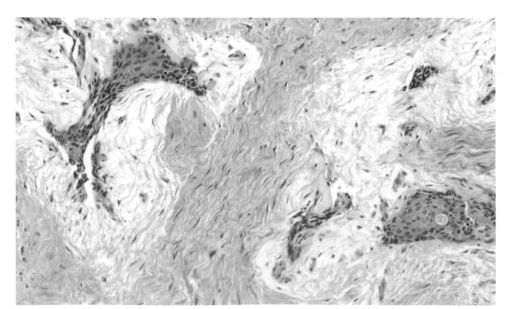

FIGURE 14-23

Medium-power view of desmoplastic ameloblastoma showing **no** evidence of Vickers and Gorlin changes, presenting as irregular islands of squamous epithelium circumscribed by edematous halos consistent with inductive effect.

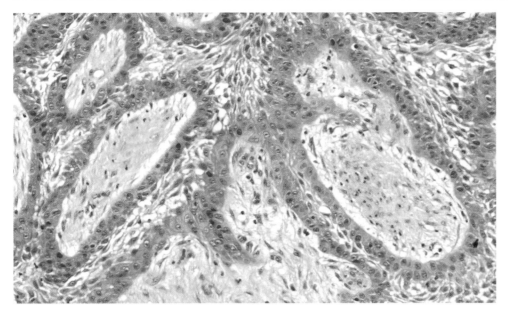

FIGURE 14-24

Medium-power view of ameloblastic carcinoma shows a condensed layer of atypical peripheral basal cells lacking columnar cells, vacuolar changes, and reverse polarization.

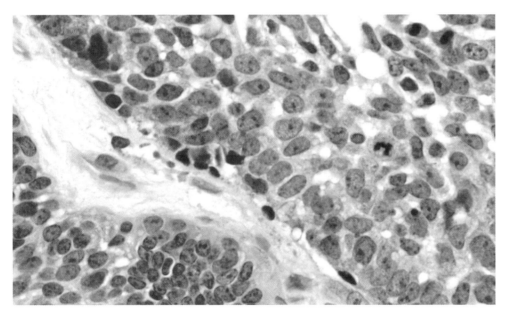

FIGURE 14-25

At high power, ameloblastic carcinoma displays a distinct connective tissue epithelial interface with unorganized basal cell layer, marked pleomorphism, and numerous mitoses.

benignity. The "true malignant" counterpart of ameloblastomas is an ameloblastic carcinoma that is a high-grade tumor, widely metastatic with a 50% mortality rate in some series. The character of ameloblastic carcinomas is reminiscent of the benign counterpart; however, they show less polarization at the connective tissue interface, a more solid cellular central area, considerable cytologic pleomorphism, and significant mitotic activity (Figure 14-24). Ameloblastic carcinomas are often solid basaloid tumors (Figure 14-25) that are locally aggressive (not slowly progressive), eroding bony margins early, as well as potentially metastatic.

■ KERATOCYSTIC ODONTOGENIC TUMOR

The keratocystic odontogenic tumor (KCOT) is a distinctive odontogenic cyst, believed to arise from the dental lamina. The lesion has been previously and continues to be called odontogenic keratocyst (OKC). This cyst is unique, however, in that it demonstrates a neoplastic-like growth potential. The change in terminology to KCOT is more in keeping with its biologic potential and is supported by molecular studies done on both sporadic and syndromic lesions.

Microscopic Findings

Histologically, nodules of odontogenic epithelium are separated by minimal stromal connective tissue. The tumor comprises two cell types. The duct-like, tubular or cord-like areas are lined by cuboidal to columnar epithelial cells (Figure 14-34), with nuclei polarized away from the central duct-like space, imparting an appearance reminiscent of ameloblastoma. The duct-like spaces are pseudolumina containing secretions of the columnar cells. The second component is a spindled to polyhedral eosinophilic cell component, which creates a nodular, nested, and swirling pattern, often containing collections of eosinophilic, amorphous amyloid-like material (Figure 14-35). These globular masses may show varying degrees of mineralization, and in their most advanced form may show distinct laminations (Figure 14-36). Minimal, loose stroma with thin-walled vessels is present, usually accentuated at the periphery.

Ancillary Studies

Ultrastructural findings reveal a fibrillar to granular quality to the eosinophilic deposits, suggesting they may represent enamel matrix or perhaps amyloid.

Differential Diagnosis

Although AOT histology is characteristic, an *ameloblastoma* must be ruled out.

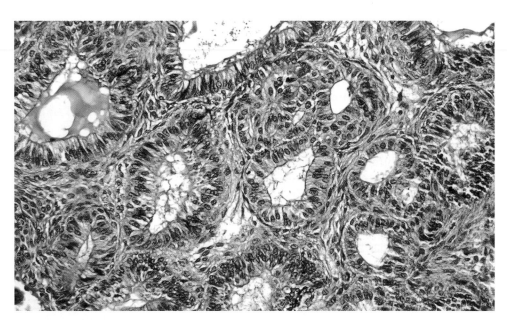

FIGURE 14-34

Nodular duct-like structures set in a spindle cell background in an adenomatoid odontogenic tumor.

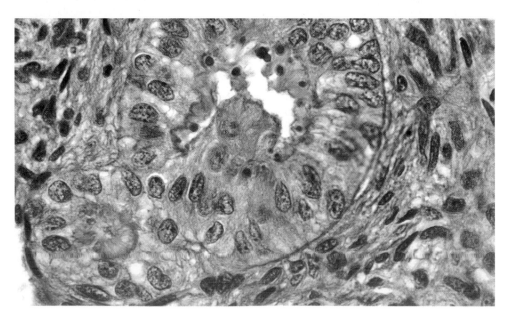

FIGURE 14-35

Gland-like spaces surrounded by cuboidal to columnar cells, surrounded by a spindle cell population, are seen in an adenomatoid odontogenic tumor.

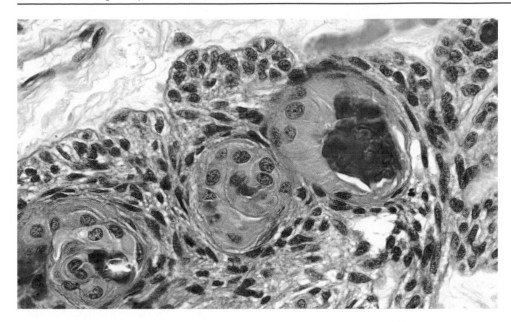

FIGURE 14-36

Calcifications adjacent to the spindle and columnar epithelial cells. Note the area of lamination, a feature helpful in confirming a diagnosis of adenomatoid odontogenic tumor.

Prognosis and Therapy

Recurrences are extremely rare. Conservative, local excision is curative, and made easier by a thick capsule.

■ CENTRAL GIANT CELL LESION

The central giant cell lesion is a localized lytic lesion of the jawbones associated with fibrosis, hemorrhage, hemosiderin-laden macrophages, reactive bone, and osteoclastic giant cells. In the past, the terms *reparative giant cell granuloma* and *central giant cell granuloma* have been used as synonyms. Currently, the WHO endorses the term "giant cell lesion."

Clinical Features

Central giant cell lesions are found in a wide age range, although the average is 20 years. Females are affected more often than males (1.5 to 2:1), and there is a definitive predilection for the mandible. Giant cell lesions of the jaw have traditionally been divided, based on clinical and radiologic features, into two categories: nonaggressive and aggressive. The WHO does not specifically recognize this division, however. Nonaggressive lesions are usually asymptomatic, incidental findings. Aggressive lesions may present with pain, paresthesias, and resorption of teeth.

CENTRAL GIANT CELL LESION—DISEASE FACT SHEET

Definition
- A localized osteolytic lesion of the jaw bones associated with fibrosis, hemorrhage, hemosiderin-laden macrophages, reactive bone, and osteoclastic giant cells

Incidence and Location
- Uncommon
- Mandible > maxilla (2:1)

Gender, Race, and Age Distribution
- Female > male (1.5 to 2:1)
- Average 20 years (>90% before 30 years)

Clinical Features
- Separated by radiographic and clinical features into nonaggressive and aggressive
- Usually asymptomatic
- Painless expansion of the jaw, paresthesias, and tooth resorption

Radiographic Features
- Range from unilocular, well-circumscribed radiolucent lesions to large, expansile multilocular lytic lesions
- Root resorption and displacement of teeth may be seen
- Intralesional bony ("wavy") septa may be seen

Prognosis and Treatment
- Long-term prognosis is good, although histology does not predict behavior
- Complete enucleation, although steroid injection, alpha-interferon injections, and calcitonin treatments are effective

RADIOLOGIC FEATURES

Central giant cell lesions present as expansile unilocular or multilocular radiolucent defects with scalloped and usually well-defined borders (Figure 14-37). Tooth displacement can be seen. Intralesional bony septa are helpful, although radiographic findings are not diagnostic.

PATHOLOGIC FEATURES

The lesion consists of oval to spindle-shaped fibroblastic cells; some lesions are highly cellular, while others are loose and myxoid. A richly vascularized stroma is associated with extravasated erythrocytes (hemorrhage), hemosiderin-laden macrophages, and giant cells (Figure 14-38). The osteoclastic giant cell population is variable,

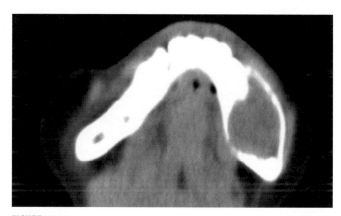

FIGURE 14-37
Computed tomography image showing a large expanding radiolucent lesion of the posterior mandible.

CENTRAL GIANT CELL LESION—PATHOLOGIC FEATURES

Gross Findings
- Red to brown hemorrhagic tissue with associated bone

Microscopic Findings
- Multinucleated, osteoclastic giant cells in a background of ovoid to spindle-shaped fibroblastic cells
- Richly vascularized; associated with extravasated erythrocytes and hemosiderin-laden macrophages
- Metaplastic bone and osteoid traverse the lesion
- Mitotic figures are common (although not atypical)

Pathologic Differential Diagnosis
- Brown tumor of hyperparathyroidism, cherubism

---

without an absolute number required for the diagnosis. While multinucleated, the number of nuclei is quite variable (Figure 14-39). Lobules of collagen and metaplastic bone traverse the lesion, although accentuated at the periphery. Mitoses are common but are not atypical. Aggressiveness is clinically and radiographically determined.

DIFFERENTIAL DIAGNOSIS

The central giant cell lesion is histologically identical to a *brown tumor of hyperparathyroidism*. Therefore, the diagnosis of this entity as *central giant cell lesion, rule out hyperparathyroidism* may be most prudent, and patient's serum calcium and parathyroid hormone levels should be checked. Histologic separation from *cherubism* may be difficult; however, the finding of eosinophilic

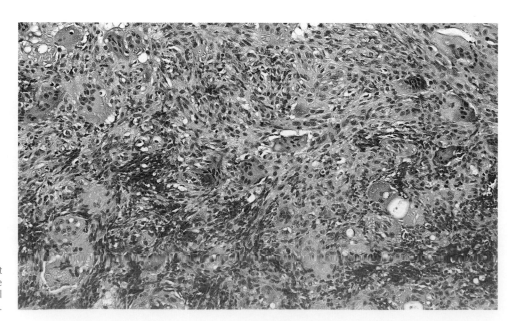

FIGURE 14-38
Many multinucleated giant cells are set within a cellular mesenchymal tissue within the bone in a central giant cell lesion. Note the extravasated erythrocytes.

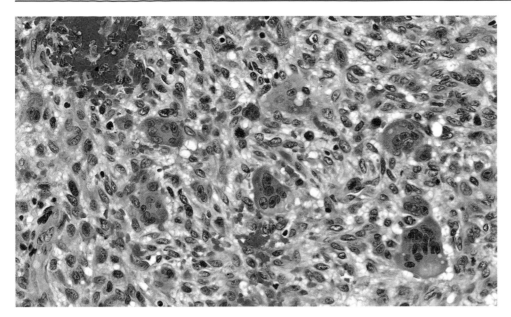

FIGURE 14-39
Multinucleated foreign-body giant cells in a stroma of ovoid to spindle-shaped cells. Note the erythrocyte extravasation in this central giant cell lesion. A mitotic figure is present.

ring-like deposits surrounding vessels plus the clinical and radiographic information, most importantly, will allow for proper separation.

PROGNOSIS AND THERAPY

Histology does not predict behavior. Recurrences are rare if there is unaffected bone at the margins of the resection. Complete enucleation has traditionally been the treatment of choice, but steroid injection, alpha-interferon injections, and calcitonin treatments have proved effective. The nonsurgical techniques require months before regression is seen.

■ ODONTOMA (COMPLEX AND COMPOUND)

Odontoma is the most common odontogenic tumor, although it may best be classified as a hamartoma, composed of enamel, dentin, pulpal tissue, and cementum. Academically, odontomas are subclassified into two types, while management is identical: *compound* when composed of rudimentary teeth-like structures and *complex* when composed of haphazardly arranged tooth structures.

CLINICAL FEATURES

Odontoma occurs more frequently than all other odontogenic tumors combined. There is no gender predilection and they develop most commonly in the first two

---

ODONTOMA (COMPLEX AND COMPOUND)—DISEASE FACT SHEET

Definition
- A tumor-like malformation (hamartoma) composed of enamel, dentin, pulpal tissue, and cementum separated into compound and complex types

Incidence and Location
- Most common odontogenic tumor
- Compound odontomas predilect to anterior maxilla
- Complex odontomas predilect to posterior mandible

Gender, Race, and Age Distribution
- Equal gender distribution
- Prevalence in the first two decades

Clinical Features
- Usually asymptomatic
- Unusually large lesions may expand the jaws, preventing normal tooth eruption

Radiographic Features
- Radiodense calcified mass surrounded by thin radiolucent rim
- Appearance of small, malformed teeth

Prognosis and Treatment
- Prognosis is good
- Conservative enucleation of odontoma and associated dental follicle or cyst

---

decades (the same time that normal teeth are developing and erupting). Most odontomas are asymptomatic, found incidentally on routine dental radiographs, while larger lesions may interfere with eruption of normal adjacent teeth, prompting radiographic investigation.

MICROSCOPIC FINDINGS

The hallmark of osteosarcoma is the production of malignant bone or osteoid from malignant mesenchymal stroma (Figure 15-3). The sarcomatous stroma varies in degree of aberrancy and cytologic character with tumor grade. Low-grade tumors are only moderately cellular with minimal pleomorphism and few mitotic figures. The tumor cells produce osteoid and bone that is irregular, lacks lamellae, and has an atypical mineralization pattern. Parosteal osteosarcomas are well-differentiated low-grade tumors, displaying almost no atypia and frequently showing focal trabecular rimming, which is not considered a typical feature of conventional osteosarcomas. High-grade tumors are very cellular with closely packed oval, spindled, or polygonal cells with nuclear pleomorphism, chromatin clumping, large nucleoli, and numerous mitotic figures (Figure 15-4). Malignant osteoid may be difficult to appreciate, because it is minimal and deposited as thin eosinophilic strands interposed between sheets of malignant osteoblasts. Tumors with heavy osteoid and bone production form broad trabeculae with isolated single osteoblasts engulfed by osteoid that is undergoing normalization with loss of cytologic atypia (Figure 15-5). Conventional osteosarcomas are histologically subclassified by their most prominent characteristic: fibroblastic (Figure 15-6), chondroblastic (Figure 15-7), or osteoblastic. Regardless of the subclassification, deposition of malignant

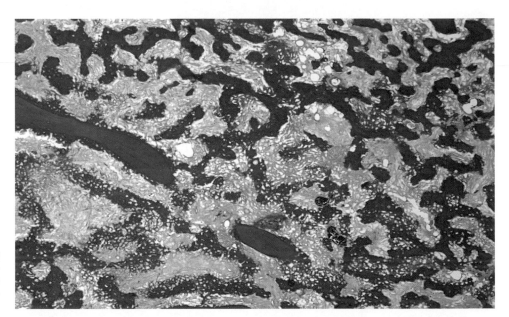

FIGURE 15-3

A medium-power photomicrograph of osteosarcoma demonstrates irregular trabeculae of tumor osteoid arising from sarcomatous stroma. The stroma is pleomorphic and disorganized.

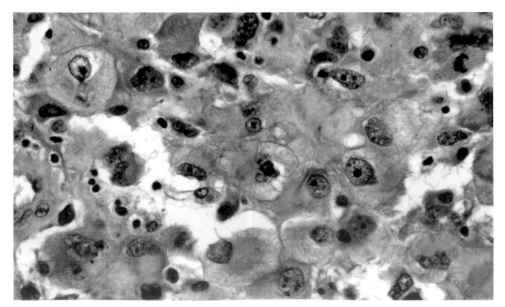

FIGURE 15-4

High-power view of a high-grade osteosarcoma. The pleomorphism and macronucleoli are striking, and the overall size of the cells is markedly increased.

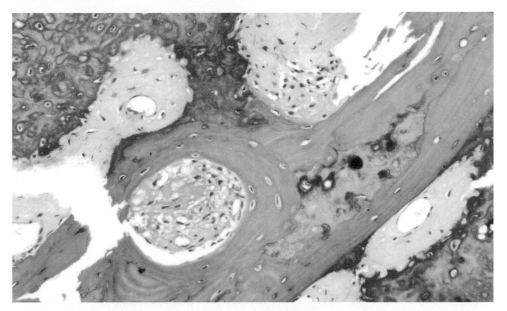

FIGURE 15-5

An aggressive osteosarcoma resorbing residual bone trabeculae with subsequent replacement by tumor bone.

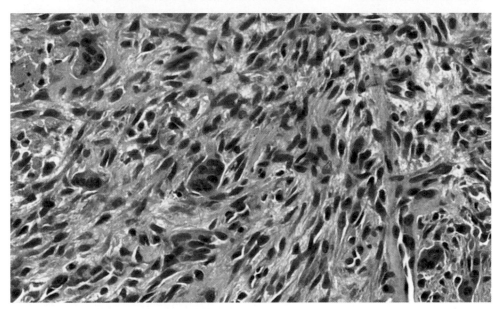

FIGURE 15-6

Fibroblastic osteosarcoma reveals a spindle cell pattern with vague storiform organization. Osseous matrix is often difficult to appreciate.

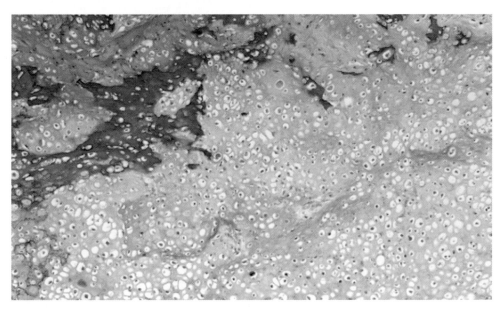

FIGURE 15-7

Chondroblastic osteosarcoma with large areas of chondroid matrix (*right*) and osseous matrix (purple/darker) (*upper left*).

bone or osteoid must be demonstrated to meet the criteria of an osteosarcoma. Telangiectatic osteosarcoma, which grossly resembles aneurysmal bone cyst, shows prominent blood-filled cystic spaces. Minimal osteoid is present, but its malignant nature is betrayed by the malignant stroma separating the cysts. Small cell osteosarcoma shows diffuse growth of small round cells with a high nuclear:cytoplasmic (N:C) ratio. Both telangiectatic and small cell osteosarcoma variants are exceedingly rare in the jaws.

ANCILLARY STUDIES

The difficulty with fine needle aspiration (FNA) of osteosarcoma is the actual sampling technique. However, once a sample is obtained, the smears are cellular, composed of pleomorphic spindled and rounded tumor cells, occasionally resembling osteoblasts and osteoclasts, multinucleated cells with metachromatic cytoplasmic granules. In fact, multinucleated tumor cells are often present (Figure 15-8). Mitotic figures may be appreciated, and amorphous background "osteoid" material may be present, staining eosinophilic with alcohol fixation and magenta with air-dried preparations. There are differing findings for other types of osteosarcoma.

DIFFERENTIAL DIAGNOSIS

Distinguishing *osteoblastoma* from osteosarcoma both radiographically and histologically is difficult. However, osteoblastoma is usually better circumscribed and has a sclerotic margin. Osteoblastoma forms thick trabeculae

from broad sheets of epithelioid osteoblasts with trabecular rimming, a feature not seen in osteosarcoma. Osteosarcoma may produce cartilage, whereas osteoblastoma produces cartilage only in areas of previous biopsy. Osteosarcoma is cytologically more pleomorphic, and while both are mitotically active, aberrant mitotic figures are not seen in osteoblastoma.

Osteosarcoma on occasion contains large numbers of reactive multinucleated giant cells, resembling *benign giant cell tumor*. Osteosarcoma with minimal osteoid and giant cells is strikingly similar to benign giant cell tumor and is separated by evaluation of the mononuclear cells, which exhibit more pleomorphism with aberrant mitotic figures.

Separation of *dedifferentiated chondrosarcoma* and *chondroblastic osteosarcoma* is challenging as each produces chondroid and osteoid. The distinguishing features are areas of low-grade chondrosarcoma in dedifferentiated chondrosarcoma, while chondroblastic osteosarcoma consists of a mixture of high-grade chondrosarcoma intermixed with osteosarcoma.

Fibroblastic osteosarcoma producing limited osteoid and malignant bone raises the differential consideration of *fibrosarcoma* and *pleomorphic sarcoma (PS; malignant fibrous histiocytoma)* (Figure 15-9). The production of malignant osteoid, however scant, favors a diagnosis of osteosarcoma over fibrosarcoma and PS. Because some pathologists accept osteoid in PS, separation from PS may be based on the more fasciculated pattern in PS.

PROGNOSIS AND THERAPY

Treatment of osteosarcoma is wide surgical resection with neoadjuvant or postsurgical chemotherapy with a

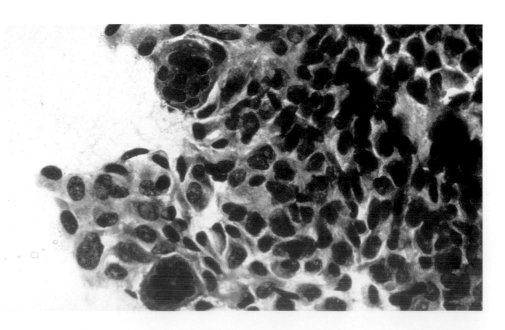

FIGURE 15-8
Malignant oval to spindle-shaped cells are arranged in a dense cluster in this fine needle aspiration. Multinucleated giant cells are seen in this osteosarcoma (air-dried, Diff-Quik stained).

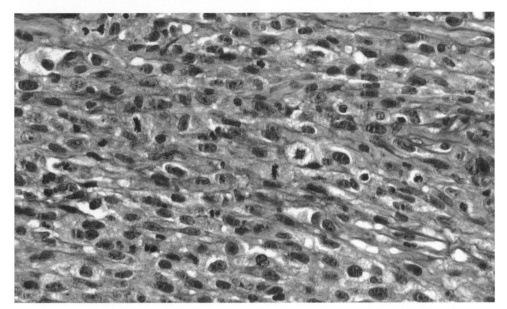

FIGURE 15-9

A high-grade fibrosarcoma composed of sheets of fibroblastic cells with sparse, fine collagen fibrils and nuclei of varying sizes with dispersed to clumped chromatin. Mitotic figures are numerous and atypical.

variety of agents. Gnathic osteosarcoma survival rates, around 80%, approximate those of extragnathic tumors in patients receiving adequate initial surgical resection. Lesions in the jaws tend to have slightly better prognosis than skeletal lesions and a lower rate of metastasis. Having said that, local recurrence and inaccessibility of the tumor frequently cause the death of patients with jaw lesions, particularly in the maxilla. The lungs are the most frequent site of metastasis and can be treated with resection of solitary metastatic lesions, resulting in a 40% salvage rate.

■ CHONDROSARCOMA

CLINICAL FEATURES

Chondrosarcomas are malignant mesenchymal tumors with hyaline cartilage differentiation as the main component and are the third most common primary malignant tumor of bone, following myeloma and osteosarcoma. The most common presenting symptoms in craniofacial bones are cortical expansion and pain, similar to their long bone counterparts. Chondrosarcoma in the head and neck is relatively rare, representing less than 10% of all chondrosarcomas and approximately 15% of sinonasal tract sarcomas.

While chondrosarcomas of long bones favor females (2:1), they are relatively equal (1:1) in their gender distribution in the head and neck. These tumors present over a broad age range, with the majority presenting in the 5th to 7th decades; the mesenchymal variant occurs earlier, between the 2nd and 3rd decades.

Mandibular tumors occur predominantly in the posterior angle and ramus. Maxillary tumors involve

CHONDROSARCOMA—DISEASE FACT SHEET

Definition

- Characterized by malignant hyaline cartilage with diverse histology, depending on grade of the lesion

Incidence and Location

- Second most common malignant mesenchymal tumor of the craniofacial bones
- 11% of all bone tumors, but 2% of malignant head and neck tumors
- Arising in central (54%), peripheral (38%), and juxtacortical (8%) location

Gender, Race, and Age Distribution

- No gender predilection
- Peak in 5th to 7th decades (mean, 55 years)
- Mesenchymal variant has younger presentation: 2nd to 3rd decades

Clinical Features

- 75% present with bony expansion and pain present for a long duration
- Malocclusion with tooth movement and developing diastema

Radiographic Features

- Mixed radiolucency with irregular opacities, central ossification and radiolucent peripheral margin
- Internal matrix production shows "rings and arcs" or stippled calcification pattern
- Widening of periodontal ligament

Prognosis and Treatment

- Wide en bloc resection with 2- to 3-cm margins
- Grade determines management and outcome:
  - Grade 1: rare metastasis, 68% to 89% 5-year survival rate
  - Grade 2: 33% metastatic rate
  - Grade 3: 70% metastatic rate
- Mesenchymal chondrosarcoma: 55% 5-year survival rate
- Pediatric patients have better prognosis
- Primary site of metastasis is the lungs

primarily the maxillary sinuses and nasal cavity and are less confined as they quickly erode the thin maxillary bone walls. Chondrosarcomas can also present in the skull base, larynx, and nasal septum.

Symptoms depend largely on the location, but the majority of these tumors present with pain and/or swelling at the affected site. Chondrosarcomas can present with headache, nasal obstruction, sinusitis, diastema, loose teeth (Figure 15-10), cranial nerve dysfunction, secondary ophthalmic aberrations, and eventual bony expansion.

RADIOLOGIC FEATURES

Radiographic findings are variable and depend on the grade of the lesion. Low-grade or grade 1 tumors are generally lytic with internal matrix production. The internal matrix production often takes the form of "rings and arcs" or stippled calcification (Figure 15-11). The lytic pattern will show a lobular pattern with endosteal scalloping that often gives a strong clue to the diagnosis on plain film or CT scan. High-grade tumors create a more diffuse radiolucency with ragged destruction of bone and extension into soft tissue.

When teeth are involved, a distinct triad of radiographic findings are seen: (1) symmetrical widening of the periodontal ligament; (2) elevation of the interdental alveolar cortical bone; and (3) tooth resorption (Figure 15-12). The borders of maxillary tumors are difficult to identify, as tumors frequently destroy maxillary indigenous bone, invading the adjacent soft tissue, nasal cavity, and sinuses. CT and MRI are helpful in determining the extent of less well-defined maxillary lesions (Figure 15-12) and can highlight the presence of internal matrix production, especially in difficult anatomic locations.

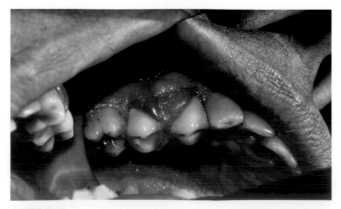

FIGURE 15-10

Chondrosarcoma creating alveolar expansion with separation of bicuspids and clinical malocclusion.

PATHOLOGIC FEATURES

CHONDROSARCOMA—PATHOLOGIC FEATURES

Gross Findings

- Pale blue to gray to white with gritty foci
- Translucent areas of hyaline cartilage and chalky calcifications
- Irregular tumor margin interface with central mucoid and cystic areas

Microscopic Findings

- Bone entrapment and destruction
- Lobules of cartilaginous matrix around atypical chondrocytes
- Increased cellularity, depending on grade of the tumor
- Enlarged, atypical nuclei, and multinucleated cells
- Higher-grade tumors have increased atypia, cellularity, and mitoses and less matrix
- Mesenchymal variant is biphasic neoplasm including a small cell component with scattered island of cartilage and "stag-horn" vascular pattern

Immunohistochemical Features

- Cartilage stains S100 protein positive
- Mesenchymal chondrosarcoma: Sox9, CD99, and Leu7 positive

Pathologic Differential Diagnosis

- Enchondroma, odontogenic myxoma, pleomorphic adenoma, chordoma, myxoid chondrosarcoma, chondroblastic osteosarcoma

GROSS FINDINGS

Grossly, chondrosarcomas are translucent light-blue to pearly white with scattered areas of gritty calcifications. Foci of recognizable hyaline cartilage in a lobular configuration with myxomatous change are commonly seen. High-grade tumors have an irregular rough interface with native bone and areas of hemorrhage and necrosis and often a paucity of cartilaginous matrix.

MICROSCOPIC FINDINGS

The most important morphologic feature in the diagnosis of chondrosarcoma is the presence of bone destruction and/or bone entrapment by the tumor (Figure 15-13). In conjunction with the radiologic appearance, the diagnosis can be reliably made. Once these determinations have been made, then attention can be turned to evaluation of the cytology, degree of cellularity, and mineralization pattern, as well as other, associated histologic patterns (i.e., spindle cells, myxoid degeneration [Figure 15 14], etc.).

The low-power architectural pattern shows cartilaginous lobules often delineated by fibrous septa with peripheral ossification, thus producing the "rings and arcs"

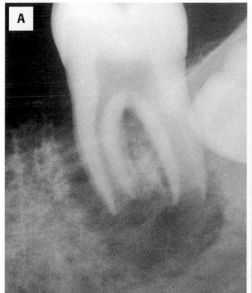
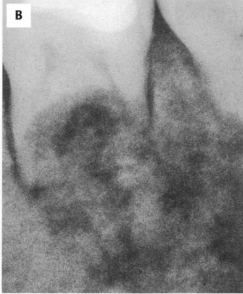

FIGURE 15-11

A, Chondrosarcoma of the mandible presenting as a radiolucent lesion involving molars with resorption and expanded periodontal ligament. **B**, Chondrosarcoma with mixed radiolucent/radiopaque appearance, "spotty calcification," and tooth resorption.

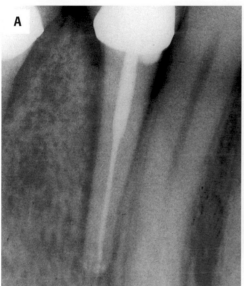
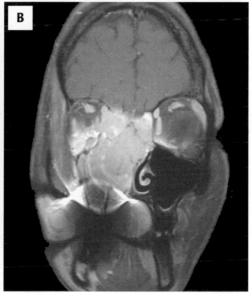

FIGURE 15-12

A, The radiographic appearance of chondrosarcoma shows fine diffuse spiculation with increased alveolar height, splaying of teeth, and widened periodontal ligament. **B**, T1-weighted magnetic resonance image demonstrating an expansile tumor of the maxillary sinus, extending into the paranasal sinuses of this mesenchymal chondrosarcoma.

mineralization pattern noted radiographically. Entrapment and resorption of native bony trabeculae are common; however, osteoid production from the tumoral cells indicates an osteosarcoma and should be addressed first (Figure 15-15). Additional histologic variants of chondrosarcoma have been described and include myxoid (Figure 15-14), dedifferentiated, clear cell, and mesenchymal chondrosarcoma.

Myxoid (or "chordoid") chondrosarcoma is distinguished by rows of cuboidal cells in a myxoid background, resembling chordoma. Dedifferentiated chondrosarcoma is characterized by the coexistence of a well-differentiated cartilaginous component and high-grade anaplastic component. The low-grade chondrosarcoma abruptly transitions

to the spindle cell sarcoma, which may include PS, rhabdomyosarcoma, fibrosarcoma, or osteosarcoma. Clear cell chondrosarcoma shows sharply defined lobules of S100 protein positive clear cells with vacuolated cytoplasm and central nuclei. These cells show chondroid features on electron microscopy. The jaw is a common site for mesenchymal chondrosarcoma, which microscopically has a biphasic appearance of islands of well-differentiated cartilage abruptly transitioning to undifferentiated stroma composed of small oval cells (Figure 15-16). In addition, these tumors are characterized by stag-horn vascular spaces reminiscent of a hemangiopericytoma ("HPC-like vascular pattern") (Figure 15-17). They are positive with Sox9, CD99, and Leu7.

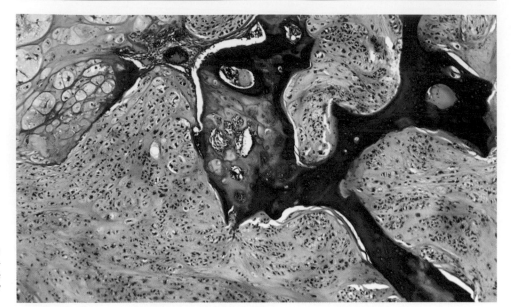

FIGURE 15-13

Low-grade chondrosarcoma (grade 1) with low to moderate cellularity. The chondroid matrix surrounds and entraps the osseous matrix, demonstrating the key diagnostic criterion for chondrosarcomas.

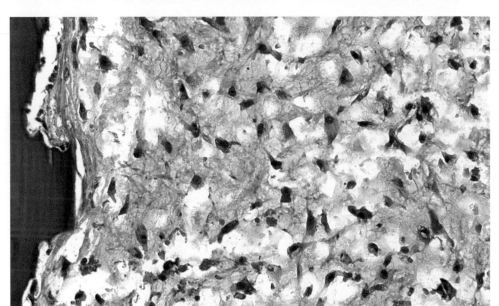

FIGURE 15-14

Grade 2 chondrosarcoma with moderate increase in cellularity and myxoid extracellular matrix. The tumor is invading the bone (*left*).

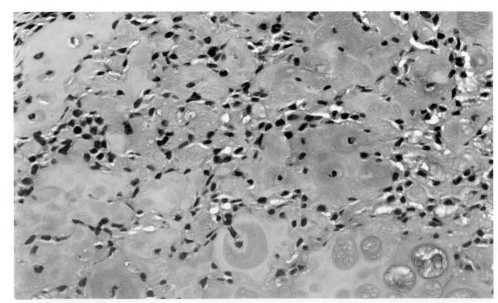

FIGURE 15-15

High-grade chondrosarcoma with marked increase in cellularity and myxoid matrix. Small foci of lower-grade chondrosarcoma (*upper left*) can assist in making the diagnosis as well as correlation with the radiographs. In small biopsy samples, staining immunohistochemically with S100 protein can be helpful.

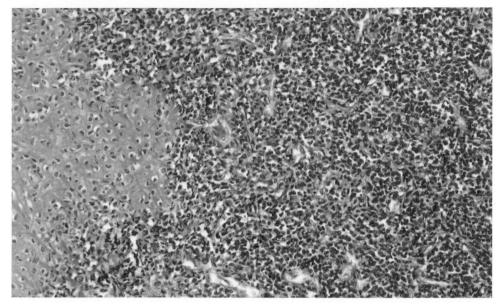

FIGURE 15-16

Medium-power view of mesenchymal chondrosarcoma with chondroid matrix (*left*) associated with small, round blue cells.

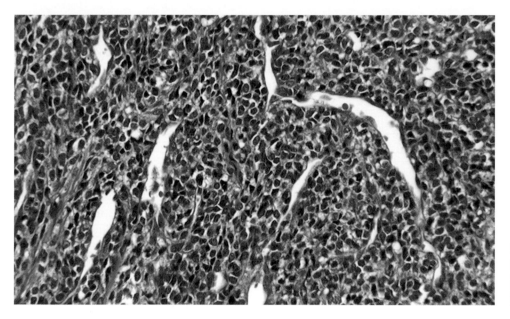

FIGURE 15-17

Hemangiopericytoma-like "stag-horn" growth is characteristic for a mesenchymal chondrosarcoma. There is no cartilage in this image.

Interestingly, ischemic change within a chondroma is frequently identified in areas that develop chondrosarcoma (Figure 15-18). Therefore, whenever ischemic change is present, careful evaluation of the whole lesion is recommended.

Grading of chondrosarcoma is important, as it generally dictates treatment and prognosis. As previously mentioned, a histologic grade is rendered only after the aggressive nature of the lesion has been established (i.e., bone destruction), thus confirming the malignant nature of the neoplasm. Increased nuclear cellularity, pleomorphism, and mitotic activity, plus necrosis, all factor into the grading of these lesions, in conjunction with the nature of the matrix being formed. Grade 1 tumors, which represent ~77% of gnathic tumors,

show increased cellularity with only scattered pleomorphic nuclei and binucleate cells in a background of predominantly hyaline matrix with little or no myxoid degeneration or change. Grade 2 tumors show moderate cellularity with easily identified enlarged atypical nuclei and lacunae containing multiple chondrocytes. There is an increase in the number of cells and the matrix is often largely myxomatous. Grade 3 tumors are highly cellular with minimal matrix and abundant pleomorphic cells with multinucleation, occasional mitotic figures, and liquefactive necrosis. These high-grade tumors can be difficult to diagnose if the cartilaginous component is scant or absent. In these cases, immunohistochemical staining with S100 protein can be of some use.

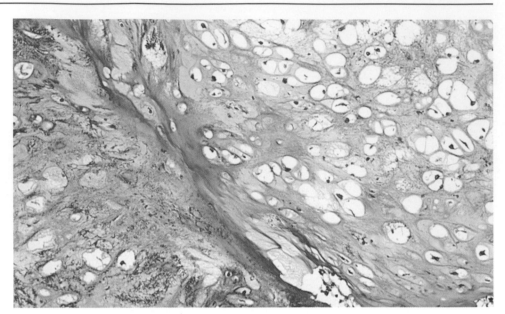

FIGURE 15-18

Left, Ischemic change with granular, eosinophilic granular degeneration. *Right,* The chondrosarcoma fills the image, showing the usual histologic features of increased cellular and architectural disarray.

ANCILLARY STUDIES

FNA of chondrosarcoma is composed of abundant, chondromyxoid matrix material surrounding atypical chondrocytes (Figure 15-19). The cells are usually enlarged with an increased N:C ratio, vacuolated cytoplasm, and nuclear atypia. The matrix material is often difficult to appreciate on alcohol-fixed preparations, which yield a pale eosinophilic appearance, in contrast to the deep magenta-colored fibrillar chondroid matrix characteristic of air-dried preparations. FNA can be of some use diagnostically, but usually the clinical and radiologic information is sufficient to establish a diagnosis.

DIFFERENTIAL DIAGNOSIS

The differential diagnosis includes a number of benign and malignant entities, including, but not limited to, enchondroma, odontogenic myxoma, pleomorphic adenoma, chordoma, myxoid chondrosarcoma, and chondroblastic osteosarcoma.

The separation of low-grade chondrosarcoma from *enchondromas* can be challenging, especially with grade 1 chondrosarcomas. However, benign cartilaginous tumors rarely, if ever, occur in the craniofacial bones. Moreover, enchondromas do not show bone entrapment or destruction unless an associated fracture is present and will often have wide areas of peripheral maturation to bone.

Chondrosarcomas with a predominant myxoid matrix may be confused with an *odontogenic myxoma*; however, they are usually easy to distinguish radiologically.

Furthermore, odontogenic myxoma is less cellular with a more uniform distribution of cytologically bland cells and the presence of odontogenic epithelium (Figure 15-20).

Pleomorphic adenoma is usually easy to distinguish on histologic sections but may prove problematic on FNA samples, which reveal varying proportions of epithelial cells, mesenchymal cells, and metachromatic stroma.

Chordoma is a diagnostic challenge, especially in lesions of the skull base. The characteristic histologic picture shows a myxoid/edematous matrix with two cell populations: chief and physaliferous. Chief cells are generally polygonal and eosinophilic and arranged in cords and nests. Physaliferous cells are larger with clear "bubbly" cytoplasm. Chordomas will stain immunohistochemically with S100 protein, similar to chondrosarcomas, but also will stain with cytokeratin and epithelial membrane antigen.

Myxoid chondrosarcoma will show cytologic atypia with bone destruction and mitotic figures.

Separation of chondrosarcoma from *chondroblastic osteosarcoma* rests almost solely on the demonstration of osteoid production arising from the cellular sarcomatous stroma in the latter. The presence of this matrix, even if very small in quantity, is sufficient to warrant the diagnosis of chondroblastic osteosarcoma.

PROGNOSIS AND THERAPY

Chondrosarcomas of the head and neck have an overall 5-year survival of ~70%. Approximately 20% of patients die of their disease due to extensive local recurrence. Recurrence is noted in ~40% of cases and depends on the location. Tumors of the skull

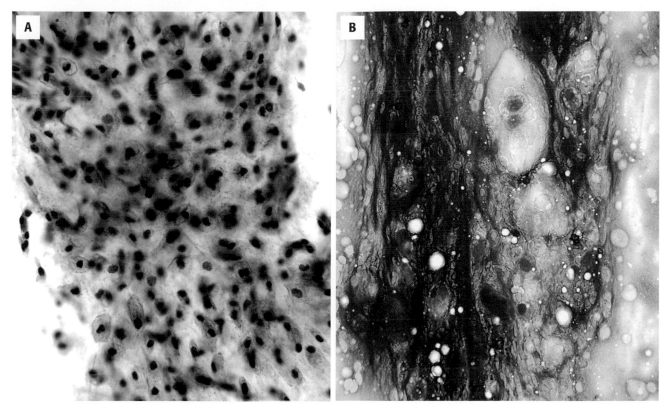

FIGURE 15-19

A, This Papanicolaou-stained fine needle aspiration (FNA) material shows a high cellularity, multinucleation, and nuclear pleomorphism in this high-grade chondrosarcoma. **B**, A low-grade chondrosarcoma on FNA has intensely magenta, fibrillar, chondroid matrix material with enlarged, binucleated cells within lacunar spaces (air-dried, Diff-Quik stained).

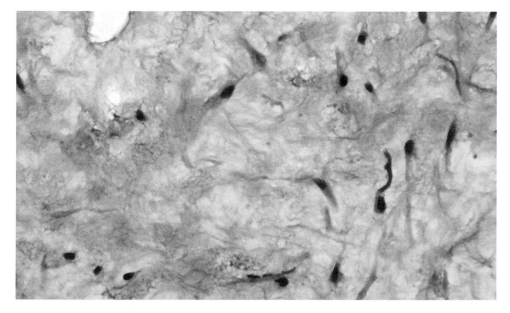

FIGURE 15-20

A myxoma is composed of slender spindle and stellate cells with delicate cytoplasmic processes and small hyperchromatic nuclei. This field does not have any odontogenic epithelium.

base show a higher recurrence from incomplete resection due to the complicated anatomy. The prognosis rests on the resectability of the primary lesion and adequacy of the margins combined with the grade of the lesion. Pediatric patients have a much better prognosis, although chondrosarcomas are significantly less common in this patient population. The prognosis of dedifferentiated chondrosarcoma depends on the grade of the spindle cell component. Metastases are not common in grade 1 and 2 tumors but can occur in 70% of grade 3 and dedifferentiated sarcomas.

■ MULTIPLE MYELOMA

CLINICAL FEATURES

Multiple myeloma is a neoplasm of plasma cells disseminated in multiple intraosseous sites. Solitary accumulations of atypical plasma cells and plasmablasts are referred to as plasmacytoma.

Approximately one-third of patients with disseminated disease will have jaw lesions, and in 30% of cases mandibular lesions are the initial presentation. Solitary lesions (plasmacytoma of bone) are rare in the jaws (2%); however, 25% of solitary plasmacytomas in other anatomic sites will progress to disseminated disease within 3 years, frequently involving the head and neck. The disease originates in hematopoietic marrow, often presenting in vertebrae, pelvis, skull, ribs, and the posterior mandible. Jaw lesions are initially painful with tooth mobility and lip paresthesia. Large lesions may lead to pathologic fractures.

Presenting symptoms include anemia, fever, weight loss, hypercalcemia, renal failure, and proteinemia and often will precede radiologic evidence of the disease. Multiple myeloma rarely occurs before 40 years, with a median age of onset of 70 years. Males are affected twice as often as females, and blacks develop multiple myeloma twice as frequently as whites. Electrophoresis of urine or serum samples in patients with multiple myeloma may be helpful in identifying increased immunoglobulin light chains (Bence-Jones proteins) in the urine and elevation of monoclonal immunoglobulin (Ig) levels. Elevated serum IgG and IgA are most commonly identified, at 55% and 25%, respectively.

RADIOLOGIC FEATURES

Multiple myeloma is generally radiographically distinctive with multiple radiolucencies in the bone. These lucencies, ranging from 0.1 to 2 cm in the jaws, reveal sharp borders without internal matrix production resulting in the classic "punched-out" appearance (Figures 15-21 and 15-22). Multiple lesions may coalesce to form large, irregular radiolucencies with less distinct irregular borders. Differential radiographic considerations include hyperparathyroidism, infection, metastases, and Langerhans cell histiocytosis.

PATHOLOGIC FEATURES

GROSS FINDINGS

Not unlike normal bone marrow, some gross specimens of multiple myeloma appear red and gelatinous,

---

MULTIPLE MYELOMA—DISEASE FACT SHEET

Definition
- Neoplasm of plasma cells disseminated in multiple intraosseous sites
- Single accumulation of clonal plasma cells is termed plasmacytoma

Incidence and Location
- Most common tumor of bone in adults >40 years
- Early lesions in vertebrae, pelvis, ribs, and skull
- Mandible involved in up to 30% of disseminated cases

Gender, Race, and Age Distribution
- Male > female (2:1)
- Blacks > whites (2:1)
- Most present in 6th to 8th decades

Clinical Features
- Pain and paresthesia
- Loosening of teeth
- Swelling in later stages with pathologic fracture

Radiographic Features
- Multiple or single "punched-out" round radiolucencies with sharp borders
- Similar to Langerhans cell histiocytosis and hyperparathyroidism radiologically

Prognosis and Treatment
- Initial response of 70%, but 10-year survival rate of <10%
- Solitary tumors have better prognosis than multifocal tumors
- Solitary tumors can be managed with radiation
- Chemotherapy

MULTIPLE MYELOMA—PATHOLOGIC FEATURES

Gross Findings
- Gray/red tumor intermixed with marrow
- "Currant jelly" appearance
- "Waxy" character when amyloid is present

Microscopic Findings
- Solid aggregations of neoplastic plasma cells
- Plasma cells vary from normal to anaplastic
- Eccentric nucleus with "cartwheel" (chromatin) appearance
- Higher-grade tumors have atypical and binucleated plasmacytoid cells with irregular clumped chromatin

Immunohistochemical Features
- Clonal expression for either κ or κ light-chain
- Positive with CD138, CD38, CD79a, CD56

Pathologic Differential Diagnosis
- Reactive inflammatory plasmacytoid odontogenic lesions, immunoblastic large B-cell lymphoma, Langerhans cell histiocytosis

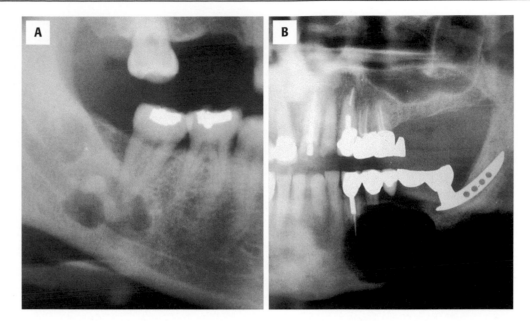

FIGURE 15-21

A, Multiple discrete oval radiolucencies of the right posterior mandible at the apex of the second molar and in the ascending ramus. **B**, Solitary plasmacytoma of the left mandible presenting as a large radiolucency with well-defined "punched-out" peripheral margin.

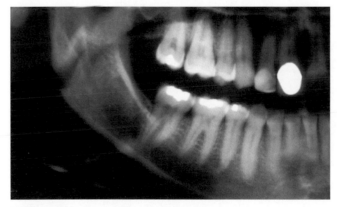

FIGURE 15-22

Multiple myeloma in the right mandible with diffuse contiguous merging lesions and pathologic fracture at angle of mandible.

which some observers have termed "currant jelly." This depends on the size of the material that is received. Some tumors, however, are firmer in consistency and resemble lymphoma in gross characteristics (i.e., white and solid). The central portions of the lesions show little evidence of residual medullary bone spicules and are easily removed by curettage.

MICROSCOPIC FINDINGS

Myeloma is histologically exemplified by sheets of atypical plasma and plasmacytoid cells (Figure 15-23), displaying eccentric nuclei with "cartwheel" or "clock face" chromatin. The atypical plasma cells show binucleation, clumped chromatin, macronucleoli, and atypical mitotic figures (Figure 15-24). The cytoplasm of these cells is usually eosinophilic due to the abundant protein being produced. Occasionally, there are globules of immunoglobulin that accumulate in the cytoplasm and stain intensely with eosin; these are called "Russell bodies." Amyloid can be noted in some of these tumors and is evidenced by extracellular accumulation of amorphous, pale pink material. The clonal plasma cells can sometimes exhibit normal morphology, making identification on hematoxylin and eosin–stained slides difficult. Immunohistochemistry can be performed to demonstrate monoclonal kappa (κ) or lambda (λ) light chains to establish the clonality of these tumors (Figure 15-25). Staining with CD138 (most sensitive and specific), CD79a, CD38, and CD56 may help with the differential diagnosis.

DIFFERENTIAL DIAGNOSIS

The main differential diagnostic consideration histologically is chronic inflammatory conditions; however, lymphoma is also in the differential. *Periapical granuloma* and *chronic periodontitis*, both chronic inflammatory conditions, have aggregated plasma cells and may be mistaken for multiple myeloma, requiring immunohistochemical separation by performing light-chain studies. Furthermore, myeloma cells react with natural killer antigen CD56, which is negative in reactive lesions. Anaplastic and plasmablastic myeloma may simulate a *poorly differentiated carcinoma*, but myeloma is keratin negative. Separation of the *immunoblastic variant of*

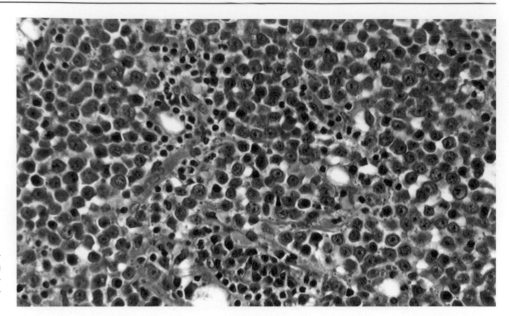

FIGURE 15-23

Moderate to poorly differentiated myeloma with closely packed cells with variability in size and minimal background stoma. There is an eccentric location to the nuclei.

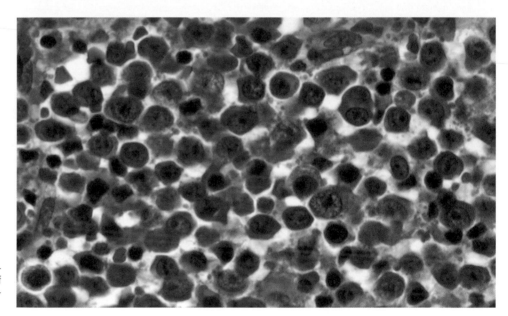

FIGURE 15-24

High-power photomicrograph of myeloma shows sheets and single cells of atypical plasma cells. Note the binucleation and prominent nucleoli.

diffuse large B-cell lymphoma from myeloma can be quite challenging due to considerable immunophenotypic overlap. Clinical evidence may be helpful, as multiple myeloma is seldom seen in lymph nodes. Lymphomas tend to be CD45RB positive, while myelomas are not.

PROGNOSIS AND THERAPY

Multiple myeloma is treated with debulking of solitary lesions, plus combination chemotherapy and local irradiation. Bone marrow transplantation can be used as first-line therapy or in patients for whom chemotherapy failed. Although initial response rates approach 70%, long-term prognosis is poor, with a median survival less than 3 years and a 10-year overall survival of 10%. There are high rates of relapse due to treatment resistance. Higher grade and stage tumors with significant marrow replacement have a worse prognosis with shortened survival. Solitary tumors generally have a better prognosis and may be treated by irradiation, particularly when the tumor is surgically inaccessible.

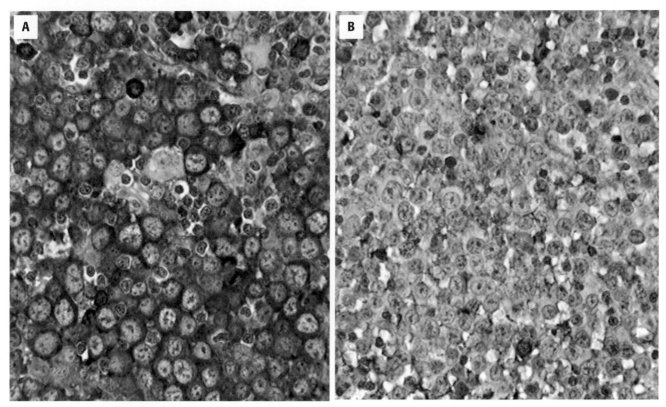

FIGURE 15-25
Immunohistochemistry shows a kappa (κ) light-chain restriction (**A**) in plasmacytoma (**B** is lambda [λ]).

■ METASTATIC NEOPLASMS

CLINICAL FEATURES

Metastatic tumors to the head and neck are rare, representing ~4% of metastases, with the majority representing carcinomas. When metastases do occur in the craniofacial bones, they generally herald widespread disease and a corresponding poor prognosis. Metastases are noted in medullary bone, developing via the venous or arterial system; periosteal lymphatics play a very small role.

Low-grade pain and progressive paresthesia are the initial symptoms, preceding any radiologic evidence of tumor. Pathologic fracture is present in up to 30% of patients, likely owing to the thin cortices of craniofacial bones. A soft tissue mass as extension of the bony metastasis is frequent (Figure 15-26). Most metastatic tumors of the jaws occur in the 5th to 8th decades (mean, 45 years), which follows the mean age of developing carcinomas in general. There does not appear to be an overall gender predilection, but some epidemiologic data correlate with the presence of the primary tumors in both males and females. The gender-specific order of frequency is as follows: female patients present with metastases from primaries originating in the breast

METASTATIC NEOPLASMS—DISEASE FACT SHEET

Definition
- Metastasis of distant primary tumors to the craniofacial bones

Incidence and Location
- 1% of all oral malignancies
- 30% are first indication of metastatic disease
- 86% are in mandible

Morbidity and Mortality
- Dependent on the underlying tumor type

Gender and Age Distribution
- Nearly equal gender distribution
- Peak in 5th to 8th decades (mean, 45 years)

Clinical Features
- Pain and paresthesia early

Radiographic Features
- Bony expansion with cortical erosion late
- Lytic radiolucent lesion with ill-defined margins

Prognosis and Treatment
- Poor prognosis as jaw metastasis is usually a late event

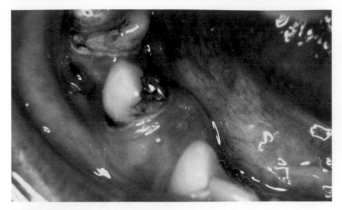

FIGURE 15-26

A metastatic carcinoma presenting as a soft tissue swelling surrounding a mandibular bicuspid with loosening and migration of teeth.

lesions (Figure 15-27). Metastatic breast carcinoma, for example, usually produces lytic lesions but additionally has the potential to produce radiopaque osteoblastic or mixed lesions (Figure 15-27). Radiopaque osteoblastic lesions are also produced by prostate carcinoma (Figure 15-28), carcinoid tumors, and medulloblastomas. Almost all metastatic tumors of the jaws are irregular lytic tumors, lacking a sclerotic border. However, metastatic tumors can be initially subtle, indistinct radiopacities, frequently not appreciated on flat radiographic films, especially given the complicated anatomy of the craniofacial bones. Advanced imaging including CT and MRI can often prove helpful in identifying these lesions.

(42%), adrenal (9%), female genitalia (8%), and thyroid (6%); male patients present with lung (22%), prostate (12%), kidney (10%), and bone (9%) metastases. Of gnathic bones, the mandible is the most frequent site of metastatic disease (86%) usually in the posterior region.

RADIOLOGIC FEATURES

The radiologic appearance of metastases depends on the characteristics of the primary lesion and can have a variety of patterns, including osteoblastic, osteolytic, or mixed. The majority of metastatic tumors are carcinomas, which usually present as lytic radiolucent

---

METASTATIC NEOPLASMS—PATHOLOGIC FEATURES

Gross Findings

- Nodular intrabony foci with soft core and irregular bony wall

Microscopic Findings

- Tumor's histologic character is dependent on and usually similar to primary tumor

Immunohistochemical Features

- Immunologic studies appropriate for primary tumor
- Cytokeratin is useful as two-thirds of metastatic lesions are carcinomas

Pathologic Differential Diagnosis

- Primary or metastatic carcinoma, sarcoma, lymphoma, melanoma

---

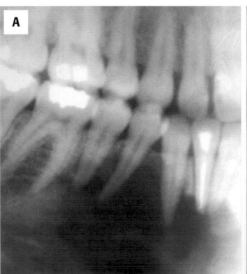
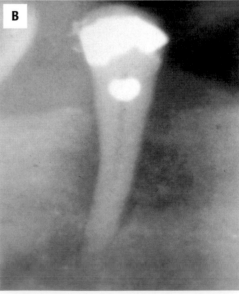

FIGURE 15-27

A, Solitary intrabony expansive lesion in the body of the mandible creating a uniform radiolucency with indistinct borders and divergence of bicuspid roots in this metastatic breast carcinoma. **B**, Radiographic presentation of metastatic carcinoma shows elevation of soft tissue surrounding the crown and a midroot diffuse radiolucency.

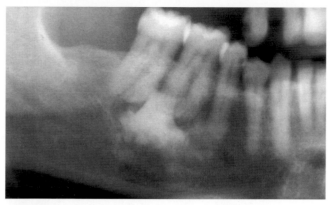

FIGURE 15-28

Metastatic prostate carcinoma of the right mandible characterized as a mixed radiolucent/radiopaque lesion with irregular peripheral radiolucent borders and a central sclerotic radiopaque mass.

PATHOLOGIC FEATURES

GROSS FINDINGS

Metastatic tumors on gross examination are nonspecific. The majority of lesions are well demarcated and easily curetted from their bony crypts. Some tumors are calcified with gritty foci, indicating possible prostate carcinoma or other osteoblastic metastases.

MICROSCOPIC FINDINGS

The histologic spectrum of metastatic tumors is diverse, usually replicating the primary site. Common tumors that metastasize to bone include prostate (Figure 15-29), renal (Figure 15-30), and lung (Figure 15-31)

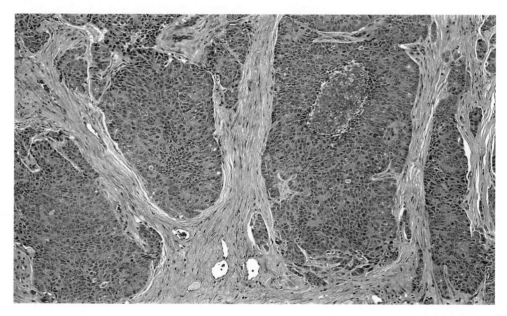

FIGURE 15-29

Metastatic prostate carcinoma shows glandular accumulations of tumor cells similar to that seen in the prostate. Note the numerous mitoses. *Upper right,* Comedonecrosis is present.

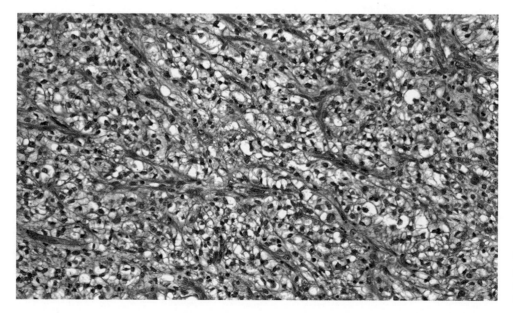

FIGURE 15-30

Metastatic renal cell carcinoma contains nests of cells with cleared cytoplasm and abundant vasculature.

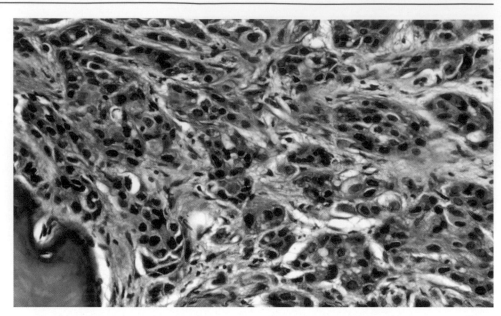

FIGURE 15-31

Metastatic lung squamous cell carcinoma with nests of large atypical cells identical to those seen in the primary.

carcinomas. When the patient has a known primary tumor, histologic comparison with the original cytologic or histologic material is essential to rule out the possibility of a second primary tumor. When samples are small or the tumor present is minute, immunohistochemistry can often be useful in helping to establish the diagnosis or suggest a primary site.

DIFFERENTIAL DIAGNOSIS

As most metastatic lesions are carcinomas, cytokeratin is a good initial screen. Undifferentiated or mesenchymal tumors may be more challenging and require a more extensive workup and clinicopathologic correlation. Occasionally, the origin of the tumor will resist identification regardless of the size of the immunohistochemistry panel or clinical investigation.

PROGNOSIS AND THERAPY

Treatment of metastatic disease is incumbent on first identifying the primary site with determination of the extent of metastatic spread. Prognosis varies with the type of tumor and the number of metastatic sites; however, presentation of a metastatic tumor in the jaws is often a late event and is likely the harbinger of incurable disease.

SUGGESTED READINGS

The complete suggested readings list is available online at www.expertconsult.com.

16

Non-Neoplastic Lesions of the Ear and Temporal Bone

■ **Carol F. Adair**

■ FIRST BRANCHIAL CLEFT ANOMALIES

First branchial cleft anomalies include fistulas, sinuses, and cysts and result from incomplete fusion of the first and second branchial arches, with persistence of the ventral component of the first branchial cleft. The most commonly used classification for first branchial cleft anomalies is the Work and Proctor two-type system. Type I lesions are ectodermal in origin with close proximity to the external auditory canal. Type II lesions contain ectodermal components of the first branchial cleft and mesodermal components of the first and second branchial arches and are more medially and inferiorly located.

CLINICAL FEATURES

Work type I branchial cleft anomalies usually manifest as periauricular cysts, rather than sinuses or fistulas. They are usually located posterior, inferior, and medial to the conchal cartilage and pinna; if a sinus tract is present, it parallels the external auditory canal. Although most are discovered in childhood, some are not diagnosed until adulthood, when they are often misdiagnosed as epidermal inclusion cysts or as abscesses, in cases of secondary infection. Females are affected twice as often as males. Incision and drainage by itself results in persistence or recurrence over years.

Work type II branchial cleft anomalies usually come to medical attention in the first year of life as a result of a draining sinus tract with otorrhea or periauricular drainage; the lesions are frequently infected at the time of diagnosis. They may present as a cystic lesion with a sinus or a fistulous tract between the neck and the ear canal (Figure 16-1). A sinus may open from a fistulous tract usually anterior to the sternocleidomastoid muscle and superior to the hyoid bone, or in the external

auditory canal. The spatial relationship to the facial nerve is variable, requiring a cautious surgical approach (Figure 16-1).

A careful physical examination with particular attention to the periauricular region and lateral neck is essential, including otologic examination to exclude a tract that communicates with the external auditory canal or, rarely, the middle ear space. High-resolution computed tomography (CT) is the preferred radiologic study for accurate delineation of the extent and course of the anomaly prior to surgery.

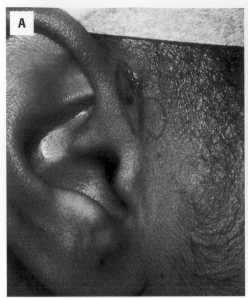
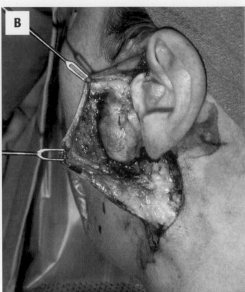

FIGURE 16-1

A, A preauricular fistula is present in a patient with a first branchial cleft anomaly. The lesion was secondarily infected and produced purulent drainage. **B**, Resection photograph of a first branchial cleft cyst. Note the close relationship to the ear.

PATHOLOGIC FEATURES

FIRST BRANCHIAL CLEFT ANOMALIES—PATHOLOGIC FEATURES

Gross Findings

- Cyst with viscous cloudy fluid
- Sinus tracts/fistulas extending from neck skin or from external auditory canal
- Abscess with purulent contents if secondarily infected

Microscopic Findings

- Cyst, sinus, or fistula lined by stratified squamous or ciliated respiratory epithelium
- Lymphoid aggregates may be present in cyst wall
- Granulation tissue or purulent material if infected, with denuded epithelium
- Work type I: epithelial component (ectodermal)
- Work type II: epithelial lining and cutaneous adnexal structures and/or cartilage (ectodermal and mesodermal)

Pathologic Differential Diagnosis

- Epidermal inclusion cyst, cholesteatoma, cystic squamous cell carcinoma, abscess, and 2nd branchial cleft anomalies

GROSS FINDINGS

Discrete cysts, sinuses, or fistulas, or a combination of structures may be seen, with the cysts frequently containing viscous cloudy fluid or, if infected, purulent material and necrotic debris. Cartilaginous components may be noticed on sectioning.

MICROSCOPIC FINDINGS

The cysts, sinuses, and fistulas may be lined by either stratified squamous epithelium or ciliated respiratory

epithelium (Figure 16-2). The cyst wall may contain lymphoid aggregates, sometimes with germinal centers (Figures 16-3 and 16-4), as commonly seen in second branchial cleft anomalies. If the lesion is infected, the epithelium may be largely denuded, replaced by heavily inflamed granulation tissue. Type II anomalies are distinguished by the presence of cutaneous adnexal structures and cartilage (Figure 16-5), the result of a mesodermal component in their development.

DIFFERENTIAL DIAGNOSIS

The pathologic differential diagnosis includes epidermal inclusion cyst, cholesteatoma, and, in adults, cystic metastatic squamous cell carcinoma. *Epidermal inclusion cysts* and *cholesteatomas* contain intracystic keratinous debris. The benign cytologic features of branchial cleft anomalies contrast with the atypia and loss of polarity encountered in *cystic metastatic squamous cell carcinoma*.

PROGNOSIS AND THERAPY

First branchial cleft anomalies are benign congenital lesions, commonly given to secondary infection. Treatment consists of complete surgical excision of the malformation, including cysts, and any associated sinus or fistula. In some cases, superficial parotidectomy may be required for complete removal. Indeed, optimal therapy is complete surgical excision. Complications of surgery include recurrence, often with infection, injury of adjacent structures such as the facial nerve, and infection or stenosis of the external

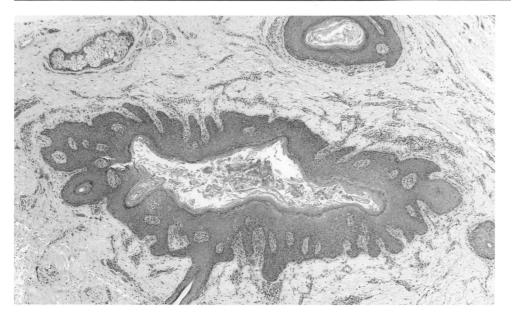

FIGURE 16-2

This series of sections (Figures 16-2 to 16-5) was taken along the course of a fistulous tract which represented a Work type II anomaly of the first branchial cleft. Near the skin surface, the tract is lined by keratinizing squamous epithelium with cutaneous adnexal structures.

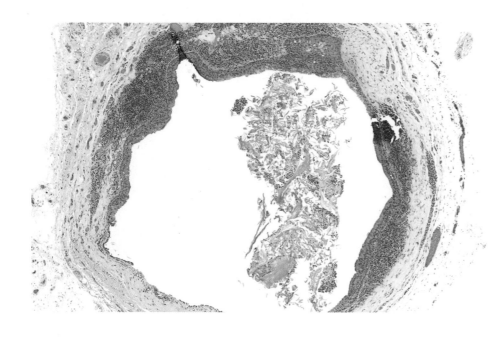

FIGURE 16-3

The lining of the deepest portion of the tract transitions to ciliated respiratory epithelium, surrounded by lymphoid tissue.

auditory canal or middle ear due to an ear canal defect.

Although there are reports in the literature of squamous cell carcinoma arising in branchial cleft cysts ("branchiogenic carcinoma"), the histologic documentation in the literature is not convincing. Most, if not all, of the cases represent cystic metastatic squamous cell carcinoma in cervical lymph nodes, with the primary usually arising in the area of Waldeyer ring (base of tongue and tonsillar region). These cystic metastases usually develop in the jugulodigastric region and usually not within the area of a first branchial cleft

anomaly. It is not uncommon for the primary tumor in the tonsil or base of tongue to be very small and inconspicuous, and in some cases, the primary site is never identified. The pathologist should not make a misleading diagnosis of "branchiogenic carcinoma" in the setting of a cystic neck lesion containing squamous cell carcinoma. Patients with cystic metastatic squamous cell carcinoma require regional radiation to include likely sites for occult primaries. Performing p16 immunohistochemistry can help confirm an oropharyngeal primary as >70% of tumors are pathogenetically related to human papillomavirus and, therefore, positive with p16.

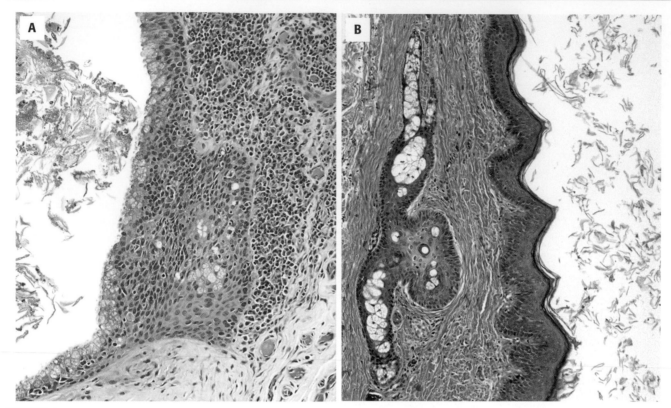

FIGURE 16-4

A, Ciliated respiratory epithelium with heavy lymphoid component. **B**, A different case showing squamous-lined epithelium with sebaceous adnexal structures in the wall.

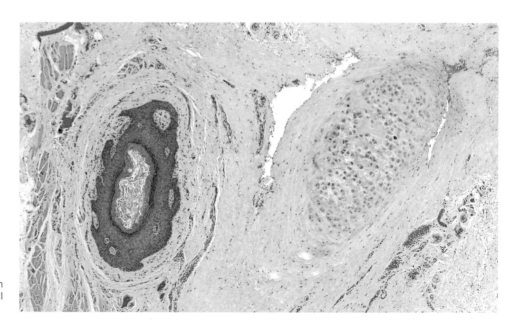

FIGURE 16-5

Cartilage appears adjacent to the tract in deeper sections of this Work type II anomaly.

■ CYSTIC CHONDROMALACIA

Idiopathic cystic chondromalacia, also known as pseudocyst of the auricle, is an uncommon degenerative cystic lesion of the auricular cartilaginous plate. There is no well-established etiology, but some possibilities include ischemic necrosis (rarely related to trauma),

abnormal release of lysosomal enzymes by chondrocytes, and an embryologic fusion defect.

CLINICAL FEATURES

Cystic chondromalacia tends to be more common in young males, although either gender and all ages may be

CYSTIC CHONDROMALACIA—DISEASE FACT SHEET

Definition

- A non-neoplastic degenerative change in the auricular cartilage resulting in a cleft-like pseudocyst within the cartilaginous plate

Incidence and Location

- Rare
- Usually involves helix or antihelix, with 80% in the scaphoid fossa

Gender, Race, and Age Distribution

- Male > female
- Higher incidence in Chinese population
- Any age, but commonly young to middle-aged adults

Clinical Features

- Usually unilateral, painless, fusiform swelling of helix or antihelix with normal overlying skin
- Often fluctuant; viscous clear fluid may be aspirated

Prognosis and Treatment

- Benign
- Usually treated for cosmetic reasons with aspiration followed by compression sutures; unroofing of anterior wall of pseudocyst followed by application of sclerosing agent

CYSTIC CHONDROMALACIA—PATHOLOGIC FEATURES

Gross Findings

- Cleft-like space centrally located within cartilaginous plate
- Cleft filled with viscous clear to olive oil–colored fluid
- Obliterated by fibrous tissue or granulation tissue in long-standing lesions

Microscopic Findings

- Central slit-like cleft in cartilage without an epithelial lining
- Cleft may contain fibrous tissue, granulation tissue with hemosiderin

Pathologic Differential Diagnosis

- Relapsing polychondritis, chondrodermatitis nodularis helicis

affected. An increased incidence has been noted in Chinese males, although cystic chondromalacia has been reported in patients of all racial backgrounds. The typical presentation is a unilateral, fusiform, slightly fluctuant, swelling of the helix or antihelix (Figure 16-6). The scaphoid fossa is the most common site. The lesion is painless and there are no changes in the overlying skin.

PATHOLOGIC FEATURES

GROSS FINDINGS

If the full thickness of the cartilaginous plate has been excised, a central, slit-like cleft can be seen in the cartilage (Figure 16-7). When incised, the cyst exudes viscous, clear to olive oil–colored fluid, usually <2 mL in volume. The cystic area, especially in long-standing lesions, may be lined by a thin, brown-tinged layer, representing old hemorrhage and granulation tissue, or may be completely replaced by fibrosis. Often the specimen is fragmented, especially if the cyst is "unroofed" (Figure 16-8), making prior knowledge of the clinical appearance helpful for diagnosis.

MICROSCOPIC FINDINGS

The cartilaginous plate contains a central cleft with no epithelial lining—hence, the term "pseudocyst."

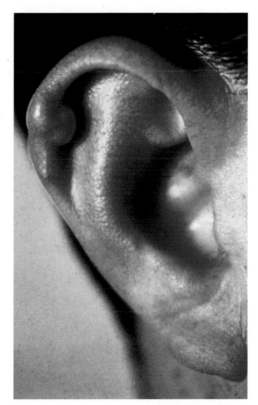

FIGURE 16-6

A young adult male has a fusiform fluctuant mass on the helix, which was histologically cystic chondromalacia. *(Used with permission from Hyams VJ. Pathology of the ear. Chicago: ASCP Press; 1976.)*

The contour of the cleft may be slightly irregular, and a thin inner rim of fibrous tissue or granulation tissue with plump fibroblasts may be seen (Figures 16-8 and 16-9). Hemosiderin deposits may be present. In long-standing cases, the fibrous tissue may obliterate the cystic space.

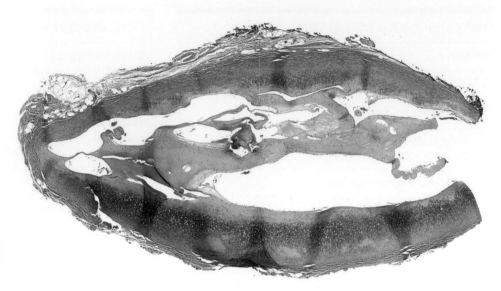

FIGURE 16-7

The cartilaginous plate contains an elongated cleft and has lost some of its normal basophilic staining in this idiopathic cystic chondromalacia.

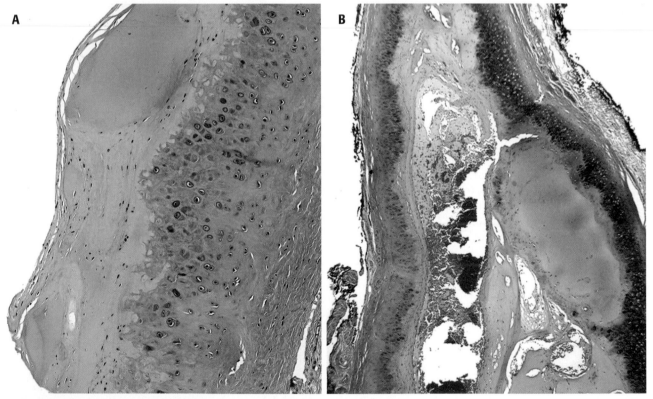

FIGURE 16-8

A, A "deroofed" lesion shows only the cartilage and some area of degeneration, but the plates are not present on both sides of the cyst. **B**, A blood-filled cyst is associated with granulation-type tissue. The cartilage plate is separated, with fluid in part of the spaces.

DIFFERENTIAL DIAGNOSIS

Cystic chondromalacia is easily distinguished from *relapsing polychondritis* by its lack of an inflammatory component, and from *chondrodermatitis nodularis helicis* by the normal skin overlying it. Both of these lesions are associated with pain.

PROGNOSIS AND THERAPY

Cosmetic concerns for this benign lesion often prompt therapeutic intervention. Treatment is usually directed at extirpation of the pseudocyst while preserving the underlying architecture of the cartilaginous plate. Incision and drainage with curettage has had variable

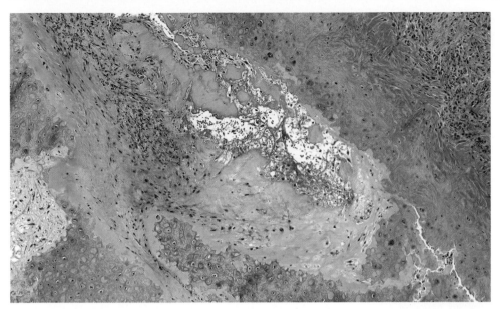

FIGURE 16-9
Granulation tissue forms the "cyst" lining, seen adjacent to the degenerating cartilaginous plate. A cystic space with debris is present.

success. Needle aspiration alone has limited value but is quite effective when combined with compression suture therapy utilizing "button" bolsters. Unroofing of the pseudocyst by removal of its anterior wall followed by application of a sclerosing agent, or by suture compression, has the lowest incidence of recurrence.

■ CHONDRODERMATITIS NODULAR HELICIS

Chondrodermatitis nodularis helicis (CDNH) is a non-neoplastic inflammatory and degenerative process of the external ear characterized by necrobiotic changes in the dermis that extend down to the perichondrium, with associated alterations in the cartilaginous plate. The dermal injury is thought to be caused by a combination of factors: local trauma, actinic damage, and the relatively tenuous vascularity of the auricle. The necrobiotic dermal collagen, and sometimes cartilaginous matrix, is extruded through a crater-like defect in the epidermis; thus, CDNH is considered to be one of the transepidermal elimination disorders. Distal narrowing of the arterioles in the perichondrium may play a role in the ischemic injury of the cartilage. Systemic diseases associated with microangiopathy may predispose individuals to CDNH; these include cardiovascular disease, diabetes mellitus, lupus erythematosus, rheumatoid arthritis, and autoimmune and connective tissue disorders.

CLINICAL FEATURES

CDNH presents as an exquisitely painful nodule, usually on the helix or antihelix; however, it may develop

CHONDRODERMATITIS NODULAR HELICIS—DISEASE FACT SHEET

Definition
- Inflammatory transepidermal elimination disorder characterized by necrobiosis of dermal collagen and degenerative changes in the cartilaginous plate

Incidence and Location
- Relatively common
- Helix most often, followed by antihelix (more common in females)

Gender, Race, and Age Distribution
- Male > female
- Usually 6th decade

Clinical Features
- Unilateral, painful, circumscribed indurated nodule with central crater filled with brown debris

Prognosis and Treatment
- Benign disorder, often removed to alleviate pain
- Intralesional steroid injection successful in 50% of cases
- Persistent or recurrent lesions adequately treated by conservative excision or deep shave biopsy

on any portion of the auricle. Lesions of the helix are twice as common as those of the antihelix. CDNH begins as a reddish, round, indurated nodule, measuring several millimeters in diameter; over a period of days to a few weeks, the nodule develops a central crater, which contains crust-like material (Figure 16-10). CDNH is more common in males; lesions of the antihelix, however, are more common in females. Most patients are in the 6th decade.

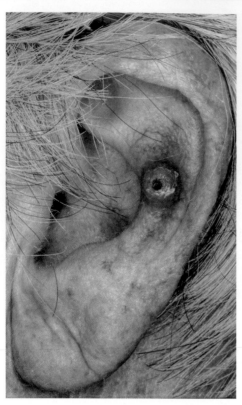

FIGURE 16-10

This firm nodule with a central crater is seen on the antihelix of an elderly woman with chondrodermatitis nodularis helicis; antihelical lesions are more common in women. *(Courtesy of Dr. S. A. Norton.)*

GROSS FINDINGS

CDNH is usually removed by shave biopsy. The nodule is firm, round, circumscribed, and nodular, with a central crater containing yellow to brown necrotic material. Most examples measure between 5 and 15 mm in diameter. Sectioning may demonstrate cartilage at the deep aspect of the biopsy, but the sharp interface between the cartilaginous plate and dermis is obscured.

MICROSCOPIC FINDINGS

There is a central crater filled with acellular necrotic debris, fibrin, and a variable number of inflammatory cells. The epidermis surrounding the crater is acanthotic with hyperkeratosis (Figure 16-11). The dermal collagen underlying the crater is homogeneous and eosinophilic, admixed with fibrin (Figure 16-12), with edema in the surrounding viable dermis. The degenerative changes extend to the level of the perichondrium and are associated with loss of the normal basophilia of the underlying cartilage, focal fibrosis with increased cellularity, and dropout of chondrocytes. The necrobiotic material and fibrin spew from the crater through a disrupted epidermis. In some cases, portions of the cartilage are also extruded through the crater. Nerve twigs are frequently "captured" by this destructive inflammatory process, perhaps accounting for the exquisite pain clinically.

PATHOLOGIC FEATURES

CHONDRODERMATITIS NODULAR HELICIS—PATHOLOGIC FEATURES

Gross Findings

- Rounded, circumscribed nodule with central crater filled with necrotic debris
- 5 to 15 mm diameter
- Cartilage may be seen at deep aspect of biopsy

Microscopic Findings

- Squamous epithelial hyperplasia surrounding central crater
- Crater filled with acellular necrotic debris, fibrin, and inflammatory cells
- Homogeneous, eosinophilic dermal collagen may extrude through the crater
- Underlying cartilage loses normal basophilia
- Interface between cartilaginous plate and dermis is blurred

Pathologic Differential Diagnosis

- Squamous cell carcinoma, actinic keratosis

DIFFERENTIAL DIAGNOSIS

CDNH is very commonly confused clinically with *squamous cell carcinoma*, occasionally leading to overtreatment. The histologic findings may be mistaken for squamous cell carcinoma or actinic keratosis because of the prominent squamous epithelial hyperplasia and underlying solar elastosis typically encountered in CDNH.

PROGNOSIS AND THERAPY

Chondrodermatitis nodularis helicis is a benign disorder, which may be treated with intralesional steroid injection, with an up to 50% cure rate. Persistent or recurrent lesions are amenable to conservative excisional biopsy or deep shave excision with excellent results. Removal of the lesion often alleviates the associated pain.

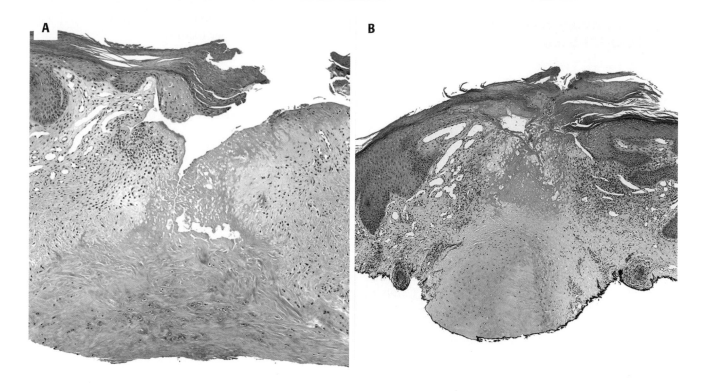

FIGURE 16-11

A and **B**, Eosinophilic degenerative dermal collagen appears ready to extrude from a central crater in chondrodermatitis nodularis helicis. The underlying interface between the cartilaginous plate and the dermis is blurred; the cartilage has lost its normal basophilia.

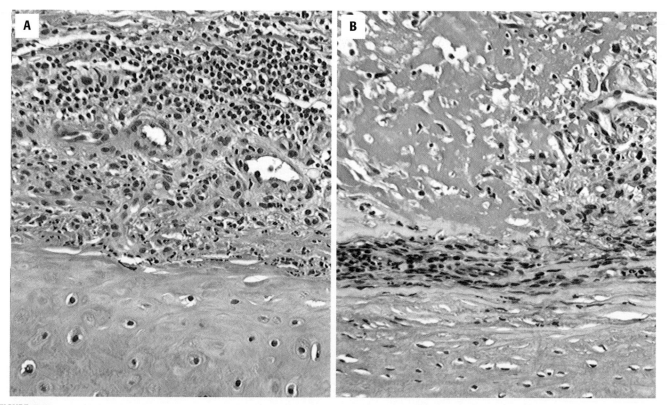

FIGURE 16-12

Deep biopsy samples of chondrodermatitis nodularis helicis may show extensive inflammation (**A**) or degenerated collagen and fibrinoid necrosis (**B**), both immediately adjacent to the cartilage.

■ ANGIOLYMPHOID HYPERPLASIA WITH EOSINOPHILIA

Angiolymphoid hyperplasia with eosinophilia (ALHE) is an uncommon benign subcutaneous vascular proliferation associated with a peculiar inflammatory infiltrate. There are some histologic similarities to Kimura disease, but the clinical features are different.

CLINICAL FEATURES

The lesions most often occur in the auricle, in and around the external auditory canal, but may also be seen on the scalp and face. The lesions are somewhat more common in females and are typically found in middle age. Some cases have been associated with pregnancy. They are characterized by intensely pruritic red-tan papules, which may bleed secondary to scratching. A minority of cases are associated with peripheral blood eosinophilia. Lymphadenopathy is rarely present.

PATHOLOGIC FEATURES

GROSS FINDINGS

ALHE generally presents with clusters of red-tan, firm papules or subcutaneous nodular lesions, usually a few millimeters in diameter. With time the papules may transform into a larger plaque.

MICROSCOPIC FINDINGS

The lesion of ALHE is a circumscribed nodular proliferation of variably sized blood vessels, capillaries to small arteries and veins, with a distinctive "epithelioid" endothelial lining (Figure 16-13). The endothelial cells are enlarged, with abundant eosinophilic cytoplasm, and large, somewhat pleomorphic nuclei. The prominent endothelial cells protrude into the vessel lumens, with a "bumpy" hobnail-like appearance. The vessels may be arranged in a lobular pattern or may be irregularly distributed within the lesion (Figure 16-13). They may be ectatic or they may have thickened walls (Figure 16-14). The background inflammatory infiltrate is often so dense that the lesion may resemble a lymph node at first glance. Closer inspection, however, fails to find the nodal architectural elements, such as sinusoids and a subcapsular sinus. The inflammatory cells include lymphocytes and histiocytes, with a variable component of eosinophils. The eosinophils are usually prominent, suggesting the diagnosis, but occasionally they are inconspicuous.

DIFFERENTIAL DIAGNOSIS

The chief differential diagnostic consideration is *Kimura disease*, which, unlike ALHE, is more commonly seen in Asian males. It is frequently associated with lymphadenopathy and with peripheral blood eosinophilia. The lesions of Kimura disease are usually larger and deeper in the subcutis or underlying

---

ANGIOLYMPHOID HYPERPLASIA WITH EOSINOPHILIA— DISEASE FACT SHEET

Definition
- An idiopathic non-neoplastic vascular proliferation with chronic inflammatory cell infiltrate, characterized by epithelioid endothelial cells

Incidence and Location
- Rare
- Usually involves the auricle or periauricular area, and sometimes the scalp or face

Gender, Race, and Age Distribution
- Slight female predominance
- No racial predominance
- Any age, but commonly middle-aged adults

Clinical Features
- Usually unilateral, multiple red-tan papules on or around the auricle; papules may coalesce into plaque
- Typically present with intense pruritis; some associated with pregnancy

Prognosis and Treatment
- Benign
- Usually treated because of pruritis, with local excision or cryotherapy

---

ANGIOLYMPHOID HYPERPLASIA WITH EOSINOPHILIA— PATHOLOGIC FEATURES

Gross Findings
- Red-tan, firm papules in clusters, to plaques
- 5 to 15 mm

Microscopic Findings
- Vascular proliferation, usually somewhat lobular
- Enlarged "epithelioid" endothelial cells with abundant eosinophilic cytoplasm and enlarged nuclei
- Hobnail pattern of endothelium protruding into vessel lumen
- Mixed lymphoid infiltrate with variable eosinophils
- Lacks lymph node architecture

Pathologic Differential Diagnosis
- Kimura disease, hemangioma

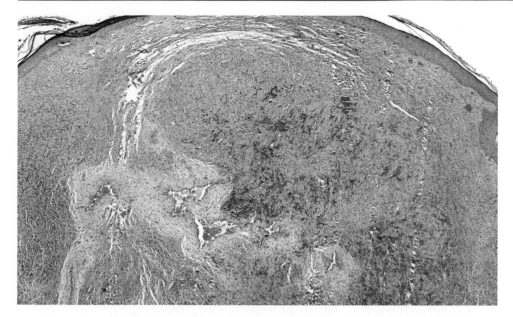

FIGURE 16-13

The low-power appearance of angiolymphoid hyperplasia with eosinophilia demonstrates a mixed lymphoid infiltrate associated with a vascular proliferation. There is an intact squamous epithelium.

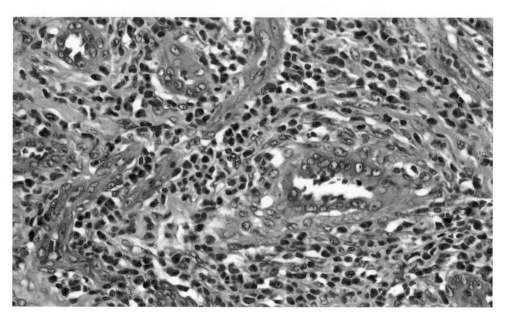

FIGURE 16-14

The vascular proliferation in angiolymphoid hyperplasia with eosinophilia is characterized by enlarged, "epithelioid" endothelial cells with abundant eosinophilic cytoplasm and large nuclei with prominent nucleoli. Note the numerous eosinophils.

soft tissue. Folliculolysis with eosinophilic abscesses and a prominent IgE immunohistochemistry is seen. The treatment for Kimura disease is similar to that for ALHE, though a more extensive excision may be required for adequate removal. *Lobular capillary hemangioma* is distinguished from ALHE by its characteristic lobular growth pattern. In addition, it lacks the heavy inflammatory infiltrate and prominent epithelioid endothelial cells of ALHE. *Angiosarcoma*, unlike ALHE, is defined by an infiltrative pattern, anastomosing and poorly formed vascular spaces, and more striking nuclear atypia with mitotic activity. A heavy inflammatory cell infiltrate is not commonly seen in angiosarcoma. Kaposi sarcoma is easily distinguished from ALHE by its spindle cell pattern and poorly

formed, slit-like vascular spaces, eosinophilic globules, and strong human herpesvirus 8 immunohistochemistry. Rarely, *metastatic thyroid papillary carcinoma* may yield a similar histologic appearance. Thyroglobulin and TTF-1 stains would help to make the separation.

PROGNOSIS AND THERAPY

ALHE is adequately treated by local excision in most cases, though spontaneous resolution has been documented. Cryotherapy has been used with some success. Occasionally, the lesions recur after treatment.

■ RELAPSING POLYCHONDRITIS

Relapsing polychondritis is a rare autoimmune inflammatory disorder with antibodies that target type II collagen. The disease is usually seen in cartilage of the ear, nose, joints, and tracheobronchial tree, often resulting in structural damage and deformity. Humoral and cell-mediated immunity seem to play a role in the destructive inflammatory process. A genetic association between relapsing polychondritis and different HLA types, particularly *HLA-DR4,* has been described. There is an increased incidence (up to 35%) of other autoimmune disorders, such as rheumatoid arthritis, Hashimoto thyroiditis, systemic lupus erythematosus, Sjögren syndrome, systemic vasculitides, inflammatory bowel disease, diabetes mellitus, and primary biliary cirrhosis. It is also associated with myelodysplastic syndromes and leukemia. Relapsing polychondritis has also been reported in HIV-infected patients without associated autoimmune connective tissue disorders.

CLINICAL FEATURES

Relapsing polychondritis has an estimated incidence of 3.5 cases per 1 million population per year in the United States. Occurring over a wide age range, the disease is most often seen in the 5th to 6th decades (mean, 47 years). Females appear to be affected more commonly than males (up to 3:1 ratio), although some studies find no gender difference.

Nearly 40% of patients are initially affected in the ear (auricle specifically), although eventually ~ 85% will have ear involvement. The ears become red to purple, swollen, and painful, except for the noncartilaginous lobule, which is spared. Inflammatory episodes may last a few days or several weeks. After repeated attacks or a prolonged episode, the cartilaginous framework is damaged, becoming "flabby" and resulting in a "cauliflower ear" deformity (Figure 16-15). When the external auditory canal and eustachian tube are involved, they may become narrowed, leading to decreased auditory acuity (conductive type) and otitis media. Other anatomic sites may also affected, with nasal chondritis (25% to 50%), producing a saddle nose deformity, and laryngotracheal disease (50%), causing obstruction, collapse, and a predisposition to pulmonary infections. Relapsing polychondritis arthropathy is the second most common clinical symptom. The typical nonerosive arthritis most often affects the knees and the small joints of the hands. Cardiovascular disease (up to 50%) presents with vasculitis and valvular dysfunction.

Biopsy is unnecessary as the diagnosis can be made clinically based on the presence of chondritis (1) in two of three sites (auricle, nose, laryngotracheal tree) or

RELAPSING POLYCHONDRITIS—DISEASE FACT SHEET

Definition
- Rare, autoimmune inflammatory disorder with antibodies to type II collagen, which lead to destruction of cartilaginous or proteoglycan-rich tissues of the auricle, nose, tracheobronchial tree, eye, heart, and blood vessels

Incidence and Location
- 3.5/1 million population per year in United States
- Auricle most common site, affected in up to 85%

Morbidity and Mortality
- Leading cause of death is airway compromise due to tracheobronchial damage
- 10-year survival of 55% to 94%
- Associated with myelodysplasia or leukemia

Gender, Race, and Age Distribution
- Female > male (up to 3:1 ratio)
- Perhaps higher incidence in whites
- 5th to 6th decades

Clinical Features
- In acute phase, the ears become red, edematous, and tender, although noncartilaginous lobule is spared
- After repeated bouts, floppy ear and/or saddle nose deformities develop
- Other symptoms relate to other anatomic sites, including laryngotracheal disease, nonerosive arthritis, ophthalmologic disease, and cardiovascular disease
- Associated autoimmune disorder in 25% to 35%; some in HIV infection
- Myelodysplastic syndrome or leukemia may be associated

Prognosis and Treatment
- Depends on severity of disease and number of anatomic sites affected, with airway compromise, secondary infections, and cardiovascular disease the most common causes of death
- Corticosteroids, nonsteroidal anti-inflammatory drugs, and immunomodulators have varying success
- Advanced age, anemia, and tracheobronchial stricture are poor prognostic factors

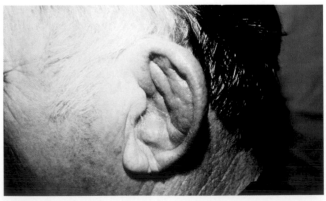

FIGURE 16-15

After multiple acute episodes of auricular chondritis, this patient's auricle is deformed and floppy as a result of destruction of the cartilaginous plate in this relapsing polychondritis. *(Courtesy of Dr. V. J. Hyams.)*

(2) in one of those sites along with two other features (ocular inflammation, audiovestibular damage, or sero-negative arthritis).

PATHOLOGIC FEATURES

GROSS FINDINGS

After long-standing or repeated episodes of active inflammation, the auricular cartilage becomes physically "floppy," owing to loss of structural integrity of the pinna.

MICROSCOPIC FINDINGS

The initial histologic finding in relapsing polychondritis is loss of the normal basophilia of the cartilage.

RELAPSING POLYCHONDRITIS—PATHOLOGIC FEATURES

Gross Findings
- Acute phase: erythematous, edematous pinna, with sparing of lobule
- After multiple episodes: floppy, deformed pinna with loss of cartilaginous structure

Microscopic Findings
- Loss of basophilia in cartilaginous plate (earliest change)
- Perichondrium infiltrated by mixed inflammation
- Damaged cartilage has moth-eaten appearance and areas are replaced by granulation tissue

Pathologic Differential Diagnosis
- Malignant external otitis, Wegener granulomatosis, and extranodal NK/T-cell lymphoma, sinonasal type

---

The perichondrium is infiltrated by neutrophils, lymphocytes, plasma cells, and eosinophils, blurring the usually sharp interface between the cartilaginous plate and the surrounding soft tissue (Figures 16-16 and 16-17). The damaged cartilage is gradually replaced by granulation tissue and fibrous tissue, with any residual cartilage demonstrating an irregular moth-eaten border (Figure 16-17). Immunofluorescence studies may show deposition of immunoglobulins and C3 at the periphery of the cartilage and within the walls of perichondral vessels.

DIFFERENTIAL DIAGNOSIS

The differential diagnosis includes *necrotizing (malignant) external otitis* (an infection due to *Pseudomonas aeruginosa*), *Wegener granulomatosis,* and *extranodal NK/T-cell lymphoma, sinonasal type* in upper aerodigestive tract locations. The ears are not usually affected by these latter disorders.

PROGNOSIS AND THERAPY

Due to the rarity of the disorder, optimal therapy is yet to be defined. Various medical therapies, including corticosteroids, nonsteroidal anti-inflammatory drugs, immunomodulators (e.g., methotrexate, azathioprine, and cyclosporine A), and tumor necrosis factor alpha antagonists (infliximab, etanercept), have all had some degree of success depending on the severity of disease. Autologous stem cell transplantation has induced complete remission of disease in some patients for whom other treatments have failed. Ear treatments are usually

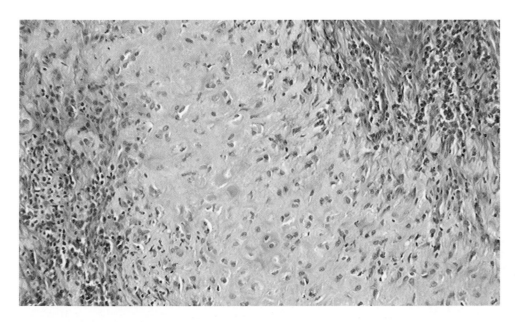

FIGURE 16-16

The interface between the cartilage and perichondrium is blurred by a mixed inflammatory infiltrate in relapsing polychondritis.

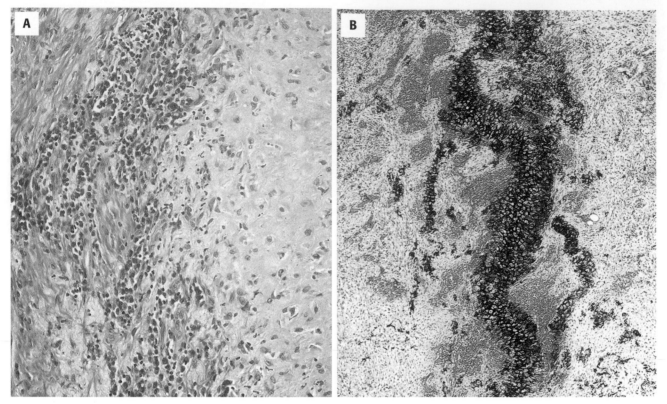

FIGURE 16-17

A, The inflammatory cells are predominantly small lymphocytes and plasma cells. The normal basophilia of the cartilage has been lost. **B**, A Movat stain highlights the extensive damage to the cartilaginous plate, which appears black. The moth-eaten appearance is typical of relapsing polychondritis.

not critical, but surgery may be needed for patients with severe airway compromise, as well as aortic grafting and valve replacement for cardiovascular disease. The leading causes of death in patients with relapsing polychondritis are airway compromise, secondary infections, and cardiovascular disease. Factors that have a negative impact on survival include advanced age at diagnosis, anemia, and tracheobronchial stricture. The 10-year survival rate varies from 55% to 94%, depending on the study.

■ LANGERHANS CELL HISTIOCYTOSIS

Langerhans cell histiocytosis (LCH) is a clonal proliferation of Langerhans cells, a dendritic antigen-presenting cell type found most commonly in the epithelium of the skin and various mucosal sites. The Langerhans cells participate in specific immune reactions by capturing foreign antigens and presenting them to the T-lymphocytes. LCH includes isolated lesions of Langerhans cell origin as well as multifocal and systemic disease. It was previously known as histiocytosis X, a general term that included eosinophilic granuloma, Hand-Schüller-Christian disease, and Letterer-Siwe disease. "Eosinophilic granuloma" referred to the

disease in general, or to an individual lesion, usually of bone. Hand-Schüller-Christian disease referred to multifocal lytic bone lesions (usually of the skull) with exophthalmos and diabetes insipidus due to pituitary involvement. Letterer-Siwe disease is a severe systemic form of the disease seen in young children, with skin, mucosal, and solid organ involvement.

CLINICAL FINDINGS

LCH is more common in males, with a peak incidence in the 2nd and 3rd decades. The majority of lesions arise in bone, particularly in the skull. Lesions of the middle ear and temporal bone may present with otorrhea, expansion of the temporal bone with a mass effect, pain, hearing loss, vertigo, otitis media, or skin ulceration.

RADIOLOGIC FEATURES

LCH may demonstrate single or multiple lesions in radiographic studies. They are seen readily on plain films, CT, or magnetic resonance imaging (MRI), as sharply circumscribed lytic lesions. Lesions of the skull characteristically

LANGERHANS CELL HISTIOCYTOSIS—DISEASE FACT SHEET

Definition

- Clonal proliferation of unique histiocyte, Langerhans cell; may be localized or systemic

Incidence and Location

- Prevalence in children: 1/200,000 population annually

Morbidity and Mortality

- Isolated bone lesions readily treated by curettage; multiple bone lesions may be difficult to control locally.
- Systemic disease with solid organ and skin involvement has poor prognosis

Gender, Race, and Age Distribution

- No gender predilection
- Most <20 years of age

Clinical Features

- Lytic lesions of skull and jaws
- Otitis media and/or destructive temporal bone involvement if localized

Prognosis and Treatment

- Dependent on extent of local involvement or systemic disease
- Localized bone lesions usually cured by surgical curettage
- Systemic disease has poor prognosis even with chemotherapy

LANGERHANS CELL HISTIOCYTOSIS—PATHOLOGIC FEATURES

Gross Findings

- Yellowish softened bone fragments in curettings

Microscopic Findings

- Prominent Langerhans cells, mononuclear, with enlarged nuclei with irregular, grooved, and convoluted contours; cytoplasm pale to eosinophilic
- Multinucleated cells with irregular nuclei
- Eosinophils increased, often prominent (eosinophilic abscesses)

Ultrastructural Features

- Langerhans cells have irregular, cerebriform nuclear contours
- Cell membranes have Birbeck granules: invaginated pentalaminar structures with fusiform distal expansion, giving "tennis racquet" appearance

Pathologic Differential Diagnosis

- Rosai-Dorfman disease, Hodgkin lymphoma, simple reactive histiocytosis

have a "beveled" margin. If multiple lesions are present, the appearance may vary; some may have a poorly defined sclerotic border, which may reflect regression of the LCH and replacement by reactive bone.

PATHOLOGIC FEATURES

GROSS FINDINGS

Since the specimens are generally either biopsy or curette samples, the gross appearance is not distinctive. The fragments may be hemorrhagic and red-brown or firm and yellow, depending on the age of the lesion.

MICROSCOPIC FINDINGS

The characteristic feature of LCH is the Langerhans cell, with its irregular, convoluted nucleus. The nuclei are somewhat bean-shaped, with grooves and indentations that give them a cerebriform appearance (Figures 16-18 and 16-19). The chromatin pattern is fine and dispersed, with slight condensation along the nuclear membrane. Nucleoli are not prominent. Mitotic activity is variable but rarely exceeds 5 per high-power field. The cytoplasm is scant to moderate in volume and may be pale or eosinophilic, and may contain hemosiderin or lipid droplets.

In addition to the Langerhans cells, the lesions contain an admixture of usual histiocytes, eosinophils, plasma cells, and neutrophils. The number of eosinophils is variable; they may be scattered individually though the lesion or may form large sheets with central necrotic patches (Figure 16-19). Charcot-Leyden crystals are sometimes seen if eosinophils are numerous. Bone, if present, is usually seen as a reactive rim at the margin of the lesion. Regressing lesions are more fibrotic, and may be more difficult to identify as LCH due to the paucity of the diagnostic cells.

ANCILLARY STUDIES

ULTRASTRUCTURAL FEATURES

Electron microscopy is rarely used in the diagnosis of LCH, since the combination of histologic features and immunohistochemistry for S100 protein and CD1a is considered confirmatory. Prior to readily accessible immunohistochemical studies, demonstration of the Birbeck granule, an elongated pentalaminar structure with a "zipper-like" pattern of cross-striations, emanating from the cell membrane, was key to the diagnosis. Some Birbeck granules have bulbous expansions, which lend them a "tennis racquet" appearance.

IMMUNOHISTOCHEMISTRY

The Langerhans cells are identified by their positive immunoreactivity for S100 protein, CD1a (Figure 16-20), and CD207 (Langerin). Reactivity for CD1a, a

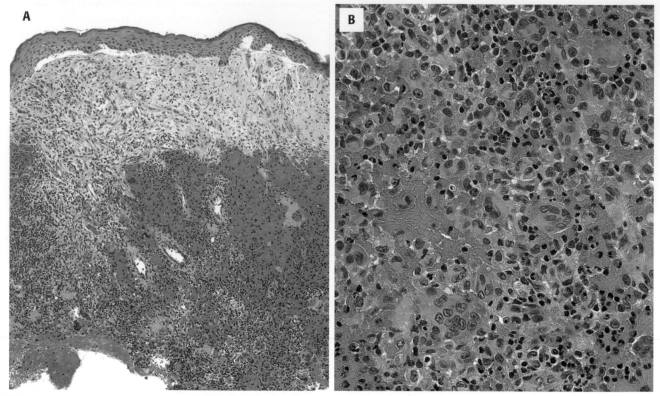

FIGURE 16-18

A, The surface epithelium is intact, overlying a rich inflammatory infiltrate with blood. Close inspection is required to correctly identify the lesional cells. **B**, The characteristic Langerhans cell with a number of giant cells and eosinophils is shown in the background.

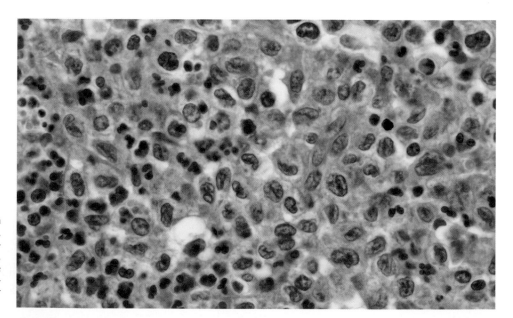

FIGURE 16-19

The Langerhans cells are admixed with a variable infiltrate of lymphocytes, plasma cells, and eosinophils. The nuclei are convoluted, folded or grooved, yielding a coffee-bean shape. In some cases, such as this one, the eosinophils are conspicuous, but in other cases their presence is subtle.

relatively specific finding, is helpful in excluding the many other entities that are S100 protein positive, such as melanocytic lesions, Rosai-Dorfman disease, and xanthogranulomas. CD68 is also positive in the lesional cells (Figure 16-21). Langerin, a transmembrane protein that mediates the formation of Birbeck granules, is also sensitive and relatively specific for LCH.

DIFFERENTIAL DIAGNOSIS

Differential diagnostic considerations based on clinical presentation include *infectious granulomatous processes, osteomyelitis, Rosai-Dorfman disease,* and *Hodgkin lymphoma.* However, the suggestive radiographic appearance

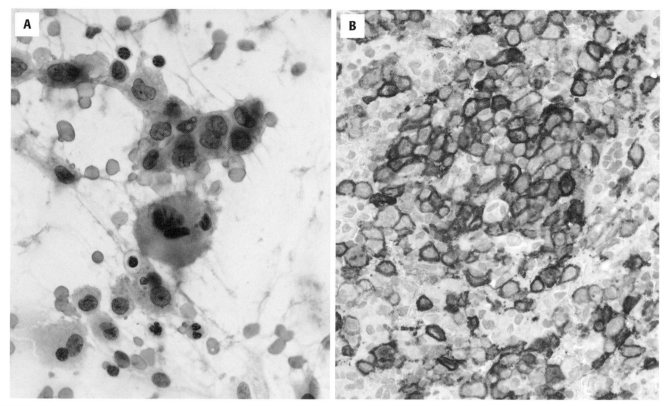

FIGURE 16-20

A, Fine needle aspirate (hematoxylin and eosin smear) demonstrates the distinctive nucleus of the Langerhans histiocyte, with a very irregular, grooved contour, lending it a cerebriform appearance. **B**, The lesional cells show a strong and diffuse cytoplasmic reaction with CD1a.

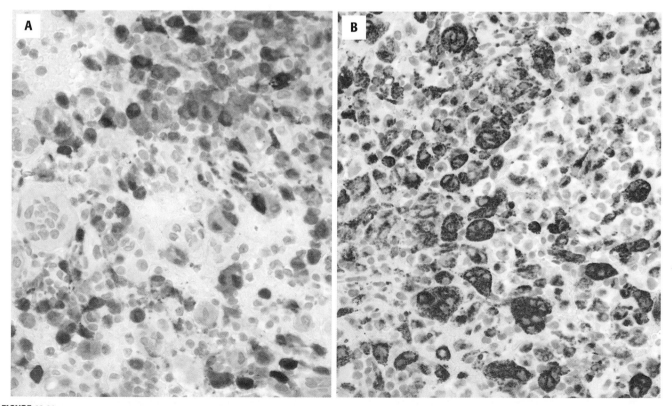

FIGURE 16-21

A, Strong and diffuse, nuclear and cytoplasmic S100 protein reaction in the Langerhans cells, while the giant cells are negative. **B**, Strong and diffuse CD68 reaction in the cytoplasm of the lesional cells and in the giant cells.

of punched-out lytic lesions of the craniofacial skeleton and identification of the Langerhans cell component by immunohistochemistry readily exclude these other lesions.

PROGNOSIS AND THERAPY

As noted earlier, some lesions spontaneously regress or "heal." Most isolated lesions of the skull are amenable to curettage or intralesional steroid injection. Low-dose radiation therapy is also useful, particularly in lesions not readily accessible surgically. Such lesions have a very good prognosis. Extensive disease in younger patients portends a less favorable prognosis, particularly in the setting of visceral involvement.

■ CHOLESTEATOMA

Cholesteatoma is a misnomer as it contains no "cholesterol" and it is not a "neoplasm." A neoplasm is simulated clinically by the propensity to destroy surrounding tissues (including bone) and to recur after excision. Collagenase production by the squamous epithelium ("matrix") is thought to result in the bone destruction. The cystic lesion, filled with keratinous debris and lined by keratinizing squamous epithelium, is found within the middle ear or mastoid region. The presence of squamous epithelium in the middle ear, which is normally lined by cuboidal or columnar glandular epithelium, is abnormal, no matter by which mechanism it arrives there. Acquired and congenital forms of cholesteatoma are recognized.

CLINICAL FEATURES

Cholesteatomas are not uncommon and usually unilateral. Older children and young adults (3rd to 4th decades) will present with a foul-smelling aural discharge and conductive hearing loss. The tympanic membrane is perforated (usually at the superior margin) in the acquired form while intact in the congenital form. Both are usually associated with a long history of severe chronic otitis media, giving an otoscopic appearance of a white-gray to yellow irregular mass associated with chronic otitis media (Figure 16-22). Facial nerve dysfunction, vomiting, severe vertigo, and very severe headaches may indicate advanced destructive disease or a suppurative infection, either one requiring immediate intervention.

CHOLESTEATOMA—DISEASE FACT SHEET

Definition

- Destructive squamous epithelial cyst of middle ear or mastoid region, usually secondary to chronic otitis media but occasionally congenital

Incidence and Location

- Common worldwide
- Origin in superior posterior middle ear and/or petrous apex but may demonstrate locally aggressive growth into adjacent structures

Morbidity and Mortality

- Chronic middle ear disease and progressive conductive hearing loss
- Intracranial extension may lead to lethal complications such as meningitis, epidural abscess, brain parenchymal abscess, or lateral sinus thrombosis

Gender, Race, and Age Distribution

- Equal gender distribution
- Any age, including congenital examples; highest incidence in 3rd to 4th decades

Clinical Features

- Long history of severe, chronic otitis media
- Progressive conductive hearing loss, otalgia, otorrhea (in part due to underlying chronic ear disease); tinnitus and vertigo less common
- Facial nerve palsy, vomiting, severe vertigo, severe headache suggests advanced destructive disease or suppurative infection
- Otoscopic appearance: white-gray to yellow irregular mass associated with chronic otitis media or perforated tympanic membrane

Radiologic Features

- Bone destruction with medial displacement of the ossicles
- No gadolinium enhancement by CT
- MRI: T1-weighted signal, low intensity; T2-weighted signal, high intensity

Prognosis and Treatment

- Surgical extirpation of the squamous epithelial lining essential
- Recurrence if incompletely excised (20%)
- Increased incidence of recurrence includes: <20 years of age, marked ossicular erosion, polypoid mucosal inflammatory disease, extensive disease
- Serious complications include labyrinthine fistula, sigmoid sinus or facial nerve canal erosion, cranial nerve dysfunction, meningitis, epidural or brain parenchymal abscess

RADIOLOGIC FEATURES

CT and MRI show a soft tissue mass displacing the ossicles medially, with a variable degree of bone destruction (Figure 16-23). Associated changes of chronic middle ear infection are common. There is usually prolongation of the signal in both T1 and T2 MRI signals, with T1-weighted signal intensity being low, while T2-weighted signal intensity is high. There may be peripheral enhancement, if degenerated.

PATHOLOGIC FEATURES

GROSS FINDINGS

Rarely is a cholesteatoma received intact for pathologic examination. The specimen usually consists of multiple fragments of flaky, white keratinous debris, accompanied by soft tissue fragments. A foul aroma and associated chronic otitis media with bone destruction may be noted at surgery, with bone fragments submitted to pathology.

MICROSCOPIC FINDINGS

Three components are essential for the diagnosis of cholesteatoma: (1) keratinous material, (2) stratified squamous epithelium with a prominent granular layer, and (3) inflamed granulation or fibrous tissue (Figures 16-24 and 16-25). The squamous epithelium is usually bland and atrophic, lacking rete pegs and without reactive changes expected in an inflammatory process. A giant cell granulomatous reaction to the keratinous material may be seen. The thin epithelium lines a sac filled with exfoliated anucleate squames. Occasionally, other disorders accompany the cholesteatoma, including cholesterol granuloma, aural polyps, tympanosclerosis, acquired encephalocele (herniation of normal brain tissue through a bony defect), and tumors (such as neuroendocrine adenoma of the middle ear).

CHOLESTEATOMA—PATHOLOGIC FEATURES

Gross Findings
- Specimen fragmented but may contain flecks of white to yellow keratinous (grumous) material
- All tissue should be processed

Microscopic Findings
- Cystic, sac-like mass
- Acellular, keratinous material
- Thin, stratified squamous epithelium with prominent granular layer
- Inflamed granulation or fibrous tissue
- Giant cell granulomatous reaction to keratinous debris and cholesterol granuloma may coexist

Immunohistochemical Features
- Strong Ki-67 immunoreactivity confirms proliferation

Pathologic Differential Diagnosis
- Squamous cell carcinoma, cholesterol granuloma

ANCILLARY STUDIES

Fluorescence in situ hybridization studies have demonstrated extra copies of chromosome 7 in over half of cholesteatomas, which correlates with proliferative activity. Additionally, this abnormality may be useful in identifying those cases that will exhibit more aggressive behavior. Other proliferation markers, such as ErbB-2 and Ki-67, may also prove to be helpful in predicting behavior in cholesteatomas.

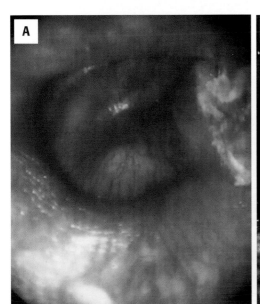 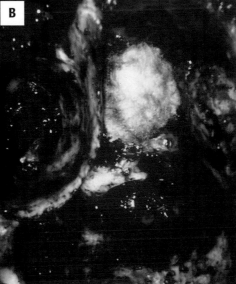

FIGURE 16-22

A, An otoscopic view demonstrates an irregular yellow to white mass behind the perforated tympanic membrane in this cholesteatoma. **B**, Surgical exposure reveals a yellow white mass that represents a cholesteatoma. Specimens received in pathology are typically fragmented.

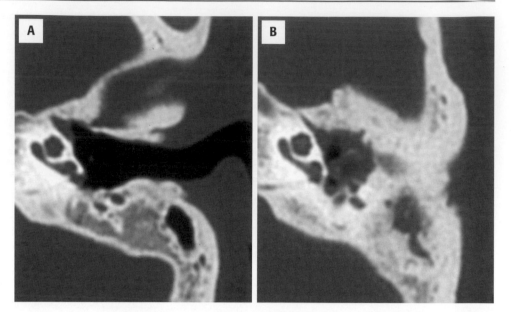

FIGURE 16-23

A, A computed tomography scan of a **normal** ear. **B**, In comparison, the scan shows a soft tissue mass in the middle ear space. The stapes is present in both views.

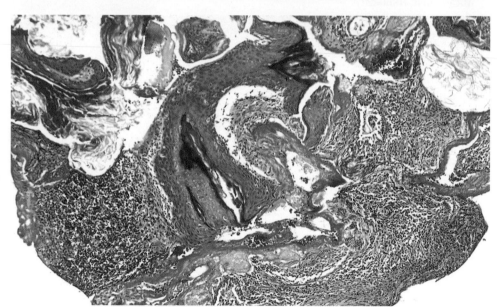

FIGURE 16-24

The essential elements of a cholesteatoma include inflamed granulation or fibrous tissue, keratinizing squamous epithelium, and acellular keratinous material.

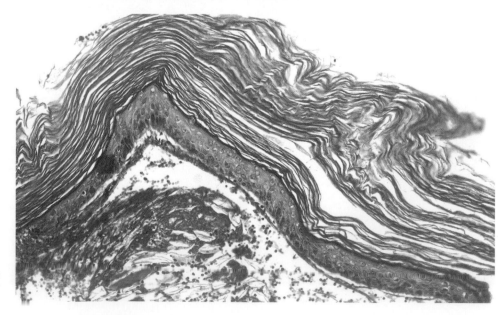

FIGURE 16-25

The squamous epithelium, or "matrix," has a granular layer in a cholesteatoma, associated with flakes of keratin and debris.

DIFFERENTIAL DIAGNOSIS

The pathologic differential diagnosis is relatively limited to *squamous cell carcinoma* and *cholesterol granuloma*. Carcinoma contains pleomorphic epithelium, not seen in cholesteatoma. Cholesterol granuloma is discussed below.

PROGNOSIS AND THERAPY

An excision or exteriorization of a cholesteatoma can be achieved by a modified radical (all ossicles left) or radical mastoidectomy (stapes left). Recurrence can occur if incompletely excised, with a rate of ~20%. Other factors associated with increased incidence of recurrence include age <20 years, marked ossicular erosion, polypoid mucosal inflammatory disease, and extensive disease. Serious complications include labyrinthitis, labyrinthine fistula, sigmoid sinus or facial nerve canal erosion, cranial nerve dysfunction, meningitis, and epidural or brain parenchymal abscess.

■ CHOLESTEROL GRANULOMA

Cholesterol granuloma of the mastoid or middle ear is a stromal reaction to hemorrhage and cholesterol crystals associated with breakdown of red blood cells and other necrotic tissues.

CLINICAL FEATURES

Cholesterol granuloma is seen at any age, with no gender preference, usually in patients with a history of chronic ear disease, such as serous otitis media or acute suppurative otitis media. Trauma or surgical procedures that produce obstruction may also predispose to these lesions. Patients present with unilateral conductive hearing loss, tinnitus, disturbances of balance, or episodes of bloody otorrhea. Otoscopic examination often demonstrates a blue to black tympanic membrane secondary to a middle ear bloody effusion. When cholesterol granulomas occur in the petrous apex, the clinical course may be more aggressive, with sensorineural hearing loss, deficits of other cranial nerves (V, VI, VII), and, in advanced cases, extension into the middle or posterior cranial fossa.

RADIOLOGIC FEATURES

Cholesterol granuloma is readily identified with CT or MRI, where it is characterized by a well-defined

intraosseous cystic lesion with associated bone remodeling. Gadolinium enhancement is not present; cholesterol granuloma demonstrates high-intensity signal with both T1- and T2-weighted images by MRI.

PATHOLOGIC FEATURES

GROSS FINDINGS

The specimen is usually fragmented, consisting of yellow-brown or red friable tissue, sometimes with overlying mucosa. The entire specimen should be processed to exclude an associated cholesteatoma or neoplasm.

MICROSCOPIC FINDINGS

The cholesterol granuloma consists of granulation tissue or fibrous tissue, with recent hemorrhage and elongated clefts (left by cholesterol crystals dissolved by processing) surrounded by multinucleated giant cells, foamy and hemosiderin-laden histiocytes, and extracellular

CHOLESTEROL GRANULOMA—PATHOLOGIC FEATURES

Gross Findings

- Fragmented, friable, yellow-brown to red friable tissue
- Processing of all material required to exclude associated cholesteatoma or neoplasm

Microscopic Findings

- Granulation or fibrous tissue with recent hemorrhage
- Elongated clefts (left by cholesterol crystals) surrounded by multinucleated giant cells, foamy and hemosiderin laden macrophages
- Extracellular aggregates of hemosiderin pigment
- Reactive epithelium, but no keratinizing squamous epithelium in pure cholesterol granuloma

Pathologic Differential Diagnosis

- Look for associated lesions: cholesteatoma, neuroendocrine adenoma of middle ear, endolymphatic sac tumor

accumulations of hemosiderin pigment (Figure 16-26). The overlying mucosa may demonstrate reactive changes, but a pure cholesterol granuloma will not include a proliferation of keratinizing squamous epithelium, which would indicate a coexisting cholesteatoma.

DIFFERENTIAL DIAGNOSIS

The cholesterol granuloma is frequently simultaneously present with other lesions, such as cholesteatoma, neuroendocrine adenoma of the middle ear, and endolymphatic sac tumor. Therefore, it is imperative to search for these other possible lesions.

PROGNOSIS AND THERAPY

Treatment of a cholesterol granuloma requires drainage and aeration of the middle ear–mastoid compartment, removing the predisposing factors for development of these lesions. Petrous apex lesions may require drainage (through a variety of techniques), depending on the presence or absence of residual hearing. Nonaggressive petrous apex lesions, often incidental, may be followed clinically and radiographically.

SUGGESTED READINGS

The complete suggested readings list is available online at www.expertconsult.com.

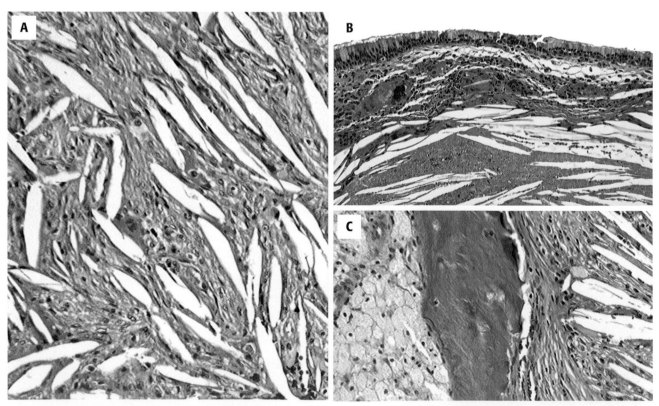

FIGURE 16-26

A, The submucosal stroma demonstrates fusiform clefts left by cholesterol crystals, which have been dissolved during processing. **B**, Many of the cholesterol crystals are engulfed by multinucleated giant cells below an intact respiratory-type epithelium. **C**, Bone with histiocytes (*left*) and cholesterol clefts (*right*).

17

Benign Neoplasms of the Ear and Temporal Bone

■ **Lester D. R. Thompson**

■ CERUMINOUS ADENOMA

Synonymously called ceruminoma, ceruminal adenoma, apocrine adenoma, or even cylindroma in the past, these terms are now discouraged as they imply a different disease type with remarkable differences in clinical behavior and treatment alternatives. "Ceruminous adenoma" is a benign glandular neoplasm of ceruminous glands (modified apocrine sweat glands) that arises solely from the external auditory canal.

CLINICAL FEATURES

Ceruminous adenoma accounts for <1% of all external ear tumors, usually affecting middle-aged (mean, 55 years) patients, without gender predilection. Patients usually present with a mass in the posterior wall of the outer one-third to one-half of the external auditory canal. There may be associated pain, hearing loss (sensorineural and conductive), tinnitus, or even paralysis of the nerves.

PATHOLOGIC FEATURES

GROSS FINDINGS

Most tumors are small (mean, 1.2 cm), nonulcerating, superficial masses found in the outer one-third to one-half of the external auditory canal, covered by intact skin. Grossly polypoid, these masses are usually fragmented during removal. As benign tumors, extension into the mastoid bone, middle ear, and base of the skull is not identified.

CERUMINOUS ADENOMA—DISEASE FACT SHEET

Definition
- Benign ceruminal gland neoplasm

Incidence and Location
- Rare
- Outer half of the external auditory canal

Morbidity and Mortality
- None

Gender, Race, and Age Distribution
- Equal gender distribution
- Wide age range, but usually 6th decade

Clinical Features
- Mass with hearing changes, pain, tinnitus

Prognosis and Treatment
- Excellent; surgery alone, although recurrences may develop

CERUMINOUS ADENOMA—PATHOLOGIC FEATURES

Gross Findings
- Nonulcerated, superficial mass in outer half of external auditory canal, mean size of 1.2 cm

Microscopic Findings
- Circumscribed mass with glandular and cystic pattern
- Dual-cell population, with inner apocrine cells showing decapitation secretion and outer basal-myoepithelial cells
- Luminal cells with cytoplasmic yellow-brown, cerumen pigment granules
- Dense, sclerotic fibrosis

Immunohistochemical Features
- CK7, CD117 positive (luminal) secretory cells
- CK5/6, p63, S100 protein positive basal-myoepithelial cells

Pathologic Differential Diagnosis
- Ceruminal gland adenocarcinoma, neuroendocrine adenoma of the middle ear (middle ear adenoma), paraganglioma

---

MICROSCOPIC FINDINGS

Ceruminous adenomas are well circumscribed but not encapsulated (Figure 17-1). Surface involvement (not *origin*) can be seen, while ulceration is absent. They are divided into three major groups based on specific histologic findings: ceruminous adenoma, ceruminous pleomorphic adenoma (chondroid syringoma), and ceruminous syringocystadenoma papilliferum (too rare to be discussed here). There is frequently a background of dense, sclerotic fibrosis that may simulate invasion. The tumors are moderately cellular, arranged in a mixture of glandular and cystic patterns each composed of a dual-cell population (Figure 17-2). The inner luminal

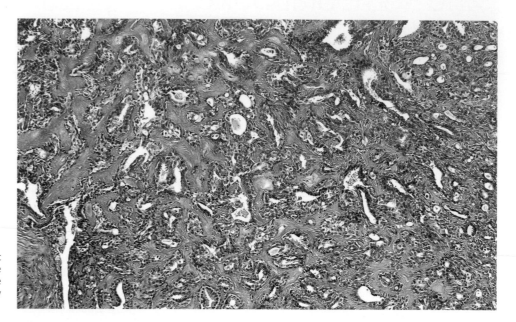

FIGURE 17-1

There is an unencapsulated neoplastic proliferation of ceruminous glands. The glandular and cystic profiles are visible even at low magnification, separated by heavy fibrosis.

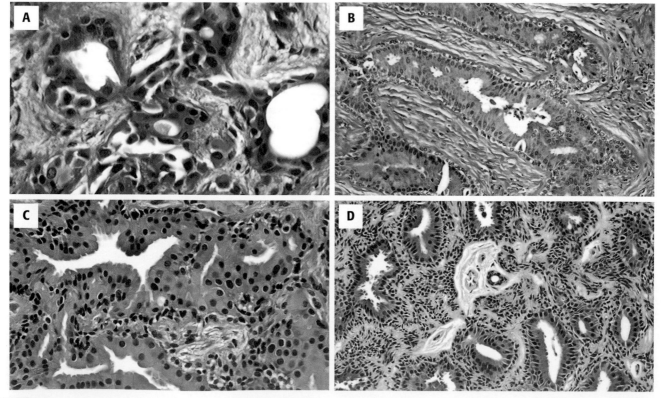

FIGURE 17-2

A variety of different patterns and histologic appearances. **A**, Inner luminal secretory cells with cerumen granules subtended by basal myoepithelial cells demonstrate the dual-cell population. **B**, Abundant eosinophilic cytoplasm is seen in the luminal cells, which show decapitation secretion. **C**, Glandular profiles with a delicate basal layer. **D**, The inner cells are surrounded by a proliferation of basal myoepithelial cells.

secretory cells have apocrine decapitation secretions or blebs and abundant granular, eosinophilic cytoplasm. Specifically, there are yellow-brown, ceroid, lipofuscin-like (cerumen, wax; acid-fast fluorescent) pigment granules within the cytoplasm of these luminal cells (Figure 17-3). These cells are surrounded by basal, myoepithelial cells lined along the basement membrane (Figure 17-2). There are usually very limited pleomorphism, occasional nucleoli, rare mitoses, and a lack of necrosis.

A *ceruminous pleomorphic adenoma* is identical to a salivary gland pleomorphic adenoma, thus showing chondromyxoid matrix material (not native cartilage) juxtaposed to, and blended with, epithelium, with the added feature of ceruminous differentiation among the epithelial and "duct-like" cells. It is important to separate a primary external auditory canal tumor from a parotid salivary gland tumor with local extension into the ear. The *ceruminous papillary cystadenoma papilliferum* has papillary projections lined by cuboidal to columnar cells, a dense plasmacytic infiltrate, and cells with ceruminous differentiation.

ANCILLARY STUDIES

Immunohistochemistry is not necessary for the diagnosis, but stains can be used to highlight the biphasic nature of the tumor cells. Although both cell types stain for epithelial membrane antigen (EMA) and pan-keratin, the luminal cells uniquely stain for CK7 and preferentially stain for CD117. In contrast, the basal-luminal cells will stain with CK5/6, p63, and S100 protein (Figure 17-4). There is no reaction with chromogranin, synaptophysin, CD56, or CK20.

DIFFERENTIAL DIAGNOSIS

This tumor type is unique to the external auditory canal, with infrequent confusion with other tumors. *Ceruminous adenocarcinoma* has an infiltrative and destructive growth pattern, greater cellularity, cribriform growth, and pronounced nuclear pleomorphism with prominent nucleoli. Mitoses and necrosis can be seen. Ceroid pigmentation, seen in the luminal cells of the benign adenoma, is notably absent. Ceruminous adenocarcinoma is also divided into types, including the adenoid cystic type and the not otherwise specified (NOS) type, which gives the most difficulty in the differential diagnosis. A *neuroendocrine adenoma of the middle ear* may expand from the middle ear into the medial aspect of the external auditory canal. This tumor also has a biphasic appearance, but the cells are plasmacytoid to cuboidal, have salt-and-pepper nuclear chromatin distribution, lack decapitation secretions, and have no ceroid granules in the cytoplasm. Furthermore, they are positive for neuroendocrine and peptide markers. A *paraganglioma* shows a classic zellballen (nested) architecture, cells with basophilic, slightly granular cytoplasm, and isolated pleomorphism. The paraganglia cells are immunoreactive with chromogranin, synaptophysin, and/or CD56, consistent with their neuroendocrine origin, while the sustentacular (supporting) cells will stain with S100 protein.

PROGNOSIS AND THERAPY

Complete excision will be curative although difficult to achieve, due to the complex anatomy of the ear. Therefore,

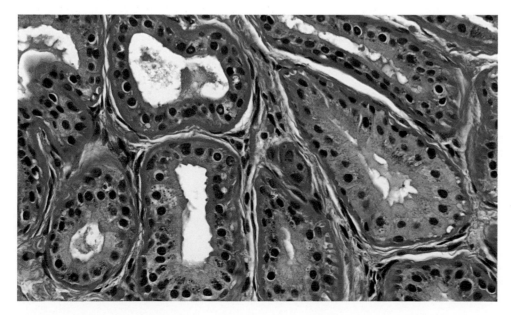

FIGURE 17-3

Yellow-brown "ceroid" lipofuscin-like material is seen in the cytoplasm of the ceruminous cells.

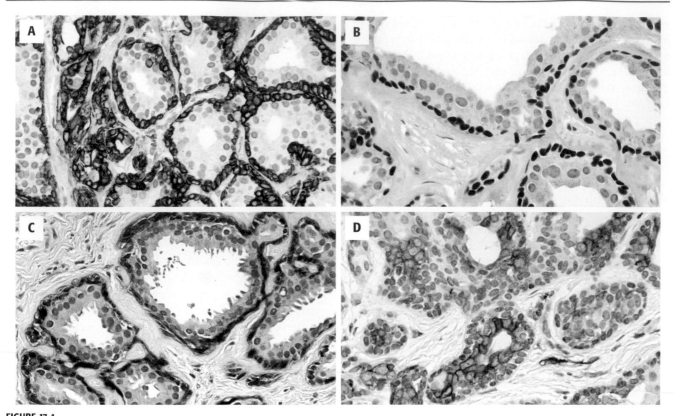

FIGURE 17-4

Differential immunohistochemical staining highlights the myoepithelial basal cells—CK5/6 (**A**), p63 (**B**), S100 protein (**C**)—while the luminal cells are highlighted by CD117 (**D**).

incomplete excision is not uncommon and is associated with an increased risk of recurrence.

■ PERIPHERAL NERVE SHEATH TUMOR (SCHWANNOMA)

Schwannoma (acoustic neuroma or neurilemmoma) is a benign peripheral nerve sheath tumor (PNST) arising within the internal auditory canal (IAC) and is the most common neoplasm of the temporal bone. The tumor arises from the myelin-forming Schwann cells, usually from the vestibular portion of the vestibulocochlear (VIII) cranial nerve, and accounts for 80% to 90% of all cerebropontine angle (CPA) tumors. About 95% of tumors are unilateral and sporadic, but if bilateral or presenting in a young patient, association with neurofibromatosis type 2 (NF2) is high.

CLINICAL FEATURES

Patients usually present in the 5th to 6th decades of life but tend to be younger (< 21 years) when NF2 associated. Progressive unilateral sensorineural (not

conductive) hearing loss and tinnitus (steam kettle–type hissing) occur in ~80% of patients, occasionally accompanied by headache, vertigo, altered balance and gait, facial pain, and facial weakness. Although the etiology is unknown in the majority of cases, occupational or recreational exposure to extremely loud noise over a prolonged period of time (~20 years) may be a risk factor in tumor development.

RADIOLOGIC FEATURES

The best radiographic diagnostic clue is a CPA mass, with a funnel-shaped widening of the IAC or small indentation of bone. Magnetic resonance imaging (MRI) shows a hyperintense mass on T2-weighted images (with gadolinium contrast) with intense enhancement into the porus acusticus.

PATHOLOGIC FEATURES

GROSS FINDINGS

The tumors are usually small (<2 cm), globular to mushroom-shaped masses frequently eccentrically

PERIPHERAL NERVE SHEATH TUMOR—DISEASE FACT SHEET

Definition
- Benign Schwann cell–derived neoplasm

Incidence and Location
- Most common cerebellopontine angle tumor (80% to 90%)
- 95% unilateral and sporadic
- If bilateral or young age, NF2 association is high

Morbidity and Mortality
- Loss of hearing, especially in NF2-associated tumors
- No mortality

Gender and Age Distribution
- Equal gender distribution
- 5th to 6th decade; younger for NF2 patients

Clinical Features
- Tinnitus (high-pitched, steam kettle–type hissing) in 80%
- Progressive sensorineural hearing loss
- Long occupational or recreational exposure to extremely loud noise

Radiologic Features
- Cerebropontine angle mass with funnel-shaped widening of the internal auditory canal
- MRI: hyperintense mass on T2

Prognosis and Treatment
- Excellent prognosis, with recurrences in up to 15%
- Surgery or serial MRI scans to follow slow-growing lesions

PERIPHERAL NERVE SHEATH TUMOR—PATHOLOGIC FEATURES

Gross Findings
- Attached to the vestibular or cochlear division of cranial nerve VIII
- Globular to mushroom shaped, usually <2 cm, rubbery yellow mass, myxoid, and cystic

Microscopic Findings
- Cellular Antoni A areas with closely backed bundles of spindled cells and Verocay bodies
- Hypocellular Antoni B areas with microcystic degeneration
- Fusiform cells with fibrillar cytoplasm
- Spindled, wavy/buckled, pointy nuclei
- Medium-sized dilated vessels with hyalinization

Immunohistochemical Features
- Diffuse, strong S100 protein and vimentin immunoreactivity
- GFAP and NSE occasionally positive
- CD34 fibroblasts within degenerated areas

Genetic Studies
- 90% of mutations in NF2 coded by *MERLIN/schwannomin* at 22q12

Pathologic Differential Diagnosis
- Meningioma and neurofibroma

---

rim of recognizable tumor. Calcification is rare. Pleomorphism, necrosis, and mitoses suggest malignancy.

attached to the vestibular division of the 8th (vestibulocochlear) cranial nerve (CN), growing centrally along the CPA ("mushroom") and peripherally along the IAC ("stalk"). When the cochlear division is involved, the nerve is stretched rather than attached. Cross sections are smooth, gray-tan to yellow, rubbery to firm, and solid to myxoid and cystic. Intratumoral hemorrhage is common.

MICROSCOPIC FINDINGS

Histologically, the tumor cells are arranged in cellular (Antoni A) closely packed bundles of spindle cells (Figure 17-5) adjacent to microcystic or loosely reticular (Antoni B) areas (Figure 17-6). When these spindled cells have their nuclei lined up in a palisade architecture, they are called Verocay bodies. The spindled or fusiform cells have fibrillary cytoplasm surrounding buckled to wavy, elongated, and pointy nuclei. Small to medium-sized vessels are characteristically ectatic with distinctive perivascular hyalinization (Figure 17-5). Mitoses are uncommon and necrosis is usually absent. However, extensive degenerative changes ("ancient schwannoma") can occur (including xanthoma-type histiocytes) and may result in only a thin

ANCILLARY STUDIES

ULTRASTRUCTURAL FEATURES

Electron microscopy (EM) reveals a single cell type (Schwann cell) characterized by thin interdigitating cytoplasmic processes that are continuous from the cell body. The Schwann cell surface is wrapped by a discrete, continuous basal lamina that contains the pathognomonic "Luse body", collagen fibrils arranged in parallel with a long-spacing (130 nm) periodicity.

IMMUNOHISTOCHEMICAL FEATURES

The neoplastic cells of schwannoma show a strong and diffuse nuclear and cytoplasmic immunoreactivity for S100 protein (Figure 17-6). Vimentin, although nonspecific, stains the cytoplasm of these cells. Glial fibrillary acidic protein (GFAP) and neuron-specific enolase (NSE) may occasionally be positive. CD34 stains a subpopulation of slender cells in the loose, Antoni B areas. Neurofilament is absent. Interestingly, the proliferation index (using Ki-67 antibody) is higher in schwannomas of NF2 patients than in sporadic, solitary lesions.

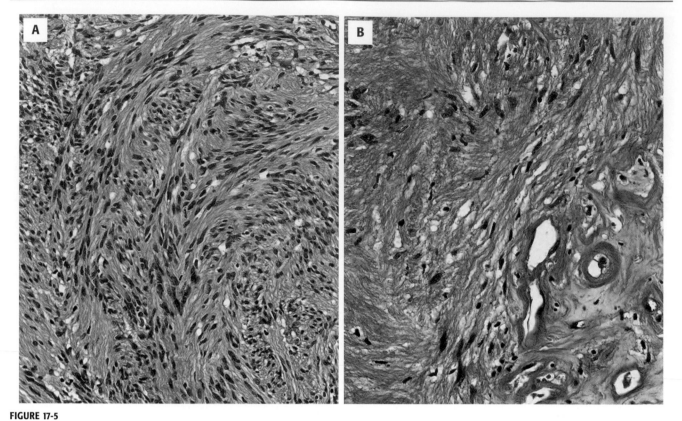

FIGURE 17-5

A, Hypercellular Antoni A area with fascicular arrangement of cells with fibrillar cytoplasm. **B**, Hypocellular Antoni B area with small vessels showing perivascular hyalinization.

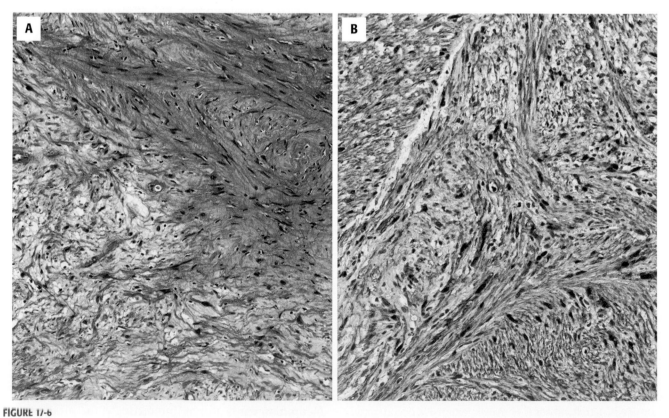

FIGURE 17-6

A, The hypocellular areas show a myxoid degeneration between the spindled cells. **B**, S100 protein positive reaction in the nucleus and cytoplasm of the lesional cells.

GENETIC STUDIES

NF2 (distinct from NF1 or von Recklinghausen disease) is an autosomal dominant disease, with >200 identified mutations involving *NF2*, a tumor suppressor gene at 22q12 that encodes the protein *MERLIN* or *schwannomin*. About 90% of mutations result in a truncated protein that cannot carry out its normal tumor suppressor function.

DIFFERENTIAL DIAGNOSIS

The uniqueness of this anatomic site (CPA) raises a limited differential that includes only meningioma and neurofibroma. Meningioma is characterized by a whorled epithelioid proliferation with psammoma bodies, intranuclear cytoplasmic inclusions, and EMA immunoreactivity. Neurofibromas are exceptionally rare in the ear and temporal bone, and lack the classic alternating Antoni A and B areas, Verocay bodies, and perivascular hyalinization.

PROGNOSIS AND THERAPY

Schwannoma is a benign tumor with a very low recurrence potential. Surgical removal by any one of various approaches (translabyrinthine, suboccipital, middle cranial fossa, or by stereotactic gamma knife surgery) is standard therapy, with the goal of preserving hearing and vestibular function. It is more difficult to preserve hearing and facial nerve function in schwannomas of NF2 patients since they tend to infiltrate the nerves to a greater extent and also grow more rapidly. However, in small tumors or elderly patients (>70 years), management can include watchful waiting using serial MR scans to monitor growth. Radiotherapy can be used but may fail in up to 15% of patients.

■ PARAGANGLIOMA

Paraganglioma is a neoplasm arising from paraganglia (chemoreceptors derived from neural crest responding to changes in blood oxygen and carbon dioxide levels) situated in the vicinity of the jugular bulb (glomus jugulare) or the medial cochlea promontory of the middle ear (glomus tympanicum), together representing nearly 80% of all head and neck paragangliomas. Paraganglioma is the preferred term for this most common neoplasm of the middle ear, but chemodectoma and glomus tumor are frequently used clinically. It is important to note that "glomus" used here is not synonymous with *glomus tumor*, which is a specific pericytic–smooth muscle vascular tumor.

CLINICAL FEATURES

Familial and solitary paragangliomas are recognized. Sporadic tumors show a strong female predilection (female:male = 5:1), while inherited or familial tumors are more common in males. There is a wide age range at initial presentation, with a mean in the 6th decade. This tumor follows the "rule of 10": 10% multicentric, 10% bilateral, 10% familial, 10% pediatric, and 10% malignant. Patients report pulsatile tinnitus (~90% of patients), hearing loss (~50% of patients; conductive rather than sensorineural), pain, and/or facial nerve paralysis, and examination reveals a vascular retrotympanic mass. Biopsy is contraindicated as it can result in profound bleeding. Rarely, catecholamine hypersecretion may be found.

PARAGANGLIOMA—DISEASE FACT SHEET

Definition
- A benign neoplasm arising from the paraganglia (chemoreceptors) of the jugular bulb or medial cochlea promontory of the middle ear

Incidence and Location
- Uncommon (represent 80% of all head and neck paragangliomas)
- Jugular bulb, middle ear
- Rule of 10%: multifocal, bilateral, familial, pediatric, and malignant

Morbidity and Mortality
- About 15% mortality

Gender, Race, and Age Distribution
- 90% are solitary tumors, more common in women
- 10% are familial tumors, more common in men
- Wide age range, mean in 6th decade

Clinical Features
- Pulsatile tinnitus (90%) and conductive hearing loss (50%)

Radiologic Features
- Angiography shows blood supply and feeder vessels
- CT: well-defined hypervascular, heterogeneous mass with bony changes
- MRI: serpentine signal voids on T1 and hyperintense areas on T2
- May find clinically occult tumors with octreotide or MIBG scintigraphy

Prognosis and Treatment
- Slow growing, but invasive
- Watchful waiting, embolization, surgery, and radiation therapy

RADIOLOGIC FEATURES

Radiographs will accurately define the location, size, and extent of the tumor. Angiography highlights feeder vessels and blood supply while also permitting presurgical embolization. MRI and computed tomography (CT) show complementary features, with the former showing an enhancing, vascular mass, and the latter highlighting bony changes, including expansion and erosion of the jugular foramen or ossicular chain. More recently, nuclear imaging, including a positron emission tomography scan with [18]fluorodeoxyglucose ([18]FDG) and octreotide and/or ^{131}I-meta-iodobenzylguanidine (MIBG) scintigraphy helps to confirm the "neuroendocrine" nature of the neoplasm, as well as identify occult or familial tumors.

PATHOLOGIC FEATURES

GROSS FINDINGS

The tumors are irregular, firm, reddish masses, ranging from 0.3 up to 6 cm and usually fragmented upon removal. The cut surface is often variegated with cystic degeneration and hemorrhage. The tympanic membrane is usually intact.

MICROSCOPIC FINDINGS

Histologically, these tumors are usually infiltrative, lacking encapsulation or circumscription, and are arranged in a characteristic clustered or zellballen architecture (Figure 17-7). These balls or nests of paraganglia are surrounded by a layer of supporting or sustentacular cells (not readily appreciable by hematoxylin and eosin staining alone) and invested by a richly vascularized

---

PARAGANGLIOMA—PATHOLOGIC FEATURES

Gross Findings
- Fragmented, irregular, reddish firm up to 6 cm mass with hemorrhage

Microscopic Findings
- Poorly encapsulated, infiltrative tumors
- Cellular tumors with clusters, alveolar or zellballen architecture
- Small, uniform cells with granular basophilic cytoplasm
- Richly vascularized stroma

Immunohistochemical Features
- Pheochromocytes: chromogranin, synaptophysin, CD56, NSE positive
- Sustentacular cells: S100 protein and GFAP positive

Genetic Studies
- Inactivating mutations in subunits of the succinate-ubiquinone oxidoreductase gene (*SDH*): *PGL1* (11q23), *PGL2* (11q13.1), *PGL3* (1q21-q23)

Pathologic Differential Diagnosis
- Schwannoma, meningioma, neuroendocrine adenoma of the middle ear

---

stroma (Figure 17-8). Tumors are moderately cellular, composed of small to intermediate-sized cells containing ample granular to basophilic cytoplasm (Figure 17-9). The nuclei are rather monotonous, although isolated marked pleomorphism can be seen. Nuclear chromatin is usually delicate to coarse. Mitoses are uncommon to rare. Multinucleated cells are occasionally present. Degenerative changes, especially after embolization, will result in cyst formation and hemorrhage, with hemosiderin-laden macrophages and fibrosis.

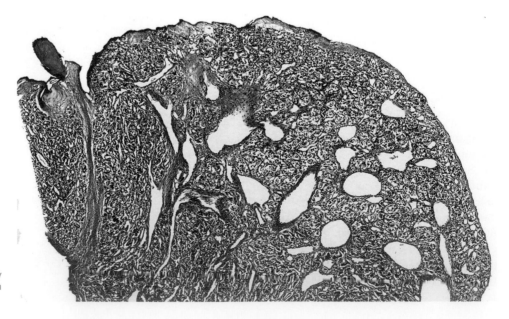

FIGURE 17-7

A polypoid tumor with a rich vascularity and a nested, alveolar (zellballen) pattern in this paraganglioma.

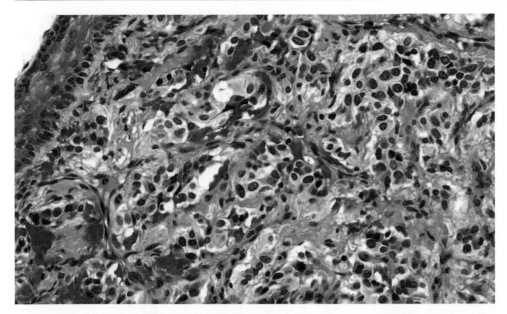

FIGURE 17-8

Nests of tumor cells are separated by a fibrovascular stroma. Note the intact surface epithelium (*upper left*).

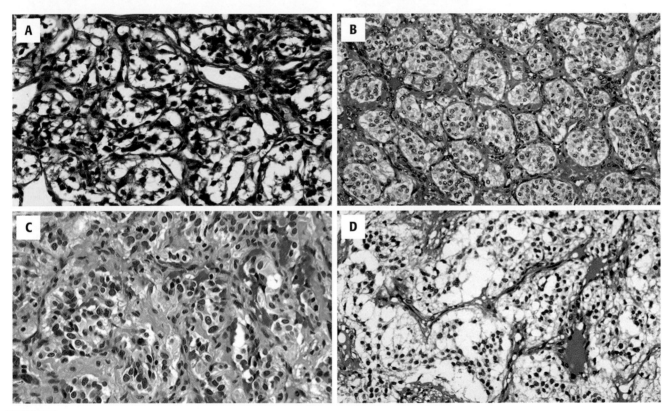

FIGURE 17-9

Paraganglioma shows a variety of different sizes of zellballen, along with variability in cytoplasmic quality (**A**, cleared; **B**, granular; **C**, basophilic; **D**, fibrillar).

ANCILLARY STUDIES

ULTRASTRUCTURAL FEATURES

Paraganglioma cells (pheochromocytes) contain cytoplasmic, membrane-bound granules with a central electron-dense core and surrounding radiolucent rim ("clear halo"), characteristic of neurosecretory granules. These vary somewhat in size (100 to 350 nm) and frequency within and between tumors, but account for the granular cytoplasm appreciated by light microscopy.

IMMUNOHISTOCHEMICAL FEATURES

The pheochromocytes will be immunoreactive with chromogranin (Figure 17-10), synaptophysin, NSE, and/or

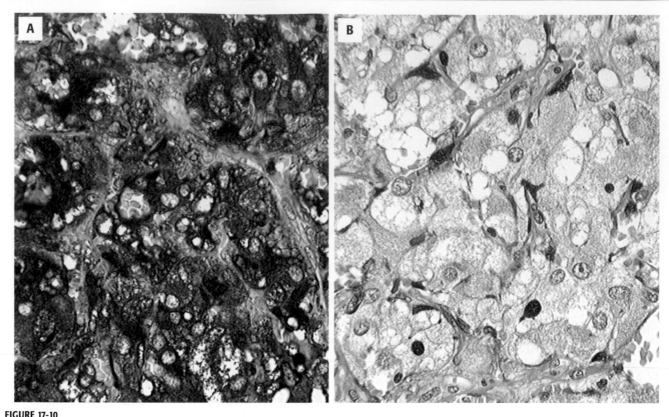

FIGURE 17-10

The paraganglia cells are strongly and diffusely immunoreactive with chromogranin (**A**), while the supporting, sustentacular cells are highlighted by S100 protein (**B**).

CD56 (membrane staining), confirming the neuroendocrine differentiation of the cells. The supporting sustentacular framework cells will react with S100 protein or with GFAP. There is no keratin, CEA, or human pancreatic polypeptide (HPP) immunoreactivity.

GENETIC STUDIES

Up to 10% of head and neck paragangliomas are familial and inherited as an autosomal dominant trait with genomic imprinting. The most common genetic loci associated with paragangliomas are within several genes encoding various subunits of the succinate-ubiquinone oxidoreductase gene (*SDH*): paraganglioma 1 (*PGL1*) at 11q23, *PGL2* at 11q13.1, and *PGL3* at 1q21-q23, which are inactivating mutations in *SDHB*, *SDHC*, and *SDHD*, respectively.

DIFFERENTIAL DIAGNOSIS

The differential is limited when considering anatomic site alone, since nearly 90% of masses in the jugular foramen are paraganglioma, with schwannoma and meningioma accounting for the remaining lesions. Nonetheless, the small size of biopsy samples from the middle ear is the principal reason for diagnostic difficulties. For

example, a minute specimen may cause confusion with neuroendocrine adenoma of the middle ear, but keratin immunoreactivity should make the distinction obvious. Moreover, necrosis due to embolization may suggest an underlying malignancy. However, the presence of embolic material in certain cases will assist in confirming the correct diagnosis.

PROGNOSIS AND THERAPY

Jugulotympanic paragangliomas are slow growing but can be locally invasive. Due to the vital structures in the region, mortality rates of 15% can be expected even though it is a benign neoplasm in 90% of cases. Watchful waiting can be used, although surgery is the standard therapy, with or without presurgical embolization. Radiation therapy plays a role in poor surgical candidates. Distant metastases are very rare.

■ MENINGIOMA

Meningioma is a common, benign neoplasm of meningothelial cells within the ear and temporal bone. This tumor arises from the arachnoid cells (arachnoid granulations, pacchionian bodies), which normally line the inner aspect of the arachnoid membrane and fill the cores of the arachnoid villi that project into the lumens of dural veins and venous sinuses. Extraneuraxial (extracranial, ectopic, extracalvarial) meningiomas are usually divided into four groups based on suggested etiologies: (1) direct extension of a primary intracranial meningioma through pressure necrosis/absorption of the bone or through an iatrogenic or natural opening; (2) extracranial metastasis from an intracranial meningioma; (3) extracranial meningioma originating from pia-arachnoid cell clusters in the sheaths of the cranial nerves (or vessels) as they exit through the foramina or suture lines of the skull; and (4) extracranial meningioma without any apparent demonstrable connection with foramina, cranial nerves, or cranial primaries. Most of the reported cases involving the ear and temporal bone fall into the first group, representing secondary extension from an intracranial lesion, a phenomenon seen in up to 20% of intracranial meningiomas. A true primary meningioma of the ear and temporal bone should only be diagnosed when there is clinical and radiographic support (i.e., a lack of any detectable intracranial mass or "dural enhancement").

Meningioma comprises ~10% of ear and temporal bone tumors, affecting predominantly middle-aged patients (mean, 50 years). There is a 2:1 female:male ratio and women tend to be older than men at presentation. Patients present with hearing loss, tinnitus, otitis, pain, headaches, dizziness, and/or vertigo. The most common locations are the internal auditory meatus, jugular foramen, middle ear, and the eustachian tube roof.

RADIOLOGIC FEATURES

Radiographic studies are performed with an eye to excluding direct central nervous system extension. MRI tends to be more yielding than CT. The tumor is usually isointense to gray matter on T1-weighted MRI, while isointense to hyperintense on T2-weighted images. A direct extension or central nervous system association should be sought and/or excluded. Specifically, en plaque lesions (flat, "carpet-like" growth along the dura) must also be actively sought and excluded.

PATHOLOGIC FEATURES

GROSS FINDINGS

Most tumors of the ear and temporal bone are relatively small (<1.5 cm), unless an intracranial component is identified. Macroscopically, the tumors are usually infiltrative into the bone through crevices and suture lines, while sparing the mucosal surface (or skin if it involves the external auditory canal). The cut

CLINICAL FEATURES

MENINGIOMA—DISEASE FACT SHEET

Definition
- A benign neoplasm of meningothelial cells

Incidence and Location
- Up to 10% of ear and temporal bone tumors
- Internal auditory meatus, jugular foramen, middle ear (cleft)

Morbidity and Mortality
- Mastoiditis
- 80% 5-year survival

Gender and Age Distribution
- Female > male (2:1) (women are usually older at presentation)
- Broad age range, mean: 50 years

Clinical Features
- Hearing loss, tinnitus, otitis, pain, headaches, dizziness, vertigo

Radiologic Features
- Direct central nervous system extension should be sought or excluded (en plaque)
- MRI: T1—isointense; T2—hyperintense
- CT: focal bone erosion, sclerosis, or hyperostosis

Prognosis and Treatment
- Good outcome (80% 5-year survival)
- 20% recurrence rate
- Wide surgical excision with clear margins

MENINGIOMA—PATHOLOGIC FEATURES

Gross Findings
- Infiltrative into bone (suture lines), sparing mucosa/skin
- Usually <1.5 cm
- Granular mass with gritty consistency and calcifications

Microscopic Findings
- Meningothelial and whorled architecture
- Syncytial and epithelioid cells with indistinct borders
- Bland, round nuclei with delicate chromatin and intranuclear cytoplasmic inclusions
- Psammoma bodies or pre-psammoma bodies

Immunohistochemical Features
- EMA focal and weak
- Keratin (CAM5.2, CK7) in pre–psammoma body pattern

Pathologic Differential Diagnosis
- Neuroendocrine adenoma of the middle ear, schwannoma, paraganglioma, meningocele

surface is gray-white and granular, with a gritty consistency due to calcifications and bony fragments that are frequently grossly visible.

MICROSCOPIC FINDINGS

The tumor cells have a syncytial, epithelioid appearance and are arranged in lobules or nests with a meningothelial and whorled architecture (Figure 17-11). In general, the cells are bland with round to oval nuclei, delicate nuclear chromatin, and intranuclear cytoplasmic inclusions (Figures 17-12 and 17-13). True psammoma bodies or "pre-psammoma" bodies are often present (Figure 17-12). Pleomorphism and necrosis are usually absent and mitoses are uncommon. Multiple patterns of growth can be seen. An infiltrative growth pattern is defined by bone and soft tissue invasion (assessed by imaging or histology) and is identified in

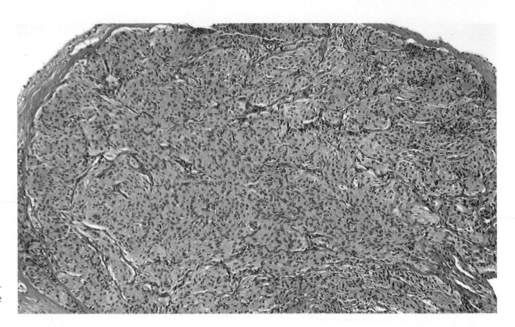

FIGURE 17-11

Typical meningotheliomatous meningioma with a whorled syncytial architecture growing in a polypoid fashion.

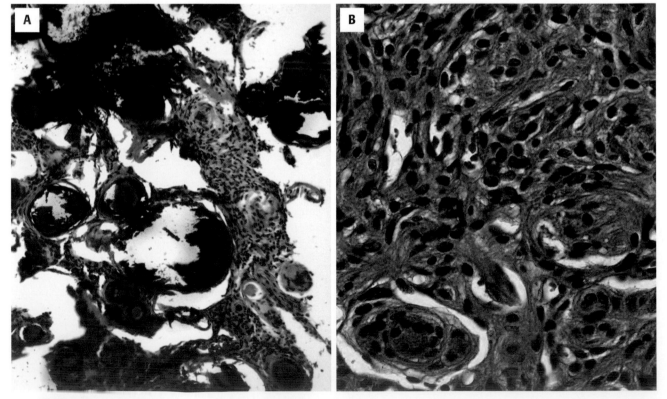

FIGURE 17-12

A, Numerous psammoma bodies are seen in this meningioma. **B**, A whorled, lobular appearance is noted, with delicate, round to oval nuclei.

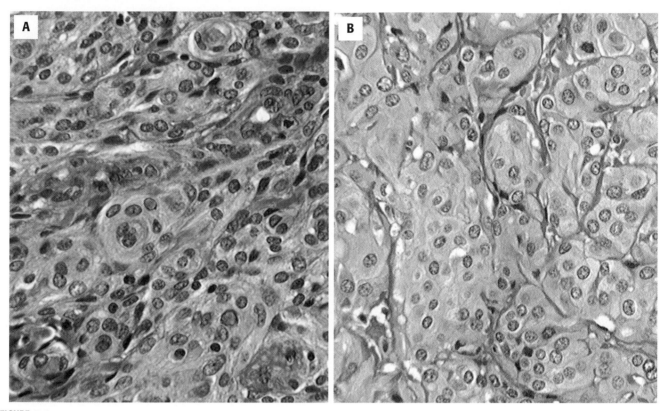

FIGURE 17-13

A variety of different growth patterns can be seen, but the meningothelial nature of the neoplasm is maintained (**A**). Note the intranuclear-cytoplasmic inclusions. A paraganglioma-like growth pattern is occasionally seen (**B**).

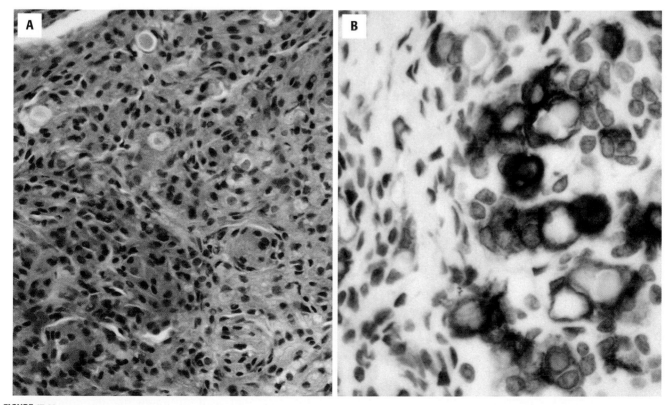

FIGURE 17-14

A, Whorled architecture with a syncytial meningothelial cell proliferation. Note the numerous "pre-psammoma bodies." **B**, Keratin will frequently stain a zone immediately around the pre-psammoma bodies.

many cases. Notably, it does not appear to have a bearing on overall patient outcome. Nearly all tumors are World Health Organization grade 1, with the meningothelial (syncytial) and psammomatous variants, respectively, the most frequently occurring.

ANCILLARY STUDIES

Nearly all meningiomas react with vimentin and have a weak, focal, but genuine reactivity for EMA, which is often helpful in making the diagnosis. It is not uncommon to also exhibit focal immunoreactivity with S100 protein, as well as keratin stains (CK7, CAM5.2) in a pre–psammoma body pattern only (Figure 17-14). The proliferation index is usually <5 % as detected with Ki-67.

DIFFERENTIAL DIAGNOSIS

The differential diagnosis for meningiomas includes neuroendocrine adenoma of the middle ear, schwannoma, paraganglioma, and meningocele. The general histologic features and immunohistochemical findings can usually separate between these tumors. A neuroendocrine adenoma of the middle ear has a more organoid growth with neuroendocrine nuclear features and strong keratin, chromogranin, and HPP immunoreactivity. A spindle cell tumor with alternating cellular (Antoni A) and hypocellular (Antoni B) areas, perivascular hyalinization, and strong and diffuse nuclear and cytoplasmic S100 protein immunoreactivity confirms a diagnosis of schwannoma. Paraganglioma shows a zellballen (nested) architecture with basophilic cells and a distinctive immunoprofile: chromogranin-positive paraganglia cells and S100 protein positive supporting sustentacular cells. A meningocele, or protrusion of the meninges through a bony defect, can occur in the middle ear and temporal bone, but these are histologically cystic lesions with a connection to the central nervous system. They can be congenital or "acquired" after surgery, infection, or trauma.

PROGNOSIS AND THERAPY

Wide excision with clear margins is required. In the case of skull base involvement, surgical approaches are complex and challenging (transpetrosal, subtemporal, transtentorial). Adjuvant radiation therapy is used in poor surgical candidates or in cases of incomplete surgical resection. Overall, there is a good 5-year survival of 80 %. However, recurrences are frequent (20 % of patients), although some of these cases may actually represent persistent or residual disease instead of true recurrence.

Despite additional surgery, occasionally patients will die with disease (although "from" disease is difficult to determine). Cerebrospinal fluid leak and hearing loss are the most common complications, while others such as mastoiditis, meningitis, and sepsis may result in patient death.

■ NEUROENDOCRINE ADENOMA OF THE MIDDLE EAR (MIDDLE EAR ADENOMA)

Neuroendocrine adenoma of the middle ear (NAME), synonymously called middle ear adenoma, carcinoid, or middle ear adenomatous tumor (MEAT), is a benign glandular neoplasm of the middle ear showing both cytomorphologic and immunohistochemical evidence of mixed mucinous and neuroendocrine differentiation.

CLINICAL FEATURES

This is an uncommon tumor (<2 % of ear tumors) usually presenting in the 5th decade, with an equal sex distribution. Patients present with unilateral disease and associated tinnitus, fullness or pressure, and conductive hearing loss, especially if the ossicular chain is involved. In early stages, otoscopy shows an intact tympanic membrane with a dark brownish-red mass behind it. The tumor may later expand to and involve the ossicular chain, thus causing conductive hearing loss, and may even penetrate the tympanic membrane. Occasionally, it may extend into the external auditory canal or into the mastoid bone and eustachian tube. Despite its neuroendocrine origin, there is no serologic evidence of peptide hyperproduction.

PATHOLOGIC FEATURES

GROSS FINDINGS

Most tumors are quite small, less than <1 cm in greatest dimension. Since they tend to encase the ossicular chain, the tumor is usually peeled away from the bone upon resection. Therefore, surgical specimens are highly fragmented and consist of whitish-yellow to gray, soft to rubbery tissue. Tumors are unencapsulated and abut the overlying intact surface epithelium.

MICROSCOPIC FINDINGS

These tumors are moderately cellular, with an infiltrative growth arranged in a variety of different patterns: glandular, trabecular, cord-like, festoon-like, solid, and single cell, although the glandular pattern predominates (Figure 17-15). The glandular pattern consists of duct-like structures with focal "back-to-back"

NEUROENDOCRINE ADENOMA OF THE MIDDLE EAR—DISEASE FACT SHEET

Definition
- Benign neuroendocrine neoplasm arising in the middle ear

Incidence and Location
- Uncommon (<2% of ear tumors)
- Middle ear

Morbidity and Mortality
- Mastoiditis
- No mortality

Gender and Age Distribution
- Equal gender distribution
- Mean, 5th decade

Clinical Features
- Unilateral conductive hearing loss, pressure, and tinnitus

Prognosis and Treatment
- Excellent, although recurrences/regrowth in ~15%
- Complete surgical excision, including ossicular chain

NEUROENDOCRINE ADENOMA OF THE MIDDLE EAR—PATHOLOGIC FEATURES

Gross Findings
- <1 cm fragmented mass within the middle ear
- Avascular, rubbery, unencapsulated gray-yellow mass

Microscopic Findings
- Many patterns: glandular, ribbon, festoon, solid, single-cell architecture
- "Infiltrative" growth is common
- Dual-cell population: inner luminal cells with eosinophilic cytoplasm and outer, cuboidal/columnar cells with indistinct cytoplasm
- Ovoid, eccentrically placed nuclei with "salt-and-pepper" nuclear chromatin distribution and no nucleoli

Immunohistochemical Features
- Keratin, CAM5.2, CK7 (the latter in luminal cells) positive
- Chromogranin, synaptophysin, CD56, human pancreatic polypeptide, preferentially outer cells

Pathologic Differential Diagnosis
- Ceruminous adenoma, paraganglioma, meningioma, metastatic adenocarcinoma

gland configuration and luminal secretions. The ducts are lined by a dual-cell population composed of an inner (luminal), flattened, slightly more intensely eosinophilic mucinous cell, surrounded by an outer (basal), cuboidal to short columnar neuroendocrine cell with eosinophilic and homogeneous to finely granular cytoplasm and indistinct cytoplasmic borders (Figure 17-16). The nuclei tend to be round to oval, eccentrically placed ("plasmacytoid"), with minimal pleomorphism and "salt-and-pepper" chromatin distribution. Nucleoli are inconspicuous and mitoses are essentially absent.

An "infiltrative" pattern is characterized by small irregular groups and strands of cells in a moderately desmoplastic stroma. This pattern gives the illusion of tumor cells dissecting the collagen bundles in an uncontrolled

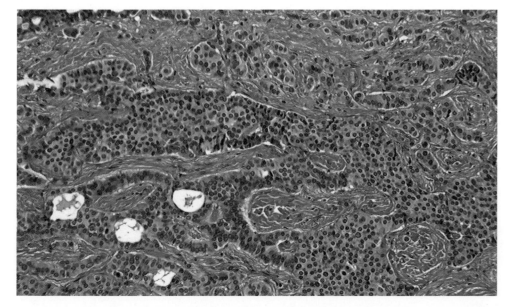

FIGURE 17-15

Neuroendocrine adenoma of the middle ear displaying multiple growth patterns, to include infiltrative (*upper right*), organoid (*upper central*), solid, trabecular, and glandular.

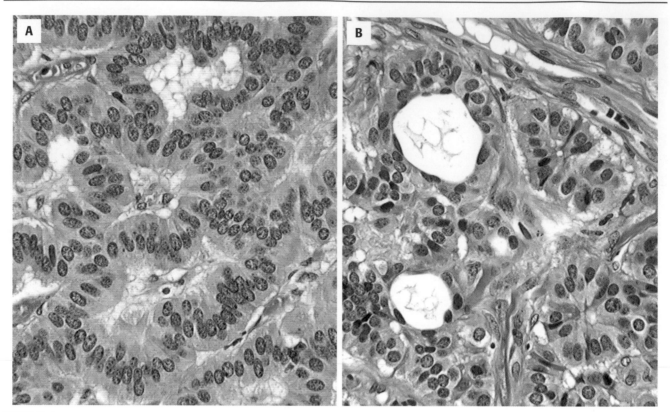

FIGURE 17-16

A, Columnar cells with oval nuclei demonstrating "salt-and-pepper" nuclear chromatin. **B**, Glandular pattern with easily identifiable inner, flattened cellular layer and an outer cuboidal-to-columnar layer. Note the lightly basophilic amorphous material within the lumen.

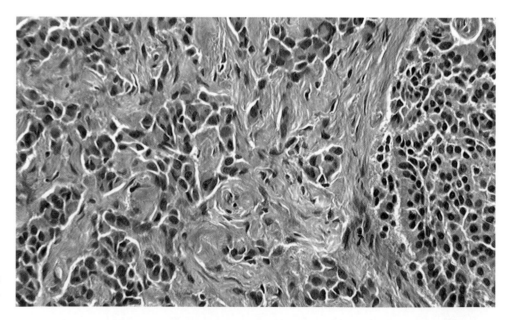

FIGURE 17-17

An "infiltrative" pattern associated with an organoid island in this adenoma. Fibrosis separates the neoplastic cells.

and aggressive fashion (Figure 17-17). The cells tend to be smaller than those within the other patterns and have a higher nuclear:cytoplasmic ratio. However, features of malignancy such as mitotic activity, pleomorphism, necrosis, and destructive invasion into bone, nerves, or lymphovascular spaces are not noted. Additional findings may include a concurrent cholesteatoma.

ANCILLARY STUDIES

ULTRASTRUCTURAL FEATURES

Electron microscopy demonstrates two distinct cell types: (1) apical cells with elongated microvilli and secretory mucus granules (type A cells) and (2) basal cells with neurosecretory granules (type B cells). Transitional forms with features of both cell types have been described.

HISTOCHEMICAL FEATURES

Mucin content can be confirmed in the gland lumen, and rarely within the cytoplasm, by periodic acid–Schiff (PAS) and Alcian blue histochemical stains. A Grimelius stain may demonstrate granular cytoplasmic positivity at the base of the cells (periphery of the acini), corresponding to the location of the neurosecretory granules by electron microscopy.

IMMUNOHISTOCHEMICAL FEATURES

The neoplastic cells have both epithelial and neuroendocrine marker immunoreactivity. These cells stain with a variety of keratin antibodies, including cytokeratin cocktail, CK7, and CAM5.2, although CK7 preferentially highlights the inner (luminal) layer of the glandular cells (Figure 17-18). Neuroendocrine marker immunoreactivity (although not systemic production) includes chromogranin, NSE, synaptophysin, CD56, and CD57 along with various hormone polypeptides (serotonin, glucagon, HPP), preferentially expressed in the outer basal cells. The cells are negative with S100 protein, EMA, GFAP, and TTF-1.

DIFFERENTIAL DIAGNOSIS

Histologically, ceruminous adenoma, paraganglioma, meningioma, and metastatic adenocarcinoma can be included in the differential diagnosis. However, the anatomic site of origin makes this a unique tumor, distinctly separable from the other lesions by histology and immunohistochemistry. Since glandular (mucosal) metaplasia of the middle ear epithelium is common in chronic inflammation, such as otitis media, adenoma would seem to be the benign neoplastic counterpart of this reactive process.

PROGNOSIS AND THERAPY

Complete surgical excision is generally curative and must include the ossicular chain to prevent recurrence. Recurrence (regrowth) is likely to develop in ~15% of patients, especially when the ossicular chain is involved but not removed. Facial nerve paralysis or paresthesias is usually mass-related compression rather than invasion. While controversial, there appears to be no well-documented metastatic potential.

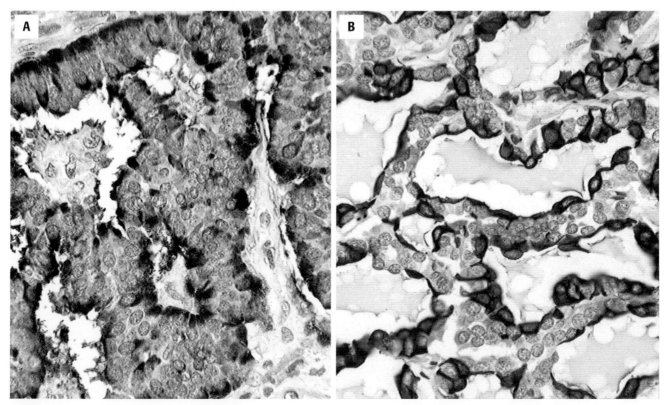

FIGURE 17-18

A, Human pancreatic polypeptide. **B**, CK7. Note the predominantly basilar staining pattern of the human pancreatic polypeptide and the inner, luminal pattern of the CK7.

■ ENDOLYMPHATIC SAC TUMOR

Endolymphatic sac tumor (ELST) is a papillary epithelial neoplasm arising within the endolymphatic sac/duct, showing a high association with von Hippel-Lindau syndrome (VHL). Growth into the middle ear is common. This tumor is intermediate, behaving in more than a benign fashion but not quite a malignant fashion, as there is no metastatic potential.

CLINICAL FEATURES

Approximately 1/35,000 to 40,000 people have VHL, of which ~10% to 15% develop ELSTs. There is a wide age range at presentation, although most patients are between 30 and 40 years, and there is no sex difference. The most common symptoms include ipsilateral hearing loss (sensorineural > conductive, although it can be mixed), tinnitus, facial nerve palsy, and vestibular dysfunction (vertigo, ataxia) resembling Ménière disease.

Many patients report a long history of symptoms, which suggests that these are slow-growing lesions.

Given the strong association with VHL, it is appropriate to assess patients who present with an ELST for the corresponding gene mutation at 3p25-26 involving VHL, which is believed to function as a tumor suppressor gene. Importantly, patients may show signs of VHL at other anatomic sites (e.g., kidney, pancreas, cerebellum). Bilateral tumors are associated with VHL.

RADIOLOGIC FEATURES

The best radiographic studies are a combination of MRI and CT. MRI shows a hyperintense (hypervascular) heterogeneous mass with T1-weighted images, while CT will show a lytic lesion with bone destruction, often with a multilocular appearance centered on the endolymphatic sac (between the internal auditory canal and sigmoid sinus). Tumor expansion into neighboring structures may also be seen.

PATHOLOGIC FEATURES

GROSS FINDINGS

The tumors will frequently expand into the posterior cranial fossa, ranging up to 10 cm in greatest dimension. Older patients tend to have larger tumors.

ENDOLYMPHATIC SAC TUMOR—DISEASE FACT SHEET

Definition
- Papillary epithelial proliferation arising within or near the endolymphatic sac

Incidence and Location
- Rare, strong association with von Hippel-Lindau syndrome (VHL)
- Temporal bone and occasionally middle ear

Morbidity and Mortality
- Locally destructive with nerve damage
- Death may result due to large, destructive lesion in vital area

Gender, Race, and Age Distribution
- Equal gender distribution
- Wide age range, mean between 30 and 40 years

Clinical Features
- Ipsilateral hearing loss, tinnitus, vestibular dysfunction, and facial nerve palsy

Radiologic Features
- MRI: hyperintense heterogeneous mass on T1-weighted images
- CT: lytic, multilocular lesion with bone destruction centered on endolymphatic sac

Prognosis and Treatment
- Good, although dependent on extent of tumor
- Recurrent if not completely excised (difficult due to site)
- Surgery; all patients with VHL should be screened for endolymphatic sac tumors

---

ENDOLYMPHATIC SAC TUMOR—PATHOLOGIC FEATURES

Gross Findings
- Large (up to 10 cm) tumor centered on the endolymphatic sac region

Microscopic Findings
- Unencapsulated with bone invasion
- Coarse, papillary projections into cystic, fluid-filled spaces
- Bland, cuboidal cells with little pleomorphism
- Glands with colloid-like material in lumens

Immunohistochemical Features
- Keratin, CK7, CAM5.2, EMA, and S100 protein immunoreactive
- Thyroglobulin and TTF-1 negative

Genetic Studies
- Germline mutations of the *VHL* tumor suppressor gene (3p25-26)

Pathologic Differential Diagnosis
- Choroid plexus papilloma, metastatic thyroid papillary carcinoma, neuroendocrine adenoma of the middle ear, metastatic adenocarcinoma (lung, kidney, and colon)

MICROSCOPIC FINDINGS

The tumors are unencapsulated, locally destructive lesions with "bone invasion" commonly identified. The classic histologic appearance consists of a cystically dilated cavity with coarse, interdigitating, papillary projections (Figure 17-19). Fibrovascular cores are seen within these papillae, which are lined by a single layer of low cuboidal to columnar epithelial cells (Figure 17-20), similar to the normal endolymphatic sac lining. These cells contain uniformly round to oval nuclei with coarse nuclear chromatin deposition and eosinophilic, granular cytoplasm with indistinct cell membranes. A histologic similarity to thyroid follicles is common (Figure 17-21), with dilated glands containing secretions. Pleomorphism, mitotic figures, and necrosis are absent.

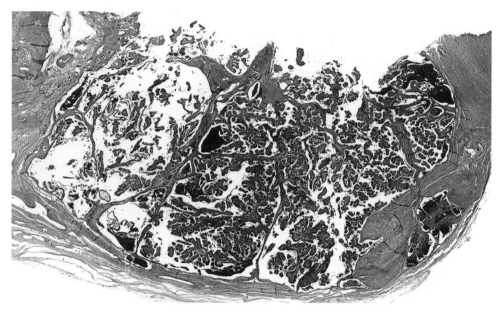

FIGURE 17-19

There is a very complex papillary architecture to this endolymphatic sac tumor.

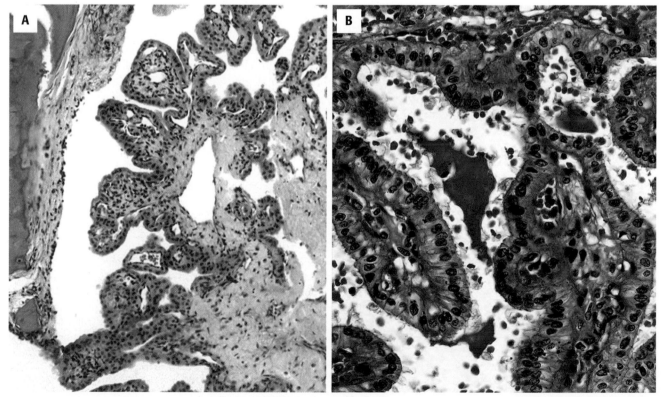

FIGURE 17-20

A, Complex, although broad papillae within a cystic cavity adjacent to bone. **B,** A single layer of cuboidal cells with small, hyperchromatic nuclei lines the papillary projections.

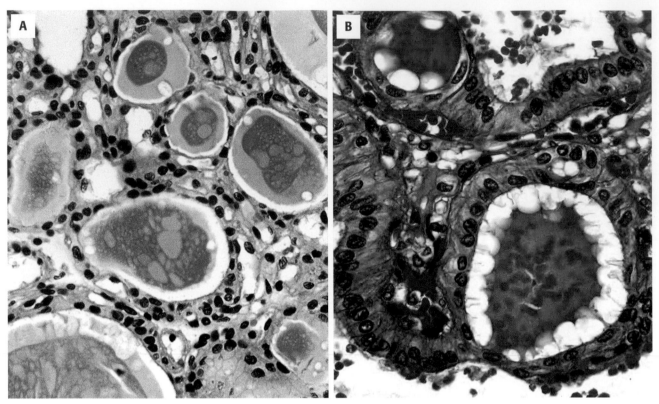

FIGURE 17-21

A and **B**, There are acini with eosinophilic secretions resembling thyroid gland follicles with colloid. However, TTF-1 and thyroglobulin would be negative.

ANCILLARY STUDIES

IMMUNOHISTOCHEMICAL FEATURES

Cytokeratin, CK7, CAM5.2, EMA, and S100 protein are immunoreactive, although the latter two are often focal and weak. GFAP may occasionally be weakly positive, while thyroglobulin and TTF-1 are always negative.

GENETIC STUDIES

Germline mutations of the VHL tumor suppressor gene (3p25-26) are usually detected in these patients, although sporadic cases may lack such abnormalities. *VHL* has multiple functions, including the upregulation of the hypoxic response (via hypoxia inducible factor [*HIF*]-1 alpha). Mutations prevent production of any functional VHL protein or result in a change of structure of VHL protein. Since individuals who have inherited one mutated copy have such a high probability of developing a second mutation in the other allele (the "two-hit" hypothesis), the inheritance pattern is autosomal dominant.

DIFFERENTIAL DIAGNOSIS

A choroid plexus papilloma is generally confined to the mid-line and is not associated with destruction of the temporal bone. Metastatic carcinomas can be distinguished with the help of immunohistochemistry. For example, reactivity with thyroglobulin and/or TTF-1 confirms a metastatic papillary thyroid carcinoma. Metastatic renal cell carcinoma (clear cell type) is usually not papillary, shows a greater degree of pleomorphism, and has extravasated erythrocytes in a pseudoalveolar pattern. In most cases, it will be immunoreactive with CD10 and PAX8. NAME is a biphasic tumor with neuroendocrine immunophenotype and does not have a papillary architecture.

PROGNOSIS AND THERAPY

Surgery is the treatment of choice and is often radical in order to completely remove the lesion, given its tendency toward infiltrative, destructive growth. Nonetheless, surgery is performed with the goal of preserving hearing. All patients with VHL should be radiographically screened for ELSTs, as the incidence can be high (up to 20%). The prognosis is dependent on the extent of the disease, with death occasionally reported due to destruction of vital structures, as a result of the indolent but progressive course.

SUGGESTED READINGS

The complete suggested readings list is available online at www.expertconsult.com.

18

Malignant Neoplasms of the Ear and Temporal Bone

■ **Lester D. R. Thompson**

■ SQUAMOUS CELL CARCINOMA (EXTERNAL AND MIDDLE EAR)

Squamous cell carcinoma (SCC) is a malignant tumor of squamous keratinocytes. Ultraviolet radiation is considered etiologic for external ear lesions, while chronic inflammation (otitis media) may be associated with middle ear tumors.

CLINICAL FEATURES

SQUAMOUS CELL CARCINOMA (EXTERNAL AND MIDDLE EAR)—DISEASE FACT SHEET

Definition
- An invasive epithelial tumor with squamous differentiation (keratinocytes)

Incidence and Location
- Common tumor (similar frequency to basal cell carcinoma)
- Pinna, external canal, and middle ear

Gender, Race, and Age Distribution
- Male > female (3:1)
- Elderly patients

Clinical Features
- Mass lesion, often with ulceration
- Pain, hearing loss and drainage of blood or pus (middle ear/external auditory canal)
- Tumor plaque, polypoid mass or ulcer with everted edges
- Obstructed external canal

Prognosis and Treatment
- Dependent on stage of disease, but usually good for external ear lesions while less so for EAC tumors
- Recurrences are common
- Death is usually due to intracranial extension
- Surgical excision and/or irradiation

The majority of SCCs of the external ear arise in older patients, with men affected much more commonly than women. The tumor arises on the pinna most frequently, with a lesser number in the external auditory canal (EAC). Lesions of the pinna are identified early due to their prominent position. In contrast, a serious problem with canal and middle ear lesions is the delay in diagnosis because of the minimal symptoms that may be present. The pinna SCCs can display a plaque-like or even polypoid mass and may become ulcerated with everted edges in the later stages (Figure 18-1).

The canal lesions present as a mass, sometimes warty, occluding the lumen and often invading deeply into the surrounding tissues (bone and internal auditory meatus). Patients present with hearing loss, discharge, bleeding, and/or pain. In the later stages, there may be dissolution of the tympanic membrane with invasion into the middle ear. Entry into the middle ear is also possible, however, in the presence of an intact tympanic membrane if the tumor passes posteriorly from the canal into the mastoid air spaces and into the middle ear (Figure 18-2). In a few cases, more often seen in younger patients, the neoplasm remains confined to the middle ear. Interestingly, concomitant cholesteatoma is usually not found.

PATHOLOGIC FEATURES

GROSS FINDINGS

The gross appearance ranges from papules to nodules to plaque-like lesions, which may be exophytic, ulcerated, or hemorrhagic.

MICROSCOPIC FINDINGS

SCC of the external ear usually shows origin from the epidermis and demonstrates significant keratinization. As at any other site, SCC is separated into well, moderately,

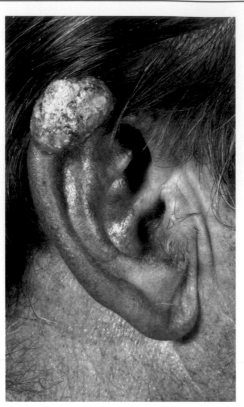

FIGURE 18-1

An oval plaque with early ulceration and exudate on the surface of this squamous cell carcinoma of the pinna.

SQUAMOUS CELL CARCINOMA (EXTERNAL AND MIDDLE EAR)—PATHOLOGIC FEATURES

Gross Findings

- Nodular or plaque-like mass arising from skin
- Invasion of elastic cartilage

Microscopic Findings

- Squamous cell carcinoma with invasion of atypical cells
- Well, moderately, or poorly differentiated
- Keratinizing or nonkeratinizing
- Multiple patterns of growth, perhaps with perineural invasion
- Stromal response with desmoplasia and inflammation
- Variant patterns may have higher risk of recurrence/death

Immunohistochemical Features

- CK5/6, CK903 (34βE12), p63, and EGFR positive
- Ber-Ep4 negative (positive in basal cell carcinoma)

Pathologic Differential Diagnosis

- Basal cell carcinoma, normal middle ear corpuscles, reactive conditions, metastatic carcinoma, atypical fibroxanthoma

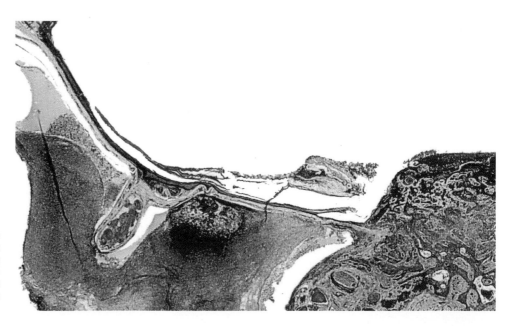

FIGURE 18-2

A low-power temporal bone section shows an intact tympanic membrane with fibrinous and necrotic material resulting from acute inflammation in association with a squamous cell carcinoma at the deep end of the external canal near the eardrum annulus, but not penetrating it.

and poorly differentiated, keratinizing and nonkeratinizing, and in situ versus invasive. The features of SCC in the ear are no different from those of other sites, similarly displaying nests, sheets, and infiltrative cords; keratin pearl formation; atypical keratinization; polarity loss; intercellular bridges; opacified cytoplasm; nuclear chromatin condensation; and increased mitotic figures, including atypical forms (Figure 18-3). Perineural invasion

is associated with a high rate of local recurrence and increased risk of metastasis. Many cases, depending on the site (external ear), will also show actinic changes (secondary to sun exposure), while middle ear tumors may show chronic inflammation or carcinoma in situ. In cases arising deeply within the ear canal, there is often dissolution of the tympanic membrane and a concomitant origin from the middle ear epidermis (squamous

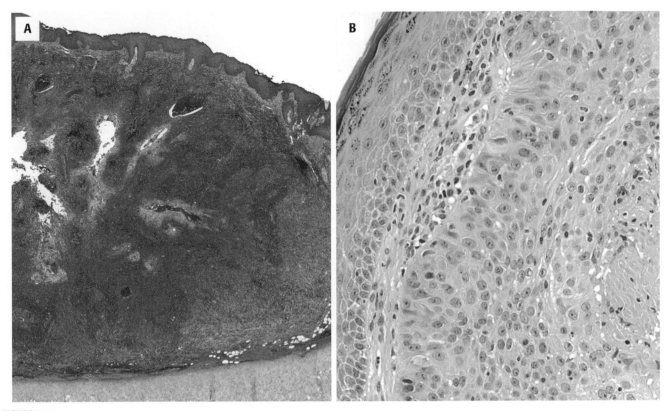

FIGURE 18-3

A, Invasive squamous cell carcinoma associated with inflammation and extension to the cartilage (lower field). **B**, A well-differentiated invasive tumor, with an area of comedonecrosis.

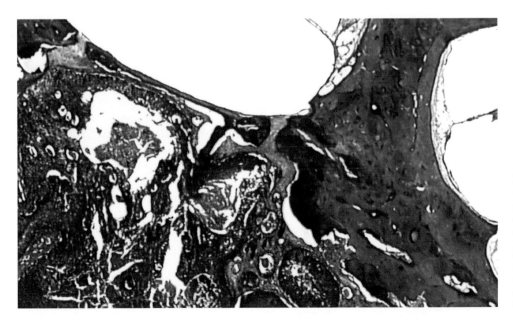

FIGURE 18-4

Low-power view of squamous carcinoma in middle ear showing sparing of otic capsule bone. The vestibule with saccule and utricle lies above. The footplate of the stapes is seen bordering the vestibule below. This thin bony plate is not invaded by the neoplasm. To the right is seen the cochlea, surrounded also by otic capsule bone. There is a little erosion of this bone by adjacent tumor.

metaplasia arising from the simple cuboidal epithelium), although passage into the middle ear is possible without damage to the eardrum (Figure 18-4). An origin directly from middle ear epithelium may also be seen.

Marked desmoplasia or reactive changes, when present, may delay the diagnosis. Other variants arising in this location include verrucous SCC, spindle cell SCC,

adenosquamous carcinoma, and adenoid squamous carcinoma, displaying similar histologic features to those of upper respiratory tract locations. Specifically, high risk patterns include spindle cell/sarcomatoid (Figure 18-5), basaloid, adenosquamous, and desmoplastic SCCs.

While cholesteatoma may be concurrently identified with SCC, SCC does *not* develop from cholesteatoma.

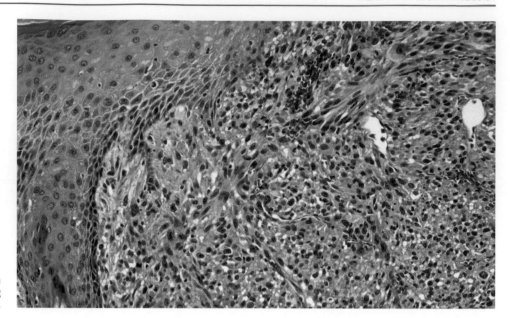

FIGURE 18-5

A spindle-cell squamous cell carcinoma shows association with the overlying surface, and a spindled cell morphology.

Spread of SCC within the middle ear is extremely rare due to the peculiar resistance of the bone of the otic capsule to direct spread of the tumor. Nonetheless, this spread begins with early erosion through the thin bony plate (up to 1 mm thick) that separates the medial wall of the middle ear at its junction with the eustachian tube from the carotid canal. Further extension along the carotid canal eventually allows for easy extension to the sympathetic nerves, making the tumor impossible to eradicate surgically. Additionally, tumor spreads through the bony walls of the posterior mastoid air cells to the dura of the posterior surface of the temporal bone.

ANCILLARY STUDIES

Immunostains are used primarily for poorly differentiated and spindle cell tumors. High-molecular-weight (HMW) cytokeratins 5/6 and 903 (34βE12) are the most sensitive markers for squamous differentiation and, along with p63, help to confirm the diagnosis in these more difficult cases.

DIFFERENTIAL DIAGNOSIS

On the pinna, there may sometimes be difficulty in distinguishing poorly differentiated SCC from basal cell carcinoma (BCC). Invocation of the usual histologic criteria for the diagnosis of the latter should enable definite diagnosis. Moreover, Ber-Ep4 is positive in BCC and negative in SCC. Middle ear corpuscles, concentrically laminated balls of collagen formed on bone-free mastoid air cell partitions, are more common in the elderly and may be difficult to separate from SCC, particularly in frozen sections. However, there is an absence of cells in the laminated corpuscles. An atypical fibroxanthoma (AFX) is usually a large, nodular tumor in heavily sun-damaged skin. There is usually profound pleomorphism, atypical mitoses, and often necrosis. However, AFX is usually negative for HMW cytokeratins and p63, while positive with CD10, CD68, and alpha-1-antitrypsin.

PROGNOSIS AND THERAPY

SCC of the external canal and middle ear is an aggressive disease with a high propensity for local recurrence. Squamous carcinoma of the pinna is less so. In both, the outlook depends on the presenting stage of the disease. Death is usually due to direct intracranial extension. Lymph node metastasis is unusual (<10%) and hematogenous spread even more rare. Optimal therapy is complete surgical excision, which may be achieved by Mohs surgery. However, topical chemotherapeutics or immunomodulators have been successfully used for external ear lesions. In advanced cases, radiation may be used.

If the middle ear is involved, the neoplasm is surgically incurable if either or both (1) the thin plate of bone between the internal carotid artery and the tympanic end of the eustachian tube and (2) the bone in the posterior wall of the mastoid, bordering the posterior cranial fossa, are breached by tumor. In the absence of these features, middle ear squamous carcinoma is often treated by "petrosectomy," which is by no means a resection of the whole petrous bone but rather a subtotal resection or extirpation of the middle ear components involved by tumor.

■ CERUMINOUS ADENOCARCINOMA

Malignant neoplasms derived from the apocrine (ceruminous glands) of the external auditory canal are rare. These neoplasms take the form of adenoid cystic carcinoma, mucoepidermoid carcinoma, and adenocarcinoma, not otherwise specified (NOS).

CLINICAL FEATURES

These rare tumors, arising from the ceruminal glands of the outer one-third to one-half of the external auditory canal, seem to occur more frequently in females than in males (1.5:1). Patients tend to be middle aged at presentation (mean, 49 years). Patients present with pain, a mass, hearing changes (conductive hearing loss), drainage, and/or neurologic deficits. Symptoms are frequently present for an average of 8 to 12 months.

CERUMINOUS ADENOCARCINOMA—DISEASE FACT SHEET

Definition
- Malignant tumor derived from apocrine glands in the cartilaginous part of the external auditory canal

Incidence
- Rare neoplasm

Morbidity and Mortality
- Hearing loss
- Mortality is variable, but ~50% dead from disease

Gender, Race, and Age Distribution
- Female > male (~1.5:1)
- Usually 5th to 6th decades

Clinical Features
- Pain, mass, hearing changes (conductive hearing loss), drainage and/or neurologic deficits

Radiographic Features
- Imaging used to exclude direct extension from parotid gland or nasopharynx

Prognosis and Treatment
- Overall, 50% at 5 years
- Frequent recurrences, direct invasion of the brain, and metastasis (lung) will often result in death
- Wide, radical resection and/or radiation

RADIOLOGIC FEATURES

Imaging studies are usually recommended to help exclude direct extension from the parotid gland or nasopharynx and to define the extent of the tumor for surgical planning.

PATHOLOGIC FEATURES

Ranging up to 3 cm (mean, 1.4 cm) in greatest dimension, these tumors are often polypoid, tend to involve the posterior canal, and are highly invasive (Figure 18-6). Although not arising from the surface epithelium, there is frequent surface epithelial involvement. Histologically, these tumors are cellular and may be arranged in a variety of different patterns: solid, cystic, cribriform, glandular, and even single cell. Uncommonly, a dual-cell population is noted but is not the dominant histology. There is usually cellular pleomorphism, with nuclear variability and prominent nucleoli. Regardless of subtype, these tumors infiltrate into the surrounding soft tissue, benign ceruminous glands, and even cartilage or bone. Perineural invasion and central comedonecrosis (Figure 18-7), features only identified in carcinoma, may be seen.

As previously mentioned, these tumors are separated into three main subtypes: (1) ceruminous adenocarcinoma, NOS; (2) ceruminous adenoid cystic carcinoma; and (3) ceruminous mucoepidermoid carcinoma (not further discussed). *Ceruminous adenocarcinoma, NOS* may be recognized by the eosinophilic

---

CERUMINOUS ADENOCARCINOMA—PATHOLOGIC FEATURES

Microscopic Findings
- Tumors are often polypoid, mean 1.4 cm
- Tumors are infiltrative with epithelial ulceration
- Range from solid to cystic, glandular or cribriform
- Increased cellularity, nuclear pleomorphism, prominent nucleoli, mitotic figures
- Cerumen granules (pigment) not present in carcinoma
- Necrosis and perineural invasion uncommon, but diagnostic of carcinoma
- Adenoid cystic type usually displays the characteristic cribriform pattern with a tendency to perineural infiltration

Immunohistochemical Features
- Keratin, CK7, and CD117 highlight luminal cells
- p63, CK5/6, and S100 protein highlight basal cells if present

Pathologic Differential Diagnosis
- Metastatic adenocarcinoma, direct extension from salivary gland carcinoma, benign ceruminous adenomas

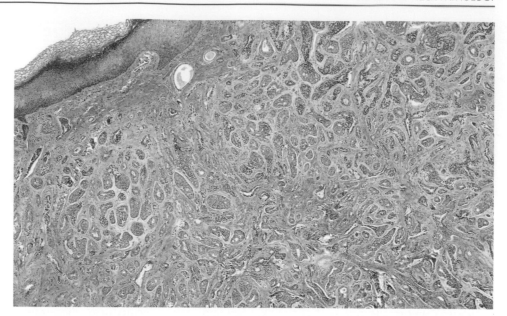

FIGURE 18-6

An invasive ceruminous adenocarcinoma is seen in association with dense fibrosis in the external auditory canal.

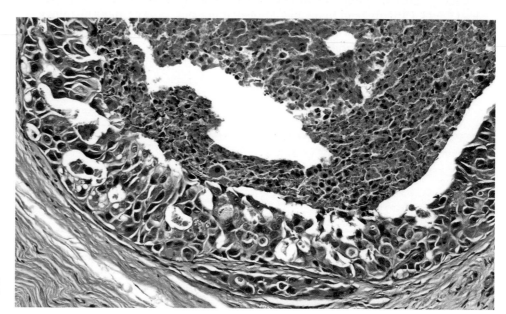

FIGURE 18-7

A high-grade ceruminous adenocarcinoma with central comedo-type necrosis. Severe nuclear pleomorphism is noted.

character of the tumor cells and increased mitotic figures, including atypical forms. Notably, the apocrine-type secretion and myoepithelial layer characteristic of benign ceruminous adenomas are not usually present in the malignant form. Moreover, the ceroid (cerumen, wax) pigment granules normally found in the cytoplasm of benign ceruminous glands are also conspicuously absent (Figure 18-8). The *ceruminous adenoid cystic carcinoma* subtype shows identical features to the same lesion growing from major and minor salivary glands and is therefore composed of masses of small cells with hyperchromatic, carrot-shaped nuclei, surrounding punched-out round spaces containing a basophilic secretion and reduplicated basement membrane (Figure 18-9).

ANCILLARY STUDIES

Immunohistochemistry may highlight the basal cells (p63, CK5/6, S100 protein) if they are present, while the luminal tumor cells are uniquely CK7 and preferentially CD117 positive.

DIFFERENTIAL DIAGNOSIS

The most important aspect of the differential diagnosis is to exclude direct invasion from a parotid gland primary, best achieved through careful imaging.

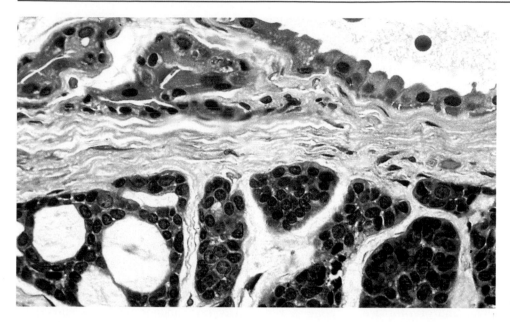

FIGURE 18-8

Benign apocrine ceruminous glands are seen above an adenoid cystic carcinoma, which is composed of small cells arranged in a cribriform pattern. Note the yellow, ceroid pigment granules within the normal ceruminous glands.

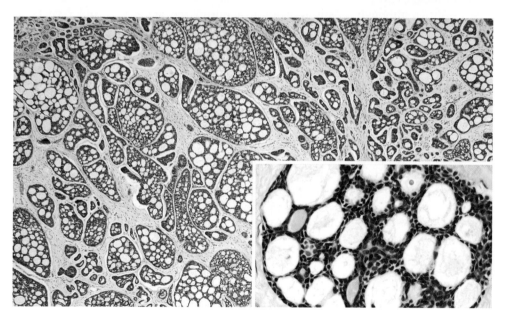

FIGURE 18-9

Multiple patterns are seen in adenoid cystic carcinoma, including the cribriform pattern (*inset*), composed of punched-out spaces filled with blue-pink amorphous material.

Metastatic adenocarcinomas (discussed later) may also be raised in the differential diagnosis, but a clinical history and unique histology should make the distinction. Separation from ceruminous adenoma is difficult on small biopsy. However, carcinomas are invasive, have pleomorphism and mitotic figures, and lack ceroid.

PROGNOSIS AND THERAPY

A wide, radical (complete) resection is required, especially for the adenoid cystic carcinoma type. Radiation is used only for palliation and usually for cases of ceruminous

adenocarcinoma, NOS and mucoepidermoid carcinoma. Multiple recurrences (especially if the margins are positive) and metastasis (lung rather than lymph nodes) may be seen. The overall prognosis is ~50% at 5 years.

■ METASTATIC NEOPLASMS

Excluding neoplasms that directly invade from a contiguous site into the ear, metastatic tumors spread via blood or lymphatic channels from a noncontiguous site. Lymphomas and leukemias, as systemic diseases, are excluded by definition. Metastases to the ear and temporal bone generally occur late in the course of the cancer producing the metastases. While unusual in surgical pathology material during life, autopsy studies show temporal bone involvement in ~20% of patients, virtually all of whom also had disseminated malignant disease.

CLINICAL FEATURES

Patients tend to be older and females are more frequently affected than males, although this is dependent on tumor type. Most lesions that metastasize to the ear and temporal bone are carcinomas and melanomas, with few sarcomas identified. Presentation is often late in the underlying disease course. Most patients are asymptomatic but may present with hearing loss, dizziness, tinnitus, facial palsy, otalgia, and/or otorrhea. Tumors are usually bilateral and multifocal. The petrous apex is the most common site (~80%), although the mastoid bone, internal auditory canal, and middle ear can also be affected.

PATHOLOGIC FEATURES

Tumors that develop as a consequence of hematogenous spread (lymphovascular invasion) include breast

(~25%; Figure 18-10), lung (~10%), kidney, gastrointestinal tract (Figure 18-11), prostate (~10%), and melanoma (~6%). Virtually any tumor, including mesenchymal tumors, can metastasize to this location. In general, metastatic deposits maintain the phenotype of the primary. Rarely are the ear and temporal bone metastases the initial presentation of the disease, and consequently an extensive clinical or histologic workup is seldom necessary. Direct extension from the parotid gland region (Figure 18-12), eustachian tube, posterior fossa (skull), and external ear may also have been seen.

ANCILLARY STUDIES

Since primary adenocarcinoma of the ear and temporal bone is vanishingly rare, adenocarcinomas should be presumed to be metastatic. Selective use of immunostains helps to confirm the metastasis and reveal the tissue of origin. In general, it is important to consider how primary ear lesions may react and to use this as a point of comparison or exclusion.

DIFFERENTIAL DIAGNOSIS

A poorly differentiated ear primary may mimic a metastatic tumor. Separation is often achieved by careful examination of architectural and histologic features, judicious use of immunohistochemistry, and correlation with clinical history and radiographic studies.

METASTATIC NEOPLASMS—DISEASE FACT SHEET

Definition
- Metastatic tumors spread by blood or lymphatic channels from noncontiguous sites (not direct invasion from adjacent neoplasms)

Incidence and Location
- About 20% of patients with disseminated malignant tumors will have ear/temporal bone metastasis
- Petrous apex most common (80%)

Gender, Race, and Age Distribution
- Gender differences based on primary site
- Usually older patients with widely disseminated disease

Clinical Features
- Usually asymptomatic
- Hearing loss, tinnitus, vertigo, facial palsy, otalgia, otorrhea
- Tumors usually bilateral and multifocal

Prognosis and Treatment
- Generally poor outcome reflecting underlying stage of primary tumor
- Surgery for symptomatic relief, with adjuvant therapy for palliation

---

METASTATIC NEOPLASMS—PATHOLOGIC FEATURES

Microscopic
- Primary adenocarcinoma is vanishingly rare, so metastasis should be excluded first
- Main sources are carcinomas of breast, lung, kidney, gastrointestinal tract, prostate, thyroid, larynx
- Melanoma and mesenchymal tumors also seen
- Histology mimics primary tumor

Immunohistochemical Features
- Selected and pertinent to primary site

Pathologic Differential Diagnosis
- Ceruminous adenocarcinoma, direct invasion from adjacent sites/organs, primary ear adenocarcinoma

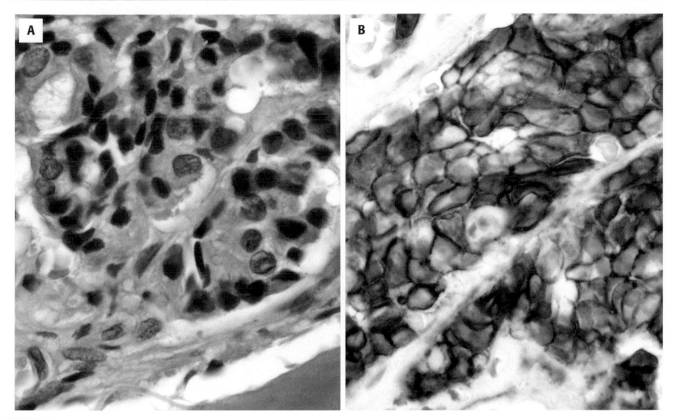

FIGURE 18-10

A, A metastatic breast carcinoma within the temporal bone. Gland formation is prominent. **B**, HER-2/neu immunoreactivity may help to support a diagnosis of breast carcinoma.

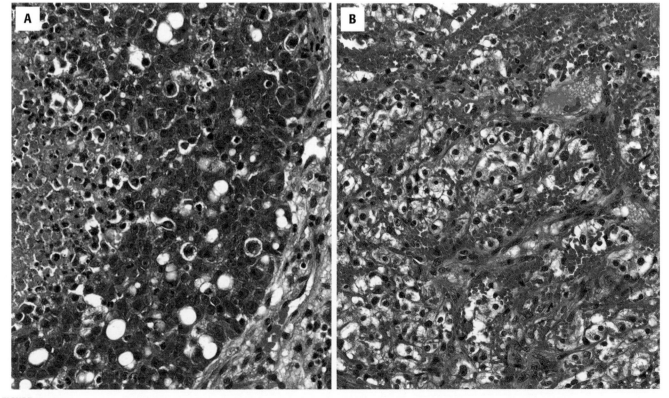

FIGURE 18-11

A, Metastatic colon adenocarcinoma usually has a different histologic appearance than primary ear/temporal bone tumors. **B**, Metastatic renal cell carcinoma, clear cell type, shows a pseudoalveolar architecture with extravasated erythrocytes.

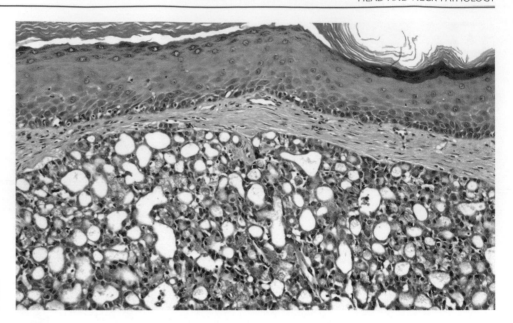

FIGURE 18-12
Direct infiltration into the ear canal from an acinic cell carcinoma of the parotid gland. Note the intact surface epithelium.

PROGNOSIS AND THERAPY

The overall prognosis matches the underlying disease; however, ear metastasis generally occurs in the setting of disseminated disease and, thus, portends a relatively poor prognosis. Surgery may be of value in selected cases for symptomatic relief, while adjuvant therapy can occasionally have a palliative effect.

SUGGESTED READINGS

The complete suggested readings list is available online at www.expertconsult.com.

19

Non-Neoplastic Lesions of the Neck (Soft Tissue, Bone, and Lymph Node)

■ **Jennifer L. Hunt**

■ BRANCHIAL CLEFT ANOMALIES

When the name "branchial cyst" is used without further qualifications, it generally refers to a cyst of second branchial cleft origin (see Chapter 16 for first branchial cleft anomalies), which accounts for 80% to 90% of all branchial anomalies. Branchial cleft cysts constitute 17% of all congenital cervical cysts in children and encompass branchial cysts, sinuses, and/or fistulas.

CLINICAL FEATURES

Patients usually present with a painless mass measuring up to 6 cm. The location is dependent on the cleft origin, and second cleft anomalies are characteristically located along the anterior border of the sternocleidomastoid muscle, from the hyoid bone to the suprasternal notch. There is no gender difference and 75% of patients are between 20 to 40 years at the time of diagnosis. The cysts are usually nontender masses, unless they become secondarily inflamed or infected. They may be bilateral, especially when associated with congenital syndromes.

RADIOLOGIC FEATURES

The radiology will characteristically show a well-circumscribed cystic mass with a smooth cavity and a dense wall (Figure 19-1).

PATHOLOGIC FEATURES

GROSS FINDINGS

Grossly, the cysts are unilocular and between 2 to 6 cm in diameter and usually contain clear to grumous material (Figure 19-1).

BRANCHIAL CLEFT ANOMALIES—DISEASE FACT SHEET

Definition
- A lateral cervical cyst that results from congenital/developmental defects arising from the primitive 2nd branchial apparatus

Incidence and Location
- 17% of all congenital cervical cysts
- Lateral neck, with most near the mandibular angle

Gender, Race, and Age Distribution
- Equal gender distribution
- 75% of patients are 20 to 40 years
- Only 1% occur in patients >50 years

Clinical Features
- Mass along the anterior border of the sternocleidomastoid muscle
- Painless mass of long duration
- May become secondarily infected, which will bring it to clinical attention

Prognosis and Treatment
- Complete excision
- Recurrence rate 2.7%

MICROSCOPIC FINDINGS

A branchial cleft cyst is usually lined by stratified squamous epithelium (90%), occasionally by respiratory epithelium (8%), or, rarely, by both (2%) (Figure 19-2). Lymphoid aggregates with or without reactive germinal centers are found beneath the epithelial lining in ~70% to 85% of cysts (Figure 19-3). However, as no true lymph node architecture is present, there will not be sinuses, medullary region, or interfollicular zones. Keratinaceous debris may be present within the cavity. Acute and chronic inflammation, foreign body giant cell reaction, and fibrosis are secondary changes in the wall of the cyst.

451

BRANCHIAL CLEFT ANOMALIES—PATHOLOGIC FEATURES

Gross Findings

- Cystic mass containing fluid up to 6 cm

Microscopic Findings

- Cysts lined by squamous epithelium (90%), respiratory (8%), or both (2%)
- Keratinaceous debris
- Lymphoid tissue nodular or diffuse (70% to 85%)
- Fibrosis and secondary changes

Fine Needle Aspiration

- Mature squamous epithelium
- Anucleate squames
- Debris, including macrophages
- Lymphoid infiltrate

Immunohistochemical Features

- Keratin positive (type dependent on lining)
- *Negative* with p16 and GLUT-1

Pathologic Differential Diagnosis

- Metastatic cystic squamous cell carcinoma, thymic cyst, bronchial cyst, thyroglossal duct cyst

ANCILLARY STUDIES

IMMUNOHISTOCHEMICAL FEATURES

The epithelial lining expresses cytokeratin of different types depending on the type of lining—pseudostratified respiratory, transitional, stratified keratinizing, or non-keratinizing. However, for the most part, p16 and GLUT-1 (glucose transporter 1) are negative in branchial cleft cyst; both of these markers can be positive in metastatic cystic squamous cell carcinoma. p16 may be focally reactive in areas of intraepithelial lymphocyte penetration in branchial cleft cysts.

FINE NEEDLE ASPIRATION

Fine needle aspiration (FNA) of a branchial cleft cyst will yield a thick, yellow, pus-like material, which microscopically is composed of anucleate squames, amorphous debris and macrophages, and variable lymphoid cells (Figure 19-4). Viable mature squamous epithelial cells and occasionally columnar respiratory epithelial cells are often noted. Epithelial atypia should not be present, and, in the right clinical setting, atypia would suggest potential malignancy.

DIFFERENTIAL DIAGNOSIS

Thymic cysts contain thymic tissue within the wall, including Hassall corpuscles (concentric island of squamous cells with central keratinization) (Figure 19-5). A *thyroglossal duct cyst* occurs in the midline and is associated with thyroid tissue. *Bronchial cysts* are more common in the subcutaneous tissue of the supraclavicular region and are lined by respiratory mucosa with smooth muscle and bronchial glands in the wall. *Dermoid cyst* can also be in the differential, although these will present in a midline location and, histologically, will show adnexal structures within the wall. The most important differential diagnostic consideration, however, particularly if the lesion is

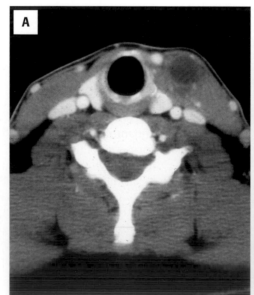
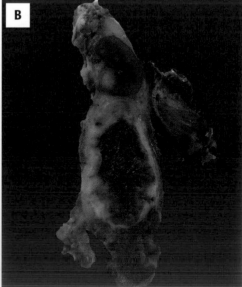

FIGURE 19-1

A, A computed tomography scan demonstrating a second branchial cleft cyst anterior to the sternocleidomastoid muscle. There is thickening of the capsule with cystic fluid. **B**, There is a thick, fibrous connective tissue wall surrounding a cyst, filled with material. Note the benign lymph node above the cyst.

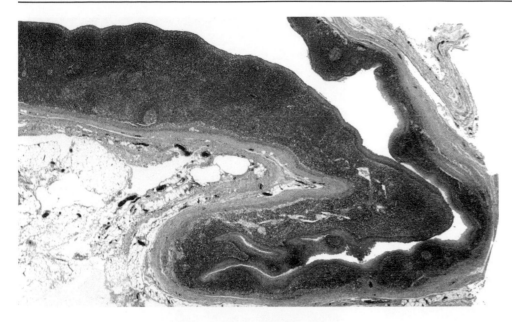

FIGURE 19-2

There is a unilocular cyst, lined by a very thin and well-defined squamous lining in this branchial cleft cyst. The epithelial lining is subtended by a rich inflammatory infiltrate, with lymphoid germinal center formation.

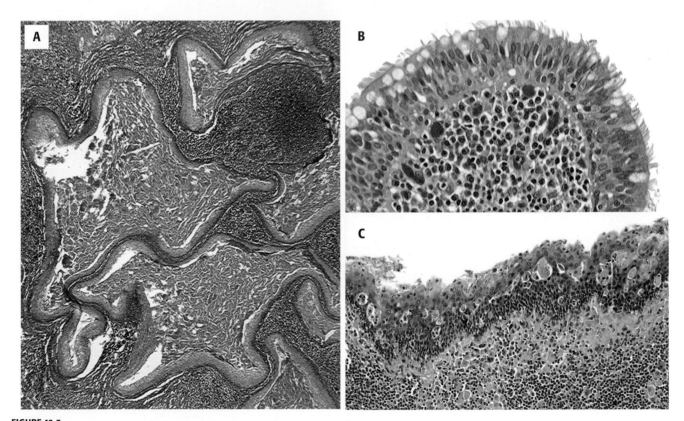

FIGURE 19-3

A, A branchial cleft cyst is often filled with keratinaceous debris. The cyst can be lined by stratified, ciliated columnar epithelium (**B**) or squamous epithelium (**C**).

in an adult, is *metastatic cystic squamous cell carcinoma*. These lesions usually have a malignant epithelial lining and may be positive for GLUT-1, p16, and human papillomavirus (HPV) (by immunohistochemistry or in situ hybridization), especially when the primary tumor is from the oropharynx (see Chapter 9).

PROGNOSIS AND THERAPY

The recurrence rate is 2.7% for cases with no history of infection or prior surgery. However, recurrence is more common in second operations or when the lesion is infected at the time of operation (14% and 21%, respectively). A complete excision of the cyst is indicated.

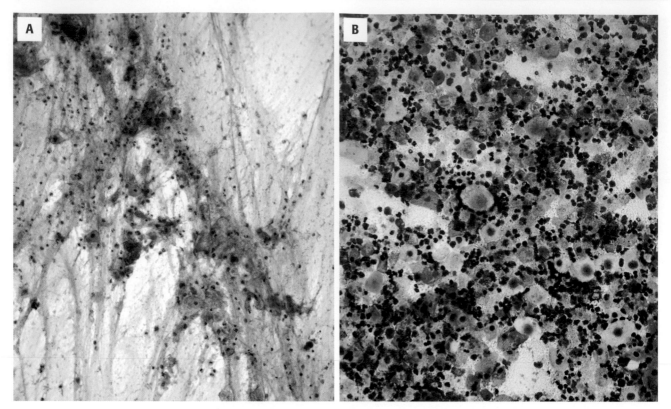

FIGURE 19-4
Keratinaceous debris with inflammatory cells are diagnostic for a branchial cleft cyst in fine needle aspiration smears, as long as there is no atypia in the epithelial component. **A**, Alcohol-fixed, Papanicolaou-stained smear. **B**, Air-dried, Diff-Quik–stained smear.

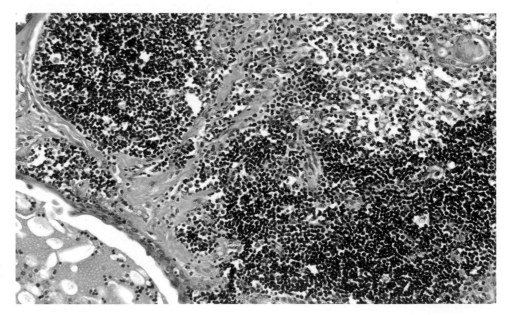

FIGURE 19-5
The wall of a thymic cyst contains lymphoid aggregates, fat, and Hassall corpuscle; these findings may sometimes mimic a branchial cleft cyst.

■ CAT SCRATCH DISEASE (GRANULOMATOUS INFLAMMATION)

Many infectious agents can affect the skin, soft tissues, and lymph nodes of the neck. Cat scratch disease (CSD) (cat scratch fever, cat scratch adenitis, Debre syndrome, Foshay-Mollaret syndrome) will be highlighted as a single example. CSD is a zoonotic infection caused by any one of a group of rickettsial microorganisms of the alpha-2 subgroup of alpha-protobacteria, specifically *Bartonella henselae,* with some taxonomic overlap with *Afipia felis* and *B. quintana. B. henselae* is a gram-negative pleomorphic rod-shaped bacillus. CSD occurs worldwide and is more common in autumn and winter, especially in dwellings where cats are kept as pets.

CLINICAL FEATURES

The characteristic clinical syndrome consists of an initial lesion that develops at the site of inoculation followed by enlargement of regional lymph nodes. The primary lesion, a cat scratch or bite, will cause skin erythema within 3 to 5 days and may be slightly painful (in some cases, this initial injury goes unnoticed). Within 3 weeks of inoculation, acute regional lymphadenopathy develops proximal to the inoculation site. The affected nodes are those that drain the primary lesion and they become enlarged and tender; occasionally, they drain to the surface, forming a fistula. Lymphadenopathy involves only one nodal region in ~85% of patients, while matted, suppurative lymph nodes are seen in ~15% of patients. Constitutional symptoms may be present and include a low-grade fever, headaches, and malaise. Most infections are in children and young adults usually <21 years. In general, most cases are self-limited, and resolve within 3 to 4 months, although lymphadenitis may persist for years. Atypical presentations include ocular, neurologic, or visceral organ involvement. Erythema nodosum, an erythematous nodular panniculitis associated with a variety of conditions, is seen in only 2% of patients. Serology for *B. henselae* antibodies does not work well, while culture is difficult to perform due to the organism's fastidious and slow growth using brain-heart infusion agar with incubation at 32° C.

PATHOLOGIC FEATURES

GROSS FINDINGS

The lymph nodes are soft and swollen and have foci of necrosis on the cut surface. They measure up to 10 cm.

MICROSCOPIC FINDINGS

The histology can be divided into three stages of progression. Histologically, early lesions show foci of swollen capillaries, which have a pink hyaline appearance and are associated with lymphoid follicular hyperplasia. As the foci of suppuration grow, they coalesce to form

---

CAT SCRATCH DISEASE (GRANULOMATOUS INFLAMMATION)—DISEASE FACT SHEET

Definition
- A zoonotic infection caused by a group of gram-negative rickettsial bacillus organisms, specifically *Bartonella henselae, Afipia felis,* and *B. quintana*

Incidence and Location
- Worldwide, most common in autumn and winter
- Found especially in dwellings where cats are kept as pets

Morbidity and Mortality
- No mortality unless patients are immunosuppressed

Gender, Race, and Age Distribution
- Equal gender distribution
- Children and young adults between 3 and 21 years (majority <18 years)

Clinical Features
- Usually associated with a cat scratch or bite
- Solitary, tender lymphadenopathy
- Constitutional symptoms including low-grade fever, malaise, and headaches

Prognosis and Treatment
- Excellent prognosis
- Supportive therapy is adequate, although ciprofloxacin has been advocated by a few
- Excision and drainage, plus antibiotics, may yield best overall results

---

CAT SCRATCH DISEASE (GRANULOMATOUS INFLAMMATION)—PATHOLOGIC FEATURES

Gross Findings
- Enlarged, swollen lymph nodes with areas of necrosis

Microscopic Findings
- Three stages of progression are generally identified:
- Early stage shows follicular hyperplasia
- Stellate abscess surrounded by histiocytes, epithelioid cells, and occasionally giant cells
- Late stage shows granulomas with central caseation

Fine Needle Aspiration
- Granulomatous inflammation with epithelioid histiocytes and occasional giant cells
- Lymphoid infiltrate
- Necrotic debris, depending on stage

Special Techniques
- Warthin-Starry stain for rod-shaped organisms
- Immunoperoxidase stain
- DNA primer for use with polymerase chain reaction
- Culture using brain-heart agar at 32° C

Pathologic Differential Diagnosis
- Primarily infectious agents (brucellosis, tuberculosis, lymphogranuloma venereum)
- May also resemble other reactive nodal conditions, including Kikuchi-Fujimoto disease
- Lymphoma

stellate abscesses (Figure 19-6), which become surrounded by histiocytes, epithelioid cells, and occasionally giant cells (Figure 19-7). Eventually, a granulomatous perimeter surrounding a central area of caseation remains. The casseous center, unlike the center of tuberculosis lesions, is rarely calcified. Obviously, these changes are nonspecific, requiring additional studies to document the causative agent.

ANCILLARY STUDIES

HISTOCHEMISTRY

Tissue Gram stain will demonstrate the bacillus, but a Warthin-Starry silver impregnation technique stains the 1 to 3 μm pleomorphic bacteria black, highlighting the organisms in the wall of the vessels in the early stages and in the suppurative areas in the latter stages (Figure 19-8). Stains are often difficult to interpret because of high background staining in the necrotic debris.

FINE NEEDLE ASPIRATION

The features on FNA are those of a granulomatous inflammation and are nonspecific. Epithelioid histiocytes, Langhans-type giant cells, inflammatory cells, and debris are present to a variable degree depending on stage (Figure 19-9). However, additional studies, including culture and/or special studies, are necessary to confirm the diagnosis.

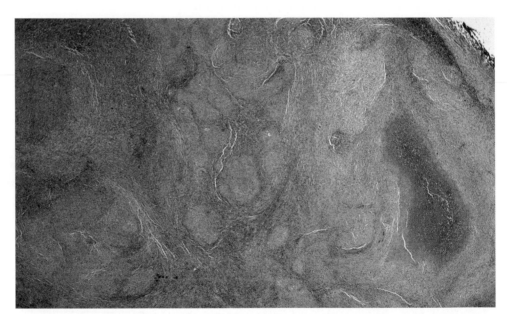

FIGURE 19-6

The characteristic stellate abscess has central necrosis surrounded by granulomatous reaction and inflammatory cells in this case of cat scratch disease.

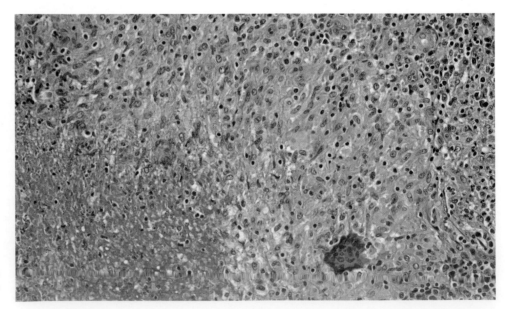

FIGURE 19-7

Epithelioid histiocytes form a palisade around an area of caseating necrosis. A single giant cell is present.

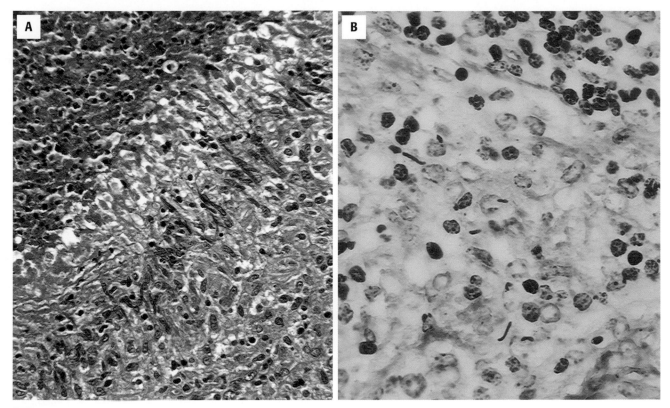

FIGURE 19-8

A, Epithelioid histiocytes palisaded around the periphery of an area of caseating necrosis. **B**, Black, rod-shaped organisms accentuated with the Warthin-Starry silver impregnation stain.

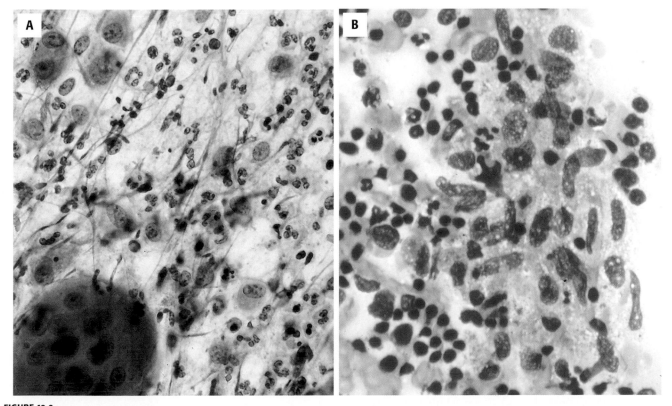

FIGURE 19-9

A fine needle aspiration usually demonstrates granulomatous-type inflammation with epithelioid histiocytes, giant cells, and mixed inflammation. **A**, Alcohol-fixed, Papanicolaou-stained smear. **B**, Air-dried, Diff-Quik–stained smear.

IMMUNOHISTOCHEMICAL FEATURES

An indirect immunoperoxidase stain has been developed to demonstrate the organisms. However, it is capricious, requiring a specific volume of cases to achieve quality, reproducible results, so it is not of much practical use.

ADDITIONAL STUDIES

DNA primers have been developed for use with a polymerase chain reaction for evaluation of CSD.

DIFFERENTIAL DIAGNOSIS

Stellate abscesses, characteristic of CSD, are also seen in a broad range of *infectious etiologies*, including mycobacterial infections, fungal infections, toxoplasmosis, tularemia, brucellosis, leishmaniasis, chancroid, granuloma inguinale, and lymphogranuloma. However, many of these are exceedingly rare or nonexistent in the head and neck region or have very specific culture findings. *Metastatic disease* will show neoplastic cells with areas of necrosis, while *lymphoma* will show specific atypical lymphoid elements with ancillary studies supporting monoclonality. *Sarcoid* shows tight, well-formed, small granulomas without necrosis, while a *branchial cleft cyst* usually lacks granulomatous or suppurative inflammation. *Kikuchi-Fujimoto disease* is a histiocytic necrotizing lymphadenitis characterized by crescentic histiocytes and marked karyorrhectic debris without neutrophils. Most helpful in diagnosing CSD is a high index of suspicion based on the clinical history leading to the demonstration of bacilli by silver impregnation or by culture.

PROGNOSIS AND THERAPY

The prognosis is excellent with supportive treatment alone. Antibiotics are generally not required to relieve symptoms, but ciprofloxacin has been advocated by a few. Excision with drainage and antibiotics yields the best overall outcome.

■ NODULAR FASCIITIS

Nodular fasciitis is a mass-forming myofibroblastic proliferation that usually occurs in the subcutaneous tissue and typically displays a tissue culture–like growth pattern. Cranial fasciitis and intravascular fasciitis are histologically related lesions. Nearly 30% of nodular fasciitis will develop in the head and neck.

CLINICAL FEATURES

NODULAR FASCIITIS—DISEASE FACT SHEET

Definition
- A mass-forming myofibroblastic proliferation, usually within subcutaneous tissues

Incidence and Location
- Most common in upper extremities and head and neck

Gender, Race, and Age Distribution
- Equal gender distribution
- Up to 35 years most commonly (rare after 60 years old)

Clinical Features
- Rapidly growing mass of up to 3 weeks' duration
- Usually <3 cm mass
- Neck, orbit, and ear
- Trauma may play an etiologic role

Prognosis and Treatment
- Excellent prognosis with <2% recurrence rate
- Complete surgical excision

Most patients give a history of a rapidly growing mass present for only a short duration (up to 3 weeks). It usually measures <3 cm and almost always <5 cm. Nodular fasciitis is almost always subcutaneous, although occasional cases are intramuscular. The upper extremities and head and neck are the most frequently affected regions. In the latter, it has been reported in the neck, face, orbit, oral cavity, and ear. Nodular fasciitis is more common in children and young adults up to 35 years. It is rare in adults older than 60 years. There is no gender predilection. Trauma is considered an etiologic factor, although the trauma may be slight or of a limited degree (seat belt pushing against the neck; cotton-tipped applicator inserted into the external auditory canal).

RADIOLOGIC FEATURES

Most of the lesions show moderate to strong enhancement on computed tomography and magnetic resonance imaging with preservation of smooth margins.

PATHOLOGIC FEATURES

GROSS FINDINGS

The lesion consists of a round to oval, nodular nonencapsulated mass, usually measuring <3 cm in greatest

NODULAR FASCIITIS—PATHOLOGIC FEATURES

Gross Findings

- Solid to cystic, nonencapsulated mass
- Usually <3 cm

Microscopic Findings

- Plump, immature fibroblasts resembling tissue culture
- Cystic spaces or areas of degeneration common
- Mitoses are abundant but not atypical
- Extravasated erythrocytes, inflammatory cells, keloid-like collagen, and giant cells often present

Fine Needle Aspiration

- Cellular smears
- Plump, spindled fibroblasts with wispy cytoplasmic extensions
- Binucleated forms may be seen
- Finely dispersed chromatin without atypia
- Blood, giant cells, and bundles of collagen occasionally present

Immunohistochemical Features

- Not necessary for diagnosis, but actins are positive
- CD68 positive histiocytes
- Negative for keratin and S100 protein

Pathologic Differential Diagnosis

- Fibrosarcoma, rhabdomyosarcoma, fibromatosis, fibrous histiocytoma, fetal rhabdomyoma

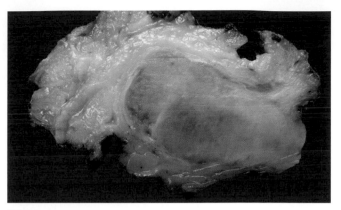

FIGURE 19-10

This focus of nodular fasciitis shows an oval, well-circumscribed but unencapsulated mass with a distinct appearance compared to the adjacent fat.

dimension (Figure 19-10). There is often attachment to the fascia. The cut surfaces may be firm and gray-white, or soft and gelatinous. Areas of cystic change are frequently noted.

MICROSCOPIC FINDINGS

Nodular fasciitis is poorly circumscribed and often assumes an irregular stellate appearance. It consists of plump, immature, relatively uniform fibroblasts, resembling the cells found in tissue culture or granulation tissue, with areas of central degeneration and extravasated erythrocytes (Figure 19-11). The fibroblasts have oval, pale staining nuclei with prominent nucleoli and are arranged in short irregular bundles and storiform fascicles (Figure 19-12). Mitotic figures are common, but atypical mitoses are never seen (Figure 19-13). Chronic inflammatory cells and giant cells are variably present. The deposition of keloid-like collagen increases with time, from small amounts in early lesions to extensive amounts in later stages of the reaction (Figure 19-13).

ANCILLARY STUDIES

ULTRASTRUCTURAL FEATURES

The elongated, bipolar fibroblastic cells have abundant rough endoplasmic reticulum and have cisternae with granular, electron-dense material. Intracytoplasmic

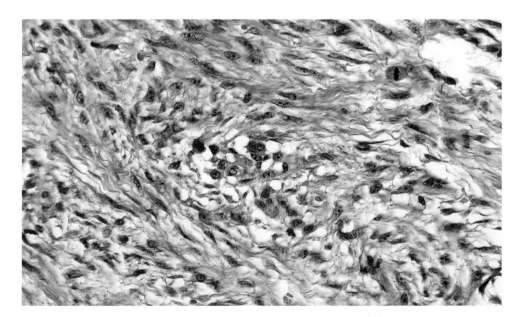

FIGURE 19-11

Nodular fasciitis shows a tissue culture–like growth with myxoid degeneration and a mitotic figure.

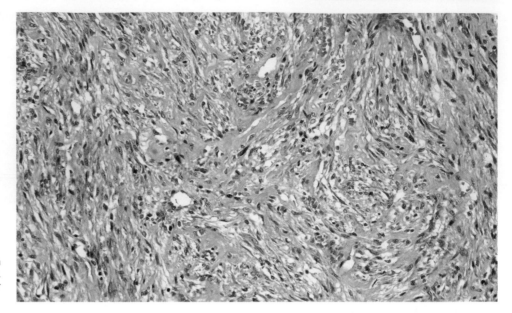

FIGURE 19-12

Tissue culture–like growth with collagen deposition and extravasated erythrocytes. A storiform growth is typical for nodular fasciitis.

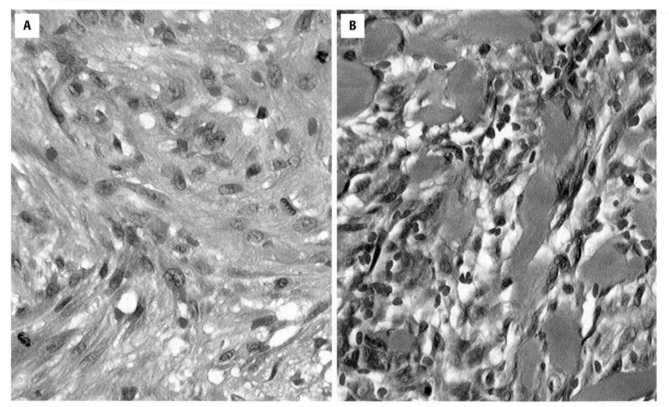

FIGURE 19-13

A, Short irregular bundles of fibroblasts with increased mitotic figures. **B**, Keloid-like collagen and increased fibroblasts with extravasated erythrocytes in nodular fasciitis.

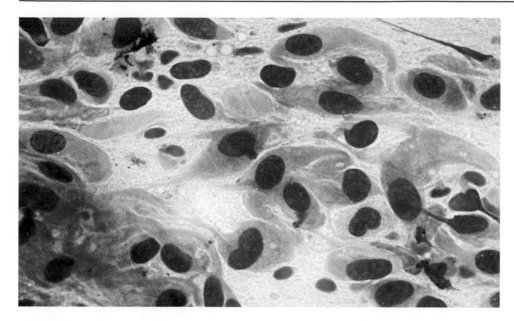

FIGURE 19-14

A fine needle aspiration of nodular fasciitis shows a cellular smear composed of single, spindle, bipolar cells in a background of myxoid material. The slightly vacuolated cytoplasm appears wispy and "tadpole"-like, while the nuclear chromatin is delicate and evenly distributed. Nucleoli are prominent (air-dried, May-Grünwald-Giemsa stain).

bundles of microfilaments are also seen. There is a fine distribution of the nuclear chromatin. Collagen fibers are seen in the background.

IMMUNOHISTOCHEMICAL FEATURES

Immunohistochemistry is not usually necessary for the diagnosis. The fibroblasts are positive with actins, while the histiocytes will be reactive with CD68. Desmin rarely may be positive, but keratin and S100 protein are typically negative.

FINE NEEDLE ASPIRATION

FNA will typically demonstrate a cellular smear composed of short, plump, spindled fibroblasts in a slightly myxoid background (Figure 19-14). The cells may be binucleated with eccentric nuclear placement. Mitotic figures are common but there is no evidence of atypia. Blood and giant cells are seen in the background, and occasionally collagen may be present.

DIFFERENTIAL DIAGNOSIS

Nodular fasciitis is often clinically worrisome because of the presentation of an enlarging mass lesion. The clinical differential diagnosis will include a variety of neoplastic conditions. Indeed, the histologic appearance can also be worrisome, and these lesions can be misdiagnosed as sarcoma (fibrosarcoma, rhabdomyosarcoma) or a variety of benign lesions. The cells in *fibrosarcoma* are densely packed without stroma and

are arranged in short, tight "herringbone" or "chevron" bundles. The individual cells differ much more in size and shape than in nodular fasciitis, and will often have numerous atypical mitoses. *Rhabdomyosarcoma* may occasionally have spindle-shaped cells, but it also tends to have pleomorphic cells with increased mitotic figures. Its unique immunohistochemical (muscle marker reactivity) and molecular profile (*FKHR* gene fusions for alveolar type) will be quite useful in this differentiation.

The benign entities in the differential diagnosis of nodular fasciitis include fibromatosis, fibrous histiocytoma, and fetal rhabdomyoma. *Fibromatosis* is less circumscribed and usually larger and often has an "invasive" growth pattern. It is characterized by slender spindle-shaped fibroblasts that are arranged in long, sweeping fascicles separated by abundant, dense collagen. Although usually not necessary, immunohistochemistry will show strong nuclear reactivity for beta-catenin. *Fibrous histiocytoma* is made up of more rounded cells that are arranged in a storiform pattern. *Fetal rhabdomyoma* has a gradient of cellularity with large cells showing cross-striations (strap cells) set in a bland but cellular stromal background (Figure 19-15).

PROGNOSIS AND THERAPY

Complete excision is the treatment of choice. Recurrences occur in ~2% of cases and usually develop shortly after surgery; this may represent a "reaction" to the trauma of surgery.

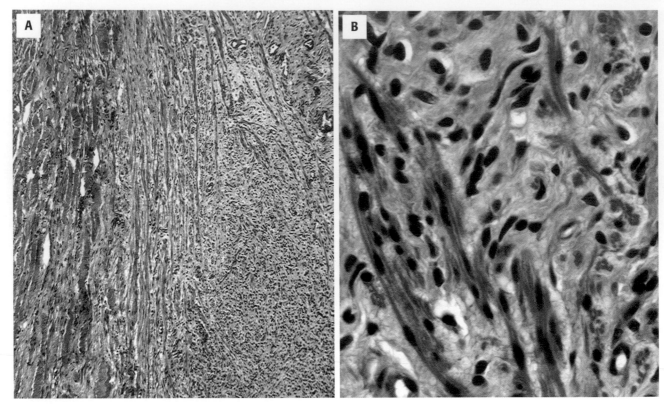

FIGURE 19-15

A, A fetal rhabdomyoma shows a gradient of cellularity, with elongated strap-like cells. There is unremarkable skeletal muscle on the far left. **B**, The large, strap-like cells with cross-striations are set in a cellular stroma of benign-appearing cells.

■ SINUS HISTIOCYTOSIS WITH MASSIVE LYMPHADENOPATHY (ROSAI-DORFMAN DISEASE)

Rosai-Dorfman disease (sinus histiocytosis with massive lymphadenopathy [SHML]) is a rare, idiopathic, histiocytic proliferation usually involving lymph nodes and following an indolent disease course. However, extranodal manifestations are frequent, especially in the upper aerodigestive tract. The histiocytes are considered to be part of the mononuclear phagocyte and immunoregulatory effector (M-PIRE) system belonging to the macrophage/histiocyte family. There is no known etiology, although immunodeficiency, autoimmune disease, or even a neoplastic process is potentially involved.

CLINICAL FEATURES

SHML is an uncommon condition that predominantly affects young black women (African and Caribbean origin), who present with massive lymphadenopathy, most commonly involving the cervical lymph nodes. However, nearly half of the affected patients will develop extranodal involvement, the majority of which (75%) occurs within the head and neck, such as the eyes, ocular adnexae, paranasal sinuses, and nasal cavity. Extranodal disease may be part of generalized disease or separate from nodal disease. Typically, these patients with head and neck involvement present with local mass-effect symptoms related to the location, such as nasal obstruction, proptosis, ptosis, stridor, pain, and/or cranial nerve deficits. Patients with SHML may also present with fever, an elevated white blood cell count, and an elevated erythrocyte sedimentation rate, but the antineutrophil cytoplasmic antibody (ANCA) and proteinase 3 are negative.

RADIOLOGIC FEATURES

The radiologic findings will depend on the location of the disease. In the sinonasal tract, for example, paranasal sinus disease can appear as a bulky, homogeneous mass, mimicking lymphoma.

PATHOLOGIC FEATURES

GROSS FINDINGS

Sinonasal tract involvement results in polypoid to nodular masses, which may be fibrotic, with a gray to yellow cut surface.

SINUS HISTIOCYTOSIS WITH MASSIVE LYMPHADENOPATHY (ROSAI-DORFMAN)—DISEASE FACT SHEET

Definition
- Rosai-Dorfman disease is a rare, idiopathic, histiocytic proliferation

Incidence and Location
- Rare
- Majority have head and neck involvement, with about 50% demonstrating extranodal disease (ocular, paranasal sinuses)

Morbidity and Mortality
- Direct mass effect into the cranial cavity

Gender, Race, and Age Distribution
- Female > male
- Predisposition in black patients
- Usually young

Clinical Features
- Nasal obstruction, proptosis, cranial nerve deficits, and mass lesion
- Cervical lymphadenopathy common
- Fever, elevated white blood cells, and erythrocyte sedimentation rate

Prognosis And Treatment
- Prognosis determined by extent and stage
- Spontaneous remission or death from complications both occur uncommonly
- Steroids conservatively manage localized disease, with surgery and/or radiation for more extensive disease

MICROSCOPIC FINDINGS

In SHML, there is a characteristic pronounced dilatation of the lymphoid sinuses, with an abundant lymphoplasmacytic infiltrate in the background (Figure 19-16). The low-power appearance of these cellular compartments

SINUS HISTIOCYTOSIS WITH MASSIVE LYMPHADENOPATHY (ROSAI-DORFMAN)—PATHOLOGIC FEATURES

Gross Findings
- Polypoid masses in the sinonasal tract, which may be fibrotic

Microscopic Findings
- Marked dilation of the lymphoid sinuses
- Abundant lymphoplasmacytic infiltrate in the background
- Pale, histiocytic cells in the sinuses demonstrating lymphophagocytosis or *emperipolesis*

Immunohistochemical Findings
- S100 protein, CD68, CD163, α-1 chymotrypsin, Leu M3, lysozyme positive
- Negative with CD1a and CD207 (Langerin)

Pathologic Differential Diagnosis
- Rhinoscleroma, lepromatous leprosy, histiocytic lymphomas

imparts a mottled appearance. Fibrosis may be associated with the dilated spaces. These sinuses are filled with abundant pale, histiocytic cells that demonstrate the nearly pathognomonic lymphophagocytosis or *emperipolesis* (Figure 19-17). There is often a clear halo around the phagocytized cells, a feature highlighted with S100 protein staining. The histiocytes tend to form clusters or nests. There is an overall lack of pleomorphism and the nuclei do not have longitudinal grooves or folds. Of note, extranodal SHML tends to be more fibrotic and may demonstrate less emperipolesis than the nodal form. Furthermore, the plasma cell population, which may have Russell bodies, may be so heavy as to obscure the histiocytes. Though axiomatic, special stains for organisms will be negative.

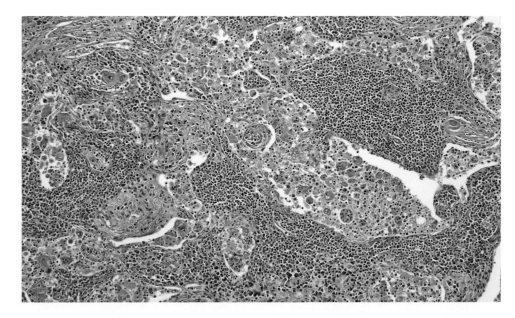

FIGURE 19-16
Lymphocytes are separated by lakes of histiocytes within expanded sinuses in this case of sinus histiocytosis with massive lymphadenopathy.

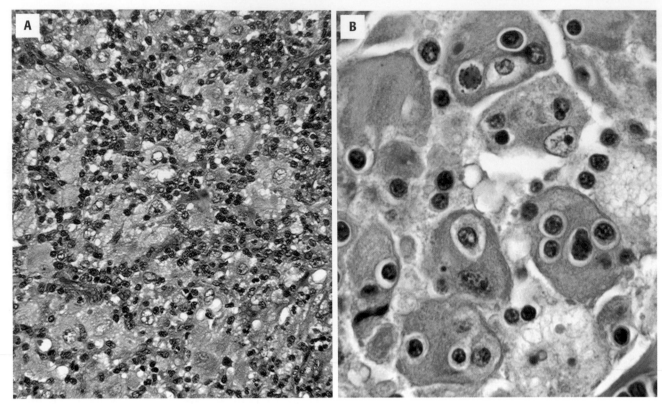

FIGURE 19-17

A, Sinus histiocytosis composed of histiocytes with phagocytosis. **B**, High power of a histiocyte with emperipolesis: Numerous plasma cell and lymphocyte nuclei are seen within the cytoplasm of the histiocyte in this example of sinus histiocytosis with massive lymphadenopathy.

ANCILLARY STUDIES

ULTRASTRUCTURAL FEATURES

The histiocytes contain fat vacuoles and lack Birbeck granules.

IMMUNOHISTOCHEMICAL FEATURES

The histiocytes of SHML are diffusely and strongly positive for S100 protein, while variably positive with macrophage antigens such as CD68, CD163, MAC387, Leu M3, lysozyme, and alpha-1-chymotrypsin. However, they are negative for CD1a and CD207 (Langerin), allowing for an important distinction to be made. Interestingly, these histiocytic cells are thought to be recently recruited blood monocytes.

DIFFERENTIAL DIAGNOSIS

The differential diagnosis includes other processes rich in histiocytes, such as rhinoscleroma, lepromatous leprosy, Langerhans cell histiocytosis, Wegener granulomatosis, and, rarely, histiocytic lymphomas. The histiocytes of the infectious diseases are smaller and not arranged within sinuses and lack S100 protein immunoreactivity. Special stains will also help to highlight respective microorganisms. B-cell lymphomas may rarely exhibit emperipolesis but will also be S100 protein negative. Wegener is a complex, largely autoimmune disease with a characteristic clinical presentation and laboratory findings.

PROGNOSIS AND THERAPY

The prognosis is determined by the extent of the disorder and "stage" of the disease. Patients may experience spontaneous remission, but occasionally, some patients may die of complications of the disorder, including infectious disease and amyloid-related organ dysfunction. Steroids may conservatively manage localized disease, but surgery (often extensive) and radiation may be necessary due to involvement of adjacent structures.

■ LANGERHANS CELL HISTIOCYTOSIS

Langerhans cell histiocytosis (LCH), formally histiocytosis X, represents a rare interrelated group of diseases including eosinophilic granuloma (EG), Hand-Schüller-Christian syndrome, and Letterer-Siwe disease. All of these lesions contain an unusual clonal histiocyte, which contains Birbeck granules on electron microscopy. Although requiring additional evaluation, new evidence suggests mutations in *BRAF* may support a neoplastic etiology.

CLINICAL FEATURES

The disease has an estimated prevalence of 1/200,000 children per year. The disease can be localized or can present with systemic findings, including multiorgan involvement. The head and neck is frequently involved in LCH, often affecting the flat bones of the skull, or the jaws, the ear, and the sinonasal tract. Though it is common for patients to present initially in the first two decades, the disease can affect a broad age range, from a few months to the 6th decade. Males are affected more frequently than females. Clinical symptoms can be very nonspecific, such as otitis media, hearing loss, bone pain, vertigo, or a destructive bone lesion.

RADIOLOGIC FEATURES

Radiographically, osseous involvement by LCH produces sharply punched-out single or multiple radiolucencies.

LANGERHANS CELL HISTIOCYTOSIS—DISEASE FACT SHEET

Definition
- A interrelated group of diseases that are manifestations of a unique histiocyte that contains Birbeck granules on electron microscopy

Incidence and Location
- Estimated prevalence in children is 1/200,000 per year

Morbidity and Mortality
- Morbidity can result from multifocal involvement of the skull
- Multiorgan involvement unresponsive to chemotherapy has a dismal prognosis

Gender, Race, and Age Distribution
- Equal gender distribution
- Usually young (<20 years)

Clinical Features
- Head and neck involvement occurs in flat bones of the skull or jaws
- Presents with otitis media and/or destructive temporal bone lesions (if the disease is localized)

Prognosis and Treatment
- Prognosis depends on stage and whether localized or systemic
- Disease progression is common if multiorgan involvement
- Surgery for localized disease has an excellent prognosis
- Combination chemotherapy and radiation for systemic disease

---

Extensive involvement of the gnathic alveolus causes the teeth to appear as if they are "floating in air."

PATHOLOGIC FEATURES

The Langerhans histiocytes are characterized as enlarged cells, containing delicate-appearing pale or eosinophilic cytoplasm, often finely vacuolated, and occasionally showing phagocytized cellular debris. The most characteristic cytologic feature, however, is the vesicular nucleus with an indented, notched, lobated, folded, grooved, reniform, vesicular, or "coffee bean"–shaped appearance, and one or two nucleoli (Figures 19-18 and 19-19). An increased number of eosinophils can be seen intermingled with the Langerhans cells and these may be concentrated in collections around areas of necrosis. Other inflammatory cells are also seen such as lymphocytes, plasma cells, and neutrophils. Multinucleated giant cells and hemorrhage may be present (Figure 19-20).

ANCILLARY STUDIES

ULTRASTRUCTURAL FEATURES

On electron microscopy, the characteristic folded, convoluted, and lobulated nuclei of Langerhans cells are readily appreciated. Cytoplasmic filipodial extensions create an uneven cell contour. Most important,

---

LANGERHANS CELL HISTIOCYTOSIS—PATHOLOGIC FEATURES

Microscopic Findings
- Langerhans cells are enlarged cells with delicate, pale cytoplasm surrounding vesicular nuclei with indented, notched, lobated, folded, grooved, or "coffee-bean" nuclei
- Increased eosinophils are often present, occasionally forming microscopic abscesses

Ultrastructural Features
- Langerhans cells have folded, convoluted, and lobulated nuclei
- Cell membrane invaginations forming Birbeck or Langerhans granules: disk shaped, pentilaminar, giving a "tennis racquet" appearance

Immunohistochemical Features
- Broadly reactive with many histiocytic markers; the diagnosis is usually confirmed with S100 protein, CD68, CD1a, and CD207 (Langerin)

Pathologic Differential Diagnosis
- Hodgkin lymphoma, extranodal NK/T-cell lymphoma, Rosai-Dorfman disease, Erdheim-Chester disease

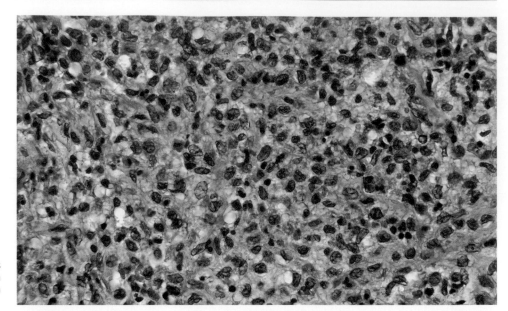

FIGURE 19-18

Langerhans cell histiocytosis demonstrates cleaved, "coffee bean"–shaped nuclei within a rich inflammatory background filled with eosinophils.

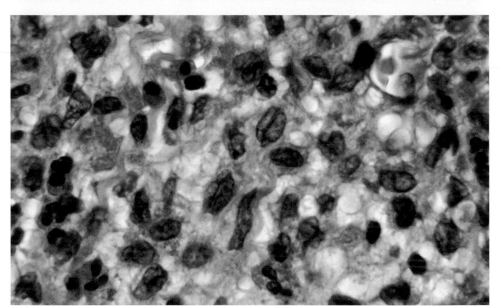

FIGURE 19-19

A cleave through the middle of the nucleus creates the characteristic lobulated "coffee-bean" appearance of Langerhans histiocytosis. Note the eosinophils in the background.

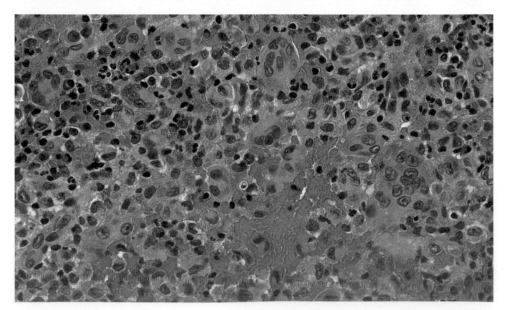

FIGURE 19-20

The Langerhans histiocytes are noted within a heavy inflammatory background including multiple giant cells and blood.

the cell contains a variable number of invaginations of the cell membrane called Birbeck or Langerhans granules. The granules are disk shaped, but when cross-sectioned, appear rod shaped. The granules are pentalaminar, showing cross-striations, often with the characteristic vesicular expansions imparting the unique "tennis racquet" appearance classically associated with the Langerhans cell (Figure 19-21).

IMMUNOHISTOCHEMICAL FEATURES

The immunohistochemical antigenic profile of Langerhans cells is remarkably wide, but in practical terms, S100 protein, CD1a, and CD68 will all yield a positive reaction (Figure 19-22). A relatively new marker, CD207, also referred to as "Langerin" (Figure 19-22) appears to have excellent sensitivity and specificity for

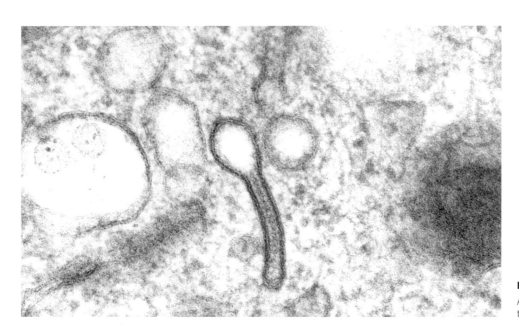

FIGURE 19-21

A Birbeck granule of Langerhans cell histiocytosis on ultrastructural examination.

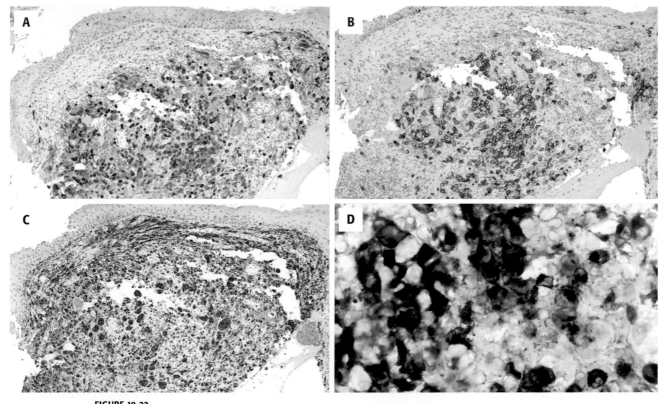

FIGURE 19-22

Immunohistochemistry of Langerhans cell histiocytosis. **A**, S100 protein. **B**, CD1a. **C**, CD68. **D**, Langerin (CD207).

the Langerhans cell histiocyte. Langerin is a type II transmembrane cell surface receptor localized in the Birbeck granules. Occasionally, sialated Leu M1, peanut agglutinin, ATPase, or T-6 antigenic determinants and HLA-DR (CD74) may be used to confirm the diagnosis. The macrophage antigens generally demonstrate a concentration in the perinuclear space and Golgi region.

MOLECULAR GENETICS

About half of LCH cases tested show an oncogenic *BRAF* V600E mutation, raising the possibility of pharmacogenomic inhibitor therapy.

DIFFERENTIAL DIAGNOSIS

The differential in the head and neck is usually limited to Hodgkin lymphoma, extranodal sinus histiocytosis with massive lymphadenopathy (Rosai-Dorfman), extranodal NK/T-cell lymphoma, and perhaps Erdheim-Chester disease. *Rosai-Dorfman* shows a different pattern of growth, has emperipolesis, and is reactive with S100 protein, while negative with CD1a and CD207. *Hodgkin lymphoma* may have a pronounced eosinophilic infiltrate but has Reed-Sternberg cells, with immunoreactivity for CD15 and CD30, but not CD1a. *NK/T-cell lymphoma* may have irregular and grooved nuclei, as well as eosinophils in the background, but will show angiocentricity and an NK or T-cell lineage. *Erdheim-Chester disease* is an idiopathic true histiocytic disorder, whose cells are S100 protein positive but CD1a negative and also lack Birbeck granules.

PROGNOSIS AND THERAPY

LCH may be a localized or systemic disease and a complex staging system is applied. Localized disease, frequently the case in the head and neck, requires conservative surgery to achieve an excellent prognosis. If no new lesions develop within 1 year, the patient is considered cured. If systemic disease is identified, combination chemotherapy is used along with radiation as necessary. Adverse prognostic findings include a young age at onset, extensive bone and/or visceral involvement, and multiple recurrences (usually within 6 months of diagnosis).

SUGGESTED READINGS

The complete suggested readings list is available online at
    www.expertconsult.com.

20

Benign Neoplasms of the Neck (Soft Tissue, Bone, and Lymph Node)

■ **Jennifer L. Hunt**

■ LYMPHANGIOMA (CYSTIC HYGROMA)

Lymphangiomas are rare congenital lymphatic malformations, with up to 70% reported in the head and neck. They are separated into three types: capillary, cavernous, and cystic (cystic hygroma). Lymphangiomas comprise ~25% of all vascular neoplasms in children and adolescents, and ~25% of cervical cysts are lymphangiomas.

CLINICAL FEATURES

LYMPHANGIOMA (CYSTIC HYGROMA)—DISEASE FACT SHEET

Definition
- A benign cystic lesion composed of dilated lymph vessels

Incidence and Location
- Represents 25% of congenital cervical cysts
- Up to 70% of lymphangiomas occur in the head and neck

Morbidity and Mortality
- Mortality 3% to 7% (via pressure destruction of adjacent vital structures)

Gender, Race, and Age Distribution
- No significant gender difference
- Most present shortly after birth and 95% by the 2nd year

Clinical Features
- Slowly enlarging, painless mass
- May produce pressure symptoms due to size
- Associated with fetal hydrops and Turner syndrome

Prognosis and Treatment
- May become secondarily infected
- Surgery is the treatment of choice; sclerosing agents and laser can be used
- Up to 50% recurrence depending on size and site of lesion (due to incomplete excision)

Approximately two-thirds of lymphangiomas are noted shortly after birth, and 95% are present by the end of the 2nd year of life. Cystic hygroma may also be detected in utero with ultrasonography. Cystic hygroma may be associated with fetal hydrops and several genetic abnormalities, most notably Turner syndrome (Figure 20-1), but also Noonan syndrome and trisomies 13, 18, and 21. In general, symptoms are related to pressure caused by the slowly enlarging mass or extension of the mass into the posterior neck or, less commonly, into the anterior compartment, cheek, mediastinum, or axilla. When located superior to the hyoid bone, they may cause dysphagia or airway compression. Ultrasound will show a cystic lesion, frequently identified prenatally, while computed tomography (CT) studies will show a nonenhancing, multilocular cystic mass.

Cavernous lymphangioma forms an ill-defined, spongy, and compressible mass and is found most commonly in the tongue, cheek, floor of mouth, and lips; it is uncommon in the soft tissues. In contrast, capillary lymphangioma is usually confined to the skin and is clinically the least significant of the three types.

PATHOLOGIC FEATURES

Cystic lymphangiomas (hygromas) vary from a single soft mass with a pseudo contour to lobulated multicystic masses (Figure 20-1). They contain clear to white-turbid fluid, described as milk-like (Figure 20-1). Histologically, they consist of dilated thin-walled spaces filled with eosinophilic, proteinaceous fluid and lined by flat endothelial cells (Figure 20-2). The intervening stroma contains scattered lymphoid aggregates and wisps of smooth muscle fibers (Figure 20-3). Fibrosis may be increased in lesions that have been present for a long duration.

ANCILLARY STUDIES

Endothelial markers (factor VIII–related antigen [FVIII-RAg], CD31, CD34, and *Ulex europaeus*) can be

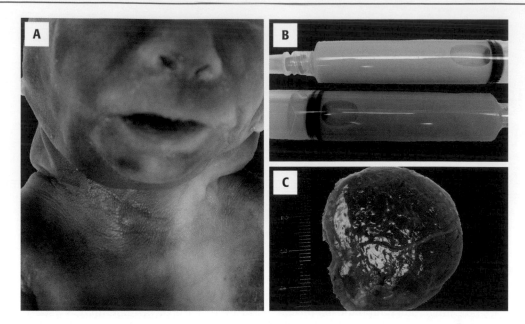

FIGURE 20-1

A, Bilateral cystic masses are noted in the posterior neck of this fetus, affected with Turner syndrome. **B**, Turbid-milky fluid removed during a fine needle aspiration of a large posterior neck cyst in a child (lymphangioma). **C**, A translucent mass, showing delicate vessels in the wall of a lymphangioma, filled with clear-watery fluid.

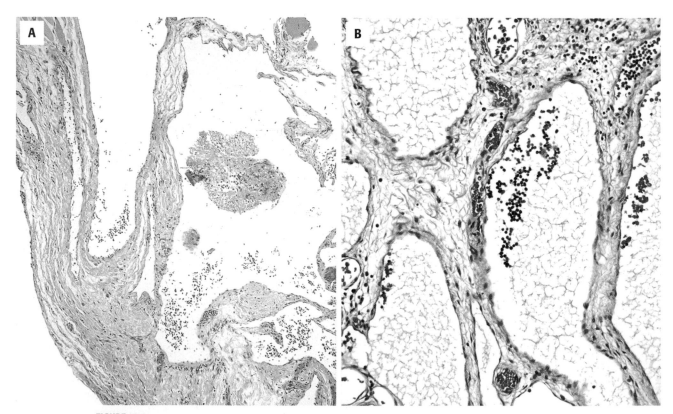

FIGURE 20-2

A, Cystic lymphangioma showing dilated lymphatic spaces. **B**, Lymphocytes are noted within the proteinaceous fluid.

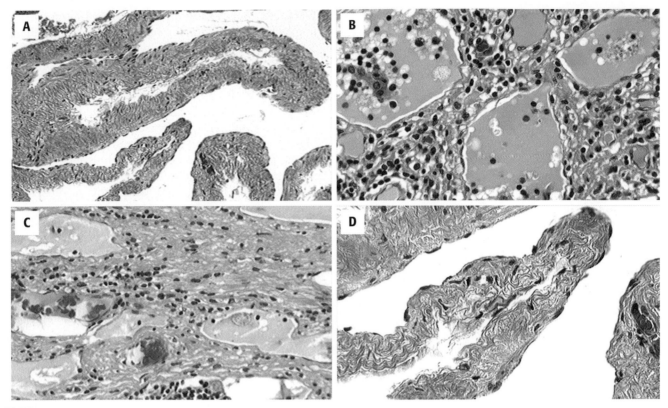

FIGURE 20-3

A, Lymphatic spaces subtended by smooth muscle. **B**, Lymphoid cells and proteinaceous fluid. **C**, Lymphoid elements with fibrosis, surrounding fluid-filled spaces. **D**, Flat, attenuated endothelial cells line the cavity.

LYMPHANGIOMA (CYSTIC HYGROMA)—PATHOLOGIC FEATURES

Gross Findings

- Sponge-like cystic mass

Microscopic Findings

- Dilated, thin-walled spaces filled with proteinaceous fluid
- Lined by flat endothelial cells
- Lymphoid aggregates in stroma
- Wisps of smooth muscle in the wall

Immunohistochemical Features

- Positive with factor VIII–related antigen, CD31, CD34, *Ulex europaeus*
- D2-40 (podoplanin) may be specific lymphatic marker (also CD9 and LYVE-1, although less common)

Pathologic Differential Diagnosis

- Cavernous hemangioma, metastatic papillary carcinoma

expressed by endothelial cells in both hemangiomas and lymphangiomas. D2-40 (podoplanin) may be a lymphatic-specific marker, along with CD9 and lymphatic vessel endothelial receptor 1 (LYVE-1), although podoplanin may be easier to interpret.

DIFFERENTIAL DIAGNOSIS

The most common differential diagnosis is with cavernous hemangioma. Lymphangioma contains proteinaceous fluid, and the surrounding tissues are usually infiltrated by lymphocytes, whereas *cavernous hemangiomas* are filled with red blood cells and lack valve structures. *Metastatic papillary carcinoma of the thyroid* may have flattened cells along the spaces, but TTF-1 or thyroglobulin will be positive. Furthermore, a lymph node architecture should be recognizable, often at the periphery.

PROGNOSIS AND THERAPY

Mortality rates are between 3% and 7%, specifically related to pressure destruction of vital structures of the neck. Lymphangiomas may occasionally become infected and may cause difficulty swallowing or respiratory distress. Surgery is the treatment of choice, while laser treatment or injected sclerosing agents (such as bleomycin) are alternative therapies. Recurrence rates range from 15% to 50% and are highest when the lymphangioma is incompletely removed. Malignant transformation is not documented.

■ TERATOMA

Teratomas are neoplasms composed of elements from each of the three germ cell layers (ectoderm, endoderm, and mesoderm). About 1 in 4,000 live births have a teratoma, with ~2% involving the head and neck, most commonly the neck, oropharynx, nasopharynx, and orbit. Specifically, cervical teratomas represent <3% of all teratomas and <1% of all neck masses in children. Teratomas are separated, histologically, into mature or immature, solid or cystic and are classified as benign or malignant depending on the degree of tissue maturation. In general, teratomas of the neck in neonates or infants are clinically benign, although they may be histologically mature or immature. By comparison, teratomas in adults are more likely to be clinically malignant and histologically immature.

CLINICAL FEATURES

More than 90% of cervical teratomas occur in neonates or infants and are rare in patients older than 1 year. They occur with similar frequency in boys and girls. In addition to a neck mass, severe respiratory distress is notable in neonates, frequently leading to airway compromise and requiring immediate surgery. Polyhydramnios and other malformations may be seen in ~20% of patients, many of whom will show an elevated α-fetoprotein concentration in amniotic fluid. Failure of midline structure development may result in fetal demise, even though the lesion is histologically benign. If detected prenatally by ultrasonographic examination, surgical planning may yield a better outcome. CT or magnetic resonance imaging (MRI) usually shows a multilocular mass (Figure 20-4). Cervical teratomas in adults are extremely rare, with patients reporting a rapidly enlarging neck mass.

PATHOLOGIC FEATURES

GROSS FINDINGS

Grossly, the tumors are encapsulated, lobulated, and usually cystic, but they can be solid or multiloculated. They measure up to 12 cm in greatest diameter.

MICROSCOPIC FINDINGS

Histologically, the tumors are composed of an assemblage of mature or immature tissues from the three embryonic germ cell layers: ectoderm, endoderm, mesoderm (Figure 20-5). The most common finding is neural tissue, arranged in islands, tubules, and rosette-like formations of immature neuroepithelium or mature glial tissue (Figure 20-6), including retinal anlage epithelium (Figure 20-7). A variety of epithelia are seen,

---

TERATOMA—DISEASE FACT SHEET

Definition
- Neoplasm composed of mature or immature elements from ectoderm, endoderm, and mesoderm

Incidence and Location
- Cervical teratomas represent 3% of all teratomas
- <1% of pediatric neck masses

Morbidity and Mortality
- High morbidity, but low mortality in neonates and infants
- High mortality in older children and adults

Gender, Race, and Age Distribution
- Equal gender distribution
- >90% occur in neonates or infants

Clinical Features
- Neck mass
- Respiratory distress
- Frequent association with congenital malformations
- Polyhydramnios seen in 20% of neonatal lesions

Prognosis and Treatment
- Prognosis is very good in neonates and infants but guarded in older children and adults
- Surgery

TERATOMA—PATHOLOGIC FEATURES

Gross Findings
- Cystic, solid, or multilocular lobulated mass

Microscopic Findings
- Mature or immature tissues from all germ cell layers
- Squamous, respiratory, glandular, and cuboidal epithelium
- Organ differentiation may be seen
- Neural tissues, including glial elements, choroid plexus, immature neuroblastema, and pigmented retinal anlage
- Bone, cartilage, muscle, and fat

Immunohistochemical Features
- α-Fetoprotein and human chorionic gonadotropin if endodermal sinus tumor and choriocarcinoma are present

Pathologic Differential Diagnosis
- Hamartoma, neuroblastoma, malignant germ cell tumors, metastatic testicular teratoma

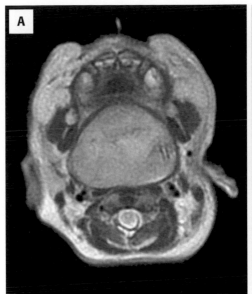
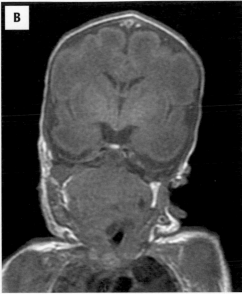

FIGURE 20-4

Magnetic resonance imaging demonstrates a large mass involving the oropharynx, nasopharynx, and neck. **A**, Axial T2-weighted image. **B**, Coronal T1-weighted image.

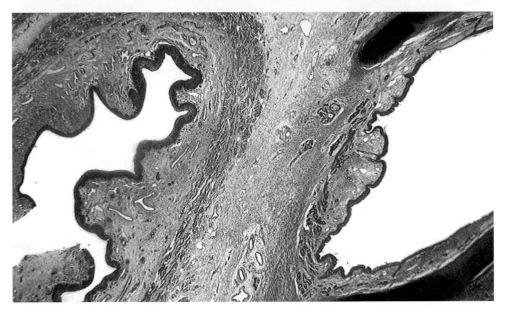

FIGURE 20-5

This benign mature teratoma contains a primitive esophagus adjacent to a primitive trachea. Other germ cell layers were noted elsewhere.

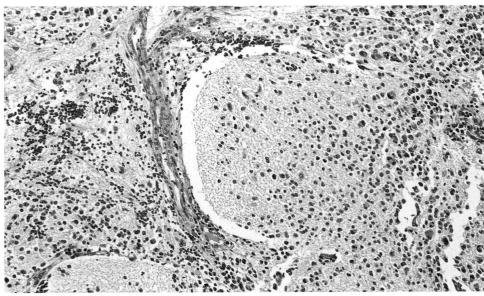

FIGURE 20-6

Teratoma containing mature glial tissue with focal fibrosis.

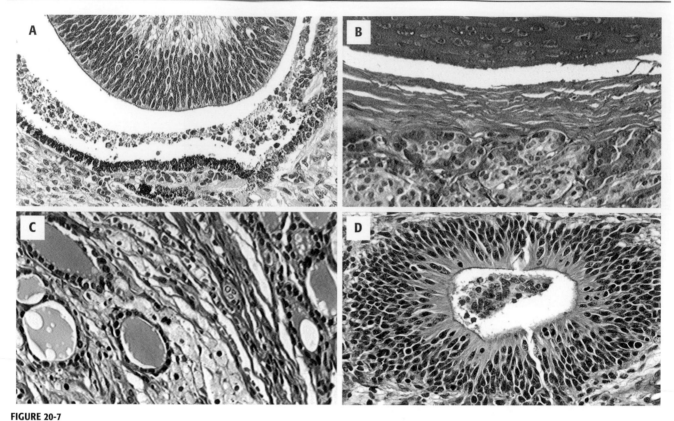

FIGURE 20-7

A, Retinal anlage epithelium. **B**, Mature cartilage adjacent to pancreatic tissue. **C**, Thyroid parenchyma with immature fat. **D**, A rosette of immature glial tissue.

including squamous, respiratory, and enteric-type mucosa, with solid organ tissues occasionally noted (pancreas, liver, thyroid) (Figure 20-7). The epithelium may line a cyst, with sebaceous units and hair frequently identified. Nodules of cartilage, fat, and muscle blend with the surrounding epithelial or glial tissues. The tissue may be mature or immature (embryonic), with the volume of immature tissues determining the overall grade of the tumor. *Benign mature* is used for tumors containing only mature elements; *benign immature* is used if there are foci of immature elements within a tumor that has a majority of mature elements; and *malignant* is used if the majority of the tumor is composed of immature elements. Foci of malignant germ cell tumor (such as endodermal sinus tumor, embryonal carcinoma, or choriocarcinoma), while uncommon, automatically place the tumor in the malignant category.

DIFFERENTIAL DIAGNOSIS

A broad differential diagnosis exists with these heterogeneous tumors when initially evaluated on small biopsy samples, offering limited sampling. Hamartoma, choristoma, ectopia, encephalocele, neuroblastoma, rhabdomyosarcoma, and malignant germ cell tumors may all be considered in the differential. However, attention to the nondescript mesenchymal background and heterogeneity of elements, including embryonic forms, provides clues to the diagnosis. A hamartoma is readily ruled out by the presence of tissues that are not indigenous to the location and/or that have an immature appearance. Depending on the age, cervical metastasis from a gonadal teratoma should also be considered in the differential diagnosis.

ANCILLARY STUDIES

Immunohistochemical stains with α-fetoprotein and human chorionic gonadotropin may be of help in findings islands of endodermal sinus tumor or choriocarcinoma, respectively, in malignant teratomas. However, immunohistochemistry is generally not necessary for diagnosis.

PROGNOSIS AND THERAPY

The prognosis of cervical teratoma in newborns and infants is excellent, although teratomas of the neck may cause significant morbidity due to their important location, despite their favorable histology. Tracheotomy or oral intubation may be required, along with a nasogastric tube for feeding. Death does occur as a result of associated developmental malformations of the vital structures of the neck. Therefore, surgery should be instituted without delay because the preoperative mortality is significant. Many advocate delivering a fetus by ex utero intrapartum treatment (EXIT) procedure to yield the best possible outcome. In adults, in whom a malignant histology is more common, the biologic behavior of the tumors is more aggressive with a poorer clinical outcome, as expected. Metastasis to lymph nodes and lung is common. Surgery with adjuvant chemotherapy and radiation is advocated, although often with mixed results.

■ SPINDLE CELL LIPOMA/PLEOMORPHIC LIPOMA

Spindle cell and pleomorphic lipomas are distinctive types of lipoma histologically on a continuum and characterized by replacement of mature fat cells by bland spindle cells, hyperchromatic round cells, and multinucleated giant cells, including the characteristic "floret cell," and associated with ropey collagen. They account for ~1.5% of all adipose tissue neoplasms, with a lipoma–to–spindle cell lipoma ratio of 60:1.

CLINICAL FEATURES

Greater than 90% of spindle cell/pleomorphic lipomas occur in men (male >>> female, 9:1), with a mean age of 55 years. Almost all of the tumors are located in the

subcutaneous tissue of the posterior neck, upper back, and shoulder girdle. Rarely, the salivary gland, lip, and maxillofacial region will be affected. Patients are usually asymptomatic but may present with a painless, mobile, subcutaneous mass, often present for many years. Characteristically, the tumors are solitary, although rarely they may be familial and multiple.

PATHOLOGIC FEATURES

GROSS FINDINGS

Spindle cell/pleomorphic lipomas range in size from 1 to 13 cm (mean, 5 cm). Grossly, they resemble an ordinary lipoma (Figure 20-8), although some are gray-white or pale-pink, and deeper tumors may be myxoid.

MICROSCOPIC FINDINGS

Microscopically, at one end of the histologic spectrum, spindle cell lipoma is composed of varying proportions of mature adipocytes and fibroblast-like spindle cells admixed with wire- or rope-like collagen fibers ("ropey collagen"), and myxoid stroma (Figures 20-9 and 20-10). The fibroblast-like cells may be arranged in a parallel fashion. Mast cells are frequently numerous. It is important to note that fat may be sparse and difficult to find in certain tumors. The myxoid stroma may be a dominant finding. Profound, but focal, nuclear pleomorphism can be seen, and is considered "degenerative" or "ancient change." Mitoses are usually absent.

SPINDLE CELL LIPOMA/PLEOMORPHIC LIPOMA—DISEASE FACT SHEET

Definition
- A distinct group of lipomas composed of spindle cells, adipocytes, and multinucleated giant cells associated with ropey collagen

Incidence and Location
- About 1.5% of all adipose tissue tumors

Gender, Race, and Age Distribution
- Male >>> female (9:1)
- Mean age: 55 years

Clinical Features
- Painless, subcutaneous, mobile mass
- Posterior neck, upper back, shoulders
- Seldom multiple

Prognosis and Treatment
- Excellent, although isolated reports of recurrence
- Surgery

SPINDLE CELL LIPOMA/PLEOMORPHIC LIPOMA—PATHOLOGIC FEATURES

Gross Findings
- Yellow to gray-white to pale-pink circumscribed mass
- Mean, 5 cm (range, 1 to 13 cm)

Microscopic Findings
- Mixture of bland spindle cells arranged in parallel, adipocytes, and multinucleated giant cells ("floret-like")
- Bands of mature, rope-like collagen fibers
- Mast cells may be numerous

Ancillary Studies
- Spindle cells of both types of lipoma express CD34
- Negative for S100 protein
- Loss of 13q and/or 16q

Pathologic Differential Diagnosis
- Well-differentiated liposarcoma, neurofibroma, schwannoma, myxoma, and nuchal fibroma

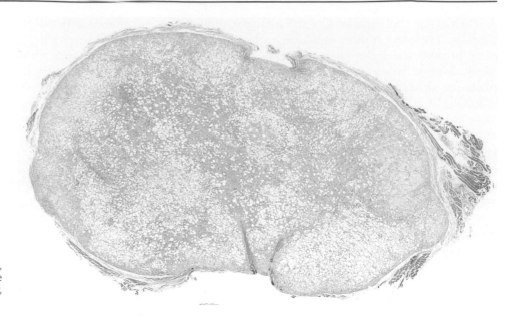

FIGURE 20-8

A well-circumscribed and encapsulated, intramuscular spindle cell lipoma. Note the myxoid appearance from low power, as well as areas of increased cellularity.

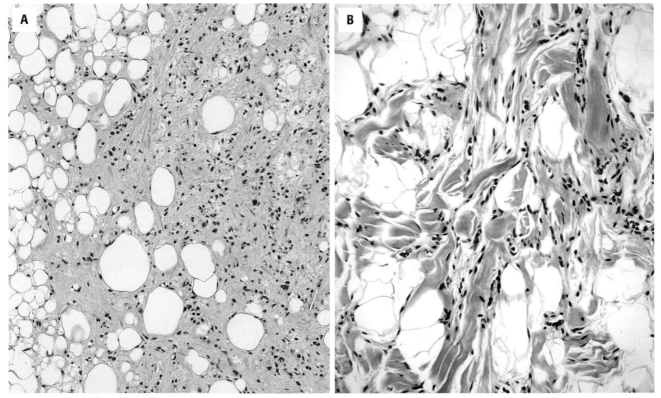

FIGURE 20-9

A, Spindle cell lipoma with bland spindle cells in a background of adipocytes. **B**, Note the areas of thick, ropey collagen fibers.

At the opposite end of the spectrum lies pleomorphic lipoma, which is characterized by small, round hyperchromatic cells and multinucleated giant cells with radially arranged "floret-like" nuclei—so named for their resemblance to petals of a flower (Figure 20-10). Cases with mixed features of spindle cell and pleomorphic lipoma occur quite often, making any distinction impossible and arbitrary. Secondary changes of fat necrosis or hyalinization can be seen and may also be associated with "aging." By definition, lipoblasts are absent.

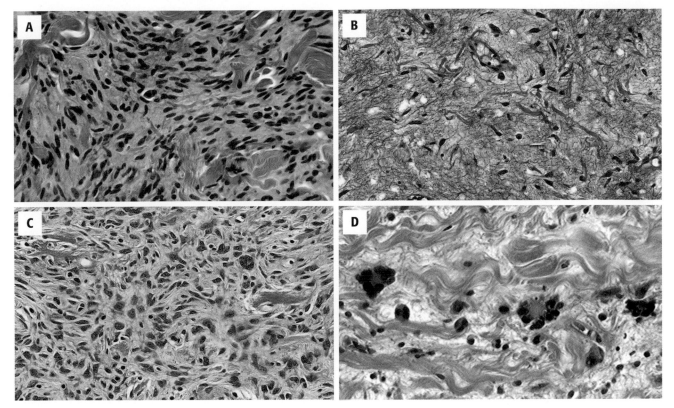

FIGURE 20-10

A, Spindled cells with collagen and isolated mast cells. **B**, Marked myxoid stroma with delicate collagen fibers and fibroblasts. **C**, Pleomorphic lipoma: Hyperchromatic nuclei are seen in cells separated by dense collagen. There are a few multinucleated cells. **D**, Floret-like ("petal") multinucleated giant cells associated with mast cells and collagenized stroma.

ANCILLARY STUDIES

ULTRASTRUCTURAL FEATURES

Electron microscopic studies have revealed spindle cells thought to represent fibroblasts or fibroblast-like cells analogous to the stellate mesenchymal cells seen in primitive fat lobules.

IMMUNOHISTOCHEMICAL FEATURES

Immunohistochemically, the spindle cells in spindle/pleomorphic lipomas express CD34 and vimentin. Rare, isolated cells may be S100 protein positive, but it is quite different from the strong reaction usually seen in ordinary lipocytes.

FINE NEEDLE ASPIRATION FINDINGS

Smears will contain large, atypical, floret-type cells within a background of mature adipocytes. Needless to say, the cells are frequently interpreted to be malignant.

GENETIC STUDIES

Loss of chromosomes 13q (13q12 and 13q14-q22) and/or 16q (16q13-qter) is characteristic of this family of lipomas (seen in ~70% of cases).

DIFFERENTIAL DIAGNOSIS

The differential diagnosis includes well-differentiated liposarcoma (due to adipocytic component) and the common neural neoplasms, neurofibroma and schwannoma (due to spindle cell component); myxoma and nuchal fibroma are occasionally a consideration. The uniformity of the spindle cells, association with mature collagen fibers, and absence of lipoblasts, coupled with the characteristic location, patient age, and overall circumscription of the lesion, all support the diagnosis of spindle cell lipoma over *liposarcoma*. *Neurofibroma*, which tends to be infiltrative, contains spindle cells that are more randomly arranged and may contain characteristic

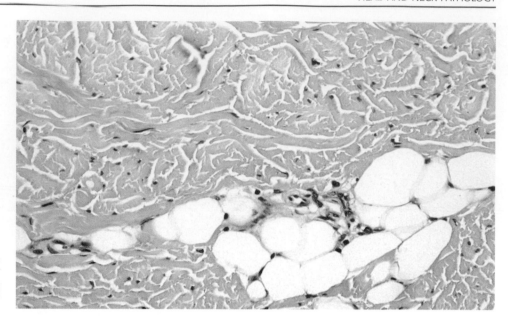

FIGURE 20-11

A nuchal-type fibroma has very heavy, dense collagen deposition with small islands of adipocytes and nerve twigs. There are no spindled tumor cells and no floret-like giant cells.

Wagner-Meissner bodies (eosinophilic-appearing touch corpuscles). Moreover, the spindle cells express S100 protein in neurofibroma but are CD34 positive in spindle cell lipoma. *Schwannoma* has buckled-wavy nuclei, cellular Antoni A areas and perivascular hyalinization. S100 protein is usually strong and diffusely immunoreactive. *Myxoma* is very hypocellular, lacks fat, and does not have thick bundles of collagen. A *nuchal-type fibroma* has fat but has a much heavier collagen deposition and has entrapped nerves (Figure 20-11).

PROGNOSIS AND THERAPY

Complete local excision is curative for both types of lipomas.

SUGGESTED READINGS

The complete suggested readings list is available online at www.expertconsult.com.

21

Malignant Neoplasms of the Neck (Soft Tissue, Bone, and Lymph Node)

■ Jennifer L. Hunt

■ METASTATIC CYSTIC SQUAMOUS CELL CARCINOMA

Metastatic cystic squamous cell carcinoma (SCC) in the neck often presents without a clinically apparent primary, and therefore a broad clinical differential diagnosis is often initially considered. Given the cystic appearance in the lateral neck, the leading contender is usually a branchial cleft cyst. About one-third of patients who have metastatic SCC in the neck have cystic metastases exclusively. However, more than half of these cystic metastases, with an initially undetected primary tumor, will eventually be tracked to primary sites in Waldeyer ring. The rich lymphatic plexus in this location can lead to early metastatic disease via the jugulodigastric lymph node chain, despite small and clinically inapparent primary tumors. Furthermore, tumors that involve the tonsils and tongue base will frequently localize to deep crypt locations, with very little clinical evidence for surface mucosal alterations.

CLINICAL FEATURES

Patients most frequently present with a short history (<6 months) of a painless mass in the upper neck involving the jugulodigastric lymph nodes. Patients may have bilateral disease (10%). There may be a history of smoking and/or alcohol abuse. Most patients are in the 6th decade of life, with a strong male predilection (4:1). Once the diagnosis of metastatic cystic SCC is established, a primary tumor is discovered in ~80% of patients, usually involving the Waldeyer ring area (base of the tongue, lingual, or palatine tonsils). Other primary sites can include the nasopharynx, esophagus, and laryngotracheal region. In up to 10% of patients, a primary is never discovered, despite an extensive workup.

RADIOLOGIC FEATURES

Computed tomography (CT) or magnetic resonance imaging (MRI) shows a cystic or multilocular mass with a thick capsule in the region of the jugulodigastric lymph nodes (Figure 21-1).

PATHOLOGIC FEATURES

GROSS FINDINGS

The neck mass ranges in size from 1.5 to 12 cm, with an average size of ~4 cm. Macroscopically, there is a thick, fibrotic capsule defining the well-circumscribed lymph node border (Figure 21-2). The cut surface is unilocular or multilocular, with the cyst(s) filled with grumous, granular, thick, tenacious, and purulent yellow-brown to hemorrhagic fluid.

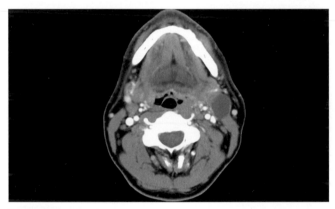

FIGURE 21-1

A computed tomography scan demonstrates a well-defined mass deep to the sternocleidomastoid muscle in the left neck. A thick capsule is noted. There is also a mass noted in the oropharynx, creating asymmetry.

METASTATIC CYSTIC SQUAMOUS CELL CARCINOMA—PATHOLOGIC FEATURES

Gross Findings

- Well-circumscribed, thickly encapsulated cystic mass
- Thick, tenacious, purulent, yellow-brown to hemorrhagic fluid
- Mean of 4 cm

Microscopic Findings

- Thick, desmoplastic fibrous connective tissue capsule
- Cystic spaces lined by ribbon-like growth
- Uniformly thick epithelium composed of bland epithelium, lacking maturation, demonstrating loss of polarity, cells with high nuclear:cytoplasmic ratio and mitotic figures
- Usually lacks keratinization and profound pleomorphism

Immunohistochemical Features

- Keratins positive, but usually not necessary for diagnosis
- Human papillomavirus (high-risk subtype) often positive
- p16 often positive

Fine Needle Aspiration Features

- Cellular smears
- Anucleate squames and debris
- Atypical squamous cells with dyskeratosis, irregular nuclear contours, nuclear hyperchromasia, and increased nuclear:cytoplasmic ratio

Pathologic Differential Diagnosis

- Branchial cleft cyst, thymopharyngeal cyst, thymic cyst, bronchial cyst

MICROSCOPIC FINDINGS

On microscopic examination, a dense, fibrous connective tissue capsule will often surround the lymph node that contains metastatic tumor. The cystic spaces are lined by a ribbon-like growth of epithelium, which

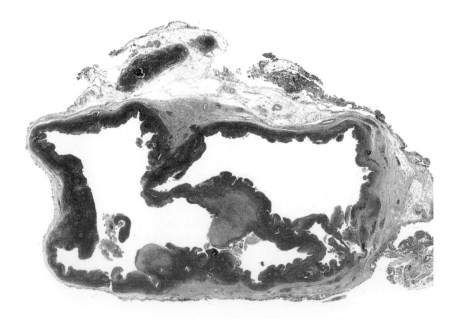

FIGURE 21-2

There is a thickened capsule at the periphery of this lymph node, which is replaced by a thin ribbon of epithelial cells around the periphery. The cyst contents were lost in processing. Note a smaller lymph node at the top of the field.

has a generally uniform thickness (Figure 21-3). The epithelium can have different morphologic features, ranging from a transitional, basaloid, and nonkeratinizing appearance to a more conventional keratinizing squamous appearance. In some areas, the lining may have an endophytic growth pattern, budding into the lymphoid stroma, while in other areas it is exophytic or papillary, with projections into the cyst spaces. The cyst contents are often washed away during fixation and histologic processing, leaving these variably sized spaces largely empty. The overall histologic appearance in many areas may be remarkably bland, recapitulating the normal squamous or transitional-type epithelium that is present in a normal deep tonsillar crypt (Figure 21-4). Nonetheless, the cells are enlarged with a high nuclear:cytoplasmic ratio, no

appreciable degree of surface maturation, and limited (if any) keratinization. Sometimes, an abrupt transition to remarkably atypical epithelium can be seen, facilitating the diagnosis, but this is not a common finding (Figure 21-5). Because of the often bland histologic appearance on initial low-power examination, these lesions require careful inspection to make the correct diagnosis.

The primary, and often occult, tumors are usually small and located deep in the tonsillar crypts or its vicinity (Waldeyer ring). Histologically, they will have a similar appearance to that of the metastatic foci described earlier. It is important to realize that Waldeyer ring can harbor nonkeratinizing, keratinizing, and basaloid SCCs, thus accounting for the variable histologic appearance of these metastatic tumors.

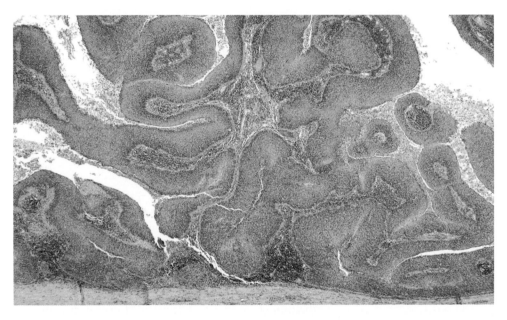

FIGURE 21-3

The ribbon-like arrangement of the metastatic squamous epithelium creates papillary infoldings into the cystic spaces of the replaced lymph node.

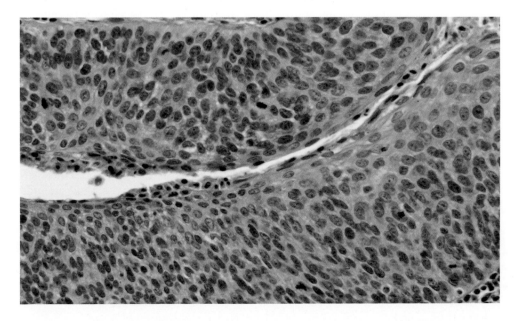

FIGURE 21-4

There is a subtle loss of polarity, a disorganization to the growth, increased mitotic figures, and an overall mild nuclear pleomorphism in this metastatic cystic squamous cell carcinoma.

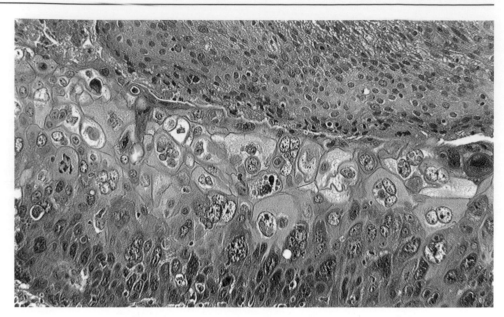

FIGURE 21-5

A monotonous, albeit atypical, epithelium is seen at the top of the field, while the opposite ribbon of epithelium shows remarkable anaplasia in this cystic squamous cell carcinoma.

ANCILLARY STUDIES

IMMUNOHISTOCHEMICAL AND MOLECULAR FEATURES

Immunohistochemistry is not necessary for the diagnosis of cystic metastatic SCC or the associated primary tumors. However, the cells are positive with a variety of keratins (AE1/AE3, CK1, CK8, CK14, and CK19), although usually not with CK7. There is an important association between oropharyngeal carcinomas and high-risk subtypes of human papillomavirus (HPV). Not only are the primary tumors positive for HPV, but the metastatic lesions are also often positive. This association has led to important diagnostic assays to assess the metastatic lesions but also to suggest a primary oropharyngeal site when HPV is positive.

HPV detection can be via direct assessment for the virus, usually using chromogenic in situ hybridization (CISH), or through amplification detection, using a polymerase chain reaction approach. CISH has the advantage of assessing cellular location, which distinguishes between episomal and integrated virus by two distinct staining patterns: punctate (dot-like) staining with integrated virus and diffuse nuclear staining with episomal virus (Figure 21-6). Because of the cellular mechanisms of HPV, p16 has also been proved to be an excellent immunohistochemical surrogate marker for the presence of HPV (Figure 21-7).

FINE NEEDLE ASPIRATION

The smears are often quite cellular and, in many cases, dominated by anucleate squamous and debris from the cystic area of the tumor. However, fragments of atypical squamous epithelium are found, as well as individual atypical keratinocytes (Figure 21-8). Nuclear atypia, cellular pleomorphism, increased nuclear:cytoplasmic ratio, and mitotic figures all help confirm the diagnosis of carcinoma.

DIFFERENTIAL DIAGNOSIS

Cystic, metastatic SCCs must be distinguished primarily from a branchial cleft cyst. *Branchial cleft cysts* will usually not have a thickened or desmoplastic capsule and will often contain clear fluid. The epithelium in branchial cleft cyst may be variable, with areas of respiratory epithelium and squamous epithelium, which may have keratinization. A focal, weak reaction with p16 may be seen in the epithelium of branchial cleft cysts. However, it is limited to areas infiltrated by inflammatory cells. For all intents and purposes, in the clinical management of patients, a primary branchial cleft carcinoma does not exist. Other benign developmental cystic lesions that may enter the differential include thymopharyngeal cyst, thymic cyst, and bronchial cyst.

PROGNOSIS AND THERAPY

Once the cystic metastasis is accurately classified, efforts toward identifying the primary should include extensive physical examination under anesthesia, panendoscopy (nasopharynx, larynx, esophagus, nasal cavity), and detailed, high-resolution CT or MRI studies of the greater Waldeyer ring area. Again, this search can be aided by assessing the metastatic lesion for the presence of HPV, either through direct viral detection or p16 immunohistochemistry. When positive, there is

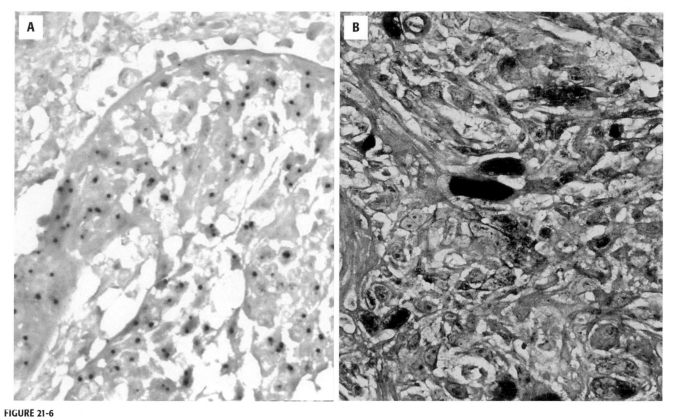

FIGURE 21-6

Human papillomavirus chromogenic in situ hybridization in oropharyngeal squamous cell carcinoma metastases. **A**, Integrated virus showing a punctate staining pattern. **B**, Episomal virus showing diffuse nuclear staining.

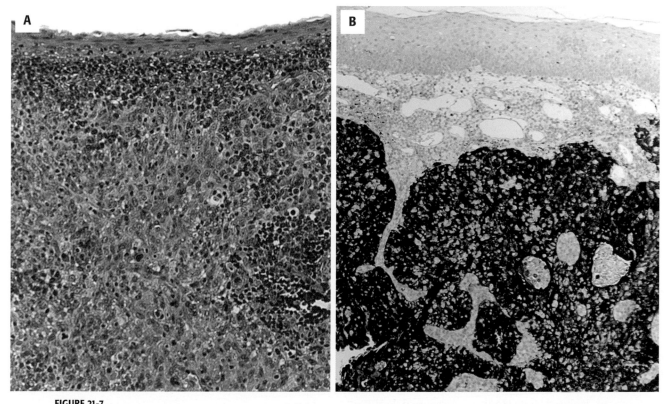

FIGURE 21-7

A, A tonsilar poorly differentiated, nonkeratinizing squamous cell carcinoma. **B**, Strong nuclear and cytoplasmic p16 immunoreactivity.

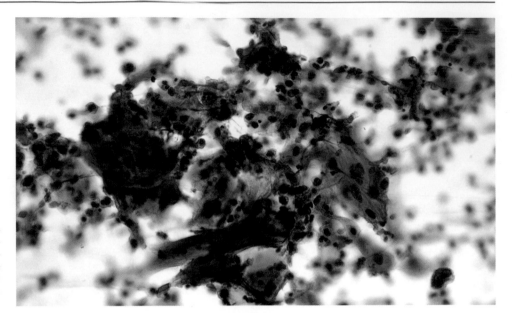

FIGURE 21-8

Atypical squamous cells with "tadpole"-like cytoplasmic extensions, nuclear hyperchromasia, and contour irregularity—helpful features on a fine needle aspirate smear for the diagnosis of squamous cell carcinoma (alcohol-fixed, Papanicolaou stained).

a strong likelihood of a primary in the oropharynx. If these studies do not provide evidence of the primary, then prophylactic lingual and palatine tonsillectomy, specifically on the ipsilateral side, should be performed, with complete embedding of the tonsils and thorough sectioning. Still, there will be an occasional patient for whom attempts at identifying the primary tumor will be defied. Radiation therapy in the region of Waldeyer ring, after the selected lymph node dissection, will yield a good long-term clinical outcome of 70% to 80% survival at 5 years. Patients with HPV (p16)-related tumors may be managed with intensity-modulated or brachy-radiation treatment to achieve a better outcome. Concurrent radiation and multiagent chemotherapy can be used, including agents such as cetuximab. A common complication of radiotherapy or chemotherapy, however, is mucositis. Overall, this type of carcinoma appears to be more indolent than conventional SCC of the tonsil (survival rates of <35% at 5 years) and HPV-related tumors are associated with a better outcome (up to 80% 5-year survival, stage dependent).

■ CHORDOMA

Chordomas are low- to intermediate-grade malignant tumors that recapitulate the notochord. They are divided into three broad categories: sacrococcygeal (60%), spheno-occipital (25%), and vertebral (15%). About 10% of all tumors are cervical. These tumors are thought to arise from vestigial remnants of the embryonic notochord tissue, which normally involutes during the 8th week of development. Isolated cases show an autosomal dominant inheritance pattern.

CLINICAL FEATURES

CHORDOMA—DISEASE FACT SHEET

Definition
- A malignant tumor of notochord origin

Incidence and Location
- Represents ~4% of malignant bone tumors
- Cervical tumors account for ~10%

Morbidity and Mortality
- 65% 5-year survival

Gender, Race, and Age Distribution
- Male > female (2:1), but not in the cervical region
- Mean age, 56 years

Clinical Features
- Neurologic symptoms referable to nerve roots
- Progressive pain
- Parapharyngeal mass if it protrudes forward

Prognosis and Treatment
- Recurrence rates up to 60%
- Approximately 65% 5-year survival, but with cervical lesions, ~60% ultimately die of disease
- Chondroid chordomas (5%) have better prognosis
- Radical, complete surgical removal yields best outcome
- Radiotherapy may be used if nonresectable
- Dedifferentiated chordomas (<5%) are associated with radiotherapy

Chordomas account for ~4% of malignant bone tumors, with ~0.05 case/100,000 population per year. It affects a broad age range, from children to the elderly, although vertebral/neck chordomas occur most frequently in the 5th to 6th decades. Cervical tumors show no gender difference, a feature unique from other anatomic sites. The most common symptoms in the neck include neurologic symptoms (nerve impingement) and progressive pain, while headaches may develop if the lesion encroaches on the skull base. Rarely, a parapharyngeal mass may occur in cervical lesions, as the mass protrudes forward. Tumors are considered slow growing and locally destructive, resulting in locoregional extension.

RADIOLOGIC FEATURES

Chordomas are typically solitary, central, lytic, expansile, and destructive lesions. CT and MRI are complementary imaging modalities, with MRI showing soft tissue changes and CT highlighting bony changes. Chordomas frequently produce an extraosseous soft tissue mass. Matrix calcification is radiographically evident in the majority (70%) of cases.

PATHOLOGIC FEATURES

GROSS FINDINGS

Chordomas are expansive, lobulated tumors with a myxoid and slippery (neural) gross appearance. Tumors of the neck involve the vertebral column, almost always destroying the vertebral disc space, with extension into

---

CHORDOMA—PATHOLOGIC FEATURES

Gross Findings
- Expansive, lobulated, glistening mass with a neural/mucoid appearance

Microscopic Findings
- Lobulated neoplasm
- Cords and island of tumor cells lying in mesenchymal mucus
- Epithelioid cells with remarkable nuclear pleomorphism
- Physaliphorous cells with "bubbly," vacuolated cytoplasm
- Island of hyaline chondroid tissue may be seen

Immunohistochemical Features
- Express keratin, epithelial membrane antigen, brachyury, and S100 protein

Pathologic Differential Diagnosis
- Chondrosarcoma, pleomorphic adenoma, carcinoma ex pleomorphic adenoma, metastatic carcinoma

---

the surrounding tissues. These tumors range in size from 1 to 10 cm (mean, 5 cm).

MICROSCOPIC FINDINGS

Three types of chordomas can be histologically identified: classic, chondroid, and dedifferentiated. The classic microscopic appearance of chordoma is a lobulated growth of cords, clusters, "hepatoid columns," and islands of polygonal tumor cells suspended in a myxoid-mucus background (Figure 21-9). The constituent dual-cell population comprises elongate epithelioid ("chief") cells and large mucus-containing ("physaliphorous") cells (Figure 21-10). Chief cells generally have round and uniform nuclei but may exhibit considerable pleomorphism. The

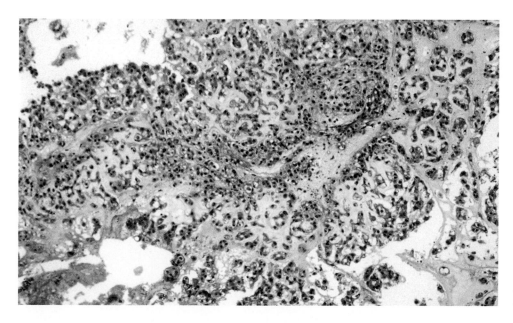

FIGURE 21-9

Lobulated growth of cords and islands of epithelioid cells with a myxoid to mucinous background.

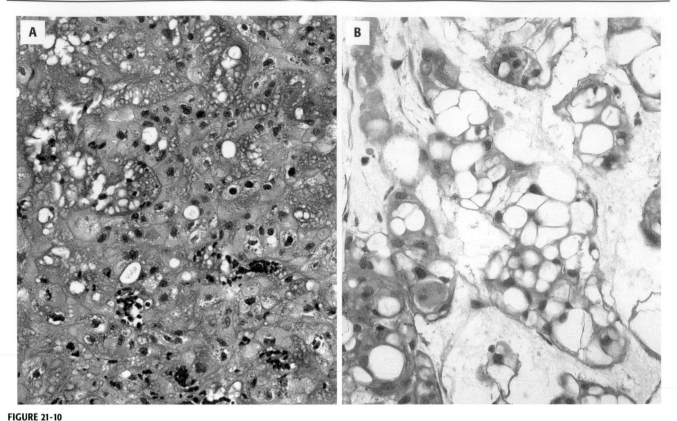

FIGURE 21-10

A, "Hepatoid" columns of epithelioid polygonal cells within a myxoid background. **B**, Physaliphorous cells in a conventional chordoma show vacuolated cytoplasm.

cytoplasm is abundant and eosinophilic but is occasionally clear. Physaliphorous cells with multivacuolated cytoplasm are characteristic for this lesion but are identified to a varying degree. About 5% of cervical chordomas contain islands of hyaline-type chondroid or cartilaginous tissue, thereby invoking the term "chondroid chordomas" (Figure 21-11). In less than 5% of chordomas, there is an association with a high-grade sarcoma (often after radiation); these constitute the "dedifferentiated" chordoma.

ANCILLARY STUDIES

ULTRASTRUCTURAL FEATURES

Electron microscopy will show large cells with abundant cytoplasm and variably sized vacuoles. There are usually characteristic mitochondrial–rough endoplasmic reticulum (RER) complexes, showing a single cisterna

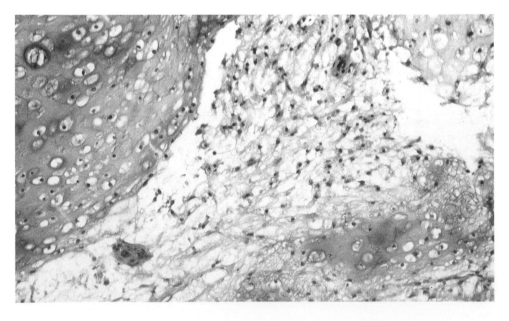

FIGURE 21-11

Islands of hyaline cartilage are noted in the background of a chordoma.

surrounded by numerous mitochondria (Figure 21-12). Intracytoplasmic lumens with scant, small, immature microvilli and cell junctions are noted, along with a fragmented basal lamina.

HISTOCHEMICAL AND IMMUNOHISTOCHEMICAL FEATURES

Mucicarmine and periodic acid–Schiff (PAS) stains highlight mucin within the physaliphorous cells. Chordomas are broadly immunoreactive with vimentin, keratin, epithelial membrane antigen (EMA), S100 protein (Figure 21-12), CAM5.2, HBME-1, CK19, and brachyury (a transcription factor; hence, showing nuclear staining). The staining of these markers can be variable, however, with strong and diffuse staining to weak and focal reactivity. The cells are negative with glial fibrillary acidic protein (GFAP).

FINE NEEDLE ASPIRATION

The smears of chordoma are usually cellular with abundant, myxoid background matrix substance, which often encircles the neoplastic cells (Figure 21-13). The predominant epithelioid cells are arranged in small clusters and short cords. They may be pleomorphic in size and shape, but the chromatin distribution is generally even and regular. The larger physaliphorous cells, with abundant bubbly cytoplasm, are sprinkled throughout but to a lesser degree (Figure 21-13). These cells are usually more easily identified on alcohol-fixed preparations.

GENETIC STUDIES

Cytogenetic studies have shown abnormalities of chromosome 21, including loss or structural rearrangement of 21(q22). In addition, through comparative genomic hybridization studies, multiple recurrent copy gains and losses have been reported, with loss of 9p21.3 (*CDKN2A* gene locus) and loss of 10q23.31 (*PTEN* gene locus) being very common.

DIFFERENTIAL DIAGNOSIS

In the neck, the main differential diagnoses are epithelial neoplasms (e.g., mucinous carcinoma, salivary gland tumors, poorly differentiated carcinoma) and chondrosarcoma, along with benign notochord tumors. The lobulation, physaliphorous cells, and diffuse, strong S100 and brachyury protein immunoreactivity distinguish chordoma

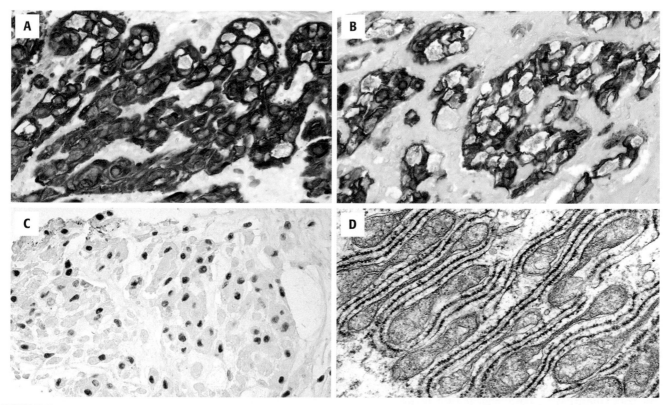

FIGURE 21-12

A, Neoplastic cells are strongly positive with keratin. **B**, Well-developed immunoreactivity for epithelial membrane antigen. **C**, Brachyury stains the nucleus of the neoplastic cells. **D**, Clusters of mitochondria line up along single rough endoplasmic reticulum cisternae creating a characteristic complex. *(Courtesy of Dr. S. Bhuta.)*

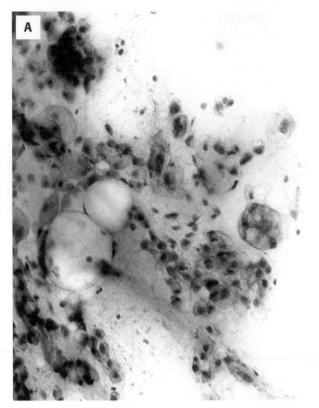
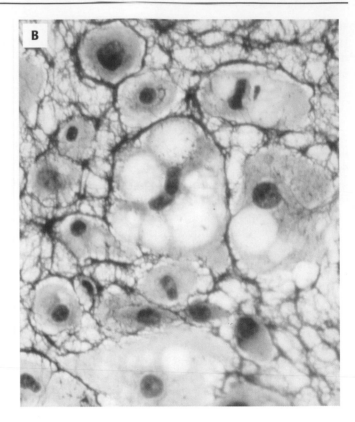

FIGURE 21-13

A, A cellular smear with epithelioid cells in a delicate background of myxoid material. There is a finely vacuolated "physaliphorous" cell in the lower center (hematoxylin and eosin stained). **B**, Epithelioid cells arranged in a magenta background of myxoid material. The center shows a physaliphorous cell (air-dried, Diff-Quik stained).

from *carcinoma*. *Chondrosarcoma* is negative for cytokeratin and brachyury and usually positive for D2-40. *Benign notochord tumors* lack intercellular myxoid matrix and bone destruction. The presence of ductal structures and the immunoreactivity for myoepithelial markers and GFAP distinguish *pleomorphic adenoma* and carcinoma ex pleomorphic adenomas from chordoma.

PROGNOSIS AND THERAPY

Chordoma is a low-grade tumor with rare distant metastases. Although it is an indolent tumor with a 65% 5-year survival, nearly 60% of patients ultimately die from disease. The site, age, gender, and completeness of surgical resection all affect the prognosis. Interestingly, the chondroid variant may have a better prognosis. Radical, complete surgical removal of the chordoma is associated with longer survival and delayed recurrences but is often difficult to achieve in the anatomic confines of the neck. For these and unresectable tumors, adjuvant radiotherapy is used. Complications (cerebrospinal fluid leak, meningitis, paralysis, fistula formation) are frequently seen after surgery.

■ SYNOVIAL SARCOMA

Synovial sarcoma (SS) is a mesenchymal spindle cell neoplasm with variable epithelial differentiation and a specific chromosomal translocation: t(X;18)(p11;q11). SS accounts for ~10% of all soft tissue sarcomas. While there is a predilection for the extremities, ~10% occur in the head and neck, usually in the neck, oropharynx, or hypopharynx. A juxta-articular location is unnecessary, as it is postulated that SS develops from a pluripotential mesenchymal cell.

CLINICAL FEATURES

Although all age groups may be affected, there is a bimodal presentation, with most patients developing the tumor as young adults (mean, 25 years) and a second peak in the 50s. Males are affected more commonly than females (3:1). Typically, the symptoms are nonspecific, manifesting as a solitary, painless mass. Occasionally, hoarseness, upper respiratory distress, and dysphagia may be present.

SYNOVIAL SARCOMA—DISEASE FACT SHEET

Definition

- A malignant tumor with variable epithelial differentiation and a specific chromosomal translocation t(X;18) (p11;q11)

Incidence and Location

- Represents ~10% of all soft issue sarcomas
- About 10% occur in the head and neck

Morbidity and Mortality

- About one-third die with tumor

Gender, Race, and Age Distribution

- Male > female (3:1)
- Median age, 25 years

Clinical Features

- Painless, solitary mass in neck or hypopharynx
- Hoarseness, upper respiratory distress, or dysphagia may occur

Radiographic Features

- Soft tissue mass on computed tomography
- Calcifications within the tumor may help with diagnosis

Prognosis and Treatment

- About 25% develop recurrence
- About 25% have metastatic disease
- About 30% die from disease, usually <4 years from diagnosis
- Clear surgical margins and calcifications portend a better prognosis
- Wide surgical excision with adjuvant multimodality therapy

SYNOVIAL SARCOMA—PATHOLOGIC FEATURES

Gross Findings

- Solid or multicystic mass with calcifications
- Partially encapsulated with variable circumscription
- Cut surface is yellow, gray-white
- Firm, gritty to soft and boggy
- Mucoid and hemorrhagic degeneration may be present

Microscopic Findings

- Biphasic has epithelial/glandular and mesenchymal spindle cell components
- Spindle cells are arranged in short, interlacing fascicles of plump cells with oval nuclei and indistinct cell borders
- Epithelioid component is glandular with cuboidal to columnar epithelial cells arranged in cords, nests, and pseudoglandular spaces
- Mitotic activity is easy to identify
- Mast cells and calcifications may be present
- Monophasic is either spindled or epithelioid

Special Studies

- Ultrastructure shows hemidesmosomes, microvilli, and intercellular junctions in the epithelioid component
- Histochemistry will show mucicarminophilic material in the cytoplasm and lumens (epithelial mucin), while Alcian blue (hyaluronidase-sensitive) mucin is seen in mesenchymal areas (mesenchymal mucin)
- Keratin and EMA positive epithelial and spindle cells, while vimentin only positive spindle cells
- Characteristic molecular t(X;18)(p11.2;q11.2) translocation

Pathologic Differential Diagnosis

- Hemangiopericytoma, fibrous histiocytoma, spindle cell carcinoma, malignant peripheral nerve sheath tumors, fibrosarcoma, leiomyosarcoma, malignant melanoma, epithelioid sarcoma, metastatic adenocarcinoma

RADIOLOGIC FEATURES

A soft tissue mass is appreciable on radiographic studies in most cases, with CT providing valuable information about the site of origin and the extent of the tumor. Irregular calcifications may be present (~20% of cases), a finding that may suggest a better prognosis.

PATHOLOGIC FEATURES

GROSS FINDINGS

Head and neck SSs range in size from 1 to 12 cm. The tumors are partially encapsulated and variably circumscribed, solid to cystic masses. The cut surface is yellow to gray-white with a firm, gritty, and friable to soft, boggy, and rubbery consistency (Figure 21-14). It usually has a whorled appearance, with areas of cyst formation, and mucoid or hemorrhagic degeneration.

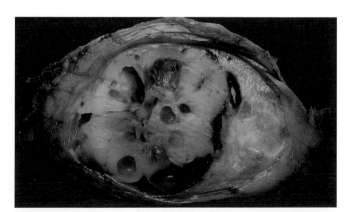

FIGURE 21-14

The synovial sarcoma is encapsulated, showing a nodular and cystic appearance.

Microscopic Findings

Tumors are separated into histologic subtypes: biphasic (both epithelial and spindled; Figures 21-15 and 21-16); monophasic spindle (Figures 21-17 and 21-18) or monophasic epithelial; and poorly differentiated. The monophasic spindled type is most common, followed by the biphasic type. At low power, the tumor shows a characteristic "marbling," with alternating light and dark areas (Figure 21-15) and contains a mesenchymal spindle and a glandular epithelioid component (Figure 21-16). The spindle cells are arranged in orderly, densely packed, short interlacing fascicles of plump cells with oval to spindle, vesicular to hyperchromatic nuclei, and scant cytoplasm with indistinct cellular boundaries, often resembling fibrosarcoma (Figures 21-16, 21-17, and 21-18).

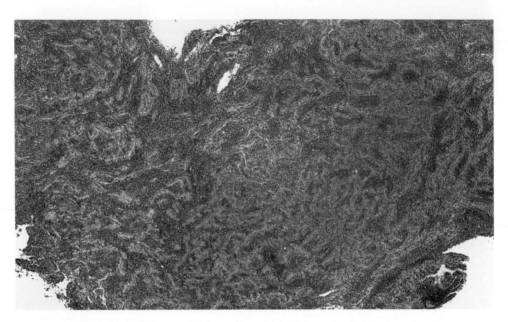

FIGURE 21-15

A biphasic synovial sarcoma shows alternating dark and light areas, a feature helpful in diagnosing this neoplasm in the differential with other tumor types.

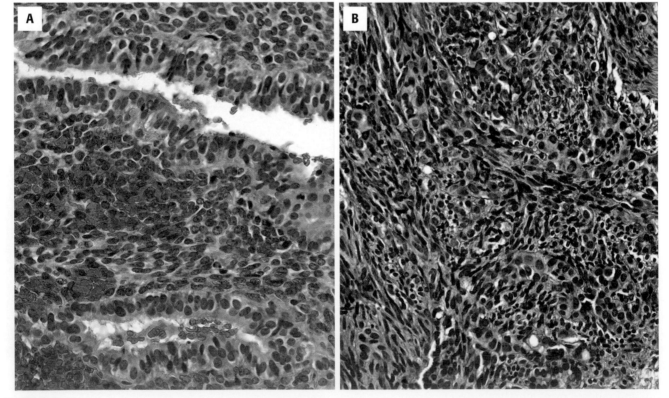

FIGURE 21-16

A biphasic synovial sarcoma. **A**, Glands are easily identified between short fascicles of spindled cells. **B**, A glandular-epithelioid component is present but is more subtle.

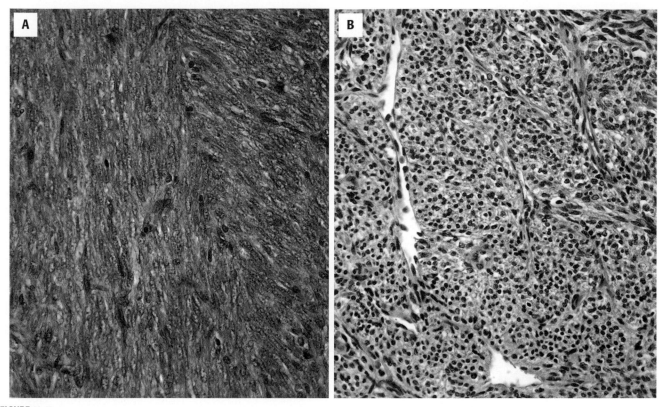

FIGURE 21-17

A, A monophasic synovial sarcoma. The tumor is composed of spindle cells arranged in fascicles. Isolated mast cells are present. **B**, The interlaced fascicles can be arranged at right angles to each other, simulating neural or smooth muscle tumors. Dilated vessels can be prominent.

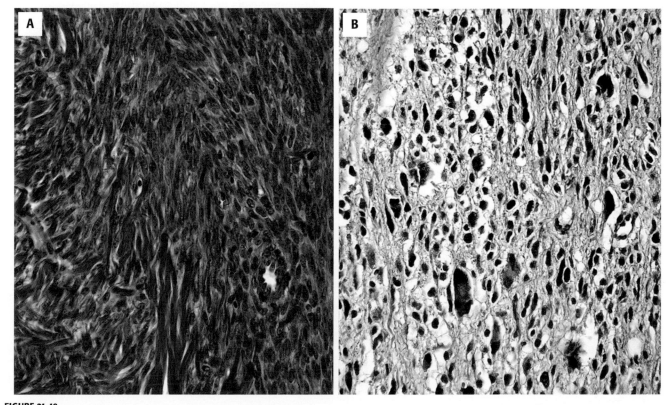

FIGURE 21-18

A, Monophasic synovial sarcoma showing relatively bland spindled cells interdigitating with collagen fibers. Mast cells are present. **B**, Cellular pleomorphism is usually seen in isolated cells, thought to represent ancient change.

The glandular component is composed of cuboidal or columnar epithelial cells arranged in cords, nests, whorls, or pseudoglandular spaces, with round to oval vesicular nuclei encompassed by abundant pale or clear cytoplasm (Figure 21-16). The monophasic SS can be purely spindled or purely epithelial (Figure 21-19). The former is composed of spindled elements arranged in whorls and fascicles of closely packed tumor cells. Mitotic activity is easily identified, although not excessive. The latter has numerous cuboidal or columnar cells arranged in glands. The spindle cells are syncytial in appearance, showing ovoid to pale staining nuclei with small nucleoli. Mast cells and exceptional calcifications can be seen in the spindle cell regions, more easily recognized in hypocellular foci or in areas of myxoid change or necrosis. A rich vascularity is often present, many times creating a hemangiopericytoma-like pattern. There is usually little wiry collagen deposition (Figure 21-18). Pleomorphic cells can be seen but are usually only isolated or in small collections within the tumor.

ANCILLARY STUDIES

ULTRASTRUCTURAL FEATURES

The epithelial elements exhibit hemidesmosomes, microvilli, intercellular junctions, tonofilaments, and an intact basal lamina. The spindle cells demonstrate poorly formed rudimentary cellular junctions, nonbranching cytoplasm, intermediate filaments, and perhaps focal short-cell processes surrounded by an external lamina.

HISTOCHEMICAL FEATURES

Mucicarmine-positive and diastase-resistant PAS-positive *epithelial* mucin can be seen within the cytoplasm of the epithelial cells, within the glandular lumens, and in intracellular areas, while hyaluronidase-sensitive Alcian blue and colloidal iron *mesenchymal* mucin can be identified in the spindle cell and myxoid areas.

IMMUNOHISTOCHEMICAL FEATURES

The epithelial and the spindle cells may express low- and high-molecular-weight cytokeratins, CK7, CK19, and EMA (Figure 21-20). Only the spindle cells are vimentin and bcl-2 positive (Figure 21-21). CD99 is positive in ~60% of cases. The spindle cells reacting with epithelial markers may show focal or weak staining. Due to vagaries of reactivity, it may be prudent to perform more than one marker. TLE1 gives a strong and diffuse nuclear reaction in both the epithelial and spindled cells (Figure 21-21). While it is not unique to SS, it can be of help.

FINE NEEDLE ASPIRATION FINDINGS

Smears from SS are usually densely cellular, showing three-dimensional tissue fragments with irregular borders. There is an accentuation of the proliferation around a capillary vascular plexus or network. Stripped or bare nuclei are often dispersed in the background. The tumor cells are small to medium and usually cytologically bland showing a spindled morphology. They are arranged in fascicles or whorls. Nuclei are ovoid to fusiform, with delicate, even chromatin distribution. If

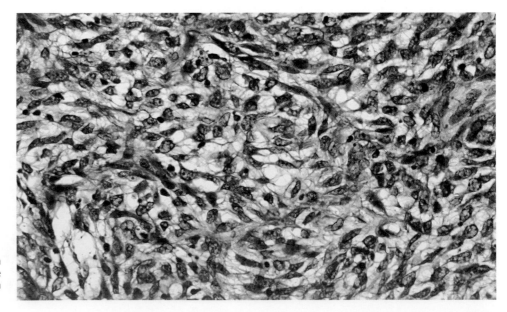

FIGURE 21-19
An epithelioid variant of synovial sarcoma still has a vaguely "spindled" appearance to the epithelioid cells. A myxoid stroma is noted.

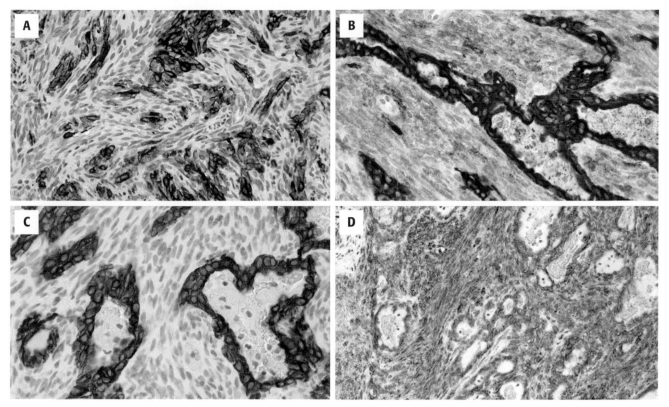

FIGURE 21-20

A variety of immunohistochemistry reactions can be seen. **A**, Pankeratin highlighting the epithelial cells. **B**, Epithelial membrane antigen is strongest in the epithelioid cells but also reactive in the spindled cells. **C**, CK7 shows a strong reaction in the epithelial component. **D**, CD99 highlights both cellular components.

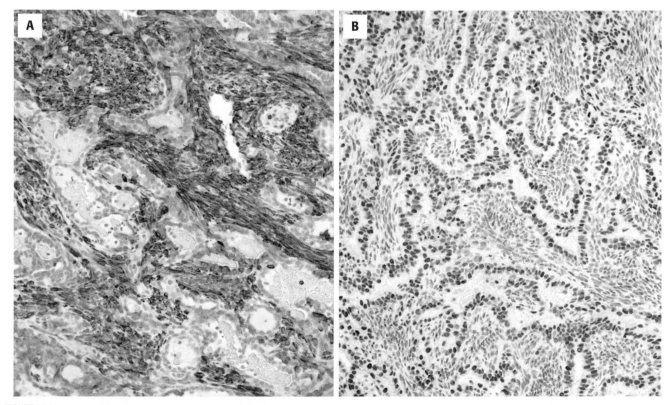

FIGURE 21-21

A, *bcl-2* shows a heavier reaction in the spindle cell population, with nonspecific staining of the glandular component. **B**, TLE1 shows a strong and diffuse nuclear reaction in both epithelial and spindled cells of synovial sarcoma.

the tumor is biphasic, then small gland-like or duct-like structures may be seen. Amorphous, acellular hyaline matrix material may be intermixed with the cells. Mast cells may be seen.

GENETIC STUDIES

By use of reverse transcriptase polymerase chain reaction or fluorescence in situ hybridization (FISH), the characteristic balanced, reciprocal translocation between chromosomes X and 18 can be identified: t(X;18) (p11.2;q11.2) (Figure 21-22). *SSX1*, *SSX2*, or *SSX4* from the X chromosome is reciprocally translocated with *SYT* from chromosome 18.

DIFFERENTIAL DIAGNOSIS

Biphasic SS presents a unique differential diagnosis, while monophasic SS may be more challenging to resolve among the numerous spindle cell neoplasms. The differential includes hemangiopericytoma, fibrous histiocytoma, spindle cell SCC, malignant peripheral nerve sheath tumors, fibrosarcoma, leiomyosarcoma, malignant melanoma, and epithelioid sarcoma. Metastatic adenocarcinoma may also be considered, particularly in cases of monophasic epithelial tumors. In general, the patient's age, specific anatomic site, unique histologic appearance, immunoprofile, and characteristic translocation will yield a definitive separation. An immunohistochemical panel may need to include keratin, EMA, vimentin, S100 protein, HMB45, CD34, desmin, and actins. Molecular assays for the translocation will often help to resolve the differential diagnosis in difficult cases. A caveat must be kept in mind: recurrent or

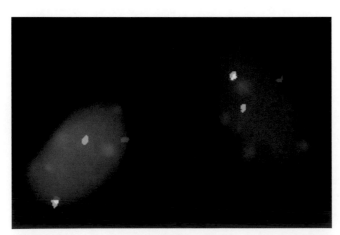

FIGURE 21-22
Fluorescent in situ hybridization (FISH) for the X;18 translocation. A FISH break-apart probe shows a single red and green signal in each cell, confirming the "break apart" or separation of the two probes normally flanking the breakpoint region. (A normal result shows a yellow fused signal indicating that the locus is intact.) *(Courtesy of Anhthu Nguyen.)*

metastatic foci may have a different histologic appearance than the primary.

PROGNOSIS AND THERAPY

Local recurrence develops in ~25% of patients, with ~25% also demonstrating metastatic disease (usually to lung). Head and neck tumor patients have a better prognosis compared to other anatomic sites. About one-third of patients die from their disease, usually within 4 years of the initial diagnosis. Interestingly, there is a suggestion that patients with calcifications in their tumors have a better prognosis than those without calcifications. There is also a better prognosis associated with small tumors, young age at presentation, and low mitotic indexes. Surgery combined with multimodality therapy (radiation and chemotherapy) is usually used. Meticulous attention to surgical margins will achieve locoregional control and thereby successful therapy.

■ METASTATIC NEOPLASM OF UNKNOWN PRIMARY

The term "occult primary tumor" refers to a primary neoplasm that has not been found in a patient with lymph node, organ, or soft tissue metastasis, even after a thorough clinical evaluation. This evaluation includes pan-endoscopy, radiographic studies, and serologic markers, usually before a lymph node biopsy, although a fine needle aspiration (FNA) or core needle biopsy is frequently the initial procedure. Neck metastasis may represent disease from a regional or distant primary neoplasm. Despite aggressive assessment, in ~10% of patients, a primary tumor will not be identified. While axiomatic, lymphomas must always be excluded, if there is a poorly differentiated neoplasm in the lymph node, as their management is unique from that of metastatic disease.

CLINICAL FEATURES

The most common symptom is a painless mass in the neck. The most frequent sites of adenopathy are upper jugulodigastric (70%), midjugular (22%), supraclavicular (18%), and posterior cervical lymph nodes (12%), with more than one site affected. The masses may be present for quite some time and are often slowly enlarging. The mean age at presentation is in the 6th decade, although this depends on the primary tumor type. When the primaries are from the upper aerodigestive system, men are affected more commonly than

METASTATIC NEOPLASM OF UNKNOWN PRIMARY—DISEASE FACT SHEET

Definition
- An unidentified primary neoplasm with cervical metastasis

Incidence and Location
- Neck lymph node metastasis is frequent, although only ~10% of patients have unknown primaries
- Upper jugular lymph nodes account for most metastatic tumors (70%)

Morbidity and Mortality
- Mortality depends on primary tumor

Gender, Race, and Age Distribution
- For upper aerodigestive tract primaries, male >> female (4:1)
- Usually adults, with a mean presentation in the 6th decade
- Other primaries are gender and age specific

Clinical Features
- Painless cervical mass
- Slow growing over several months
- Primary sites include Waldeyer ring, nasopharynx, larynx, and esophagus, while lung, gastrointestinal tract, breast, pancreas, and prostate account for carcinomas outside of the head and neck region
- Melanoma and sarcoma also present as metastatic tumors

Prognosis and Treatment
- Prognosis is determined by the underlying primary but is usually poor as metastatic disease is already present
- Initial fine needle aspiration evaluation guides therapy, which includes lymph node dissection and radiation

METASTATIC NEOPLASM OF UNKNOWN PRIMARY—PATHOLOGIC FEATURES

Gross Findings
- Solid or cystic mass
- Up to 10 cm in size (mean, ~3 cm)

Microscopic Findings
- Tumor type determines the lymph node appearance
- Squamous cell carcinoma, adenocarcinoma, undifferentiated carcinoma, melanoma, sarcoma, and lymphoma are all considerations, with carcinomas most common

Special Studies
- Variable depending on the histologic type
- Screening panel to include keratin, p63, CD45RB, S100 protein, HMB45, actin, and desmin with follow-on targeted antibodies

Pathologic Differential Diagnosis
- Developmental cysts, infections, reactive hyperplasia, lymphoma, ectopic nests in the lymph node

and the histologic features are highly variable based on the tumor of origin. However, the most common metastatic primary sites in the cervical lymph nodes are SCC (60%), adenocarcinoma (20%; Figure 21-23), undifferentiated carcinoma (12%), and melanoma (5%; Figure 21-24); other, miscellaneous tumor types comprise the remainder (3%). Adenocarcinomas, undifferentiated carcinoma, and thyroid carcinomas are more common in the supraclavicular and scalene lymph nodes.

ANCILLARY STUDIES

HISTOCHEMICAL AND IMMUNOHISTOCHEMICAL STUDIES

Histochemical studies, such as mucicarmine (Figures 21-23 and 21-24), may help to confirm the tumor type (i.e., adenocarcinoma). In many cases, a targeted immunohistochemical panel will help to suggest a primary site. Keratin, p63, CD45RB, S100 protein, HMB45, actin, and desmin are often used as initial screening studies, to help narrow the selection of additional antibodies. Naturally, the clinical history, including the patient's gender, age, physical examination, and laboratory studies will also help to direct the immunohistochemical workup.

FINE NEEDLE ASPIRATION

FNA is an excellent screening study; it is a rapid, inexpensive, and safe procedure that can be performed at the time of the patient's initial presentation. When it comes to metastatic tumors, separation can usually be made between squamous and adenocarcinoma, with

women (4:1), with many patients reporting a history of heavy smoking and drinking. Non–head and neck carcinoma primary sites (gender dependent) include lung, gastrointestinal tract, breast, pancreas, and prostate, while melanoma and sarcomas round out the list.

PATHOLOGIC FEATURES

GROSS FINDINGS

The lymph nodes may be solid, unicystic or multicystic, white, gray to dark, and hemorrhagic. The size ranges up to 10 cm in greatest dimension (mean, ~3 cm). The primary tumor type will frequently dictate the lymph node appearance.

MICROSCOPIC FINDINGS

Nearly every known malignancy may at some time result in metastatic deposits in cervical lymph nodes

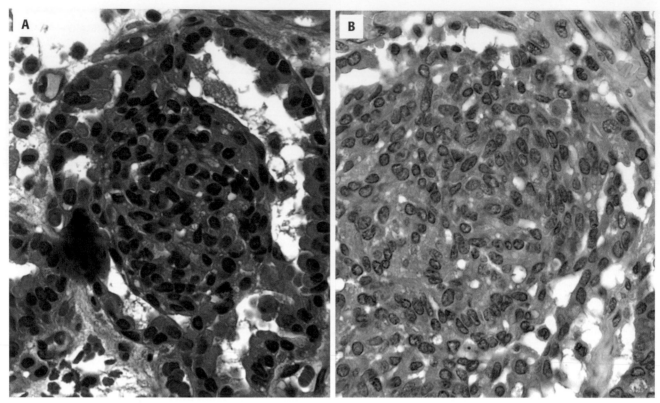

FIGURE 21-23

A, A metastatic adenocarcinoma from the breast demonstrates small gland lumen and a suggestion of intracytoplasmic vacuoles of mucin. **B**, Mucicarmine stain highlights the mucin vacuoles.

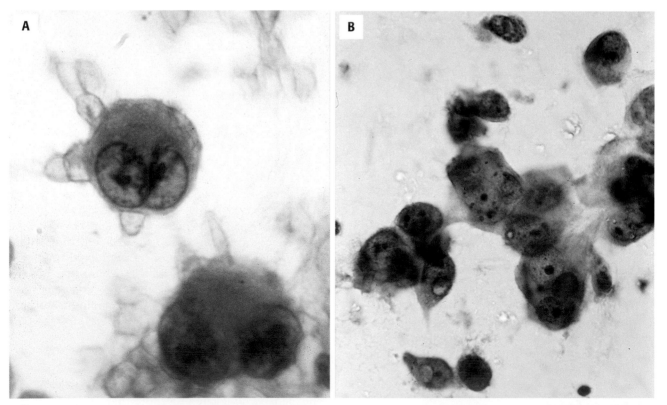

FIGURE 21-24

A, Large, binucleated atypical individual cells raise the differential diagnosis of a melanoma, sarcoma, or Hodgkin lymphoma. This case represented metastatic melanoma, but without cytoplasmic pigmentation, immunohistochemical analysis would be necessary, along with the clinical history (alcohol-fixed, Papanicolaou stained). **B**, A mucicarmine stain highlights the intracellular mucin in this metastatic lung adenocarcinoma (mucicarmine stain).

additional histochemical or immunohistochemical studies performed on the smears as directed by the cytologic findings. More generally, a diagnosis of lymphoma, carcinoma, melanoma, or sarcoma as major categories is also helpful for directing the search in a specific direction, eliminating the need for more invasive and costly procedures while also enhancing treatment planning.

DIFFERENTIAL DIAGNOSIS

The differential diagnosis usually encompasses benign and reactive versus neoplastic lesions; however, given the lymph node location, any identified epithelial neoplasm is reasonably assumed to be malignant. Benign entities are also in the differential and include branchial cleft cysts, developmental cysts, ectopia, infections, and reactive inflammatory lymphoid hyperplasias, most of which can usually be easily separated.

PROGNOSIS AND THERAPY

The prognosis is determined largely by the underlying primary, although the presence of metastases at the time of diagnosis already portends a poorer prognosis. Rare exceptions do exist, however. Lymph node dissection and radiation can often palliate tumor progression.

SUGGESTED READINGS

The complete suggested readings list is available online at www.expertconsult.com.

22

Non-Neoplastic Lesions of the Thyroid Gland

■ **Carol F. Adair**

■ THYROGLOSSAL DUCT CYST

Persistence of the tract that represents the migratory path of the thyroid anlage from the foregut (foramen cecum) to its normal position in the midline neck can give rise to fistulous tracts, sinuses, or cysts anywhere along the tract. Thyroglossal duct cysts represent the most common midline mass in children but may also be found in adults and in the elderly.

CLINICAL FEATURES

Thyroglossal duct anomalies are found in up to 7% of adults. Approximately two-thirds present as cysts and one-third are fistulas. Fistulas or sinus tracts usually reflect secondary trauma or infection. Occurring equally in the genders, two-thirds are diagnosed in children or young adults. Approximately 75% of thyroglossal duct cysts are found in the midline of the neck, at or immediately below the hyoid bone. Other locations include intralingual (2%), suprahyoid or submental (25%), and suprasternal (13%). Slightly off-midline examples may be seen; in such cases, the presence of a fibrous tract or cord emanating from the hyoid bone is a helpful finding.

Most patients discover an asymptomatic midline mass on their own (Figure 22-1), although sometimes there is pain, a draining sinus or fistula, or dysphagia. The cysts may fluctuate in size, especially if infected. Thyroglossal duct cysts move vertically with swallowing or protrusion of the tongue. On radiographic studies, they usually present as a cystic mass, often with bright signal on magnetic resonance imaging (MRI) studies. They are usually midline, with the point of origin frequently identified.

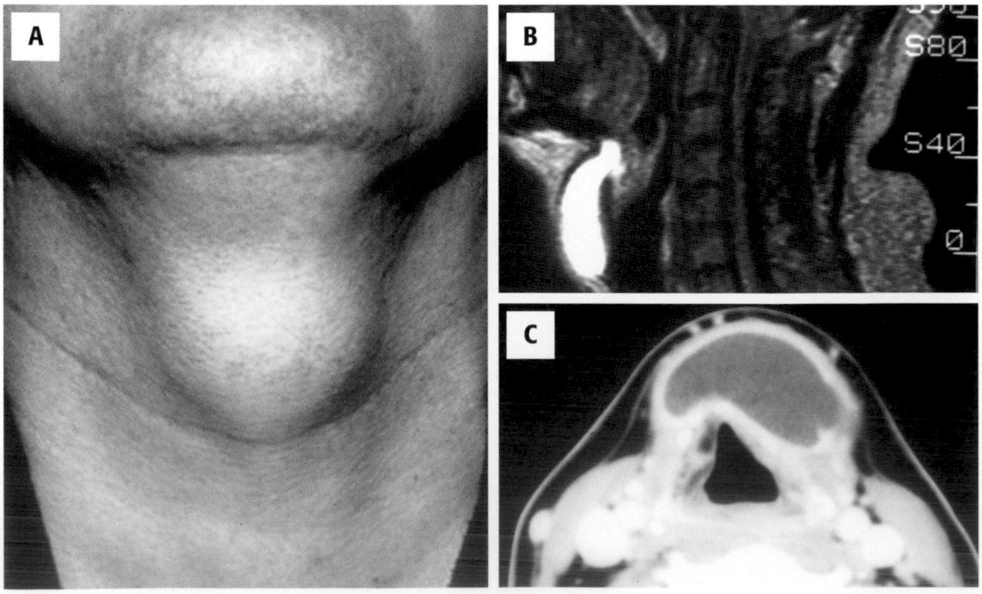

FIGURE 22-1

A, A mass in the midline, encompassing the hyoid bone, which moves with swallowing. **B**, Magnetic resonance image showing a bright signal of the fluid-filled thyroglossal duct cyst as it extends from the foramen cecum. **C**, Computed tomography scan showing a large fluid-filled cyst anterior to the larynx. Note a slight "shift" to the left of midline.

THYROGLOSSAL DUCT CYST—DISEASE FACT SHEET

Definition

■ A persistent tract representing the embryologic migratory path of the thyroid anlage in the anterior neck

Incidence and Location

■ Up to 7% of adults
■ 75% in anterior midline of neck at or immediately below hyoid bone; remainder found in intralingual, suprahyoid (submental), and suprasternal loci

Morbidity and Mortality

■ May become secondarily infected
■ Thyroid carcinoma, usually papillary type, develops in 1% of cases; associated with favorable prognosis

Gender and Age Distribution

■ Equal gender distribution
■ Most common in children or young adults

Clinical Features

■ Asymptomatic midline neck mass
■ Draining sinus or fistula and pain, if infected

Prognosis and Therapy

■ 4% to 6% recurrence rate with Sistrunk procedure
■ Preferred treatment is Sistrunk procedure

THYROGLOSSAL DUCT CYST—PATHOLOGIC FEATURES

Gross Findings

■ Cyst filled with mucoid or purulent material
■ Fibrous tract from area of foramen cecum to hyoid bone
■ One-third present as fistulas, usually due to infection
■ Solid areas sampled to exclude neoplasm

Microscopic Findings

■ Cyst lined by respiratory or squamous epithelium
■ If infected, granulation tissue may replace epithelium
■ Fibrosis and chronic inflammation in cyst wall
■ Thyroid tissue identified in up to two-thirds of cases
■ If carcinoma is present, 90% are papillary type

Fine Needle Aspiration

■ Thick mucoid or purulent material, sparsely cellular with inflammatory material the rule

Pathologic Differential Diagnosis

■ Epidermoid cysts, degenerated adenomatoid nodules

PATHOLOGIC FEATURES

GROSS FINDINGS

The surgical specimen usually consists of the thyroglossal duct cyst, measuring up to 4 cm, as well as the fibrous tract extending to the foramen cecum and the central 1 to 2 cm of the hyoid bone (Figure 22-2). The cyst may contain clear mucoid fluid or, if infected, purulent material. Solid or firm areas should be carefully sampled to exclude an associated neoplasm.

MICROSCOPIC FINDINGS

The thyroglossal duct cyst is normally lined by respiratory epithelium, but squamous metaplasia is quite common (Figures 22-3 and 22-4). If the cyst has been infected, the lining epithelium may be replaced by granulation tissue, sometimes with granulomatous elements such as foamy histiocytes and multinucleated

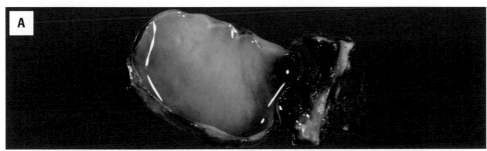

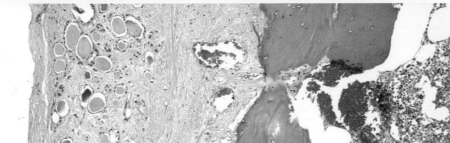

FIGURE 22-2

A, This thyroglossal duct cyst is from a Sistrunk procedure and includes the cyst, the tract of the thyroglossal duct, and the midsection of the hyoid bone. **B**, Thyroid parenchyma is noted at the left side, while a portion of bone and marrow is noted immediately adjacent.

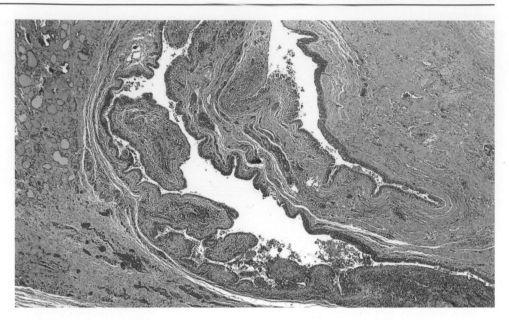

FIGURE 22-3

Thyroglossal duct cyst. The cyst is lined by epithelium and is surrounded by fibrous tissue with chronic inflammation and a small amount of thyroid tissue (*left side*).

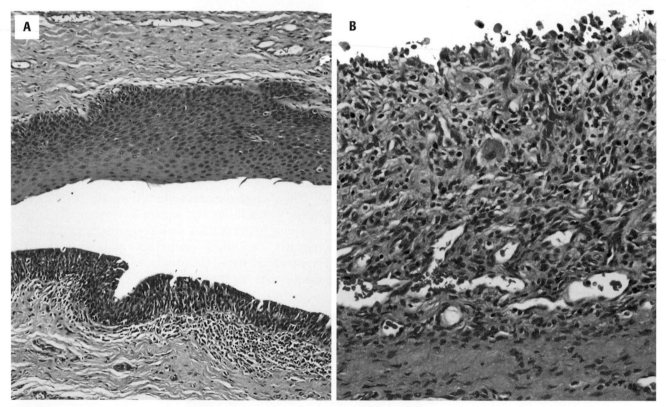

FIGURE 22-4

A, The cyst lining may be either squamous epithelium (*upper*) or respiratory type (*lower*). **B**, Infection may cause denudation of the epithelial lining, which is replaced by granulation tissue.

giant cells (Figure 22-4). Fibrosis and chronic inflammation are common in the cyst wall. Thyroid tissue is not invariably present but is found in up to two-thirds of cases with careful examination.

The associated thyroid tissue may harbor any inflammatory, hyperplastic, or neoplastic alteration that can be seen in the normal follicular epithelial component of the thyroid gland. Up to 1% of thyroglossal duct cysts will have an associated carcinoma, with papillary carcinoma representing ~90% of cases. Thyroglossal duct cysts in elderly patients are much more likely to harbor malignancies. Interestingly, no examples of medullary carcinoma have been documented, presumably due to the different embryologic origin of the C cells of the thyroid from the ultimobranchial body.

ANCILLARY STUDIES

FINE NEEDLE ASPIRATION

Fine needle aspiration (FNA) is not widely used in the diagnosis of thyroglossal duct cyst because of the limited cytologic findings, but it is useful in documenting other lesions that may form midline neck masses. Aspirates consist of thick mucoid or purulent material and are sparsely cellular; inflammatory cells tend to outnumber the benign squamous or respiratory epithelial cells.

DIFFERENTIAL DIAGNOSIS

Epidermoid cysts of the thyroid or degenerated cystic *adenomatoid nodules* may be considered in the differential diagnosis; but the midline location and respiratory and/or squamous epithelial lining are key elements in making the diagnosis of thyroglossal duct cyst. When a thyroid carcinoma arising in a thyroglossal duct cyst is under consideration, the possibility of a metastatic tumor from the thyroid proper should be excluded.

PROGNOSIS AND THERAPY

The preferred treatment for a thyroglossal duct cyst is the Sistrunk procedure, which requires resection of the entire tract of the thyroglossal duct, along with the cyst or fistula and the central 1 to 2 cm of the hyoid bone. The recurrence rate after this procedure is 4% to 6%; if the hyoid bone segment is not removed, the recurrence rate increases above 25%. Well-differentiated thyroid carcinoma arising in a thyroglossal duct cyst has an excellent prognosis with the Sistrunk procedure. Total thyroidectomy is not usually required, except in high-risk patients, or in the instance of carcinoma arising in the thyroglossal duct cyst.

■ STRUMA OVARII

The term "struma ovarii" refers to ovarian teratomas in which thyroid tissue is the predominant or only tissue component. The thyroid tissue is benign; however, primary thyroid neoplasms of follicular cell derivation as well as carcinoid tumor may arise in struma ovarii.

CLINICAL FEATURES

Most cases of struma ovarii are discovered in the 5th decade, but they may occur over a wide age range.

STRUMA OVARII—DISEASE FACT SHEET

Definition

■ An ovarian teratoma in which the predominant or only component is benign thyroid tissue

Incidence and Location

■ <5% of ovarian teratomas represent struma ovarii
■ Localized to the ovary; some cases with peritoneal implants
■ Usually unilateral, but may be bilateral

Morbidity and Mortality

■ Some with hyperthyroidism; almost all benign; rare cases with thyroid carcinoma in struma ovarii usually pursue indolent course, only rarely metastasizing

Gender and Age Distribution

■ Females
■ Peak incidence, 5th decade

Clinical Features

■ Pelvic/ovarian mass, often cystic; rarely hyperthyroidism

Prognosis and Therapy

■ Almost all cured by oophorectomy; even papillary thyroid carcinoma or carcinoid in struma ovarii usually cured by oophorectomy

---

Most present simply as an ovarian mass and are no different clinically from other teratomas. Rarely, however, struma ovarii produces hyperthyroidism. Ascites is sometimes present.

The rare papillary thyroid carcinoma (malignant struma) or carcinoid tumor (strumal carcinoid) arising within struma ovarii is typically an incidental histologic finding, with no prior clinical features to raise suspicion.

PATHOLOGIC FEATURES

GROSS FINDINGS

The thyroid tissue of struma ovarii usually is found in association with a dermoid cyst and appears as a solid red to brown soft tissue mass. Gelatinous colloid may be visible, and cystic areas are not uncommonly observed. Unless the lesion is completely composed of thyroid tissue, other elements of a dermoid cyst are seen, particularly keratinous cystic areas. As with any ovarian teratoma, bone, cartilage, and a wide array of epithelial components may give the lesion a variegated appearance. The size is highly variable.

MICROSCOPIC FINDINGS

The thyroid tissue usually has the appearance of normal thyroid or nodular goiter, with large follicles lined by flattened follicular cells and filled with abundant colloid

STRUMA OVARII—PATHOLOGIC FEATURES

Gross Findings

- Cystic and/or solid ovarian mass, may contain cartilage, keratinous debris and other elements common to dermoid cysts/teratomas
- Thyroid tissue red-brown, often with green-brown colloid in cystic areas
- Solid areas sampled carefully to exclude carcinoid or carcinoma

Microscopic Findings

- Benign thyroid usually with large colloid-filled follicles and flattened epithelium
- Proliferative examples with small follicles, hyperplastic epithelium, and increased cellularity
- Carcinoma usually with papillary-type nuclear features
- Carcinoid with trabecular or insular growth pattern, enlarged nuclei with coarse chromatin, often admixed with benign thyroid follicles

Immunohistochemical Results

- Struma: thyroglobulin, TTF-1, PAX8 positive
- Carcinoid: chromogranin, synaptophysin, calcitonin, CEA positive

Pathologic Differential Diagnosis

- Primary ovarian epithelial neoplasms, particularly benign and borderline mucinous neoplasms, and metastatic carcinoma

(Figure 22-5). In such instances the tissue is readily recognized. Some examples, however, are more proliferative, with highly cellular areas including microfollicular, solid, or trabecular growth patterns (Figure 22-6). Clear cells or oxyphilic cells may predominate, making the thyroid origin of the tissue difficult to discern. The nuclei are generally round and regular, with a dense chromatin pattern.

Papillary thyroid carcinoma arising in struma ovarii has the same distinctive nuclear features as it does as a primary thyroid tumor. Furthermore, it may have a follicular or a papillary architectural pattern.

Carcinoid tumor may also arise within struma ovarii. The carcinoid usually forms a solid mass, and it may be yellow-white in color and grossly distinctive from the background thyroid tissue; however, its presence may not be noted until histologic examination. The carcinoid tumor is most often admixed with the thyroid tissue and has an insular or trabecular growth pattern. Sometimes, the transition between a proliferative struma ovarii and carcinoid tumor is extremely subtle and immunohistochemical stains are needed to clearly separate the two entities (Figure 22-7).

ANCILLARY STUDIES

IMMUNOHISTOCHEMICAL STUDIES

The thyroid tissue of struma ovarii is positive for thyroglobulin, PAX8, and TTF-1; sometimes these stains are needed to confirm the diagnosis in proliferative examples of struma ovarii, which may resemble other primary ovarian neoplasms.

Strumal carcinoid is immunoreactive with chromogranin, synaptophysin, CD56, and carcinoembryonic antigen (CEA). The carcinoid cells are negative for thyroglobulin and TTF-1, but there may be diffusion of the thyroglobulin from adjacent or admixed thyroid tissue.

DIFFERENTIAL DIAGNOSIS

Struma ovarii is usually easily recognized, but proliferative examples may be mistaken for other *primary ovarian tumors*, such as those of surface epithelial origin (particularly

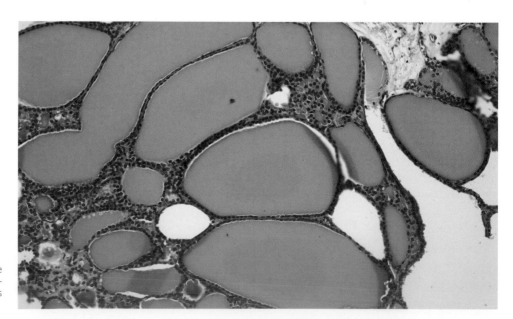

FIGURE 22-5

Struma ovarii, typical pattern, with large follicles and abundant colloid, resembling nodular hyperplasia. This pattern is easily recognizable.

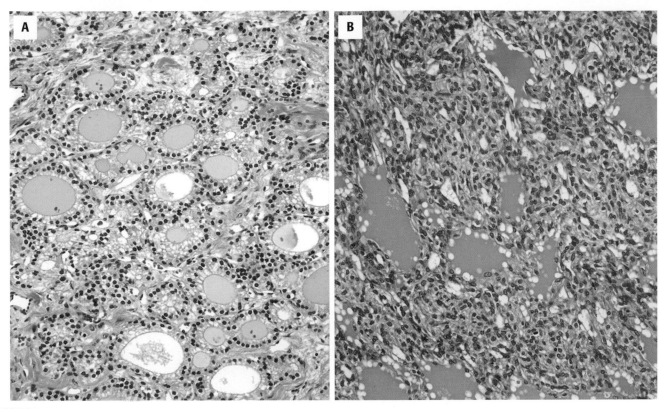

FIGURE 22-6
A and **B**, Proliferative patterns of struma ovarii, with increased cellularity and less prominent colloid, may be difficult to recognize, especially on frozen section slides.

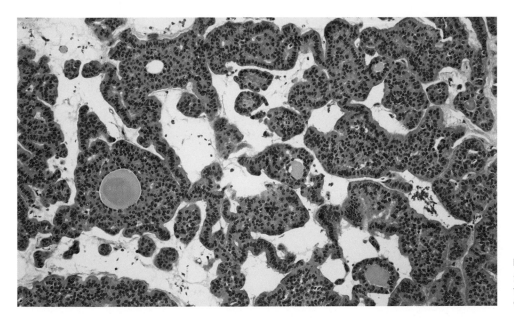

FIGURE 22-7

Strumal carcinoid, with a trabecular pattern of carcinoid, admixed with the follicles of struma ovarii.

the mucinous ovarian tumors) and gonadal stroma tumors, as well as *metastatic carcinoma* to the ovary. The presence of eosinophilic colloid-like material and a somewhat uniform follicular/glandular pattern that is unlike those typically seen in primary ovarian tumors should suggest the correct diagnosis. In a difficult case, thyroglobulin and TTF-1 immunostains are quite helpful.

PROGNOSIS AND THERAPY

Struma ovarii is treated as any other teratoma, namely, by surgical removal. Even those cases with papillary thyroid carcinoma or strumal carcinoid are almost always cured by resection. Aggressive behavior is very uncommon. There are, however, rare cases of histologi-cally benign-appearing struma ovarii that have metasta-sized to the peritoneum and lymph nodes, but even these cases typically follow a benign or indolent course.

■ ULTIMOBRANCHIAL BODY REMNANTS AND OTHER INTRATHYROIDAL INCLUSIONS

Small remnants of the ultimobranchial apparatus, known as "solid cell nests," are associated with the embryologic development of the C-cell (calcitonin-producing) popula-tion of the thyroid. They are encountered as an inciden-tal finding, usually in the posterior medial and posterior lateral lobes but never in the isthmus.

CLINICAL FEATURES

Solid cell nests are of no clinical significance but are fairly common. They are identified in ~25% of thyroid resection specimens; their discovery is largely related to the generosity of sampling of "normal" thyroid tissue.

PATHOLOGIC FEATURES

Ultimobranchial remnants are quite small, most measur-ing no more than 0.1 mm. They are represented by a cluster of small epithelial nests or a small lobulated struc-ture and may be solid or partially cystic (Figure 22-8). Occasionally, several foci may be found in a gland. The epithelial cells are small and ovoid to polygonal, with slightly elongated nuclei; they are designated "main cells." The chromatin is finely granular and evenly dis-persed. A longitudinal nuclear groove is often present

(Figure 22-9). The overall histologic pattern is very simi-lar to immature squamous metaplasia, but keratinization and intercellular bridges are not visible. Occasional cells with clear cytoplasm may be scattered through the epi-thelium; degenerative changes are thought to account for the occasional presence of mucicarmine-positive material in ultimobranchial remnants. A minor population of cells with clear cytoplasm represents C cells.

ANCILLARY STUDIES

Although immunohistochemical studies are certainly not necessary for making a diagnosis, the staining pattern of ultimobranchial remnants is fairly distinctive. Main cells are positive for p63, bcl-2, CK19, and galectin-3. The C cells are positive for calcitonin, CEA, and galectin-3. Neither cell type is positive for thyroglobulin.

DIFFERENTIAL DIAGNOSIS

Ultimobranchial remnants are sometimes mistaken for incidental microscopic *papillary carcinoma*. Although nuclear grooves are frequent in ultimobranchial rem-nants, these lesions lack the other nuclear features of papillary carcinoma (overlapping nuclei, ground-glass chromatin pattern, intranuclear inclusions) as well as an adjacent stromal desmoplastic reaction.

These remnants may also resemble *squamous metapla-sia*. While not necessarily within the differential diagnosis, *endodermally derived tissues* may be encountered in the thyroid gland, including cartilage, parathyroid gland (Figure 22-10), thymic tissue, and salivary gland tissue (Figure 22-11). These "inclusions" are usually of no clinical

---

ULTIMOBRANCHIAL BODY REMNANTS—DISEASE FACT SHEET

Definition
- Small remnant of the ultimobranchial apparatus, associated with development of thyroid C cells

Incidence and Location
- Incidental finding in ~25% of thyroid specimens
- Posteromedial and posterolateral areas of lobes; *never* in isthmus

Clinical Features
- Patients present with unrelated thyroid nodule(s)

Prognosis and Therapy
- No clinical significance

ULTIMOBRANCHIAL BODY REMNANTS—PATHOLOGIC FEATURES

Microscopic Findings
- Small nests or lobulated aggregates of polygonal epithelial cells, usually ~0.1 mm
- Some examples are partially cystic
- No keratinization or intercellular bridges
- Nuclei ovoid, with evenly distributed chromatin, and frequent longitudinal nuclear grooves
- Occasional clear cells and mucoid material may be seen

Immunohistochemical Results
- May stain with chromogranin, synaptophysin, calcitonin, carcino-embryonic antigen (small size limits study)

Pathologic Differential Diagnosis
- Incidental papillary thyroid carcinoma, squamous metaplasia

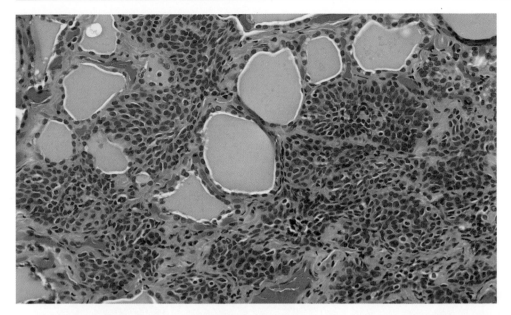

FIGURE 22-8

This ultimobranchial body remnant is a solid cell nest, adjacent to normal thyroid parenchyma, and is an incidental finding. Note the "pavemented" appearance.

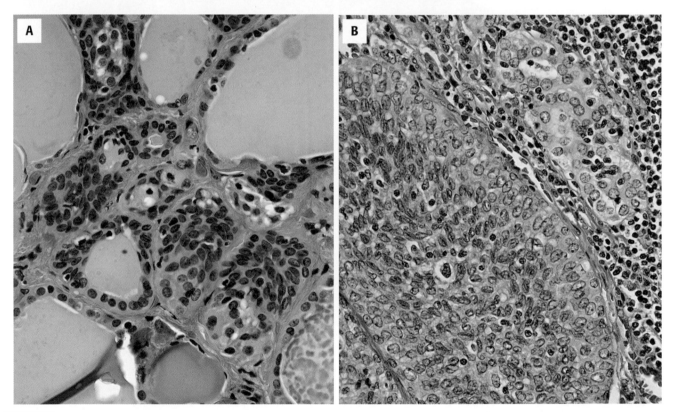

FIGURE 22-9

A, The ultimobranchial body epithelium is reminiscent of immature squamous metaplasia. Note the lack of keratinization and intercellular bridges. **B**, The nuclei are ovoid, often with a longitudinal groove. This collection is quite cellular, adjacent to a thyroid follicle within lymphocytic thyroiditis.

significance, typically representing incidental findings in surgical resection specimens. *Thymic tissue* retains its lobulated appearance, has small cystic islands of squamous epithelium (Hassall corpuscles) with an abundant lymphoid component which may be mistaken for lymphocytic thyroiditis or a lymph node (Figure 22-11). *Parathyroid tissue*, particularly if it is hyperplastic or neoplastic, can be difficult to distinguish from a cellular adenomatoid nodule or follicular thyroid neoplasm. *Oxyphilic change*

makes separation a challenge. *Parathyroid cells* are usually smaller than follicular epithelial cells, and the nuclei are very small, round, and hyperchromatic, with rather coarse chromatin that suggests a neuroendocrine cell type. A cytologic preparation (particularly a "scrape prep") is especially useful in the differential diagnosis of parathyroid versus thyroid nodules; they are highly recommended in all intraoperative consultations on parathyroid and thyroid lesions.

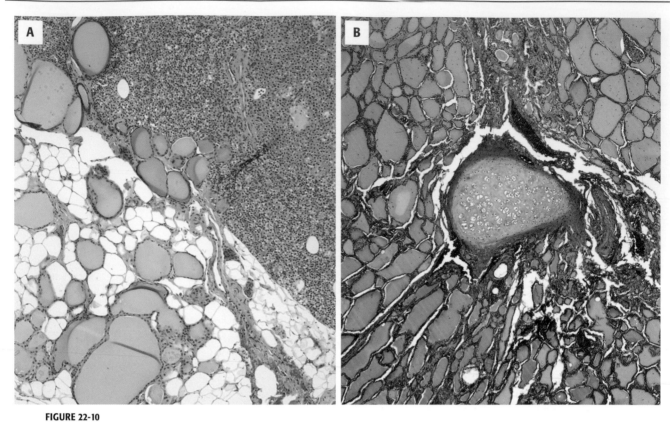

FIGURE 22-10
There are often inclusions identified within the thyroid gland. Here is an intrathyroidal parathyroid (**A**) and a small fragment of cartilage (**B**).

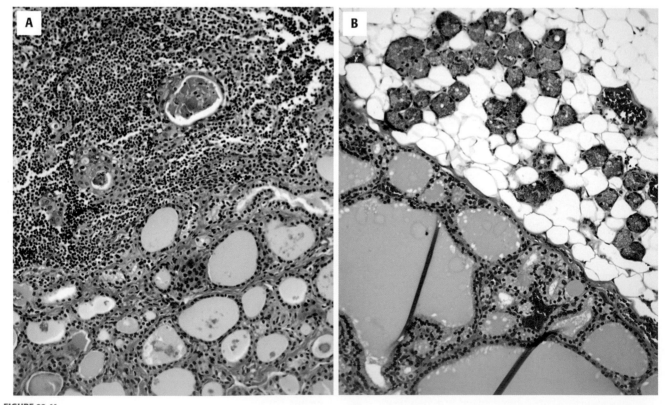

FIGURE 22-11
Thymic tissue (**A**) is noted in direct continuity with the thyroid gland. Salivary gland tissue (**B**) is noted adjacent to unremarkable thyroid parenchyma. These are normal tissue elements without any tissue reaction.

PROGNOSIS AND THERAPY

No therapy is necessary as this is an incidental finding.

■ ACUTE THYROIDITIS

Acute inflammation with a neutrophilic inflammatory infiltrate in the thyroid parenchyma is rare; it may be associated with either a localized or systemic infection due to bacterial, fungal, or viral agents such as rubella and cytomegalovirus. Predisposing factors include neck trauma or immunosuppression.

CLINICAL FEATURES

Most examples of acute thyroiditis represent secondary involvement due to generalized sepsis or spread from an adjacent head and neck site of infection, such as suppurative pharyngitis. Patients usually are febrile and complain of chills, malaise, and pain and swelling of the anterior neck. Dysphagia or hoarseness may also be noted. While most patients are euthyroid, occasional patients demonstrate clinical and laboratory evidence of hyperthyroidism or hypothyroidism.

ACUTE THYROIDITIS—DISEASE FACT SHEET

Definition
- Acute inflammation of the thyroid parenchyma, associated with a local or systemic viral, bacterial, or fungal infection

Incidence and Location
- Rare
- Most cases associated with immunosuppression or trauma

Morbidity and Mortality
- Part of generalized sepsis or spread from traumatic entry

Clinical Features
- Most cases due to generalized sepsis or extension from an adjacent head and neck site
- Fever, chills, malaise, pain, swelling of anterior neck
- Dysphagia or hoarseness occasionally
- Most patients are euthyroid; occasionally hypothyroid or hyperthyroid

Prognosis and Therapy
- Prognosis related to underlying condition
- Cultures to determine causative agent
- Aggressive antibiotic or antifungal therapy with surgery reserved for abscess drainage or injury debridement

---

PATHOLOGIC FEATURES

GROSS FINDINGS

The thyroid is seldom removed for acute thyroiditis. A specimen is usually submitted as part of an incision and drainage of an abscess or debridement following neck trauma. The gland is erythematous and soft and may contain pockets of purulent exudate or areas of necrosis.

MICROSCOPIC FINDINGS

The key feature is the presence of polymorphonuclear leukocytes infiltrating the thyroid parenchyma. Microabscesses, foci of necrosis (Figure 22-12), and vasculitis may be seen. Identification of a causative organism may be possible with histochemical stains, such as tissue Gram stains, Gomori methenamine silver or periodic acid–Schiff (PAS) stains for fungi, or mycobacterial stains (Ziehl-Neelsen). Immunosuppressed patients may develop an acute, rather than the typical granulomatous, infectious thyroiditis in response to fungal or mycobacterial organisms. Tissue cultures are invaluable in identifying the organism and in determining its sensitivity to antibiotic therapy.

DIFFERENTIAL DIAGNOSIS

Subacute (granulomatous) thyroiditis also has a neutrophilic infiltrate in its early phase, but it is folliculocentric with accompanying histiocytes, lymphocytes, and multinucleated giant cells. No infectious agent is identified.

PROGNOSIS AND THERAPY

The prognosis is favorable in the absence of underlying predisposing factors such as immunosuppressive states or extensive neck trauma that may carry their own risk of poor outcome. Appropriate treatment requires identification of the infectious agent, preferably by culture,

---

ACUTE THYROIDITIS—PATHOLOGIC FEATURES

Gross Findings
- Thyroid erythematous, soft, with pockets of purulent exudate or necrosis

Microscopic Findings
- Infiltration of parenchyma by neutrophils
- Microabscesses, foci of necrosis, vasculitis common
- Organisms may be identified on histology in some cases

Pathologic Differential Diagnosis
- Subacute (granulomatous) thyroiditis

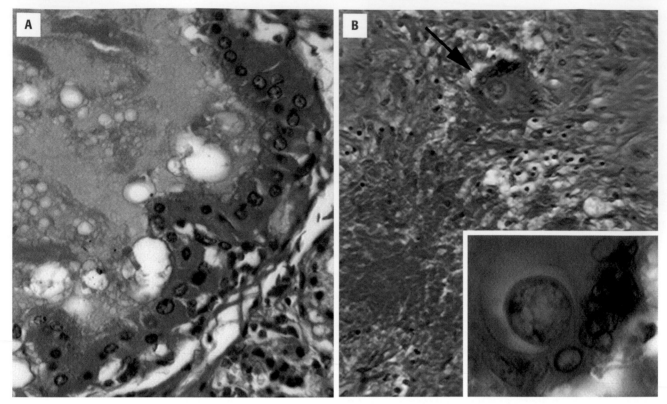

FIGURE 22-12
A, The thyroid follicular epithelium is oncocytic with organisms identified within the colloid. **B**, Coccidioidomycosis organisms are identified in a background of necrosis in this case of acute thyroiditis.

and initiation of effective antibiotic therapy. If abscesses or areas of infarction are present, surgical incision and drainage or debridement may be necessary.

■ GRANULOMATOUS THYROIDITIS

Also known as de Quervain thyroiditis (named after Fritz de Quervain, 1868-1940) or subacute thyroiditis, granulomatous thyroiditis is a self-limited inflammatory disorder widely thought to be related to a systemic viral infection. Association with viral epidemics such as mumps, influenza, coxsackievirus, and measles has been reported. Some cases have also been associated with Epstein-Barr virus and with immunosuppressive therapy. Although seasonal variation has been noted in the past, some recent studies show only a modest increase in cases during the spring and summer. An autoimmune component is also postulated due to the presence of thyroidal autoantibodies in some patients.

CLINICAL FEATURES

The annual incidence in the United States is estimated at 5/100,000 population. Women are more commonly affected than men, with a female:male ratio of 3.5:1. The

mean age of onset is in the 5th decade (range, 14 to 87 years). The most common presenting symptom is pain in the thyroid region, sometimes radiating to the jaw. Other complaints include dysphagia, sore throat, low-grade fever, arthralgia, myalgia, tremor, excessive sweating, and weight loss. Physical examination is notable for pain on palpation of the thyroid. The entire gland is usually involved; however, the changes may be localized to one lobe or to a distinct nodule. Thyroid function often varies with disease activity. In the early phase, patients may be hyperthyroid due to destruction of follicles and release of thyroglobulin. Consequently, serum thyroid-stimulating hormone (TSH) is suppressed, total and free T_4 and T_3 are elevated, and radioactive iodine uptake is decreased. Rarely, a life-threatening thyrotoxicosis or "thyroid storm" occurs early in the disease. With disease progression, thyroid epithelium is destroyed, resulting in hypothyroidism. However, most patients regain normal thyroid function after resolution of the disease.

PATHOLOGIC FEATURES

GROSS FINDINGS

Surgery is unnecessary, but the rare resection specimen shows asymmetric enlargement of the thyroid, vague nodularity, and a somewhat firm consistency.

GRANULOMATOUS THYROIDITIS—DISEASE FACT SHEET

Definition
- Self-limited inflammatory disorder thought to be related to systemic viral illness and possible autoimmune factors
- Also called de Quervain thyroiditis, subacute thyroiditis

Incidence and Location
- About 5/100,000 population/year
- Seasonal increase in spring and summer may occur

Gender and Age Distribution
- Female >> male (3.5:1)
- Peak in 5th decade (range, 14 to 87 years)

Clinical Features
- Pain in the thyroid region, tender to palpation
- Other complaints include dysphagia, "sore throat," fever, arthralgia, myalgia, tremor, excessive sweating, weight loss
- Entire gland usually involved, but may be localized
- Thyroid function varies: hyperthyroidism may occur early; hypothyroidism may develop in mid-phase
- Most patients euthyroid after resolution

Prognosis and Therapy
- Usually self-limiting disease which resolves in months, although may recur (years after initial disease)
- 5% remain hypothyroid
- Treatment includes aspirin, nonsteroidal anti-inflammatory drugs, steroids, and beta-blocking agents if hyperthyroidism present

GRANULOMATOUS THYROIDITIS—PATHOLOGIC FEATURES

Gross Findings
- Rarely removed, but shows asymmetrically enlarged, firm, vaguely nodular gland

Microscopic Findings
- Nodular, but whole gland affected
- *Early stage:* follicle-centered with groups of follicles disrupted by lymphohistiocytic infiltrate with neutrophils aggregated in follicle lumens
- *Late stage:* multinucleated giant cells more prominent and neutrophils absent, with extensive destruction of follicular epithelium, obscuring follicle-centered disease
- *Resolution:* follicular regeneration, little fibrosis remains

Fine Needle Aspiration
- Aggregates of lymphocytes, histiocytes, plasma cells, multinucleated giant cells
- Neutrophils may be prominent in early phase
- Giant cells may contain colloid fragments
- Colloid and follicular epithelial cells usually scant

Pathologic Differential Diagnosis
- Sarcoidosis, mycobacterial or fungal granulomatous infection, palpation thyroiditis, postoperative granuloma

MICROSCOPIC FINDINGS

Histologic features are usually seen throughout the gland. The inflammatory infiltrate is distributed in a relatively nodular fashion and includes lymphocytes, plasma cells, foamy histiocytes, epithelioid histiocytes, multinucleated giant cells, and neutrophils (Figure 22-13). A variable background of fibrosis is also present. In the hyperthyroid phase of the disease, the inflammatory process is centered on the follicle. A group of follicles is surrounded and disrupted by a lymphohistiocytic infiltrate; aggregates of neutrophils within the follicle lumens are very characteristic of this phase (Figure 22-14). Multinucleated giant cells, often containing engulfed colloid, become more prominent in the hypothyroid phase. The inflammatory infiltrate is largely composed of lymphocytes, plasma cells, and histiocytes during this phase (Figure 22-15). Much of the follicular

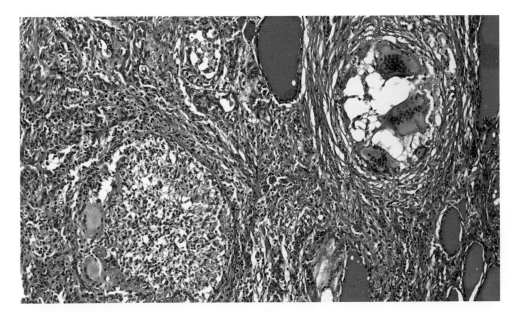

FIGURE 22-13

The thyroid is affected by nodules of a follicle-centered inflammatory infiltrate including lymphocytes, plasma cells, histiocytes, giant cells, and neutrophils. The follicles are destroyed by the process. Note the "follicle abscess" (*left*) and the giant cells (*right*).

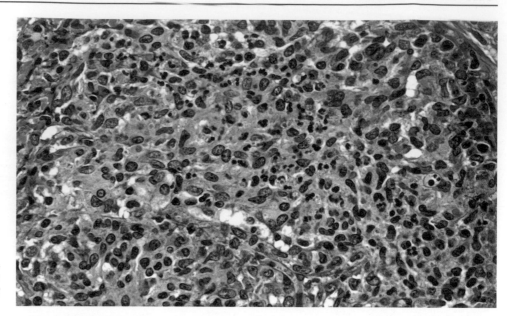

FIGURE 22-14

The destroyed follicle contains an admixture of histiocytes and lymphocytes with neutrophils, characteristic for the early phase of the disease.

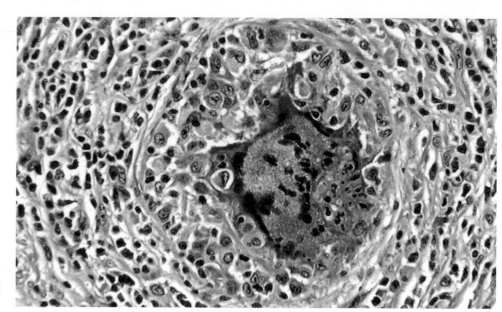

FIGURE 22-15

The follicular epithelium is replaced by a layer of histiocytes with a large giant cell, more prominent in the later phases of the process.

epithelium has been destroyed by this stage, making it less obvious that the process was centered on the thyroid follicle. With time, the gland recovers, with regeneration of the follicles and, in most cases, resolution of the fibrosis and inflammatory infiltrate.

ANCILLARY STUDIES

FINE NEEDLE ASPIRATION

In most patients, the diagnosis of granulomatous thyroiditis can be made on clinical evidence alone. Occasionally, FNA may be requested, particularly in the minority of patients without thyroid pain. The aspirate contains a mixed inflammatory infiltrate, including lymphocytes,

plasma cells, foamy and epithelioid histiocytes, and multinucleated giant cells (Figures 22-16 and 22-17); neutrophils are seen in the early phase of the disease. Follicular cells vary in number with the phase of disease: early-phase aspirates often contain small sheets of follicular cells or isolated cells (Figure 22-16). Colloid may be present within small acinar groups or as isolated fragments. Abundant thin colloid, as seen in normal glands or in adenomatoid nodules, is not present.

DIFFERENTIAL DIAGNOSIS

The pathologic differential diagnosis of granulomatous thyroiditis includes other granulomatous processes,

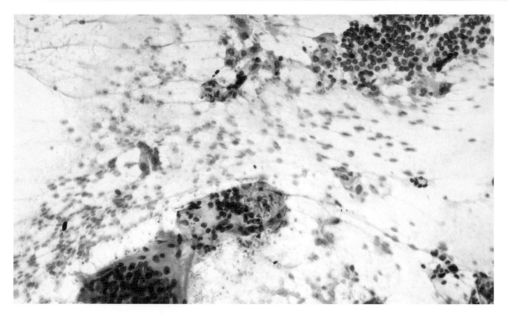

FIGURE 22-16

A fine needle aspiration demonstrates a sheet of benign follicular epithelium with a mixed inflammatory infiltrate, which includes lymphocytes, histiocytes, and multinucleated giant cells (alcohol-fixed, Papanicolaou stain).

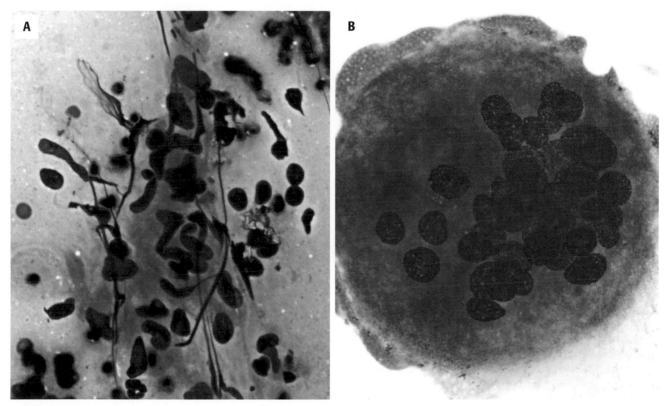

FIGURE 22-17

A, Aggregates of epithelioid histiocytes suggest the granulomatous nature of this process. **B**, A multinucleated giant cell. While typical of this type of granulomatous thyroiditis, giant cells are not specific as they may be seen in adenomatoid nodules, lymphocytic thyroiditis, and papillary thyroid carcinoma (air-dried, Diff-Quik stained).

which may involve the thyroid, including infectious processes, sarcoidosis, palpation thyroiditis, and postoperative granulomas. *Tuberculosis* or *fungal thyroiditis* is usually characterized by necrotizing granulomas (Figure 22-18), in contrast to granulomatous thyroiditis. *Sarcoidal granulomas* are small and compact, and are usually located in the interstitium, rather than centered on the thyroid follicles. *Palpation thyroiditis* lacks neutrophils and is very patchy in its distribution. *Postoperative granulomas* are a recognized procedural phenomenon supported by the clinical history.

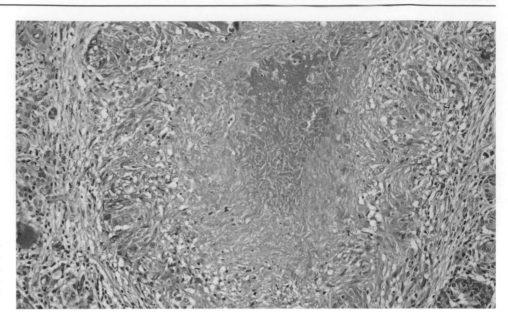

FIGURE 22-18

The patient has disseminated tuberculosis with extensive granulomatous inflammation in the thyroid. The central necrosis distinguishes these granulomas from those seen in subacute thyroiditis, palpation thyroiditis, and sarcoidosis.

PROGNOSIS AND THERAPY

Most patients with granulomatous thyroiditis experience a self-limiting disease that resolves within several months. Treatment modalities include aspirin, nonsteroidal anti-inflammatory drugs, prednisone (for more severe symptoms), and, if thyrotoxicosis is present, beta-adrenergic blocking agents such as propranolol. A small number of patients experience recurrence of disease years after the initial episode. Permanent hypothyroidism occurs in ~5% of patients with granulomatous thyroiditis.

■ PALPATION THYROIDITIS

Palpation thyroiditis is an incidental finding of no clinical significance in most instances, usually found in thyroid glands removed surgically for other reasons. It is thought to result from the traumatic rupture of follicles caused by vigorous palpation of the gland preoperatively. Occasionally, traumatic injuries to the thyroid (e.g., martial arts blows) may yield a similar finding. These lesions are tiny granulomatous foci, centered on thyroid follicles.

CLINICAL FEATURES

Clinical findings in patients who have histologic evidence of palpation thyroiditis are only very rarely related to this condition. Most patients have a palpable

---

PALPATION THYROIDITIS—DISEASE FACT SHEET

Definition

- Microscopic granulomatous foci, follicle-centered, seen as an incidental finding in resected thyroid gland, thought to result from rupture of follicles due to palpation

Clinical Features

- The palpation thyroiditis is of no clinical significance
- Patients almost always have a thyroid nodule(s)
- Palpation thyroiditis may be very prominent in "completion thyroidectomy" specimens
- Serum thyroglobulin not elevated

---

nodule (over 80%), which may represent a thyroid neoplasm, an adenomatoid nodule, or thyroiditis (the reason there was palpation in the first place). Thyroid function is usually normal, unless related to the nodule or underlying thyroid disease. Serum thyroglobulin is not usually elevated. There are, however, examples of palpation thyroiditis with hyperthyroidism—generally following neck surgery for an unrelated reason—manifested by atrial fibrillation in elderly patients. The hyperthyroidism appears to result from excessive manipulation of the thyroid gland intraoperatively.

PATHOLOGIC FEATURES

GROSS FINDINGS

There are no gross findings related directly to palpation thyroiditis. However, the thyroid usually contains a

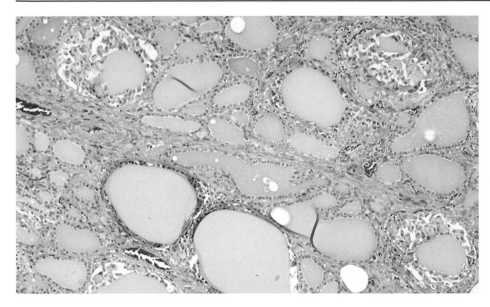

FIGURE 22-19
Scattered foci of palpation thyroiditis are centered on a few follicles in each location.

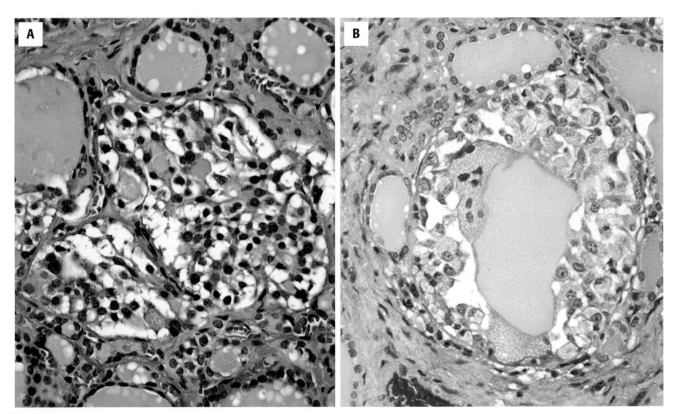

FIGURE 22-20
A, Early palpation thyroiditis with foamy histiocytes colonizing the follicles. **B**, More fully developed lesions have mononuclear histiocytes and lymphocytes, with occasional multinucleated giant cells.

nodule that prompted the vigorous palpation and subsequent surgery.

MICROSCOPIC FINDINGS

Lesions of palpation thyroiditis are widely scattered throughout the gland, usually involving only a single follicle or, at most, a few adjacent follicles (Figure 22-19). The affected follicle contains mononuclear histiocytes with foamy pale cytoplasm, an occasional multinucleated histiocyte, and a few lymphocytes (Figure 22-20). Most of the tiny granulomas are located within follicles, but they may also be found adjacent to a ruptured follicle. There is a minimal fibrous response to these lesions. No acute inflammatory cells or necrosis is present.

DIFFERENTIAL DIAGNOSIS

The differential diagnosis includes the other causes of granulomatous change in the thyroid, including *subacute thyroiditis* (larger aggregates of follicle-centered granulomas, with neutrophils and histiocytes), *sarcoidosis* (tight, small, compact granulomas within the interstitium), and *tuberculosis and fungal infections* (destructive granulomas with possible necrosis).

PROGNOSIS AND THERAPY

The patient's outcome is not affected by the presence or absence of palpation thyroiditis but is entirely dependent on the nature of the abnormality which prompted the surgery.

■ RIEDEL DISEASE (RIEDEL THYROIDITIS)

Riedel thyroiditis (Riedel struma; ligneous thyroiditis; named after Bernhard Moritz Carl Ludwig Riedel, 1846-1916) is a rare, fibrosing form of chronic thyroiditis without a known etiology, although an autoimmune disorder is postulated. The thyroid gland is replaced by dense fibrous tissue, often extending beyond the thyroid gland to involve the soft tissues of the neck. In some cases, a similar process is seen in other sites, such as the retroperitoneum, mediastinum, eyes, hepatobiliary tree, lung, and, especially, the pancreas ("autoimmune pancreatitis"). These fibrosclerosing disorders are characterized by elevated serum IgG4 titers, and increased density of IgG4-positive plasma cells in tissue sections.

CLINICAL FEATURES

Riedel thyroiditis is noted in <0.3% of thyroidectomy specimens. The disease is much more common in women (female:male ratio is 5:1). There is a peak in the 5th decade, although identified over a wide range of 23 to 77 years. An enigmatic association with smoking has been noted. Interestingly, nearly one-third of patients with Riedel thyroiditis develop another fibrosing disorder within a 10-year period, supporting the common pathogenesis and systemic nature of this disease. In fact, this idiopathic fibrosclerotic disease process includes retroperitoneal fibrosis, sclerosing cholangitis, mediastinal fibrosis, orbital pseudotumor, pulmonary fibrosis, subcutaneous fibrosclerosis, fibrous parotitis, diffuse pancreatic fibrosis (autoimmune pancreatitis), Dupuytren contractures, and Peyronie disease, among others.

In thyroid disease, patients present with a firm goiter (thyroid enlargement) often associated with pressure symptoms, such as discomfort in the anterior neck, dysphagia, dyspnea, or stridor. The infiltrative nature of the disease may cause damage to the recurrent laryngeal nerve (vocal cord paralysis and hoarseness) or to the sympathetic trunk (Horner syndrome). Advanced fibrosis in the neck may produce vascular compromise such as superior vena cava syndrome, or hypoparathyroidism secondary to parathyroid gland destruction. In fact, while most patients are euthyroid at the time of diagnosis, up to 40% develop hypothyroidism over a period of 10 years. Although variable, thyroglobulin and thyroid peroxidase antibodies are slightly elevated in up to two-thirds of patients. The concurrence of other thyroid autoimmune diseases, as mentioned above, will, of course, affect the laboratory profile.

RIEDEL DISEASE—DISEASE FACT SHEET

Definition

- Rare fibrosing form of chronic thyroiditis with extensive replacement of thyroid parenchyma by dense fibrosis

Incidence and Location

- <0.3% of thyroidectomy specimens
- Fibrosing disorder may also affect retroperitoneum, lung, mediastinum, biliary tree, pancreas, kidney, subcutis

Morbidity and Mortality

- Vascular compromise, recurrent laryngeal nerve damage, hypoparathyroidism

Gender and Age Distribution

- Female >> male (5:1)
- Peak in 5th decade (range, 23 to 77 years)

Clinical Features

- Most present with very firm goiter
- Symptoms include dysphagia, hoarseness, stridor, Horner syndrome, fever, neck pain
- Most euthyroid at diagnosis
- Mass may be mistaken for malignant neoplasm

Prognosis and Therapy

- Benign, self-limited disease
- About one-third develop another fibrosing disorder within 10 years
- 40% develop hypothyroidism over 10 years
- Poor outcome is associated with fibrosis in other organs
- Corticosteroid and tamoxifen useful in control or reversal of disease
- Surgery may be necessary for symptoms of compression

RIEDEL DISEASE—PATHOLOGIC FEATURES

Gross Findings

- Diffuse enlargement of thyroid with adherence to strap muscle and perithyroidal soft tissue
- Surgical margins "ragged" due to difficult dissection
- Cut surface white, with a woody texture

Microscopic Findings

- Extensive fibrosis predominates over inflammatory infiltrate with extension into soft tissue without a specific interface
- Patchy infiltrate of lymphocytes, plasma cells, monocytes, neutrophils, and occasional eosinophils
- Rare, peripheral entrapped thyroid follicles
- *Occlusive phlebitis* with small to medium-sized veins infiltrated by inflammatory cells with thickened walls and myxoid change

Fine Needle Aspiration

- Paucicellular to acellular aspirates
- Scant material with atypical spindle cells is misleading

Pathologic Differential Diagnosis

- Undifferentiated thyroid carcinoma, diffuse sclerosing variant of papillary carcinoma, solitary fibrous tumor, fibrous variant of Hashimoto thyroiditis, Hodgkin lymphoma, sarcoma

RADIOLOGIC FEATURES

While other radiographic techniques are nonspecific, MRI demonstrates homogeneous hypointensity on both T1- and T2-weighted images, findings distinct from all the other forms of thyroiditis and thyroid neoplasia.

PATHOLOGIC FEATURES

GROSS FINDINGS

The thyroid is usually diffusely abnormal without normal tissue; rarely will only one lobe be affected. The gland is pale tan to white, with a woody consistency. The surgical margins of the specimen are typically ragged due to extension of the fibrosing process into perithyroidal soft tissue (Figure 22-21). Remnants of strap muscle may be adherent to the gland's surface.

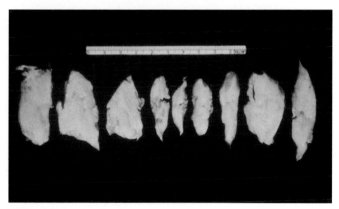

FIGURE 22-21

The thyroid gland in Riedel thyroiditis is pale and woody. The surgical border of the gland is quite ragged following a difficult dissection resulting from extrathyroidal extension of the fibrosing process. *(With permission from Wenig BM, et al. Atlas of endocrine pathology. Philadelphia: WB Saunders; 1997.)*

MICROSCOPIC FINDINGS

There is a distinctive fibroinflammatory process extensively involving the gland, extending into the perithyroidal soft tissue and strap muscles (Figure 22-22). The interface between thyroid gland and soft tissue of the neck is lost. The fibrosis typically predominates over the inflammatory infiltrate, which consists of patchy aggregates of lymphocytes, plasma cells, monocytes, neutrophils, and eosinophils (Figure 22-23). Giant cells, granulomas, and germinal centers are not present. If residual thyroid tissue is present, rare entrapped follicles

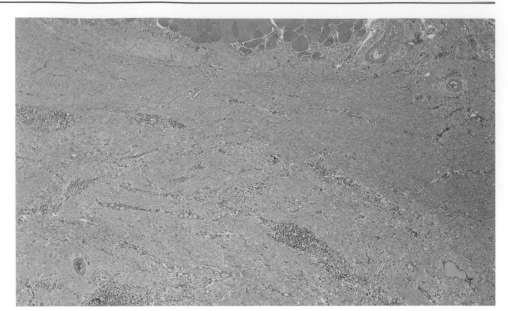

FIGURE 22-22

A low-power view of Riedel thyroiditis demonstrates the dense fibrosis obscuring the architecture of the thyroid and extending into the perithyroidal soft tissue. Note the skeletal muscle at the upper edge.

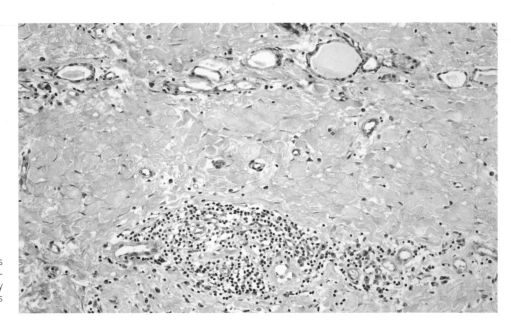

FIGURE 22-23

The lobular pattern of the thyroid has been destroyed by the fibroinflammatory process in Riedel thyroiditis. Only scattered residual follicles remain in this gland.

may be identified in the sclerotic periphery (Figure 22-24). Oxyphilic follicular epithelial metaplasia is absent. A characteristic vascular alteration, *occlusive phlebitis* (Figure 22-25), is pathognomonic of Riedel thyroiditis. Small and medium-sized veins are infiltrated by a sparse infiltrate of lymphocytes and plasma cells. The vessel walls are thickened, often with myxoid change.

ANCILLARY STUDIES

IMMUNOHISTOCHEMICAL RESULTS

Immunohistochemical studies are not necessary for the diagnosis. However, it is of interest that T cells

predominate in Riedel thyroiditis, in contrast to the fibrous variant of Hashimoto thyroiditis in which B cells predominate. IgG4-positive lymphocytes are also present in increased number compared to IgG control lymphocytes, but the interpretation is fraught with difficulty.

FINE NEEDLE ASPIRATION

FNA is typically unsuccessful, with paucicellular to acellular aspirates due to the densely fibrotic gland. The scant material may, in fact, be misleading. Rare atypical spindle cells, sometimes with intranuclear cytoplasmic intrusions (pseudoinclusions), should not be overinterpreted as anaplastic carcinoma.

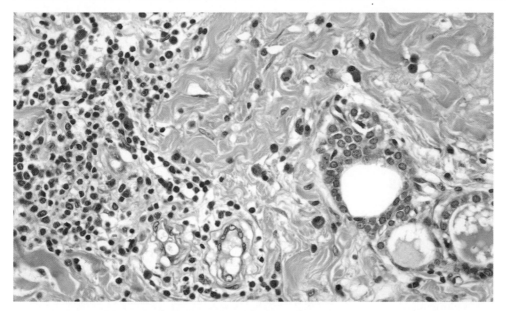

FIGURE 22-24

The inflammatory infiltrate in Riedel thyroiditis includes lymphocytes, plasma cells, and occasional eosinophils. Note the atrophic appearance of the follicular epithelium.

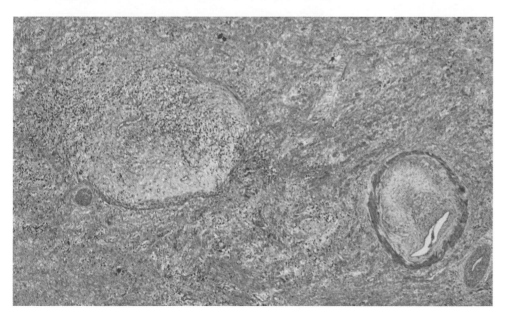

FIGURE 22-25

Occlusive phlebitis is characteristic of Riedel thyroiditis. Several small and medium-sized veins demonstrate thickening of the vessel walls with myxoid degeneration and a chronic inflammatory infiltrate.

DIFFERENTIAL DIAGNOSIS

Riedel thyroiditis must be separated from undifferentiated carcinoma, solitary fibrous tumor, fibrous variant of Hashimoto thyroiditis, diffuse sclerosing variant of papillary carcinoma, Hodgkin lymphoma, and sarcoma. The paucicellular variant of *undifferentiated thyroid carcinoma* includes areas of infarction or necrosis, highly atypical spindle or epithelioid cells with a high mitotic rate, and at least focal positive staining for cytokeratin. *Solitary fibrous tumor* is circumscribed and lacks the inflammatory infiltrate of thyroiditis. Immunohistochemical studies for CD34, CD99, and bcl-2 are positive. The *fibrous variant of Hashimoto thyroiditis* has significant deposition of dense fibrous tissue with effacement of the thyroid architecture and follicular atrophy. However, the process is limited to

the thyroid gland, unlike extrathyroidal extension seen in Riedel thyroiditis. The *diffuse sclerosing variant of papillary carcinoma* demonstrates numerous psammoma bodies, lymphocytic thyroiditis, and areas of tumor with the diagnostic nuclear features of papillary carcinoma. *Hodgkin lymphoma* (nodular sclerosis type) should have Reed-Sternberg cells and lacunar cells positive for CD15 and/or CD30 and an appropriate background of inflammatory elements. *Sarcomas* will have cytologic atypia, necrosis, and mitotic figures.

PROGNOSIS AND THERAPY

Riedel thyroiditis is a benign, and often self-limiting, disease. The chief morbidity is related to hypothyroidism, since the local effects of the goiter can be addressed surgically if necessary. Other potential complications include hypoparathyroidism and nerve injury related either to the disease or to the difficulty of surgery in these patients. In those individuals with multifocal systemic fibrosclerosis, other organ systems may be affected by life-threatening disease. Corticosteroid therapy has been successful in the majority of patients in controlling disease progression or in complete or partial reversal of symptoms.

■ CHRONIC LYMPHOCYTIC THYROIDITIS (HASHIMOTO THYROIDITIS)

Widely known by its eponym, Hashimoto thyroiditis (named after Hakaru Hashimoto, 1881-1934), chronic lymphocytic thyroiditis (previously struma lymphomatosa) is an autoimmune chronic inflammatory disorder of the thyroid associated with diffuse enlargement of the gland and several thyroid autoantibodies. A fibrous variant is associated with marked fibrosclerosis and atrophy of the thyroid epithelium. The mechanism of autoimmunity is not clearly understood. However, major histocompatibility complex class II proteins, HLA-DR, HLA-DP, and HLA-DQ, are expressed by the follicular epithelial cells in patients with chronic lymphocytic thyroiditis; these proteins are necessary for presentation of antigen to CD4 T cells. The activated helper T cells, in turn, stimulate autoreactive B cells to be recruited into the thyroid, where they secrete autoantibodies. The key target antigens for this autoimmune reaction are thyroglobulin, thyroid peroxidase, and the thyrotropin receptor. Thyrotropin receptor antibodies may contribute to hypothyroidism by blocking the binding capacity for TSH. The activated helper T cells also recruit cytotoxic CD8 T cells, which may be responsible for the destruction of follicular epithelial cells, which ultimately leads to hypothyroidism in many patients.

CLINICAL FEATURES

The actual incidence of chronic lymphocytic thyroiditis is difficult to determine as many cases are subclinical. Whereas some degree of lymphocytic thyroiditis is present in autopsy series in 40% to 45% of women and in 20% of men, high titers of antithyroid peroxidase antibodies are found in ~1% of the population (increasing with age) to suggest an approximate incidence. A familial association is seen, while there is also an increased incidence in individuals with Down syndrome, Turner syndrome, and familial Alzheimer disease. HLA-DR3 and HLA-DR5 have been linked to the disease. Other autoimmune diseases may be found in patients with Hashimoto thyroiditis, including pernicious anemia, diabetes mellitus, Addison disease, Graves disease, chronic active hepatitis, and Sjögren syndrome.

CHRONIC LYMPHOCYTIC THYROIDITIS (HASHIMOTO)— DISEASE FACT SHEET

Definition
- Autoimmune chronic inflammatory disorder of the thyroid associated with diffuse enlargement and thyroid autoantibodies

Incidence and Location
- Incidence difficult to determine due to high number of subclinical cases, although ~1% of population has autothyroid antibodies
- Familial cases well-documented

Morbidity and Mortality
- Chief morbidity due to hypothyroidism
- Increased risk of thyroid lymphoma (up to 80-fold increase)

Gender and Age Distribution
- Female >> male (5 to 7:1), except for fibrous variant
- Highest incidence in the United States and Japan related to iodine intake
- Peak in middle age (mean, 59 years), but wide age range

Clinical Features
- Diffusely enlarged, nontender gland
- Enlargement usually gradual
- Hypothyroidism common, but rarely hyperthyroidism
- Other associated autoimmune disorders

Laboratory Findings
- Serum thyroid antibodies are elevated (various types)

Prognosis and Treatment
- Increased incidence of thyroid lymphoma
- Thyroxin replacement for hypothyroidism and antithyroid drugs for hashitoxicosis
- Surgery if symptomatic or for suspicious nodules

Hashimoto thyroiditis can be found over a wide age range, although it shows a peak in middle age. Women are much more frequently affected, with a female:male ratio of 5 to 7:1. An exception to this is the fibrous variant of Hashimoto thyroiditis, which is more common in older men. The risk of the disease seems highest in countries with the highest iodine intake (United States and Japan). Furthermore, amiodarone and lithium are associated with an increased risk of both hypothyroidism and development of thyroid autoantibodies.

Patients with lymphocytic thyroiditis have a gradual, diffuse enlargement of a firm, nontender thyroid gland, usually two to three times the normal weight. Occasionally, patients with the fibrous variant of Hashimoto thyroiditis have rapid enlargement of the gland; however, this finding should raise the suspicion of thyroid lymphoma in a patient with a history of autoimmune thyroiditis.

Hypothyroidism is common but not invariably present at the time of presentation. Rare patients present with hyperthyroidism, known as hashitoxicosis. Laboratory evidence of Graves disease may or may not be present;

the histologic features in such cases are identical to those of other cases of chronic lymphocytic thyroiditis.

Laboratory assessment requires testing for serum thyroid antibodies (antithyroglobulin, antithyroid microsomal antibodies, antithyroid peroxidase antibodies), although antithyroglobulin is less commonly elevated and is least useful. In population studies, 50% to 75% of subjects with positive thyroid antibodies are euthyroid, 25% to 50% have subclinical hypothyroidism, and 5% to 10% have overt hypothyroidism. Thyrotropin assay is routine in suspected Hashimoto thyroiditis, to assess for hypothyroidism. Severe hypothyroidism is commonly associated with the fibrous variant of the disease.

Juvenile Hashimoto thyroiditis, usually seen in adolescents and young adults, may present with hypothyroidism or hyperthyroidism; the patients often have a strong family history of thyroid disease. Some patients also have hypoadrenalism (Schmidt syndrome), hypoparathyroidism, diabetes mellitus, or hypogonadism.

RADIOLOGIC FEATURES

Radiologic imaging is not necessary in the diagnosis of autoimmune thyroiditis and may, in fact, be misleading. Radioactive iodine uptake is usually normal or increased in Hashimoto thyroiditis, suggesting Graves disease, even in patients with hypothyroidism.

PATHOLOGIC FEATURES

GROSS FINDINGS

Thyroidectomy is often performed because of a thyroid nodule. The gland is diffusely enlarged and pale

---

CHRONIC LYMPHOCYTIC THYROIDITIS (HASHIMOTO)—PATHOLOGIC FEATURES

Gross Findings

- Diffusely enlarged gland, may be lobulated or nodular
- Pale white cut surface resembles lymphoid tissue
- Nodules or fibrous bands common in long-standing disease

Microscopic Findings

- Diffuse, dense lymphoplasmacytic infiltrate, often with well-developed germinal centers
- Follicular atrophy with decrease in colloid
- Oxyphilic, or "Hürthle," cell metaplasia (follicular cells with intensely granular eosinophilic cytoplasm)
- Squamous metaplasia is common
- Fibrous variant shows dense lymphoid infiltrate, extensive fibrosis, and minimal residual follicular epithelium

Fine Needle Aspiration

- Mixed, polymorphic lymphoplasmacytic infiltrate
- Occasional multinucleated giant cells and histiocytes
- Oxyphilic epithelial cells in small clusters and sheets
- Scant colloid in most cases

Pathologic Differential Diagnosis

- Papillary thyroid carcinoma, extranodal marginal zone B-cell lymphoma, Riedel thyroiditis, nonspecific lymphocytic thyroiditis

---

gray to white, with a consistency of lymphoid tissue (Figure 22-26). If the disease is long-standing, it may contain distinct nodules and bands of fibrous tissue. The fibrous variant is very firm and fibrotic, with a multinodular cut surface resembling cirrhosis of the liver.

MICROSCOPIC FINDINGS

The histologic features of classic Hashimoto thyroiditis include diffuse and rather dense infiltration of the

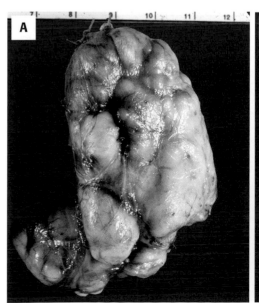
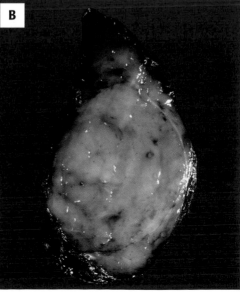

FIGURE 22-26

A, The thyroid is enlarged, with a lobulated appearance in lymphocytic thyroiditis. The pale white tan color reflects the dense lymphoid infiltrate. **B**, The cut surface of lymphocytic thyroiditis bears a striking resemblance to lymph node tissue.

PATHOLOGIC FEATURES

GROSS FINDINGS

The thyroid gland is diffusely and symmetrically enlarged and beefy red (Figure 22-36). The cut surface gives

---

DIFFUSE HYPERPLASIA (GRAVES DISEASE)—PATHOLOGIC FEATURES

Gross Findings

- Diffuse thyroid enlargement with beefy red gland
- Average weights range from 50 to 150 g
- Treatment may result in nodules and prominent fibrosis

Microscopic Findings

- Highly cellular gland with little colloid
- Hyperplastic, redundant follicular epithelium with papillary infoldings; follicle lumens stellate
- Follicular cells columnar, with eosinophilic granular cytoplasm
- Follicular cell nuclei round and only slightly enlarged and are basally oriented
- If colloid present, scalloping is seen (small vacuoles along apical border of epithelial cells)
- Accentuation of lobular pattern of gland, with increased fibrosis in interlobular septae
- Patchy lymphocytic infiltrate
- After treatment, follicles regain colloid; mild hyperplastic changes persist
- Following radioactive iodine, gland may become nodular, with increased fibrosis and atypia of follicular epithelial cells

Fine Needle Aspiration

- Highly cellular smears
- Minimal or no colloid
- Sheets of follicular epithelial cells
- Follicular cells have abundant granular cytoplasm ("flame cells"), nuclei with compact chromatin

Pathologic Differential Diagnosis

- Papillary carcinoma, toxic nodular goiter (Plummer disease), Hashimoto thyroiditis, follicular carcinoma (post-treatment)

---

an impression of hypervascularity. Average weights range from 50 to 150 g. If the patient has been treated or if the Graves disease is long-standing or "burnt-out," the gland may contain multiple nodules or patches of fibrosis.

MICROSCOPIC FINDINGS

The low-power appearance of the gland is remarkable for accentuation of the normal lobular pattern of the thyroid. This is due to increased fibrous tissue in the interlobular septae (Figure 22-37). A patchy lymphocytic infiltrate is present in the perifollicular stroma (Figure 22-38); the density varies from case to case: It is sparse in some patients, but conspicuous, with germinal centers in others, related to the autoimmune nature of the underlying process.

An important microscopic feature of Graves disease is the diffuse nature of the pathologic findings (Figure 22-39): *the entire gland is affected.* The thyroid follicles are lined by columnar epithelial cells with basally located round nuclei with relatively dense chromatin; the cytoplasm is granular and eosinophilic (Figure 22-40). The hyperplastic follicular epithelium forms infoldings into the lumen of the follicle, producing a stellate outline (Figure 22-41). These infoldings may resemble papillae, and must not be mistaken for evidence of papillary carcinoma (Figure 22-42). Vacuoles are noted along the apical aspect of the follicular cells, giving the colloid a "scalloped" appearance.

In cases of *treated* Graves disease, the histologic appearance depends on the type and duration of treatment. Potassium iodide causes involution, with follicular cells reverting to their normal cuboidal or flattened appearance, alternating with areas retaining some of the features of hyperplasia (Figure 22-43). Radioactive iodine therapy may produce a nodular gland, with nodules that are often quite cellular and may exhibit striking nuclear atypia (Figure 22-43). The periphery of such nodules should be scrutinized for evidence of capsular or vascular invasion that would identify them as follicular carcinomas. Fibrosis and areas of follicular atrophy are frequently present.

ANCILLARY STUDIES

IMMUNOHISTOCHEMICAL FEATURES

Immunohistochemical studies are not required for the diagnosis of Graves disease, but HLA-DR positivity is typically demonstrable in the follicular epithelial cells as well as in the lymphoid cells.

FINE NEEDLE ASPIRATION

Cytologic examination of diffuse hyperplasia is treacherous and seldom attempted in patients with active

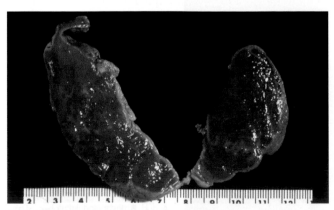

FIGURE 22-36

This thyroidectomy specimen from a child with hyperthyroidism is enlarged and hyperemic, with a "beefy red" appearance. *(With permission from Wenig BM, et al. Atlas of endocrine pathology. Philadelphia: WB Saunders; 1997.)*

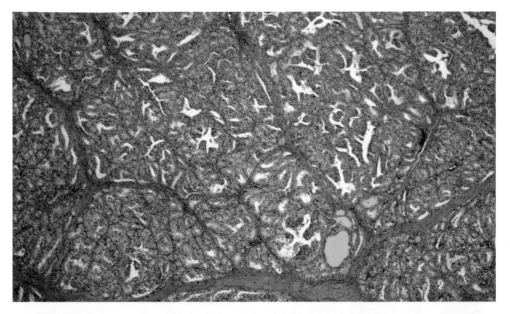

FIGURE 22-37

The gland is intensely cellular, with little colloid. Note the prominence of the somewhat fibrotic interlobular septae, which are usually inapparent in a normal thyroid gland.

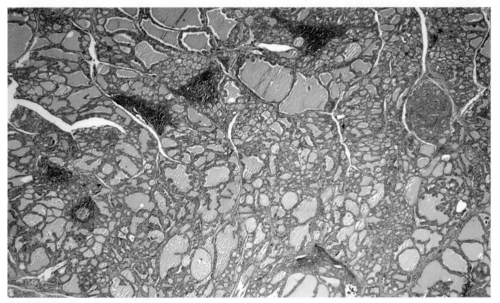

FIGURE 22-38

Patches of lymphoid cells are noted in this hyperplastic gland. Because Graves is an autoimmune disorder, inflammation is not uncommon. A microscopic papillary carcinoma is present (*right upper*).

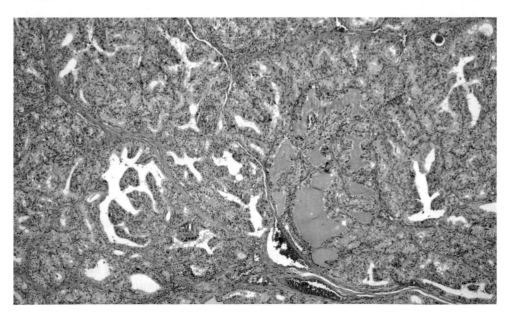

FIGURE 22-39

The hyperplastic epithelium is redundant, giving the follicle lumen a stellate outline. Papillary structures are present in some of the hyperplastic follicles. Colloid is present in several of the follicles.

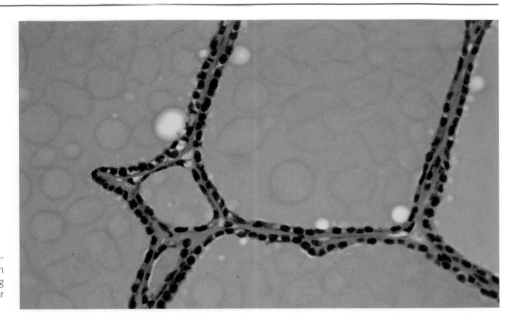

FIGURE 22-49

The classic adenomatoid nodule is composed of large follicles distended with colloid (showing cracking or caking artifact) and lined by flattened follicular epithelium.

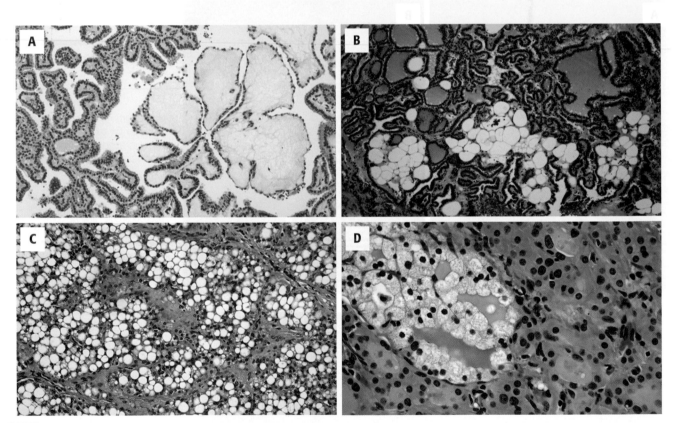

FIGURE 22-50

A, Papillary structures in adenomatoid nodules may be edematous and bulbous or fine and arborizing. **B**, Papillary structures with fat and colloid. **C**, Clear cell change within the cytoplasm of the follicular epithelium. **D**, Oncocytic cells, focally showing early clear cell change. Colloid is present.

(occasionally) (Figure 22-50). It is important to realize that oxyphilic cells may exhibit some of the nuclear features of papillary carcinoma, including nuclear enlargement, vesicular chromatin, and irregular nuclear contours, but these are set in the architecture of a nodule (Figure 22-51).

Some adenomatoid nodules, usually those with cystic change, develop papillary structures (Figure 22-52). The cells lining these papillae, unlike papillary carcinoma, usually have small round nuclei with dense chromatin; the polarity of the cells is maintained, with the nuclei aligned evenly at the base of the epithelium.

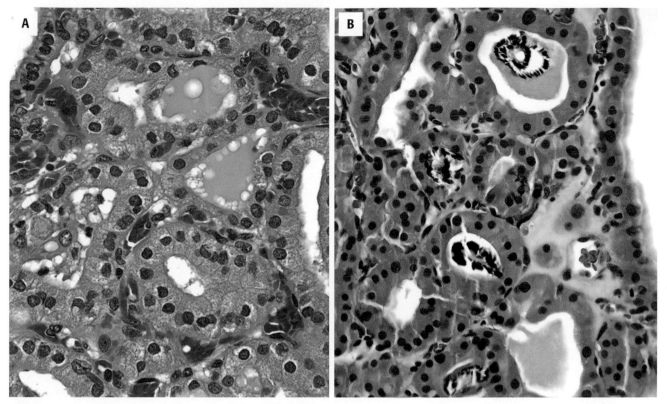

FIGURE 22-51

A, Granular cytoplasm surrounds nuclei that are focally irregular. The nuclear chromatin is coarse and heavy. **B**, Oncocytic cytoplasm is well developed in this case. Note the calcifications within the colloid. These calcifications are not psammoma bodies.

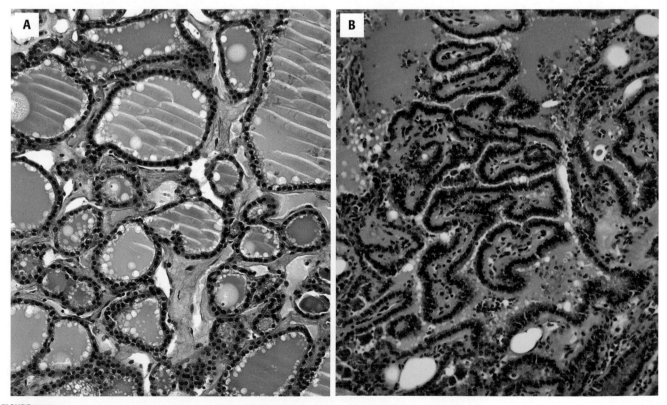

FIGURE 22-52

A, This cystic adenomatoid nodule shows abundant colloid, with cracking artifacts. **B**, This nodule shows a well-developed papillary architecture, but the cells are small and the nuclei are round with well-preserved basal orientation.

Hemorrhage and cystic degeneration often go hand in hand (Figure 22-53). Hemosiderin may be seen deposited in granulation tissue or fibrous scar tissue in areas of degeneration. Hemosiderin-laden macrophages are often seen in the cystic areas and in adjacent parenchyma. In areas of marked hemorrhage, small granules of hemosiderin may be present in the cytoplasm of follicular cells, giving them a red-brown appearance (Figure 22-54). A chronic inflammatory infiltrate may be present. A variety of metaplastic changes may be seen, including fatty, squamous, cartilaginous, and osseous metaplasia.

A phenomenon that occasionally causes confusion, particularly during frozen section examination, is the parasitic nodule (Figure 22-55). This represents a nodule

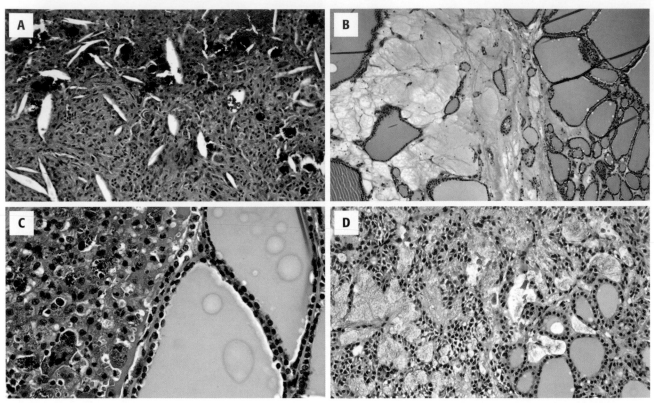

FIGURE 22-53

A, Hemorrhage, hemosiderin-laden macrophages, cholesterol clefts, and a reactive fibrosis in a degenerated adenomatoid nodule. **B**, Edematous change is frequent in nodules. **C**, Hemosiderin-laden macrophages nearly completely replace the colloid in part of this nodule. **D**, Myxoid degeneration can sometimes be seen in adenomatoid nodules.

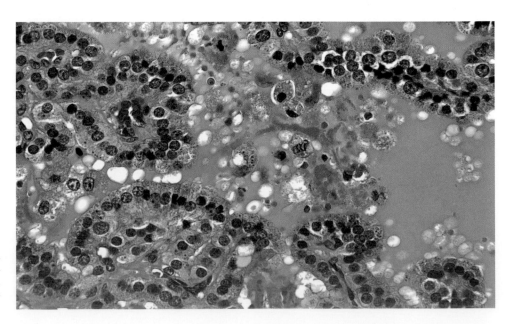

FIGURE 22-54

Hemosiderin is noted within the histiocytes but is also present within the cytoplasm of the follicular epithelial cells. This is a common occurrence in nodules but very rare in papillary carcinoma.

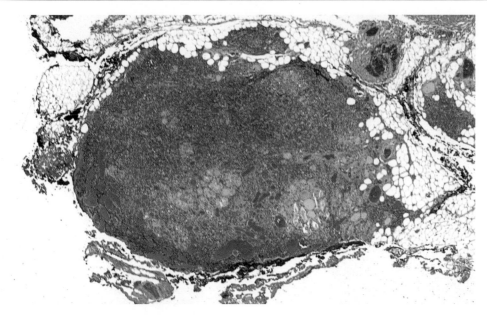

FIGURE 22-55

This patient had a multinodular goiter with a background of lymphocytic thyroiditis. Small fragments of inflamed thyroid epithelium, detached from the gland, may resemble lymph nodes intraoperatively and histologically.

of thyroid tissue which has become separated from the thyroid gland, often demonstrating either adenomatoid nodules or nodular Hashimoto thyroiditis. The attachment to the thyroid is by an inconspicuous cord of fibrous tissue, often overlooked intraoperatively. The histologic appearance is usually that of an adenomatoid nodule; however, in cases associated with a dense lymphocytic infiltrate, they may resemble lymph node, especially when submitted as such during intraoperative assessment. As parasitic nodules lack the structures of a lymph node (subcapsular sinus, sinusoids, etc.), the misdiagnosis of metastatic papillary carcinoma in a lymph node can be averted.

ANCILLARY STUDIES

FINE NEEDLE ASPIRATION

The cytologic features of the usual adenomatoid nodule include abundant, usually thin, colloid and relatively low cellularity with hemosiderin-laden macrophages (Figure 22-56). The follicular epithelial cells from the large follicles ruptured by the aspiration process are usually found as large flat sheets, with evenly spaced, round nuclei, in a honeycomb pattern. The nuclei of the follicular cells have dense chromatin and are not crowded or overlapping (Figure 22-57). In lesions with degenerative changes, the follicular cells may be somewhat oxyphilic. Reactive or reparative follicular cells may be present; they are elongated, and may demonstrate nuclear enlargement and prominent nucleoli. Occasionally, aspirates of cellular adenomatoid nodules that have little colloid are indistinguishable from those of follicular neoplasms, based on cytologic examination alone. These are considered to be indeterminate or "suggestive of neoplasm"; surgical removal of the nodule is usually required in such cases.

DIFFERENTIAL DIAGNOSIS

The chief differential diagnostic problems arise when adenomatoid nodules are cellular or when papillary hyperplasia is present, requiring separation from follicular neoplasms and papillary carcinoma. Cellular adenomatoid nodules may have a pseudocapsule associated with degenerative changes; prominent cystic degeneration is more often found in adenomatoid nodules than in follicular neoplasms, although FNA may induce such changes in neoplasms. Examination of the nodule's periphery for capsular or vascular invasion is necessary to exclude a minimally invasive *follicular carcinoma*. Once invasion is excluded, the distinction between an adenomatoid nodule and a follicular adenoma is of no clinical significance, and may, in fact, be impossible. A true neoplasm usually has smooth muscle–walled vessels in the fibrosis, but this is not always identifiable. Adenomatoid nodules with extensive papillae lack the nuclear features of *papillary carcinoma* and have an orderly, polarized arrangement of their cells and are called "adenomatoid nodules, cystic with papillae."

PROGNOSIS AND THERAPY

Multinodular goiters are not life threatening, and treatment is usually sought for cosmetic or comfort issues. There is no increased incidence of thyroid carcinomas in patients with multinodular goiters. The therapeutic approach to multinodular goiter includes medical therapy (thyroxin administration for suppression of the gland), radioactive iodine ablation, and thyroidectomy. Radioactive iodine ablation is not widely used in the United States for treatment of multinodular goiter, but

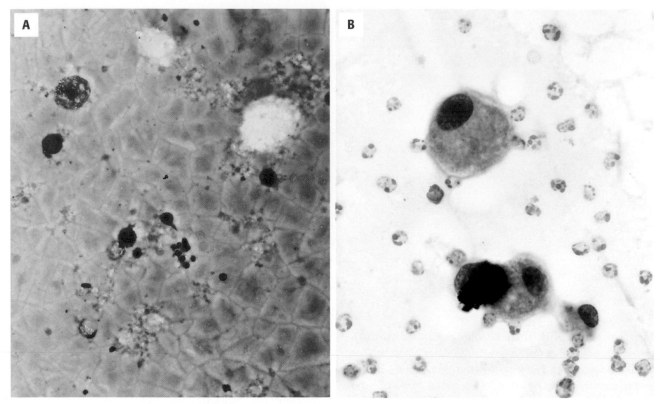

FIGURE 22-56

A, Colloid is abundant in fine needle aspiration samples of typical adenomatoid nodules. The colloid often has a wavy or cracked appearance (air-dried, Diff-Quik stained). **B**, Cystic degeneration or hemorrhage results in the presence of hemosiderin-laden macrophages in many cases (alcohol-fixed, Papanicolaou stain).

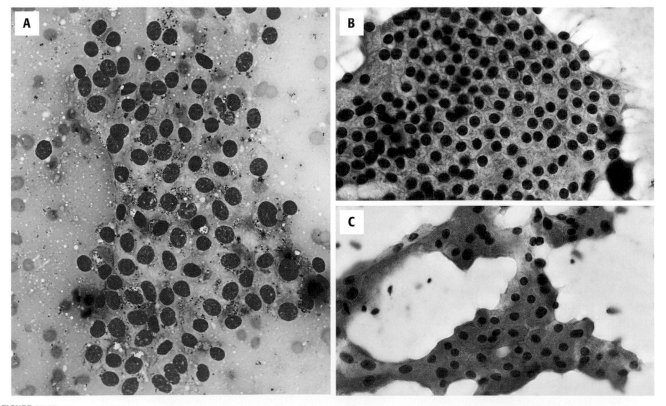

FIGURE 22-57

A, The follicular epithelium appears as flat sheets, in this case with hemosiderin present within the cytoplasm (air-dried, Diff-Quik stained). **B**, The sheets of follicular epithelium usually have a "honeycomb" appearance due to their polarity and distinct cell borders (alcohol-fixed, Papanicolaou-stained). **C**, This cellular adenomatoid nodule has scant colloid, high cellularity, and oxyphilic change; separation from a neoplasm is often impossible by fine needle aspiration smears alone (alcohol-fixed, Papanicolaou stain).

may be useful in patients who are not surgical candidates or for those with toxic multinodular goiter. Hypothyroidism is a risk in any patient treated surgically for multinodular goiter.

■ DYSHORMONOGENETIC GOITER

Dyshormonogenetic goiter represents a hyperplastic thyroid with hypothyroidism resulting from an inherited defect in one of the biochemical steps of thyroid hormone production. Several major enzyme defects are known, and include thyroglobulin synthesis, iodine transport (sodium-iodide symporter; Pendrin), iodide oxidation and organification (thyroperoxidase), coupling of MIT (mono-iodotyrosine) and DIT (di-iodotyrosine), and iodide recycling. These defects result in absent or severely decreased thyroid hormone synthesis, which leads to increased but futile secretion of TSH in response to functional hypothyroidism; the end result is thyroid hyperplasia with no improvement in thyroid function. The genetic mode of transmission is usually autosomal recessive.

CLINICAL FEATURES

Dyshormonogenetic goiter is rare, with a prevalence estimated to be 1 in 30,000 to 50,000 population. It is the second most frequent cause of permanent congenital hypothyroidism. However, only patients with the most severe impairment in thyroid hormone production present clinically in infancy with cretinism. Approximately two-thirds of patients are known to have hypothyroidism prior to recognition of the goiter, which tends to develop later in life.

The average age at presentation is 16 years, but ranges from neonates to adults. There is a slight female predominance. Laboratory studies show a low to absent T_4 and/or T_3 and high TSH. A family history of hypothyroidism and/or goiter is elicited in 20% of patients. Pendred syndrome is an association of dyshormonogenetic goiter with familial deaf-mutism due to sensorineural deafness; it is very rare, involving *SLC26A4* at 7q31.

PATHOLOGIC FEATURES

GROSS FINDINGS

The thyroid gland is enlarged, asymmetric, and nodular, with weights up to 600 g. The nodules resemble adenomatoid nodules, but colloid does not exude from the cut surfaces (Figure 22-58). The nodules tend to

---

DYSHORMONOGENETIC GOITER—DISEASE FACT SHEET

Definition
- Thyroid hyperplasia with hypothyroidism resulting from a number of inherited defects in thyroid hormone production

Incidence and Location
- Rare (estimated 1 in 30,000 to 50,000)
- Family history of hypothyroidism in 20%

Gender and Age Distribution
- Female slightly > male
- Mean, 16 years (wide age range)

Clinical Features
- Permanent congenital hypothyroidism
- Severe impairment presents in infancy; may be associated with cretinism; partial defects in hormone synthesis may present later in life
- Hypothyroidism recognized prior to goiter in two-thirds
- Diffuse thyroid enlargement, often nodular with time
- Rarely Pendred syndrome (familial deaf-mutism and dyshormonogenetic goiter)

Prognosis and Treatment
- No increased risk of thyroid carcinoma
- Lifelong treatment with thyroxin necessary
- Symptomatic goiter treated with total thyroidectomy

DYSHORMONOGENETIC GOITER—PATHOLOGIC FEATURES

Gross Findings
- Thyroid enlarged, asymmetric, nodular
- Weights up to 600 g
- Nodules have more opaque appearance

Microscopic Findings
- Most often nodules are hypercellular, with microfollicular or solid patterns, and little, if any, colloid
- Some glands may have hyperplastic appearance similar to Graves disease, with empty follicles
- Fibrosis often prominent and may distort the borders of the nodules
- Cytologic atypia may be striking, especially in parenchyma between nodules

Fine Needle Aspiration
- Highly cellular aspirate, with small sheets and clusters of follicular epithelial cells
- Little or no colloid
- Follicular cells often have cytoplasmic oxyphilia and marked nuclear atypia, with enlarged, hyperchromatic, and irregularly shaped nuclei
- Impossible to exclude a follicular neoplasm based on cytology alone

Pathologic Differential Diagnosis
- Follicular neoplasm, diffuse hyperplasia, radiation thyroiditis

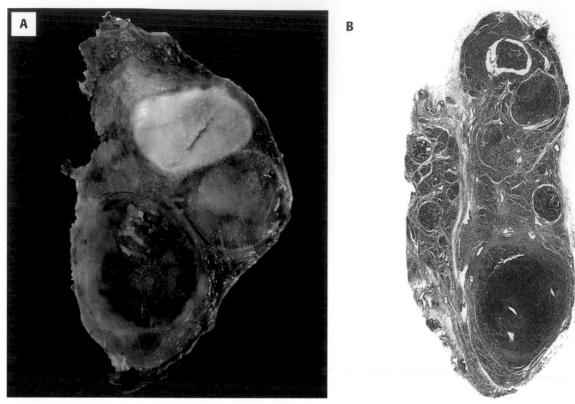

FIGURE 22-58

A, The thyroid gland shows a multinodular appearance. Each nodule is different, lacking easily identified colloid. **B**, There is nearly absent colloid in this low-power view of the thyroid gland, showing multiple nodules.

have a more opaque appearance in contrast to the some-what translucent appearance of adenomatoid nodules.

MICROSCOPIC FINDINGS

All of the thyroid tissue has an abnormal histologic appearance (Figure 22-59), different from the relatively normal thyroid seen between adenomatoid nodules.

The nodules of dyshormonogenetic goiter vary in their appearances, probably as a result of the different en-zyme defects and the duration of the disease (age of patient) at the time of diagnosis (Figure 22-60). The most common finding is the presence of hypercellular nodules with solid or microfollicular patterns. Papillary and insular patterns may also be observed. Colloid is usually scant if it is present at all (Figure 22-61). Fibrosis

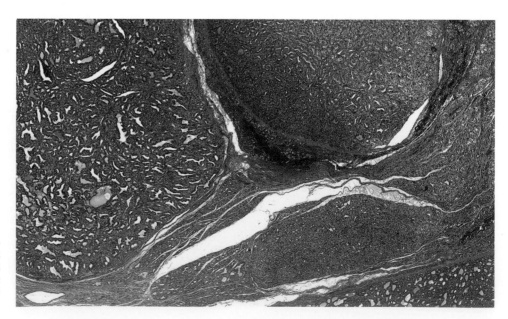

FIGURE 22-59

This example of dyshormonogenetic goi-ter bears a striking resemblance to Graves disease, with diffuse hyperplastic changes throughout the gland, creating multiple asymmetric nodules. However, the tissue between the nodules is also abnormal.

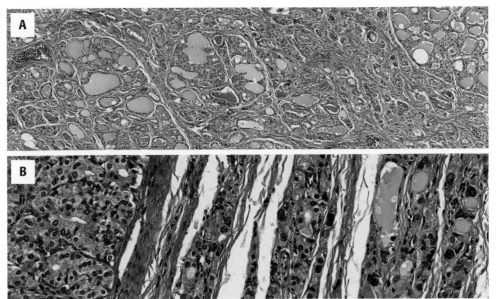

FIGURE 22-60

A, There are multiple "nodules" of tissue, showing variably stained colloid. Note the microfollicular arrangement and abnormal intervening tissue. **B**, The nodule (*far left*) lacks atypia, while remarkable nuclear atypia is noted in between the nodules.

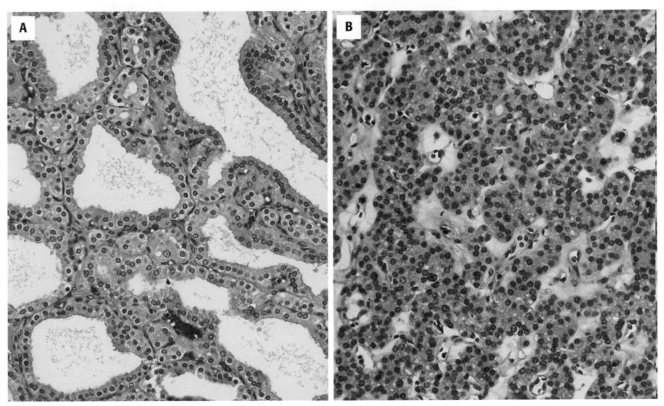

FIGURE 22-61

A, There is a complete lack of normal colloid. **B**, The nodules may be quite cellular, so as to suggest a follicular neoplasm.

is often a prominent finding and may be so extensive that it distorts the contours of the nodules, suggesting an invasive pattern as seen in follicular carcinoma. Cytologic atypia is present in many cases, and may be quite striking, similar to that seen in radiation thyroiditis (Figure 22-62), with an accentuation of this finding in the cells between the nodules.

ANCILLARY STUDIES

FINE NEEDLE ASPIRATION

The aspirates are remarkably cellular, with little or no colloid, and often with prominent nuclear atypia. These findings make exclusion of a follicular neoplasm impossible,

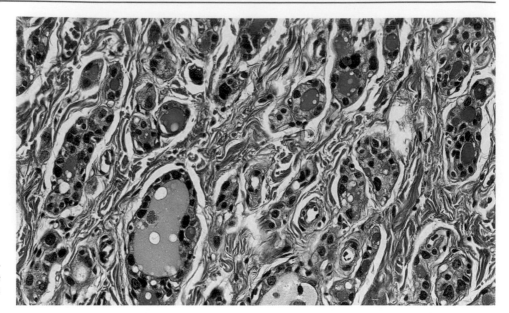

FIGURE 22-62

Cytologic atypia is common in dyshormonogenetic goiter. It should not be overinterpreted as suggesting malignancy. All of this area is between nodules.

even if the history of dyshormonogenetic goiter is known. Aspiration cytology in these cases is useful primarily for ruling out papillary thyroid carcinoma.

DIFFERENTIAL DIAGNOSIS

The differential diagnosis includes follicular carcinoma, diffuse hyperplasia (Graves disease) and radiation thyroiditis. A *follicular carcinoma* is cellular, often with an irregular contour and the presence of definitive invasion. However, the cellularity, fibrosis, and cellular atypia make a diagnosis of follicular carcinoma extremely challenging in the setting of dyshormonogenetic goiter. Only when there is *definitive* invasion should the diagnosis be made. *Diffuse hyperplasia* has clinical hyperthyroidism, often has lymphoid aggregates, and usually has colloid present. *Radiation thyroiditis* may demonstrate cellular nodules with cytologic atypia and increased fibrosis within the gland. An accurate clinical history should readily make the distinction between dyshormonogenetic goiter and these two entities.

PROGNOSIS AND THERAPY

Patients have a favorable outcome with thyroid hormone replacement therapy. There is no increased risk of thyroid carcinoma. Treatment of the hypothyroidism associated with dyshormonogenetic goiter is the primary goal. For symptomatic goiter, total thyroidectomy is the procedure of choice.

■ AMYLOID GOITER

Amyloid goiter represents a symptomatic mass or clinically detectable thyroid enlargement due to extracellular deposition of amyloid. The amyloid deposits may be related to primary systemic amyloidosis or to secondary amyloidosis associated with chronic inflammatory disease (such as rheumatoid arthritis, Crohn disease, familial Mediterranean fever) or neoplastic diseases (plasma cell dyscrasia/myeloma, Hodgkin lymphoma).

CLINICAL FEATURES

Amyloid goiter is very rare, without a known gender predilection. It occurs over a wide age range, from adolescents (especially with juvenile rheumatoid arthritis or familial Mediterranean fever) to the elderly (with hematolymphoid neoplasia). The majority of cases are associated with secondary amyloidosis. Patients usually detect a palpable mass, which, if symptomatic, may have caused dysphagia, dyspnea, and hoarseness. Patients are usually euthyroid.

PATHOLOGIC FEATURES

GROSS FINDINGS

The thyroid is variably enlarged and firm, with a pale tan, "waxy" cut surface; nodules may be present.

AMYLOID GOITER—DISEASE FACT SHEET

Definition
- Amyloid goiter represents thyroid enlargement due to the intercellular deposition of amyloid

Incidence and Location
- Extremely rare

Gender and Age Distribution
- Equal gender distribution
- Wide age range

Clinical Features
- Most cases associated with secondary amyloidosis
- Palpable mass
- May have dysphagia, dyspnea, and hoarseness
- Patients are usually euthyroid
- Associated disease: juvenile rheumatoid arthritis and other rheumatologic disease, familial Mediterranean fever, hematolymphoid neoplasms

Prognosis and Treatment
- Prognosis largely related to underlying disorder (especially hematolymphoid malignancy)
- Compressive symptoms may be relieved by thyroidectomy

AMYLOID GOITER—PATHOLOGIC FEATURES

Gross Findings
- Thyroid diffusely enlarged with a firm, pale, tan, waxy cut surface
- Nodules may be present

Microscopic Findings
- Amyloid deposits usually diffuse, but occasionally nodular
- Extracellular accumulation of acellular homogeneous eosinophilic material with "smudgy" appearance
- Angiocentric deposits and amyloid in walls of blood vessels common
- Atrophy of follicular component of thyroid, with scattered follicles entrapped in amyloid deposits
- Groups of fat cells scattered through gland
- Squamous metaplasia is common
- Chronic inflammatory infiltrate, sometimes with multinucleated giant cells

Immunohistochemical Features
- Most cases are positive for amyloid AA, while cases associated with plasma cell dyscrasia may be positive for amyloid AL

Histochemical Features
- Crystal violet: amyloid metachromatic
- Thioflavin T positive
- Congo red deposits rose-colored, with apple-green birefringence with polarization

Pathologic Differential Diagnosis
- Fibrous variant of Hashimoto thyroiditis, Riedel thyroiditis, adenomatoid nodules, lymphoplasmacytic neoplasm

MICROSCOPIC FINDINGS

The amyloid deposition is usually diffuse, but nodular deposits may occur. Amyloid appears as extracellular, acellular, homogeneous eosinophilic material, classically accentuated in and around vessels (Figure 22-63). Adipose tissue and squamous metaplasia are frequent coexistent findings (Figure 22-64). Follicles are often remarkably elongated and lined by squamous epithelium. Not uncommonly, a chronic inflammatory cell infiltrate, and sometimes multinucleated giant cells, may be present.

ANCILLARY STUDIES

ULTRASTRUCTURAL FEATURES

Electron microscopy is rarely necessary for the diagnosis, but shows masses of nonbranching filaments ranging in size from 50 to 150 Å.

HISTOCHEMISTRY

Amyloid can be demonstrated with crystal violet (metachromatic amorphous material), thioflavin-T and Congo red. The Congo red stain is most commonly used and exhibits apple-green birefringence when polarized (Figure 22-65).

IMMUNOHISTOCHEMICAL FEATURES

Most examples of amyloid goiter are positive for amyloid AA (amyloid A protein, an acute-phase reactant associated with chronic inflammatory conditions) immunohistochemistry, though cases associated with plasma cell dyscrasias may be positive for amyloid AL (amyloid light chain). Light chain restriction may be seen if the patient has a plasma cell dyscrasia or lymphoplasmacytic lymphoma.

DIFFERENTIAL DIAGNOSIS

Amyloid is usually distinctive, with the adipose tissue an initial clue to the diagnosis. Collagenous tissue seen in the *fibrous variant of Hashimoto thyroiditis* or *Riedel thyroiditis* will stain differently with histochemical stains. A *neoplastic plasma cell* or *lymphoplasmacytic neoplasm* may not be obvious in the setting of amyloid goiter; immunohistochemical stains for assessing immunophenotype and clonality (κ and λ) are useful in this regard. *Adenomatoid nodules* may have fatty infiltration, but do not have amyloid present.

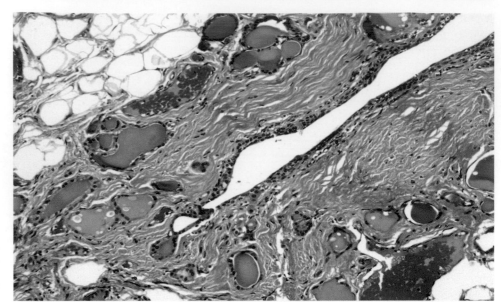

FIGURE 22-63

The thyroid is diffusely infiltrated by inter-cellular deposits of amorphous eosino-philic amyloid, crowding out the thyroid follicles. Fat cells and squamous metapla-sia are frequently observed.

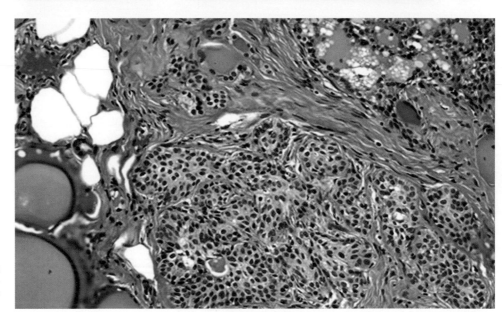

FIGURE 22-64

Squamous metaplasia and adipose tissue with eosinophilic material in the back-ground. Squamous metaplasia and fat are strongly associated with this disorder.

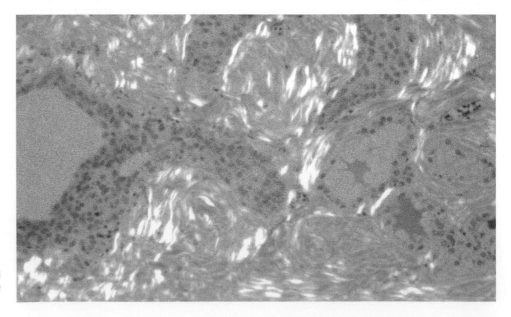

FIGURE 22-65

Congo red stain highlights the amyloid deposits with "apple-green" birefringence when polarized.

PROGNOSIS AND THERAPY

Both prognosis and therapy are dependent on the underlying cause of amyloid goiter: primary systemic amyloidosis, or secondary to chronic inflammatory disease or neoplasia. If there are compressive symptoms, thyroidectomy may be necessary. The more ominous findings are involvement of other organs, such as the heart, kidneys, or liver.

SUGGESTED READINGS

The complete suggested readings list is available online at www.expertconsult.com.

23

Benign Neoplasms of the Thyroid Gland

■ **Lester D. R. Thompson**

Most thyroid neoplasms are benign, with the vast majority accounted for by follicular adenoma (FA). While FA may be difficult to separate from adenomatoid nodule, many authors do not make this distinction in a multinodular gland. Even though there are variants of FA, they are of no clinical consequence but are diagnosed to exclude the lesions raised in the differential diagnosis. Fine needle aspiration (FNA) is an excellent screening tool to diagnose follicular lesions and separate them from other thyroid disease and neoplasms, but FNA will not reproducibly or accurately separate FA from follicular carcinoma. Furthermore, intraoperative consultation cannot reliably separate FA from follicular carcinoma, and therefore is not helpful. Finally, how much of the periphery should be sampled to adequately assess the capsule for invasion? It is my practice to submit at least one section per 1 cm of tumor diameter, but I try to submit the whole periphery if possible. If the tumor looks macroscopically homogeneous after being bivalved, then the center of the tumor is not of interest. The tumor is serially sectioned, with 2 to 3 mm thick sections created. Then, only the very periphery of the tumor to capsule to parenchymal interface is embedded. As many as five sections, 3 mm thick and up to 3 cm long, can be placed side by side in the 2.5 cm wide cassette. With this technique, most tumors can be placed in four to eight blocks, allowing for complete evaluation of the capsule (Figure 23-1).

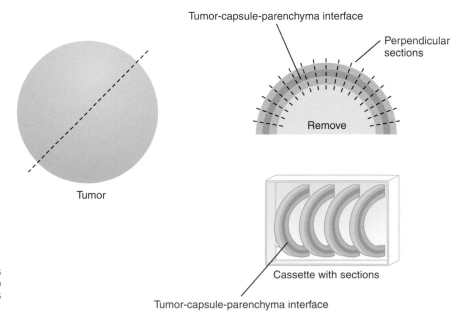

FIGURE 23-1

The tumor is cross-sectioned. The central portion is removed. Serial sections are cut perpendicular to the tumor-capsule-parenchymal interface. Sections are submitted to ensure the interface is examined.

■ FOLLICULAR ADENOMA

FA is a benign encapsulated neoplasm of follicular epithelial differentiation and is the most common neoplasm of the thyroid gland. About 3% to 8% of adults have a solitary nodule, of which nearly 75% represent FAs.

CLINICAL FEATURES

The most common tumor of the thyroid gland, FA is often discovered incidentally during routine physical exam as a solitary, painless, mobile mass, or during radiographic studies for other reasons; sometimes patients present with a history of a slow-growing nodule present for months to years. Iodine deficiency, radiation (γ radiation specifically), and inherited syndromes (Cowden, Carney) may have an etiologic relationship to FA development, which is thought to be a monoclonal proliferation. Women are affected more frequently than men (4 to 5:1). Patients present over a wide age range, but there is a peak in the 5th to 6th decades. Patients are typically euthyroid and only rarely develop hyperfunction or hypofunction. Neck pain

or pressure may be reported if bleeding into the tumor has occurred or due to compressive symptoms in large tumors. Initial management includes an FNA with or without ultrasonography guidance.

RADIOLOGIC FEATURES

Imaging studies cannot reliably separate benign from malignant neoplasms, but ultrasound (US) is the best study, helping to identify the size, location, and character of the nodule (Figure 23-2). US may aid in guiding an FNA for deep-seated or nonpalpable masses. Since adenomas are encapsulated, they are easily identified by a well-defined echo-poor halo at the periphery of an otherwise solid, homogeneous isoechoic mass. Color Doppler gives a "spoke and wheel" appearance of peripheral blood vessels extending toward the center of the lesion. Nuclear imaging studies are invariably "cold," although a functional or "hot" nodule can be seen (Figure 23-2). Computed tomography tends to be nonspecific, showing a hypodense intrathyroid mass, showing enhancement with contrast (Figure 23-3).

PATHOLOGIC FEATURES

FOLLICULAR ADENOMA—DISEASE FACT SHEET

Definition
- Benign encapsulated tumor with evidence of follicular cell differentiation

Incidence and Location
- About 5% of population has palpable thyroid nodule (up to 20% if ultrasound is used)

Morbidity and Mortality
- None (although hypoparathyroidism or recurrent laryngeal nerve damage may occur during surgery)

Gender and Age Distribution
- Female >> male (4-5:1)
- Wide age range, but usually 5th to 6th decade

Clinical Features
- Painless neck mass, often present for years
- Solitary nodule involving only one lobe

Radiologic Features
- Ultrasound shows size, character, and location and aids in fine needle aspiration
- Echo-poor halo at the periphery in a solid, isoechoic mass

Prognosis and Therapy
- Excellent
- Surgery (lobectomy)

FOLLICULAR ADENOMA—PATHOLOGIC FEATURES

Gross Findings
- Solitary, well-demarcated encapsulated spherical mass
- Interior of tumor distinct from remaining thyroid parenchyma
- Mean size: 3 cm

Microscopic Findings
- Surrounded by intact, easily identified capsule (no invasion)
- Smooth muscle–walled vessels present in capsule
- Histology "inside" mass is distinct and separate from parenchyma
- Colloid is usually present
- Cells are slightly enlarged with low nuclear:cytoplasmic ratio
- Variants include trabecular, oncocytic, fetal, clear cell, signet-ring cell

Immunohistochemical Results
- TTF-1, thyroglobulin, keratin, PAX8

Fine Needle Aspiration
- Cellular smears with ample colloid (usually)
- Follicular groups without nuclear features of papillary carcinoma
- Cannot separate between adenomatoid nodule, follicular adenoma, and follicular carcinoma

Pathologic Differential Diagnosis
- Cellular/dominant adenomatoid nodule, follicular carcinoma, papillary carcinoma, trabecular neoplasm (hyalinizing trabecular tumor), metastatic carcinoma

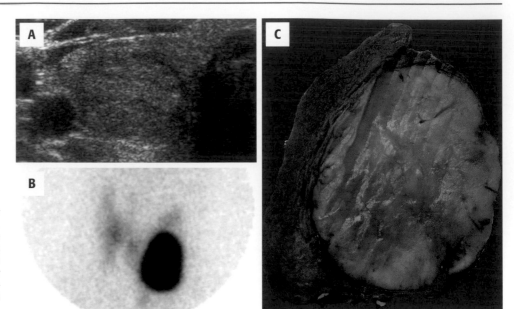

FIGURE 23-2

A, Ultrasound shows an echo-poor halo at the periphery of a solid nodule. **B**, A "hot" nodule in the left lobe of the thyroid gland demonstrates increased uptake of the radiolabeled [123]I. **C**, A single, encapsulated follicular adenoma with a different cut appearance than the surrounding thyroid parenchyma.

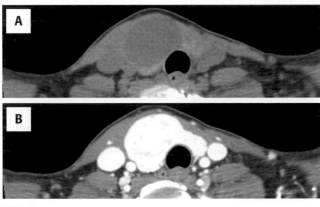

FIGURE 23-3

A, Computed tomography scan showing a well-defined nodule in the right thyroid gland, brightly enhancing with contrast (**B**).

GROSS FINDINGS

FAs are solitary, well-demarcated, and encapsulated masses identified in one lobe or the isthmus (Figure 23-2). The capsule is usually thin but distinct (Figure 23-4); a thick capsule should raise suspicion for a follicular carcinoma. Adenomas are usually round to spherical, measuring ~1 to 3 cm on average, although quite variable depending on clinical presentation (palpable versus incidental radiographic finding). The cut surface is rubbery to firm with a homogeneous solid appearance. Gray-white lesions are usually more cellular, while brown-tan lesions tend to have more colloid. Cystic change, degeneration, calcification, and infarction are common and may alter the physical appearance.

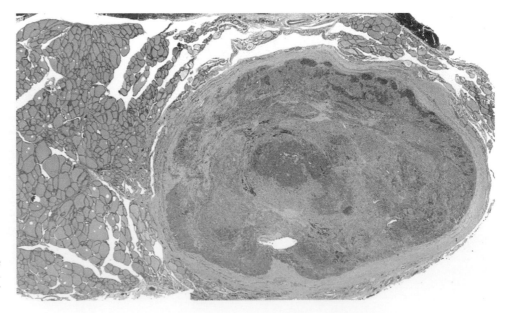

FIGURE 23-4

A variably thick fibrous connective tissue capsule surrounds a follicular adenoma. Central degeneration is a result of previous fine needle aspiration.

Sections are cut perpendicular to the capsule, with an attempt to submit as much of the peripheral zone as is practical.

MICROSCOPIC FINDINGS

A well-defined, variably thick fibrous connective tissue capsule encloses the neoplastic cells, separating them from the compressed or atrophic thyroid parenchyma (Figures 23-5 and 23-6). If the capsule is very thick, additional sections should be evaluated to exclude a carcinoma. Small to medium-sized, smooth muscle–walled vessels can usually be seen within the fibrous connective tissue (Figure 23-7). A reticulin or elastic stain can highlight fibers in a true capsule. No invasion is present by definition, although entrapped epithelium

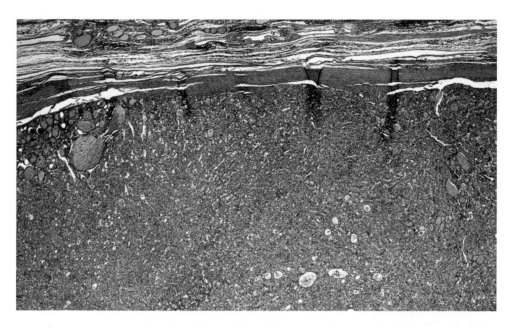

FIGURE 23-5

A cellular follicular adenoma is surrounded by a thin but well-formed capsule. Compressed parenchyma is noted at the periphery.

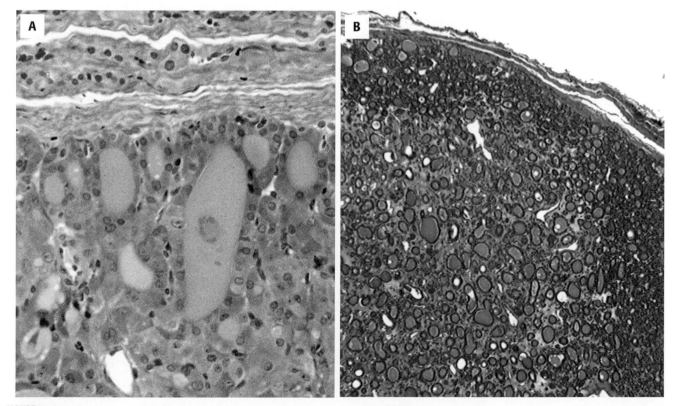

FIGURE 23-6

A, A capsule separates the tumor from the thyroid parenchyma. Abundant colloid is present within this "macrofollicular variant" follicular adenoma. **B**, Most of the follicles are of similar size and shape (normofollicular), but there is a thin capsule at the periphery.

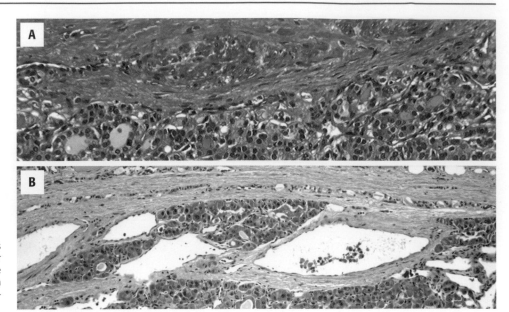

FIGURE 23-7

A, A smooth muscle–walled vessel is identified within the capsule of a follicular adenoma. **B**, Multiple vessels within the wall have entrapped follicles between them, but this does not represent invasion in this follicular adenoma.

can be seen. FNA may result in iatrogenic defects in the capsule, but these are usually associated with a linear tract, extravasated erythrocytes, hemosiderin-laden macrophages, "reactive" fibrosis, and endothelial hyperplasia (Figure 23-8). The site of puncture often has a "sharp edge" of transgression, suggesting a mechanical device rather than biologic aggression.

The cells are arranged in a variety of patterns with a variable amount of colloid, usually distinctive from the surrounding parenchyma. While the patterns of growth have been given "type" or "variant" designations (normofollicular [Figure 23-9], macrofollicular, microfollicular, fetal, embryonal, solid, trabecular [Figure 23-10], insular, organoid), these terms are of no clinical consequence. The follicles are usually uniform with a single architectural pattern predominating. Colloid may be highlighted by a periodic acid–Schiff (PAS) stain if it is limited. Delicate capillaries are easily identified, but intratumoral fibrosis is uncommon. While the cells are slightly enlarged, there is a low nuclear:cytoplasmic ratio with well-defined cell borders in the cuboidal to columnar cells. The nuclei are usually aligned in an orderly arrangement along the basal aspect of the cell. Ample cytoplasm, ranging from eosinophilic, oncocytic (Figure 23-11), amphophilic, granular to clear (Figure 23-12), surrounds round and regular nuclei with coarse to heavy nuclear chromatin distribution. Nucleoli are inconspicuous, although they may be prominent and centrally placed in an oncocytic FA. Nuclear pleomorphism can be seen but is usually focal. Mitotic figures

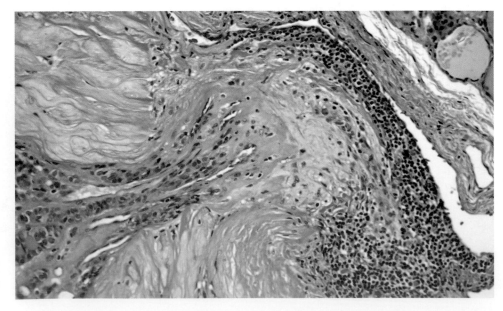

FIGURE 23-8

Note the sharp edge of transgression, with follicular cells associated with lymphocytes and histiocytes in this post–fine needle aspiration site.

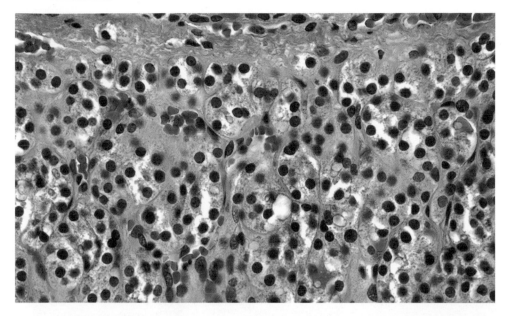

FIGURE 23-9

A normofollicular architecture showing scant colloid. The cells are cuboidal with round nuclei.

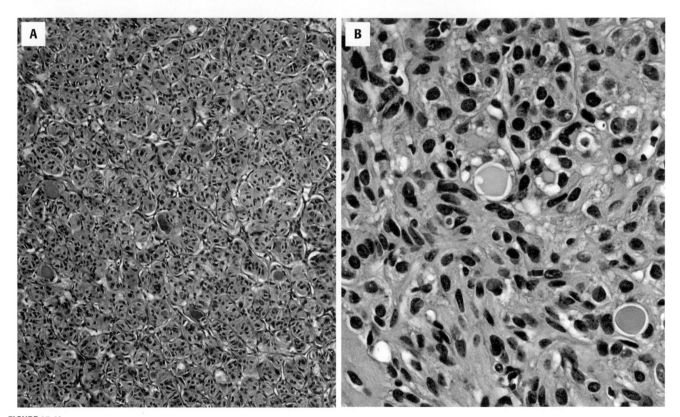

FIGURE 23-10

A, A trabecular-to-insular architecture is noted in this adenoma with scant colloid. **B**, The lesional cells show a spindled architecture with easily identified colloid.

are inconspicuous but may be increased in the post-FNA setting. Degenerative and cystic changes include edema, fibrosis, hemorrhage, cyst formation, and calcification, but tumor necrosis is not identified. Infarction, especially in oncocytic tumors, may be associated with FNA or decreased blood supply. Viable tumor cells may be limited to the periphery. Fat is rarely noted (lipid-rich adenoma) within the tumor cells and presents as intracytoplasmic, oil red O–positive vesicles. This is distinct

from lipoadenoma, in which mature fat is interspersed between the follicular epithelial cells. Squamous metaplasia may be seen but is more common in papillary carcinoma.

Oncocytic (oxyphilic, Hürthle cell, Ashkenazi cell), clear cell, and signet-ring cell variants (Figure 23-12) are recognized but are of no clinical value. The *oncocytic adenoma* tends to have a mahogany brown cut surface with central scarring. The tumor typically has less colloid

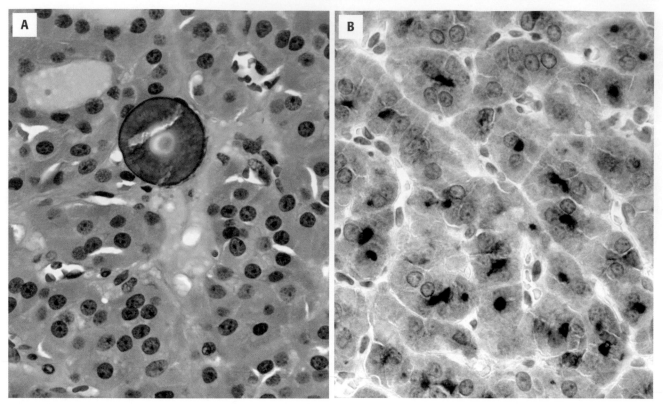

FIGURE 23-11

A, Colloid has become inspissated and calcified, but the nuclei are round and regular in this oncocytic follicular adenoma. **B**, Thyroglobulin may help to confirm the follicular derivation of tumors with limited to absent colloid production.

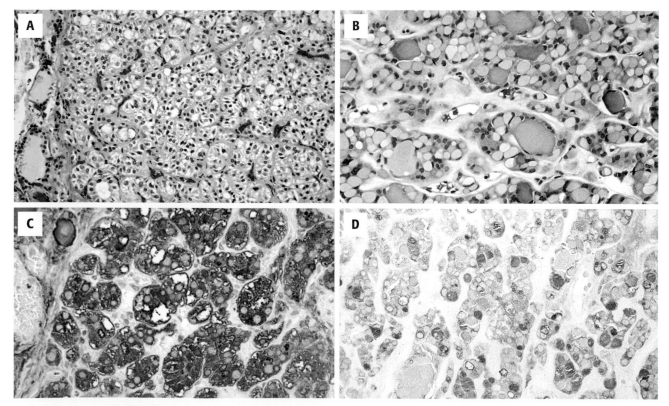

FIGURE 23-12

A follicular adenoma is composed exclusively of clear cells (**A**), although colloid production can still be identified (**C**). **B**, Signet-ring adenoma is composed of cells with a large cytoplasmic vacuole that compresses the nucleus. **D**, Thyroglobulin highlights the vacuoles in a signet ring adenoma.

production, frequently resulting in inspissated colloid that can mimic psammoma bodies (Figures 23-6, left, and 23-11, left). Tumor cells tend to have a greater degree of nuclear pleomorphism, with vesicular nuclear chromatin and prominent nucleoli. The cytoplasm often has a "glassy" opaque appearance. However, oncocytic adenoma is a histologic description only and *does not* imply a different biologic potential. To be qualified as a *clear cell variant*, the tumor should be predominantly or exclusively composed of cells with clear cytoplasm (Figure 23-12). The nuclei are usually centrally situated and are hyperchromatic. *Signet-ring cell adenoma* is extremely rare but has cells with large intracytoplasmic vacuoles which compress the nucleus to the side (Figure 23-12). These vacuoles contain diastase-resistant, PAS-positive material, which is strongly thyroglobulin immunoreactive, suggesting an abnormal thyroglobulin accumulation. Metastatic adenocarcinoma may rarely give a similar histologic appearance.

ANCILLARY STUDIES

IMMUNOHISTOCHEMICAL RESULTS

Immunohistochemistry is seldom necessary for the diagnosis, but in cases where the diagnosis is in question,

the neoplastic cells will be thyroglobulin (Figures 23-11 and 23-12), TTF-1, PAX8, and keratin immunoreactive (CAM5.2, AE1/AE3, CK7). Oncocytic tumors must be interpreted with caution due to high background and nonspecific staining.

FINE NEEDLE ASPIRATION

FNA is the first-line evaluation technique. Unfortunately, FNA does not separate between a cellular or dominant adenomatoid nodule, FA, or follicular carcinoma with any degree of reliability or reproducibility. After adequacy is assessed (five or six follicular epithelial groups of at least 10 epithelial cells per group), a follicular neoplasm may be favored over adenomatoid nodule (colloid goiter). Features that favor a neoplasm are syncytial groups with a microfollicular arrangement in a cellular smear in which there is increased cellularity compared to the amount of colloid, and uniform, monotonous cells that vary little from one another (Figure 23-13). The epithelial groups are arranged as small spherical aggregates surrounding a colloid droplet. Oncocytic adenomas have large, polygonal cells with granular cytoplasm. The nucleoli tend to be more prominent. Adenomatoid nodules tend to have cellular variability and often have extensive degenerative changes present. The diagnosis of "follicular neoplasm or suspicious for a

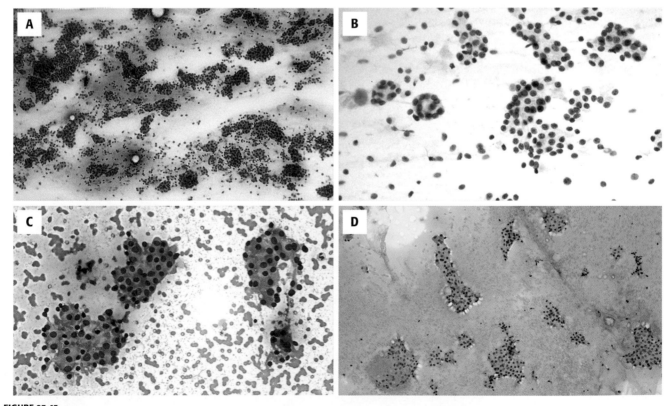

FIGURE 23-13

Fine needle aspiration smear of "thyroid follicular epithelial proliferation, favor neoplasm." Cellular smears, with syncytial groups of uniform and monotonous cells. Scant colloid is present (**A** and **C**, air-dried, Diff-Quik stain; **B** and **D**, alcohol-fixed, Papanicolaou stain). Note the oncocytic appearance of the cells in **C** and **D**.

follicular neoplasm" will result in appropriate surgery for a solitary thyroid mass (equivalent to Bethesda System for Reporting Thyroid Cytopathology: Group IV).

GENETICS

Numerical chromosome changes can be seen, with trisomy 7 seen in ~15% of FAs, while tetrasomy is seen in ~45% of oncocytic adenomas. Translocations involving 2p21 (*THADA*) and 19q13 (*ZNF331/RITA*) are seen in ~10% and ~20%, respectively, of FA. Activating point mutations of *RAS* genes (specifically *NRAS* and *HRAS*) are most prevalent and detected in ~30% of cases. Somatic mutations in mitochondrial DNA (mtDNA) are found in oncocytic tumors.

DIFFERENTIAL DIAGNOSIS

The differential diagnosis includes cellular or dominant adenomatoid nodules, follicular carcinoma, papillary carcinoma, medullary carcinoma, hyalinizing trabecular tumor, and metastatic carcinomas. Definitive separation between FA and *adenomatoid nodule* is arbitrary and sometimes semantic, as both are benign lesions requiring no difference in management. With that said, adenomatoid nodules are usually multiple, lack a capsule with smooth muscle–walled vessels, and usually have much more abundant colloid and degenerative changes than an adenoma. Oncocytic cells can be seen. Without capsular or vascular invasion, a diagnosis of *carcinoma* cannot be rendered in follicular neoplasms. However, features that raise the suspicion of carcinoma include a remarkably thickened fibrous capsule, increased cellularity (especially at the periphery of the tumor), increased mitotic activity, atypical mitotic figures, and tumor necrosis. Still, invasion must be present to call the tumor a follicular carcinoma. The designation "atypical adenoma" may be used in these circumstances where a definitive separation is impossible (Figure 23-14). To date, cytogenetic and molecular studies cannot reliably separate follicular tumors. Oxyphilia often results in nuclear contour irregularities and intranuclear cytoplasmic inclusions (any cell with abundant cytoplasm is prone to intranuclear cytoplasmic invaginations), both features seen in *papillary carcinoma*. However, additional architectural and cytomorphologic features of papillary carcinoma must be present before making the diagnosis: intratumoral fibrosis, thick, eosinophilic colloid, large cells, loss of polarity, and the characteristic nuclear features of crowding, grooves, chromatin clearing, and pseudo inclusions. *Clear cell tumors*, such as medullary carcinoma, parathyroid neoplasms, or metastatic renal cell carcinoma (CD10, RCC), can usually be separated on immunohistochemical grounds. *Hyalinizing trabecular tumor* shows a trabecular growth pattern with perpendicular arrangement of nuclei, grooves, and pseudo inclusions and demonstrates a distinctive membranous staining pattern with Dako Ki-67.

PROGNOSIS AND THERAPY

There is an excellent long-term clinical prognosis without recurrences or metastasis when removed by conservative surgery (lobectomy alone). Hypoparathyroidism and recurrent laryngeal nerve damage may result from surgery.

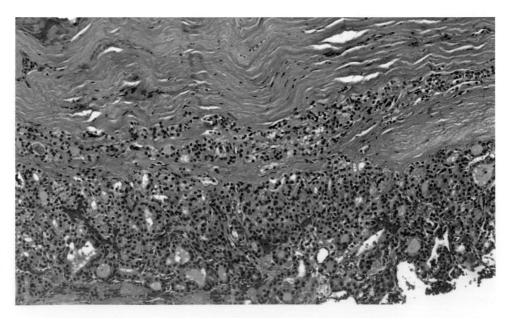

FIGURE 23-14

A very thick fibrous connective tissue capsule with irregularities in the contour, focal areas of "entrapment" and an increased cellularity at the periphery are worrisome for a follicular carcinoma, but not quite definitive for invasion. "Atypical adenoma" may be employed as the diagnosis.

■ TERATOMA

Tumors of the cervical region are regarded as thyroid teratomas if:

- The tumor occupies a portion of the thyroid gland
- There is direct continuity or close anatomic relationship between the tumor and the thyroid gland
- A cervical teratoma is accompanied by total absence of the thyroid gland

In a given case, it may be difficult to rule out the possibility that the thyroid tissue found adjacent to the teratoma may represent either normal thyroid gland secondarily replaced by a primary teratoma or just a component of the teratoma. The tumors histologically display mature or immature tissues from all three embryonic germ cell layers: ectoderm, endoderm, and mesoderm. The percentage of each element is used to separate the tumors into mature, immature, and malignant types.

CLINICAL FEATURES

Teratoma is a rare tumor comprising <0.1% of all primary thyroid neoplasms. Patients range from newborn to 85 years at initial presentation, although the peak and median is the "newborn" period. The average age, however, is skewed by *older* patients who usually have *malignant* teratomas. In fact, >90% of the tumors in the neonatal group will be benign teratomas, whereas ≥50% of the children/adult group will have malignant teratomas. There is no gender predilection. All patients present with an anterior neck mass, often reaching a significant size. Patients may also experience dyspnea, difficulty breathing, and/or stridor. Benign teratomas, whether mature or immature, may result in the patient's death due to tracheal compression or maldevelopment of the neck organs.

RADIOLOGIC FEATURES

Radiographic images can be obtained in utero, at the time of birth, or in the adult patient. Ultrasonographic techniques provide the best information and are easiest to perform in utero or in the neonatal period. A multicystic mass lesion of the thyroid gland is most frequently identified. Computed tomography images show an inhomogeneous mass arising in the thyroid gland and compressing the upper airway in either the benign or malignant teratomas (Figure 23-15). The presence of enlarged, peripherally enhancing lymph nodes in the neck suggests a malignant teratoma.

PATHOLOGIC FEATURES

GROSS FINDINGS

The tumors average 6 to 7 cm but can be quite large. The outer tumor surface is lobulated and smooth with a variable consistency, from firm to soft and cystic (Figure 23-15). It may be well circumscribed to widely infiltrative. A gray-tan to translucent cut surface is common. Small, multiloculated cysts may contain white-tan creamy material, mucoid glairy material, or dark brown hemorrhagic fluid with necrotic debris. "Brain" tissue is frequent, while black pigmentation (retinal anlage) is less common. Bone and cartilage can be recognized macroscopically.

MICROSCOPIC FINDINGS

Teratoma, choristoma, hamartoma, heterotopia, epignathus, and dermoid are all unique lesions, and while semantic, these separations are well accepted. Teratoma should

TERATOMA—PATHOLOGIC FEATURES

Gross Findings

- Mean size: 6 to 7 cm
- Lobulated, smooth with variable consistency
- Multiloculated cysts with white-tan creamy material, mucoid glairy material, or dark hemorrhagic fluid with necrotic debris
- "Brain" tissue is usually present
- Gritty material represents bone or cartilage

Microscopic Findings

- Thyroid parenchyma should be identified
- Mature or immature tissues from all germ cell layers
- Squamous, respiratory, glandular, and cuboidal epithelium
- Organ differentiation may be seen
- Neural tissues, including glial elements, choroid plexus, immature neuroblastema, and pigmented retinal anlage
- Bone, cartilage, muscle, and fat
- Separated into benign, immature, and malignant based on degree and extent of immature neuroectodermal elements

Immunohistochemical Results

- Variable for each specific element within teratoma
- Immature glial elements can be highlighted with S100 protein, GFAP, NSE, and NFP

Fine Needle Aspiration

- Cellular smears with various elements often misdiagnosed as "contamination" or "missed lesion"
- Immature/malignant neural elements are called "malignant" but not specific for teratoma

Pathologic Differential Diagnosis

- Benign: epignathus, choristoma, hamartoma, heterotopia, dermoid
- Malignant: Ewing sarcoma, lymphoma, rhabdomyosarcoma, small cell carcinoma

only be applied to a tumor with *tri-lineage* differentiation. Thyroid parenchyma should be identified somewhere within the mass to qualify as a thyroid teratoma (Figure 23-16), although in malignant teratomas residual thyroid follicles are frequently scarce or absent. Tumors display a wide array of tissue types and growth patterns within a single lesion (Figure 23-17). A host of small cystic spaces are lined by a variety of different epithelia (Figure 23-18): squamous, pseudostratified ciliated columnar (respiratory), cuboidal (with and without goblet cells), glandular, and transitional epithelia. Pilosebaceous and other adnexal structures are seen in association with squamous epithelium. True "organ" differentiation (pancreas, liver, lung) is uncommonly noted. Nearly all cases contain neural tissue, which consists of mature glial elements, choroid plexus, pigmented retinal anlage, or immature neuroblastemal elements, resembling embryonic tissue. Neuroblastic elements often arranged in sheets or rosette-like structures (Homer Wright or Flexner-Wintersteiner) are characterized by small to medium-sized cells with dense hyperchromatic nuclei and mitoses (Figure 23-19). Mitotic figures are common in these immature areas. Cartilage, bone, striated skeletal muscle (Figure 23-20), smooth muscle, adipose tissue, and loose myxoid to fibrous embryonic mesenchymal connective tissue are seen intermixed with the neural and epithelial elements.

The maturation of the neural-type tissue determines the grade. Benign mature teratomas contain only mature elements (grade 0; Figure 23-21). The term "benign, immature teratoma" encompasses tumors with a limited degree of immaturity: (1) embryonal-type tissue in only 1 low-power field (grade 1) and (2) tumors with >1 but <4 low-power fields of immature foci (grade 2). "Malignant teratomas" contain >4 low-power fields of immature tissue (Figure 23-22), along with mitoses and cellular atypia (grade 3). The presence of embryonal

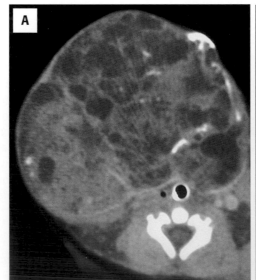
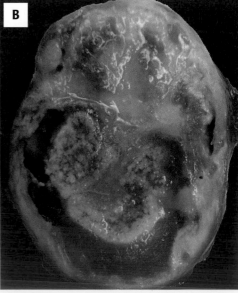

FIGURE 23-15

A, This computed tomography scan demonstrates a large multicystic thyroid teratoma in the anterior neck that completely replaces the thyroid gland. **B,** The teratoma has a multinodular appearance and has completely replaced the thyroid gland. Cystic and calcified areas are noted with myxoid-mucinous areas.

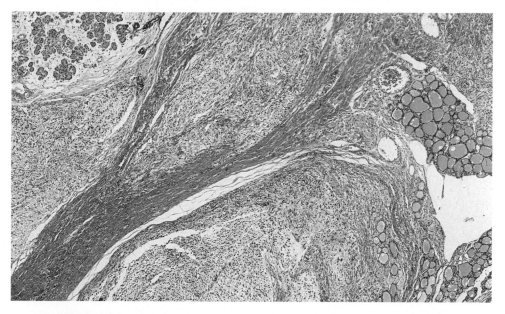

FIGURE 23-16

Benign mature teratoma. Mature thyroid follicular epithelium is compressed to the periphery by mature glial tissue and salivary gland tissue.

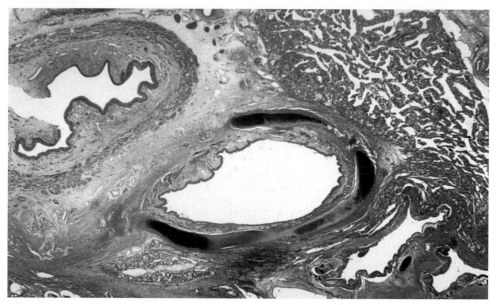

FIGURE 23-17

A mature "esophagus," "trachea," and "lung" are seen in this mature thyroid teratoma, forming an "epignathus"-type lesion.

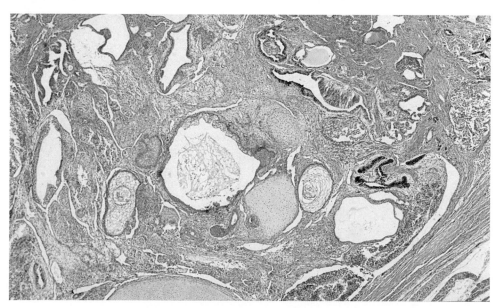

FIGURE 23-18

Multiple cystic spaces are lined by squamous, cuboidal, and respiratory type epithelium in this benign mature teratoma. Neural tissue and pigmented retinal anlage are also noted.

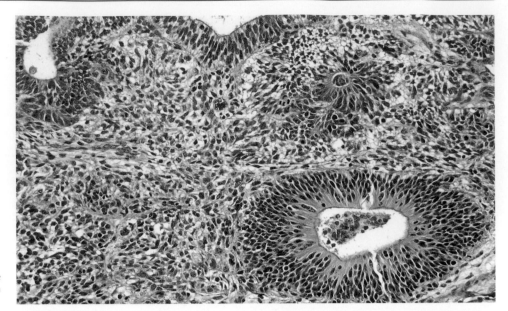

FIGURE 23-19

Benign immature teratoma. Immature neuroectodermal tissue arranged in Flexner-Wintersteiner rosettes.

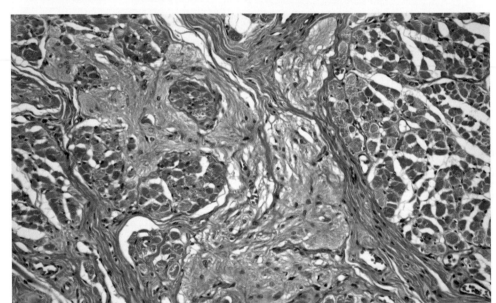

FIGURE 23-20

This benign mature teratoma has a haphazard arrangement of skeletal muscle with mature glial tissue.

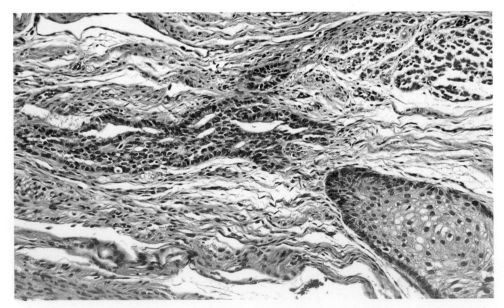

FIGURE 23-21

Benign mature teratoma. Mature squamous epithelium, cuboidal epithelium, cartilage, and mature skeletal muscle are haphazardly arranged.

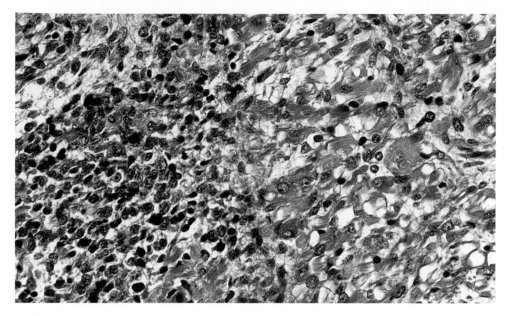

FIGURE 23-22

Malignant teratoma. This tumor has immature neuroectodermal and rhabdomyosarcomatous differentiation.

carcinoma or yolk sac tumor would place a teratoma into the malignant category by definition.

ANCILLARY STUDIES

IMMUNOHISTOCHEMICAL RESULTS

Immunohistochemistry for S100 protein, glial fibrillary acidic protein, neuron specific enolase, neural filament protein, desmin, myogenin, or MYOD1 may be of value for the characterization of the various immature elements.

FINE NEEDLE ASPIRATION

Smears will demonstrate various cellular components, often misinterpreted to represent a contamination or a "missed" lesion. In malignant teratomas, the FNA smears will show a "neuroepithelial" small round blue cell appearance when taken from the immature/malignant neural elements. These cells are frequently interpreted as "malignant cells" rather than giving a specific diagnosis of malignant teratoma.

DIFFERENTIAL DIAGNOSIS

Choristoma is used for histologically normal tissues in a location other than the site at which it is normally detected. *Hamartoma* refers to a disorganized collection of normal mature tissues for the anatomic area. *Heterotopias* are normal tissue in an abnormal location (misplaced or displaced). *Epignathus* is used for tumors of the palate, sometimes considered to be a parasitic

fetus in which the tumor contains nearly all of the tissues seen in a complete fetus. *Dermoid cyst* ("resembling skin") generally contains only ectodermal and mesodermal elements, specifically skin and hair.

The majority of thyroid teratomas are easily recognizable as such on clinical, radiographic, and pathologic grounds. However, when immature elements predominate, extraskeletal Ewing sarcoma, small cell carcinoma, lymphoma, and rhabdomyosarcoma enter the differential diagnosis. The diagnosis of teratoma under these circumstances is largely dependent on the identification of other tissue elements, the immature/malignant neural tissues, and a confirmatory immunohistochemical panel.

PROGNOSIS AND THERAPY

The outcome for thyroid teratomas is dependent largely on the age of the patient, the size of the tumor at initial presentation, and the presence and proportion of immaturity. Even though histologically benign teratomas (whether mature or immature) do not invade or metastasize, they can still result in the patient's death due to tracheal compression or a lack of development of vital neck structures during fetal growth. Prompt surgical intervention, including in utero procedures (ex utero intrapartum treatment [EXIT] procedure), may be necessary to yield a good patient outcome. Age at presentation and tumor histology are strongly correlated: neonates nearly always have benign or immature teratomas and do not die from disease (but may die with disease); children and adults tend to have malignant teratomas and may die from disease. Recurrence and dissemination are known to occur in about one-third of patients with malignant teratomas, nearly all of whom are adults. Lymph node metastasis is usually followed by lung disease. These patients are managed with radiation and chemotherapy, although it is generally considered palliative with an almost uniformly fatal outcome. Staging is not usually applied since the local effect is more prognostically significant than other features.

■ HYALINIZING TRABECULAR TUMOR

Also known as a paraganglioma-like adenoma, hyalinizing trabecular tumor (HTT) is a very rare follicular neoplasm with trabecular growth and intratrabecular hyalinization that seems to have a molecular link to papillary thyroid carcinoma (*RET/PTC* rearrangements, but not *BRAF*). A few cases have occurred following radiation exposure.

CLINICAL FEATURES

Women are affected much more commonly than men (female:male, 6:1) with a wide age range at initial presentation, although the mean age is 50 years. Patients usually have an asymptomatic neck mass, incidentally discovered during routine physical exam or discovered in multinodular glands removed for a different reason. Patients are usually euthyroid. Ultrasonography shows a solid nodule, with hypoechoic or heterogeneous echogenicity.

PATHOLOGIC FEATURES

GROSS FINDINGS

A solitary, encapsulated to well-circumscribed thyroid tumor that is usually small, with a mean size of 2.5 cm. The cut surface is usually solid with a slight yellow tinge, delicately lobulated and occasionally showing patulous vessels. Calcifications are uncommon.

MICROSCOPIC FINDINGS

The cellular and solid tumors are surrounded by a well-formed, but thin, fibrous connective tissue capsule. Vascular and/or capsular invasion are almost always absent. The cells are arranged in trabecular and insular

---

HYALINIZING TRABECULAR TUMOR—DISEASE FACT SHEET

Definition
- Hyalinizing trabecular adenoma is a follicular cell tumor with a trabecular growth pattern and heavy intratrabecular hyalinization

Incidence and Location
- Rare

Morbidity and Mortality
- None (although trabecular pattern can be seen in follicular carcinoma)

Gender and Age Distribution
- Female > > male (6:1)
- Usually presents in 5th to 6th decades

Clinical Features
- Palpable, solitary mass
- Usually asymptomatic and incidentally found
- Rare association with radiation

Prognosis and Therapy
- By definition, excellent
- Reports of lymph node metastases may suggest a relationship with papillary carcinoma

---

HYALINIZING TRABECULAR TUMOR—PATHOLOGIC FEATURES

Gross Findings
- Solitary, solid, encapsulated neoplasm
- Usually small, mean: 2.5 cm

Microscopic Findings
- Thin fibrous connective tissue capsule
- Trabecular to insular growth pattern
- Scant to absent colloid
- Calcific bodies
- Medium-sized to large polygonal to fusiform cells, arranged perpendicular
- Variable cytoplasm, sometimes containing yellow paranuclear bodies
- Prominent nuclear grooves and perinucleolar halos
- Prominent intranuclear cytoplasmic inclusions
- Hyalinized stroma separating neoplastic cells into trabeculae
- Cytoplasmic, round, refractile, yellow bodies/vacuoles

Immunohistochemical Results
- Thyroglobulin, TTF-1, and CK7 immunoreactive
- Membrane MIB-1 (Ki-67) immunoreactivity

Fine Needle Aspiration
- Cellular aspirates
- Elongated nuclei may be misinterpreted as papillary carcinoma
- Lumpy basement membrane material

Pathologic Differential Diagnosis
- Papillary carcinoma, follicular adenoma, follicular carcinoma, medullary thyroid carcinoma, paraganglioma

patterns (Figure 23-23), resulting in straight to curvilinear bands of tumor cells two to four cells thick. The nests are formed by a dense, heavily hyalinized, eosinophilic fibrovascular stroma. The basement membrane material may resemble amyloid but is Congo red negative. Colloid is limited to absent. The nuclei are arranged perpendicular to the long axis of the trabeculae and fibrovascular stroma (Figure 23-24). The cells are medium to large, polygonal to fusiform, with variable cytoplasm surrounding the oval to elongated nuclei. Intranuclear cytoplasmic inclusions are common, with easily identified nuclear grooves (Figure 23-25). Perinucleolar halos are common. Distinctive, small, round, refractile, slightly yellow intracytoplasmic bodies are seen in a paranuclear distribution (Figure 23-26). Lymphocytic thyroiditis may be present in the background thyroid parenchyma.

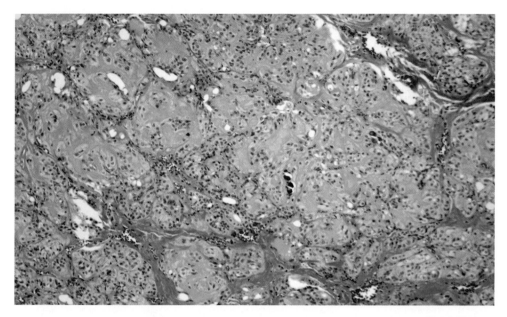

FIGURE 23-23

A well-circumscribed hyalinizing trabecular tumor with cells arranged in trabeculae separated by fibrous connective tissue and showing basement membrane material within the groups.

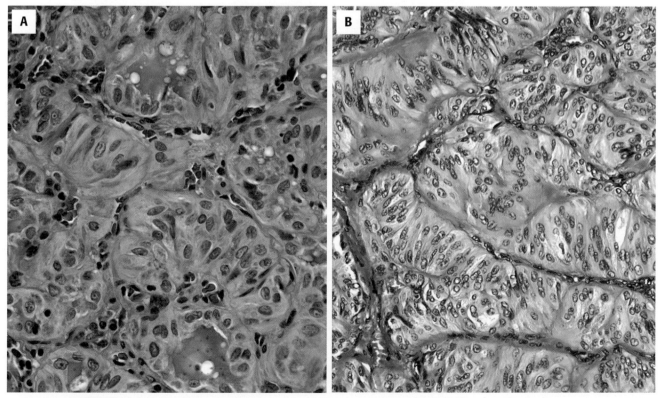

FIGURE 23-24

A and **B**, The fusiform cells are arranged perpendicular to the fibrovascular stroma in these hyalinizing trabecular adenomas.

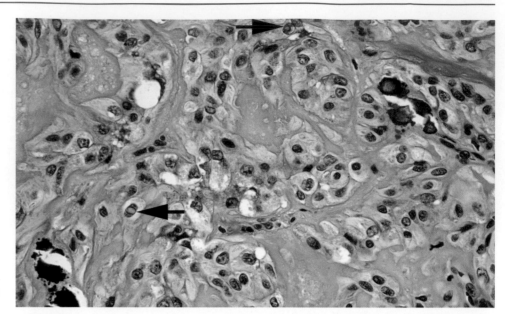

FIGURE 23-25

Multiple intranuclear cytoplasmic inclusions (*arrows*) and perinucleolar halos are seen. Calcifications are also noted.

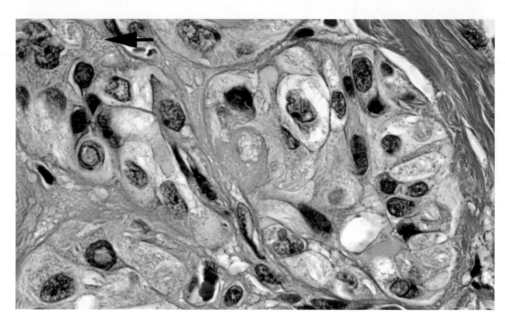

FIGURE 23-26

Intranuclear inclusions are noted. There are also slightly yellow, paranuclear cytoplasmic bodies (*arrow*), a unique feature in this tumor.

Occasional calcospherites (psammoma bodies) may be seen within the tumor (Figure 23-25).

ANCILLARY STUDIES

ULTRASTRUCTURAL FEATURES

Nests and cords of cells surrounded by basal lamina are seen, with cells showing short microvilli. The nuclei have irregular contours with multiple indentations and intranuclear grooves and pseudo inclusions and contain bundles of intermediate filaments in the cytoplasm. There are large, membrane-bound lysosomes, containing vacuoles, granular material, and regularly stacked membranes or "fingerprint" bodies. There are lumpy accumulations of basement membrane material.

IMMUNOHISTOCHEMICAL RESULTS

The neoplastic cells are thyroglobulin (Figure 23-27), TTF-1, CK7, keratin, and vimentin reactive, while nonreactive with chromogranin, calcitonin, and S100 protein. Strong membranous Ki-67 (MIB-1, Dako antibody) staining is distinctive (Figure 23-27).

FINE NEEDLE ASPIRATION

Cellular aspirates are often misinterpreted as papillary carcinoma due to the similar nuclear features. Aspirates are cellular with cohesive clusters of cells with abundant cytoplasm. Nuclei are elongated with evenly dispersed chromatin, intranuclear cytoplasmic inclusions, and nuclear grooves. The dense, lumpy basement membrane material between cells may help

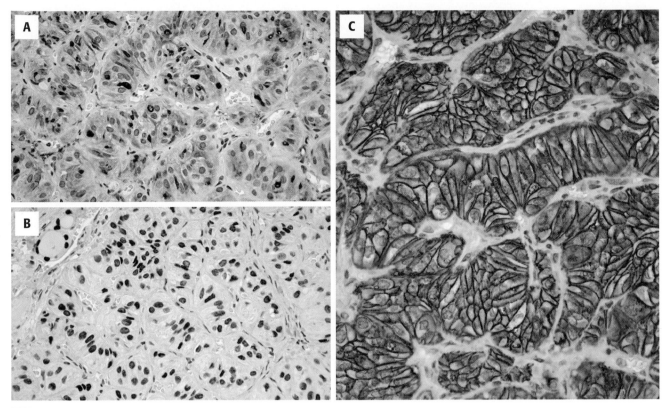

FIGURE 23-27

A, There is cytoplasmic immunoreactivity with thyroglobulin, along with highlighting the colloid. **B**, Strong, diffuse nuclear TTF-1 reactivity. **C**, The MIB-1 (Dako antibody) gives a unique membranous reaction for Ki-67.

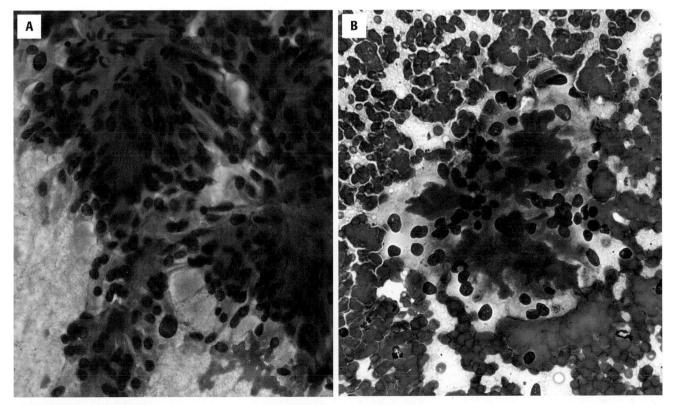

FIGURE 23-28

A, Fine needle aspiration shows a cellular smear with intranuclear cytoplasmic inclusions in the round to regular nuclei (alcohol-fixed, Papanicolaou stained). The dense, basement membrane material can be seen in both images, although highlighted magenta-purple with the Diff-Quik preparation (**B**).

with the diagnosis, but may be difficult to appreciate (Figure 23-28). When present, this material is often radially oriented around cells, accounting for the hyalinized nature of this tumor.

DIFFERENTIAL DIAGNOSIS

The differential diagnosis includes papillary carcinoma, medullary carcinoma, paraganglioma, FA, and follicular carcinoma. *Paraganglioma*, rare in the thyroid, can be readily ruled out by their characteristic immunophenotype (neuroendocrine markers positive with S100 protein staining in sustentacular cells). Trabecular pattern of growth can be seen in papillary, medullary, and follicular neoplasms. *Follicular carcinoma* with trabecular architecture, by definition, will have invasion. The nuclei are not usually arranged perpendicular to the axis. Interestingly, recent molecular *RET/PTC* studies of HTT have shown a possible link with *papillary carcinoma*, and so the separation may sometimes be challenging. A trabecular growth, lack of colloid, extensive intratrabecular stromal hyalinization, and the cytoplasmic yellowish bodies/vacuoles are not usually present in papillary carcinoma. *Medullary carcinoma* lacks colloid, but has amyloid, and is reactive with calcitonin, chromogranin, and CEA.

PROGNOSIS AND THERAPY

Complete but conservative surgery yields an excellent prognosis. Isolated case reports of lymph node metastases may suggest that the relationship with papillary carcinoma needs further exploration.

SUGGESTED READINGS

The complete suggested readings list is available online at www.expertconsult.com.

24

Malignant Neoplasms of the Thyroid Gland

■ **Lester D. R. Thompson**

Thyroid neoplasms account for ~1% of all cancers (7.9/100,000 population), but they represent the most common malignancy of the endocrine system, posing a substantial diagnostic challenge to pathologists. In general, thyroid cancer afflicts young to middle-aged adults with environmental, genetic, and hormonal factors often playing an etiologic role. Iodine is essential for normal thyroid function and consequently radioactive iodine can be used in treatment. Women are affected by thyroid lesions nearly four times as frequently as men. Fine needle aspiration (FNA) has contributed significantly to the assessment of thyroid nodules, especially ultrasound-detected masses, with a corresponding decline in use of nuclear scintigraphy. FNA is satisfactory or unsatisfactory, making certain to meet the adequacy criteria as established by the Bethesda system. Lesions are then separated into benign, follicular lesion of undetermined significance, neoplasm, suspicious for malignancy, malignant, and nondiagnostic. There is a sensitivity for cancer of 65% to 98%, specificity of 72% to 100%, and a positive predictive value of 90% to 96%. The false negative rate is from 1% to 11%, while the false positive rate is <1%. Most of the tumors are of thyroid follicular cell derivation and, for the most part, carry an excellent long-term prognosis.

■ PAPILLARY CARCINOMA

"A malignant epithelial tumour showing evidence of follicular cell differentiation and characterized by distinctive nuclear features" is the somewhat vague World Health Organization (WHO) definition of papillary carcinoma of the thyroid (PTC). However, with a constellation of architectural and cytomorphologic features, accurate diagnosis of papillary carcinoma is achievable.

CLINICAL FEATURES

Papillary carcinoma represents ~85% of all malignant thyroid neoplasms and occurs largely in young to middle-aged adults with a 4:1 female:male ratio. Women are

---

PAPILLARY CARCINOMA—DISEASE FACT SHEET

Definition
- A malignant epithelial tumor showing evidence of follicular cell differentiation and characterized by distinctive nuclear features

Incidence and Location
- Thyroid malignancies represent ~1% of all carcinomas
- ~85% of thyroid malignancies are papillary carcinoma

Morbidity and Mortality
- Recurrent laryngeal nerve damage and hypoparathyroidism

Gender and Age Distribution
- Female >> male (4:1)
- Age: 20 to 60 years

Clinical Features
- Associated with radiation
- Usually a palpable mass lesion, often with neck lymph nodes
- Uncommonly dysphagia or hoarseness

Radiologic Features
- Ultrasound shows a solid or cystic mass and guides fine needle aspiration
- Computed tomography is useful to determine extent of the mass and lymph node disease
- Nuclear scintigraphy seldom used

Prognosis and Therapy
- Excellent long-term prognosis (>98% 20-year survival)
- Surgery (lobectomy or thyroidectomy) with radioactive iodine

usually affected between 20 and 40 years, while men are between 40 and 60 years. Even though rare, papillary carcinoma is still the most common pediatric thyroid malignancy. Whites are affected more commonly than blacks. Curiously, there is about a 20% prevalence of PTC (autopsy studies), supporting the overall excellent long-term prognosis and highlighting the difficulty in deciding appropriate patient management. There is a close link with radiation exposure, an association much more highly developed in children (especially for the solid variant of PTC). There is also a higher incidence of carcinoma in regions with high dietary iodine intake, in patients who have preexisting benign thyroid disease, and in some inherited disorders (Carney complex; familial adenomatous polyposis [FAP]). Patients present with a solitary, painless thyroid mass or with cervical lymphadenopathy (metastatic disease in ~30%). Dysphagia, stridor, and cough are usually seen in patients with large tumors due to compression. There are many "incidental" papillary carcinomas (discussed later), which are frequently discovered during routine radiographic studies for unrelated reasons or in patients with other thyroid diseases. FNA is the initial study of choice for a thyroid nodule, with excellent positive predictive value. Thyroid function studies are not useful in the initial evaluation of patients as there is rarely functional compromise. However, serum thyroglobulin levels can be used to monitor disease status (if elevated).

RADIOLOGIC FEATURES

Ultrasound will usually establish the size and whether the lesion is solid or cystic, while also being a valuable adjunct for guiding FNA. Punctate microcalcifications are frequently present (Figure 24-1), with high central blood flow on color Doppler. While nuclear scintigraphy was widely used to demonstrate functionality ("cold," without uptake; "hot," increased uptake) in comparison to the uninvolved thyroid parenchyma, it has been almost completely replaced by ultrasound and FNA as the techniques of choice in initial evaluation of a thyroid nodule. Computed tomography (CT) or magnetic resonance imaging (MRI) is valuable in highlighting enlarged, cystic lymph nodes, which may suggest metastatic disease (Figure 24-1), showing increased signal intensity on T1-weighted images and may reveal punctate calcifications.

PATHOLOGIC FEATURES

GROSS FINDINGS

Most clinical tumors are discrete, ill-defined but circumscribed, often with an irregular and infiltrative border (Figure 24-2). Ranging from microscopic foci to 20 cm, extension beyond the thyroid gland capsule can be identified along with infiltration into the surrounding thyroid parenchyma. Gritty, dystrophic calcification is common, as well as cystic change with hemorrhage. Multifocality is occasionally identified macroscopically. The cut surface can be shaggy to papillary, with irregular areas of fibrosis. The best sections to submit capture the "tumor-to-capsule-to-parenchyma" interface, including approximately one section per centimeter of tumor size.

MICROSCOPIC FINDINGS

The diagnosis of papillary carcinoma is made by using an assemblage of architectural and cytologic features,

FIGURE 24-1

A, Computed tomography scan of a large thyroid tumor with extensive infiltration into the soft tissues of the neck and cystic change in lymph nodes. **B**, An irregular mass within the thyroid with mixed echogenicity, showing punctate calcifications, characteristic for a papillary carcinoma.

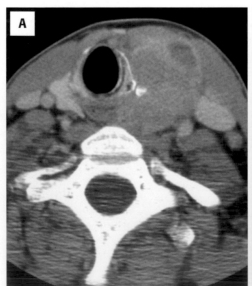
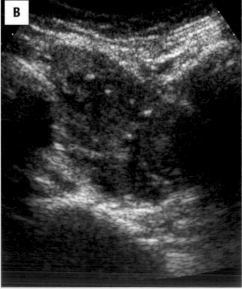

PAPILLARY CARCINOMA—PATHOLOGIC FEATURES

Gross Findings

- Discrete, gray-white, firm mass with irregular borders, although often circumscribed
- Calcifications give a "gritty" cut surface
- Extrathyroidal capsular extension can be seen
- Up to 20 cm

Microscopic Findings

- **Architecture:** variable growth patterns, complex papillae, elongated and twisted follicles, invasive growth, psammoma bodies, "bright eosinophilic" colloid, intratumoral sclerosis, crystals and giant cells in colloid
- **Cytology:** enlarged cells, increased nuclear:cytoplasmic ratio, nuclear enlargement, nuclear overlapping and crowding, loss of polarity, nuclear contour irregularities and grooves, folds or "crescent moons," pale nuclear chromatin, nuclear chromatin clearing, intranuclear cytoplasmic inclusions
- Intratumoral fibrosis, psammoma bodies, colloid scalloping

Immunohistochemical Results

- TTF-1, thyroglobulin, CK7, CK19
- **Panel:** HBME-1, galectin-3, CITED1 positive

Fine Needle Aspiration

- Cellular aspirate with papillary and monolayered sheets, cuboidal cells with enlarged and overlapped nuclei, powdery nuclear chromatin with nuclear grooves and intranuclear cytoplasmic inclusions, and ropey, "bubble-gum" colloid

Pathologic Differential Diagnosis

- Adenomatoid nodules, diffuse hyperplasia (Graves disease), dyshormonogenetic goiter, follicular adenoma, follicular carcinoma, medullary carcinoma, metastatic tumors

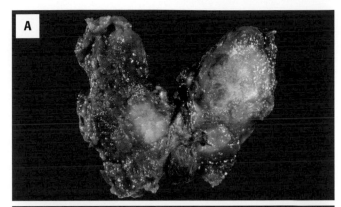
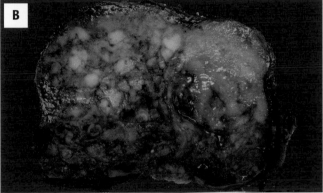

FIGURE 24-2

A, Three separate primary tumors are noted, with the largest lesion in the left upper lobe. There is an infiltrative border of these sclerotic tumors. **B**, A large, irregular, multilobular mass nearly completely replaces the thyroid lobe. Note the areas of more fleshy tumor compared to cystic areas of degeneration. This tumor fits within the columnar variant of papillary carcinoma. (**A**, Courtesy of Dr. J. A. Ohara.)

with no single feature being diagnostic. The exact number of features necessary for the diagnosis is undefined, but the nuclear features must be present to be diagnostic. Multinodular and multifocal tumors are common (Figure 24-3). An irregular and invasive border is common, with both capsular and lymphovascular invasion usually easily identified. The architectural features include variable growth patterns (papillary, solid, trabecular, microfollicular or macrofollicular, cystic); elongated and/or twisted follicles; complex, arborizing, delicate, narrow papillae; intratumoral dense fibrosis; "bright," hypereosinophilic, intense colloid (distinct from surrounding thyroid parenchyma); and psammoma bodies (concentrically laminated calcific bodies) (Figures 24-4 to 24-9). If a single tumor has many different growth patterns, suspicion for papillary carcinoma should be raised.

The cytomorphologic and nuclear features are vital in the diagnosis of papillary carcinoma and are usually constant even between the variants. These features include: enlarged cells with a high nuclear:cytoplasmic ratio; nuclear enlargement of oval to elongated nuclei; variability in size and shape, with nuclear overlapping and crowding; and loss of polarity and disorganized nuclear arrangement within the cell, with a haphazard position of the nucleus within the cell. The nuclear crowding creates a "herd," "lake," or "egg-basket" appearance. The nuclear chromatin is pale ("ground glass") with chromatin margination or condensation and clearing ("Orphan Annie" nuclei; Figure 24-6). If slides are left on the heating block for too long or in an aqueous solution during processing, "false" intranuclear bubbles are created. Formalin fixation gives the clearing, since it is not seen in frozen section material or in alcohol fixatives (SafeFix, HistoChoice). Nuclear grooves and folds, creating a "crescent-moon," triangular, angulated or convoluted shape ("coffee bean," "popcorn") are characteristic (Figure 24-5). Nuclear irregularities are more difficult to assess on frozen section material. Intranuclear cytoplasmic inclusions (pseudoinclusions) are recognized by the contents of the inclusion having an appearance similar to the cytoplasm—and not an artifactual "vacuole" formed secondary to fixation (Figure 24-10). The nucleus is rounded with a sharply demarcated thick nuclear membrane. Nucleoli, if present, are usually small and inconspicuous and

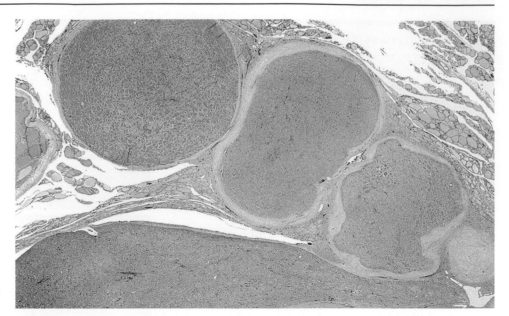

FIGURE 24-3

Multiple nodules of papillary carcinoma are surrounded by dense fibrosis.

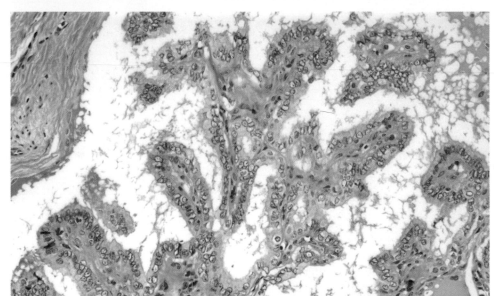

FIGURE 24-4

Delicate and complex papillary fronds lined by cells with an increased nuclear: cytoplasmic ratio, disorganized placement of the nuclei within the cell, and nuclear crowding and overlap.

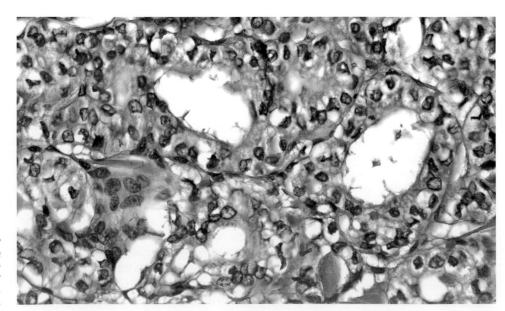

FIGURE 24-5

The classic features seen in papillary carcinoma: irregular placement of the nuclei around the follicle, nuclear crowding, nuclear contour irregularities, nuclear "crescent-moon" formation, nuclear grooves, nuclear folds, and nuclear chromatin clearing.

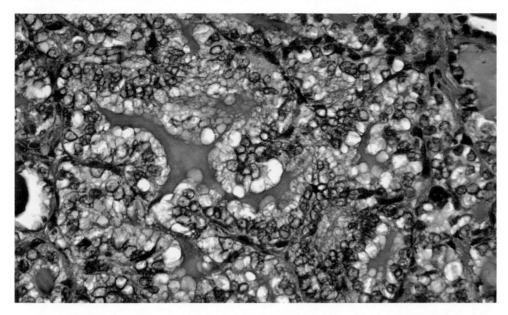

FIGURE 24-6

There is nuclear crowding and overlapping within hypereosinophilic colloid that shows peripheral scalloping. There is well-developed nuclear chromatin clearing (optical clearing: Orphan Annie nuclei).

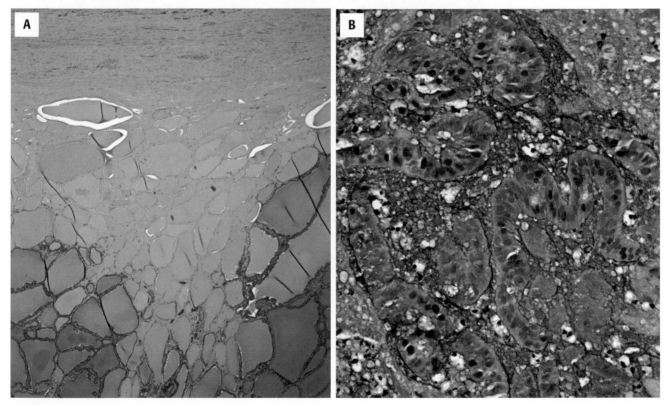

FIGURE 24-7

A, "Mummification" of the cells, at the periphery of the tumor, creating a wedge shape is an uncommon, but unique feature of papillary carcinoma. **B,** Tumor infarction results in ghost cell outlines, still showing papillae, but no longer viable tumor cells.

seem to touch the nuclear membrane rather than being centrally located (Figure 24-8). The cytoplasm is variable and usually not helpful in the diagnosis, although variants are named according to the cytoplasm (clear, oncocytic). Giant cells in the colloid and the presence of crystals are "soft" criteria seen less frequently (Figure 24-9). Squamous metaplasia, cyst formation, and degeneration are

not uncommon, with infarction seen after FNA (Figure 24-7). Psammoma bodies are ***not*** the same as dystrophic calcification of colloid in the center of a follicle. Psammoma bodies (Greek for "salt-like") represent apoptotic cells that form the nidus for concentric lamellation of calcium (Figure 24-10). Present in up to 50% of cases, they are often identified within lymphovascular

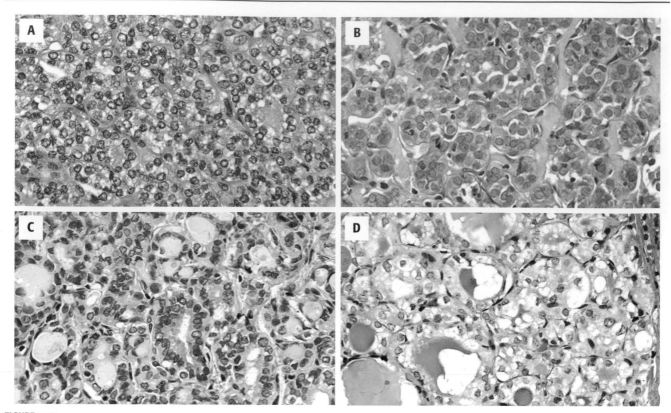

FIGURE 24-8

Cytomorphologic features. **A**, Nuclear crowding and nuclear chromatin clearing. **B**, Fine, ground-glass nuclear chromatin. **C**, Nuclear overlapping, nuclear chromatin irregularities and loss of nuclear polarity. **D**, Pale nuclear chromatin in irregular nuclei surrounding follicles with scalloped, dense colloid.

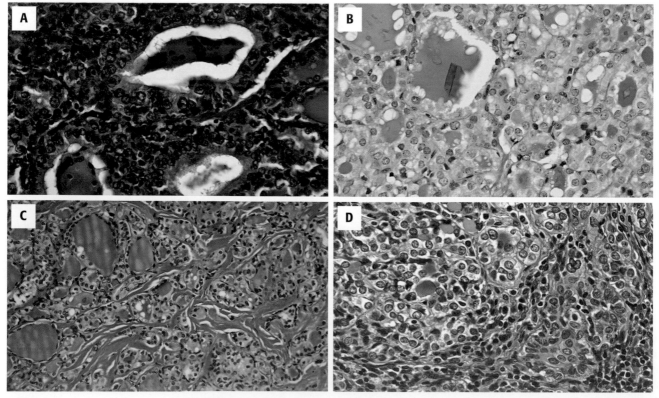

FIGURE 24-9

Associated findings in papillary carcinoma. **A**, Giant cells within the colloid. **B**, Crystals within the colloid. Nucleoli are noted along the nuclear membrane. **C**, Dense fibrosis separating the tumor cells. **D**, Squamous metaplasia within a papillary carcinoma (*lower right corner*).

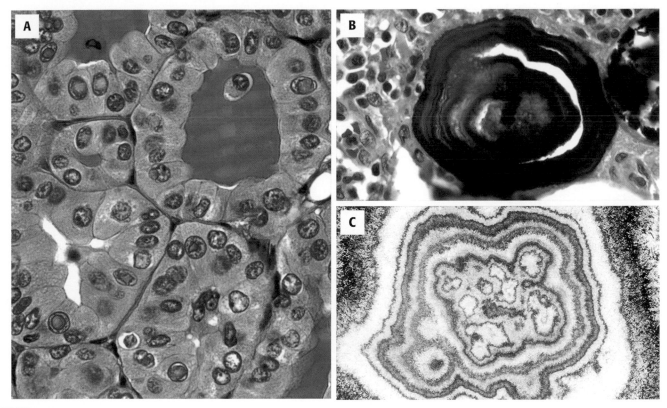

FIGURE 24-10

A, Multiple intranuclear cytoplasmic inclusions contain material the same color as the cytoplasm. **B**, Light microscopic appearance of a psammoma body with concentric laminations. **C**, Electron micrograph of a psammoma body showing concentric lamination and crenated nuclei in the center. (**C**, *Courtesy of Dr. C. S. Heffess.*)

channels, diagnostic of intraglandular spread. Likewise, their presence in lymph nodes is practically pathognomonic for metastatic disease.

Separation of multifocal versus intraglandular spread of papillary carcinoma can be difficult. Intraglandular spread is suggested when the tumor is within a septa, within a lymphovascular channel, and has no stellate fibrosis at the periphery (Figure 24-11). Intratumoral fibrosis is an acellular, sclerotic, dense, eosinophilic fibrosis found in up to 90 % of cases. The fibrosis is often irregular to stellate, a feature that is useful during gross examination to select areas for microscopic examination. Mummification (peripheral cell death) is infrequently seen but is quite characteristic for papillary carcinoma. A heavy lymphocytic response is frequently seen both adjacent to and within the tumor (Figure 24-12). Fatty metaplasia, spindled tumor cells, and limited colloid can be seen. Papillary carcinoma is not graded, as nearly all are considered well-differentiated. The variants are described in the next section.

ANCILLARY STUDIES

IMMUNOHISTOCHEMICAL RESULTS

Immunohistochemistry is seldom of value in diagnosing papillary carcinoma, although it may play a role in

metastatic disease. The neoplastic cells are strongly and diffusely immunoreactive with keratin, CK7, thyroglobulin, and TTF-1, while other markers (HBME-1 [Figure 24-13], galectin-3, S100 protein, CK19 [Figure 24-13], *RET*) yield variable results. In challenging cases, there is good sensitivity and specificity when using a panel approach: HBME-1, galectin-3, and CITED1. However, for >98 % of cases, immunohistochemistry is unnecessary. p27 (lost) and cyclin D1 (upregulation) show differential staining in tumors that are more likely to metastasize.

FINE NEEDLE ASPIRATION

FNA is considered the test of choice for the diagnosis and management of thyroid nodules, having an excellent sensitivity, specificity, and positive predictive value. An initial pass using a 25-gauge needle—without suction—yields excellent material uncontaminated by blood. In general practice, ~70 % of thyroid FNAs are benign, 10 % are indeterminate, 15 % are unsatisfactory, and 5 % are malignant.

Aspirates from papillary carcinomas are usually diagnostic, meeting the adequacy criteria (at least 6 follicular groups with >10 follicular cells per group) and are characteristically cellular, with monolayered sheets (syncytium) and three-dimensional clusters of enlarged cells (Figure 24-14). The nuclei are enlarged

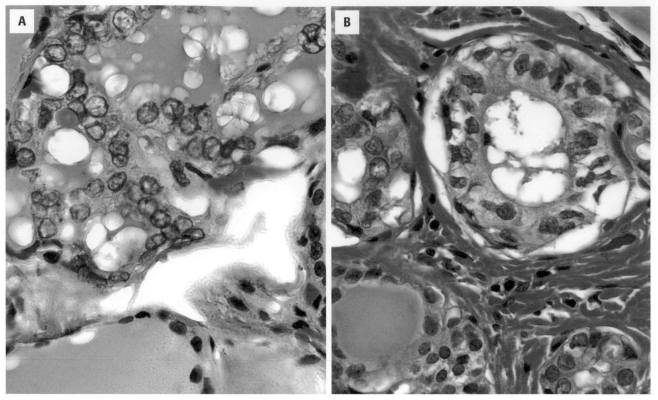

FIGURE 24-11

Intraglandular spread with foci of papillary carcinoma confined to the septa (**A**) and within lymphovascular channels surrounded by fibrosis (**B**). Benign thyroid parenchyma is noted in the lower portions of each figure as a point of comparison.

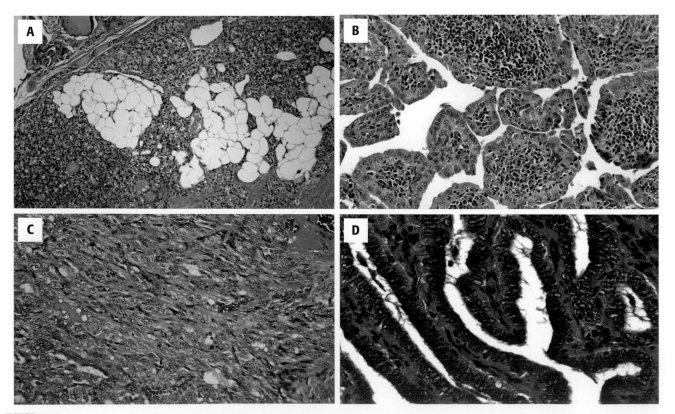

FIGURE 24-12

Uncommon features in papillary carcinoma. **A**, Fatty metaplasia. **B**, Lymphocytes and plasma cells, sometimes referred to as "Warthin" variant of papillary carcinoma. **C**, Tumor cell spindling. **D**, No colloid is seen in this tumor with marked nuclear overlapping and stratification.

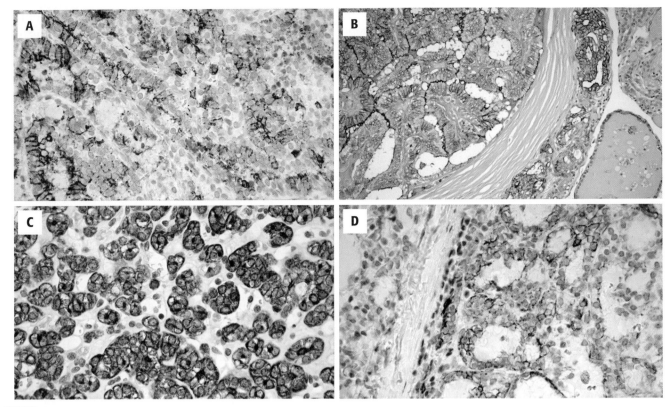

FIGURE 24-13

A and **B**, HMBE-1. Note the variable membrane and cytoplasmic expression in the tumor cells, including an area of invasion. **C** and **D**, CK19. There can be strong cytoplasmic reactivity to only delicate, partial membranous staining.

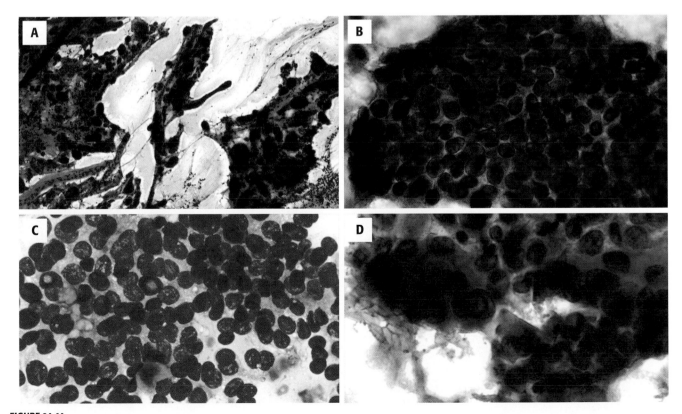

FIGURE 24-14

A and **B**, Three-dimensional clusters in a cellular smear. A syncytium of cells with enlarged nuclei and nuclear grooves (alcohol-fixed, Papanicolaou stain). **C** and **D**, Three-dimensional papillae around a central fibrovascular core showing an intranuclear cytoplasmic inclusion (air-dried, Diff-Quik stain).

and overlapped with irregular borders, but with a powdery/dusty, delicate nuclear chromatin on alcohol-fixed preparations. Nuclear folds or grooves and intranuclear cytoplasmic inclusions are also common. The cytoplasm is often pale or foamy, but not distinctive on FNA. Colloid is often scant and thickened ("chewing gum" or ropey), with occasional multinucleate giant cells and rarely psammoma bodies. The features of papillary carcinoma are best appreciated with alcohol-preserved Papanicolaou preparations rather than with air-dried material.

MOLECULAR ANALYSIS

Results are quite dependent on technique, immuno-histochemistry, patient age, radiation history, and the specific histologic variant. Rearrangements or mutations involving *BRAF* (part of the RAF family of protein kinases), *RET* gene, and *RAS* are structural genetic alterations identified to a variable degree in PTC. Specifically, these mutations result in activation of the mitogen-activated protein kinase (MAPK) pathway, which regulates cell growth, differentiation, and survival. Point mutations in the *BRAF* gene are identified in up to 60% of papillary carcinomas (valine-to-glutamate substitution at residue 600: V600E), while

RET/PTC1 or *RET*/PTC3 is in a highly variable frequency from 0% to 80% of cases. *RAS* mutations are seen in up to 15% of tumors, but almost exclusively in follicular variant tumors, in tumors that are encapsulated, and in tumors with a low rate of lymph node metastases. Each mutation/rearrangement has distinct phenotypic and biologic properties. Therefore, until there is greater standardization, molecular studies at present do not add to the diagnosis. One caveat may be in inherited papillary carcinoma syndromes, such as familial adenomatous polyposis coli or Cowden syndrome, where genetic studies may help in patient management.

DIFFERENTIAL DIAGNOSIS

The principal differential diagnosis includes a number of disorders with papillae, including adenomatoid nodules (Figures 24-15 and 24-16), diffuse hyperplasia (Graves disease), and dyshormonogenetic goiter, while follicular adenoma (FA), follicular carcinoma, medullary carcinoma, and metastatic tumors are also considered. In general, the papillae of all of these other lesions are short, simple, nonbranching, and often

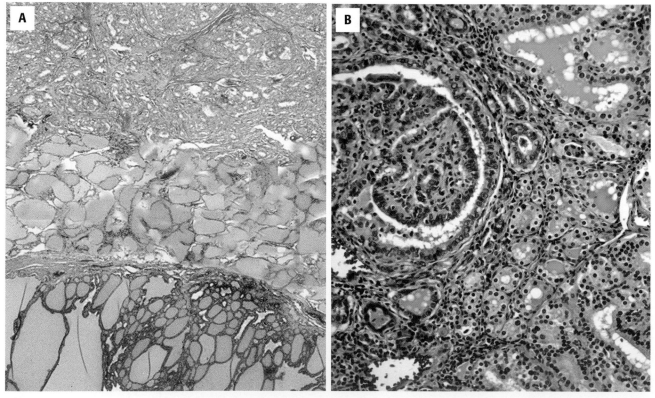

FIGURE 24-15

A, Adenomatoid nodule (*lower half*) and papillary carcinoma (*upper half*) frequently coexist. There are differences in architecture and cytology, even at this low magnification. **B**, A papillary carcinoma (*upper right*) has a completely different appearance than the background of diffuse hyperplasia.

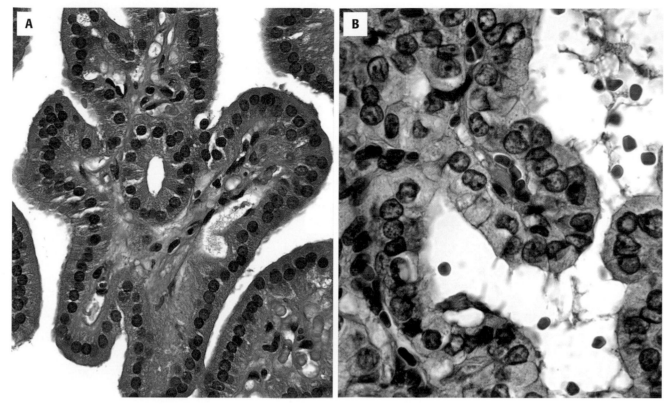

FIGURE 24-16

A, An adenomatoid nodule has small cells in an orderly arrangement around the follicles with coarse/heavy nuclear chromatin distribution. **B**, Papillary carcinoma has large cells with an increased nuclear:cytoplasmic ratio, irregular placement of the nuclei, nuclear contour irregularities, nuclear grooves and folds, and delicate to fine nuclear chromatin distribution (same magnification).

"thick." The nuclei are round, regular, basally located, and hyperchromatic. Intracytoplasmic hemosiderin pigment is nearly always lacking in papillary carcinoma. Although a nuclear feature or two may be present in these other lesions, there is both a qualitative and quantitative difference in their appearance. Many lesions that have oncocytic cytoplasm may induce nuclear enlargement, but other features of papillary carcinoma are lacking. It is worth noting that alcohol fixatives will often cause nuclear enlargement and "optical clearing," and so caution must be used when making a diagnosis of papillary carcinoma when non–formalin-based fixatives have been used.

PROGNOSIS AND THERAPY

Papillary carcinoma spreads preferentially by lymphatic channels, with the regional lymph nodes affected most commonly, and in a significant proportion of cases (Figure 24-17). Intraglandular spread, including the contralateral lobe, is common. However, the prognosis is excellent, with >98% 20-year survival rate and a <0.2% mortality rate. Extrathyroidal extension into the adjacent fat or skeletal muscle places the tumor in the American Joint Committee on Cancer (AJCC) stage pT3 (2010 criteria). Age (<45 years) and gender (female) are the most important prognostic factors, although tumor size, extrathyroidal extension, and metastasis are significant for patients >45 years. Surgery is the treatment of choice, although the extent of surgery (lobectomy, subtotal, or total thyroidectomy) remains controversial. Recurrent laryngeal nerve damage and hypoparathyroidism are known surgical complications. Radioablative iodine therapy is incorporated after a total thyroidectomy. However, the tumor needs to show uptake of the radiolabeled iodine to be therapeutically sensitive. Lymph node sampling is advocated only if there is clinical or radiographic enlargement, although central compartment lymph node removal has been recommended.

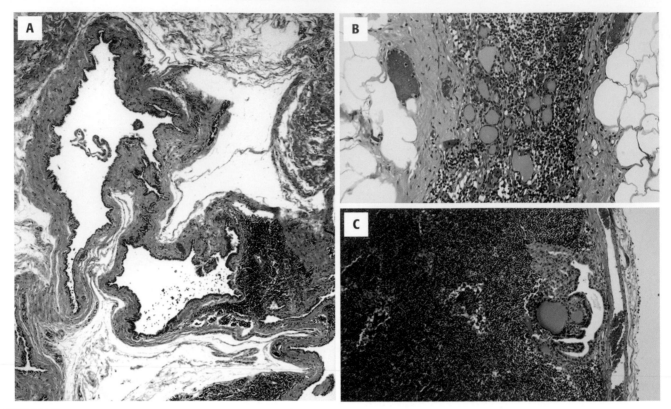

FIGURE 24-17

A, A predominantly cystic metastasis can sometimes simulate a lymphangioma or branchial cyst. **B**, Almost "normal"-appearing follicles within a lymph node. However, this represented metastatic disease from a ipsilateral primary papillary carcinoma. **C**, Papillary projections and colloid of metastatic papillary carcinoma in a lymph node.

HISTOLOGICAL VARIANTS OF PAPILLARY CARCINOMA

Variants of papillary carcinoma have specific features that may be associated with a different patient outcome or cause difficulty with the differential diagnosis. In general, the changes should be the dominant finding to qualify as a histologic variant.

FOLLICULAR VARIANT

Usually encapsulated, the tumor must be *exclusively* composed of small, tight follicles with scant, hypereosinophilic colloid. Papillae are absent or vanishingly rare (Figure 24-18), although if enough sections are submitted papillary structures may be found. The

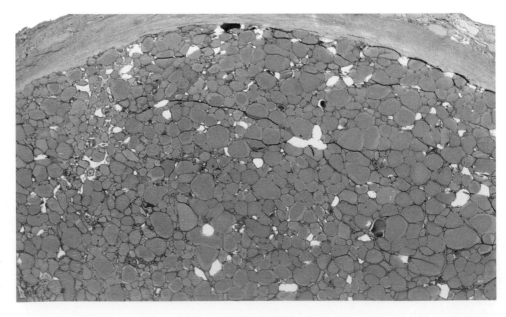

FIGURE 24-18

A very thick capsule surrounds a tumor that shows a monotonous, medium-sized follicular tumor with hypereosinophilic colloid.

HISTOLOGIC VARIANTS OF PAPILLARY CARCINOMA

Follicular Variant

- Almost exclusively small follicles with scant, bright colloid
- Classic nuclear features of papillary carcinoma

Macrofollicular Variant

- Enlarged follicles with remaining features similar to follicular variant although nuclei are often flattened
- Abortive, rigid papillae may be seen
- Separation from adenomatoid nodule is imperative

Oncocytic Variant

- >70% papillary architecture
- Enlarged cells with abundant oncocytic cytoplasm, apically oriented enlarged nuclei, increased number of intranuclear cytoplasmic inclusions
- Degenerative changes common

Clear Cell Variant

- Clear cytoplasm, although occasionally oncocytic and clear cells are combined
- Must be separated from medullary and metastatic renal cell carcinoma

Diffuse Sclerosing Variant

- Diffuse, bilateral involvement, extensive fibrosis, innumerable psammoma bodies, extensive intravascular growth and extrathyroidal extension, florid squamous metaplasia, dense lymphocytic thyroiditis, solid or papillary growth of papillary carcinoma cells

Tall Cell Variant

- >70% of tumor area composed of cells which are at least three times as tall as they are wide, usually oncocytic cytoplasm, sharply defined cellular borders, increased intranuclear cytoplasmic inclusions, centrally placed nuclei within the cell

Columnar Cell Variant

- Prominent papillary growth, parallel follicles ("railroad tracks"), scant colloid, syncytial architecture with prominent nuclear stratification, coarse nuclear chromatin, subnuclear cytoplasmic vacuolization, squamous metaplasia as "morules," and increased mitotic figures

Solid/Insular Variant

- Solid or insular pattern with nuclear features of papillary carcinoma

Cribriform-Morula Variant

- Patients with familial adenomatous polyposis
- Multiple encapsulated tumors, mixed patterns, cribriform dominant
- Morules or whorls of squamous cells without keratinization

Size Variation

- Incidentally found, <1 cm papillary carcinoma with a proclivity for thyroid subcapsular location—designated "microcarcinoma"

nuclear features determine the diagnosis in this variant. Specifically, the nuclei are large with pale to powdery to cleared nuclear chromatin and an increased number of nuclear grooves and intranuclear inclusions (Figure 24-19). Internal sclerosis or fibrosis is seen (Figure 24-20). This variant has no impact on patient management and has an identical outcome to conventional papillary carcinoma.

MACROFOLLICULAR VARIANT

An uncommon variant that is difficult to recognize as it has an architectural resemblance to adenomatoid nodules or hyperplastic nodules (Figure 24-21). The tumor is composed of predominantly large/macrofollicles with a subtle increased cellularity, often accentuated at the periphery (Figure 24-22). The colloid is often scalloped or vacuolated. The nuclei are often flattened and hyperchromatic, although classic papillary nuclei are scattered throughout the tumor (Figure 24-23). Abortive, "rigid," or straight papillary structures will extend into the center of the colloid-filled follicle, usually lined by the atypical cells. This variant seems to metastasize less frequently than classic papillary carcinoma but is otherwise similar in treatment and outcome.

ONCOCYTIC VARIANT

The macroscopic appearance is of a deep brown ("mahogany") encapsulated neoplasm, which tends to be large and have cystic change. More than 70% of the tumor should have complex, arborizing papillary structures (Figure 24-24) with fibrovascular stromal cores lined by enlarged cells with abundant oncocytic (oxyphilic, Ashkenazi, Hürthle) cytoplasm. The oncocytic cytoplasm is compact and "glassy" with a fine granularity, representing an increased number of mitochondria. The enlarged nuclei tend to be apically oriented and slightly more hyperchromatic than classic papillary carcinoma (Figure 24-25), with numerous intranuclear cytoplasmic inclusions (the latter a common finding in any tumor with abundant cytoplasm). Psammoma bodies are occasionally present. Degenerative changes are common. The cells are frequently immunoreactive with CK19, but this finding is nonspecific (Figure 24-25). The diagnosis by FNA is very difficult, but clear nuclei with grooves and inclusions may help to separate it from a follicular neoplasm. Oncocytic cells can be seen in the tall cell variant of papillary carcinoma, from which it should be separated. The patient outcome and management for the oncocytic variant are identical to classic papillary carcinoma.

CLEAR CELL VARIANT

This is a very uncommon variant that is predominantly composed of cells with clear cytoplasm. Papillary or follicular patterns may predominate. Occasionally, a

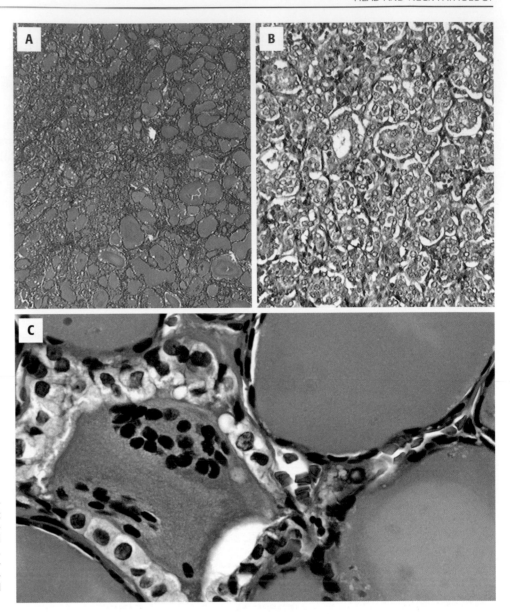

FIGURE 24-19

A, Small, tight follicles with hypereosinophilic colloid in this follicular variant of papillary carcinoma. **B**, Nuclear chromatin clearing and overlap with small tight follicles and no colloid production. **C**, Nuclear features of papillary carcinoma can be isolated to just a few follicles at a time. The whole tumor is still papillary carcinoma.

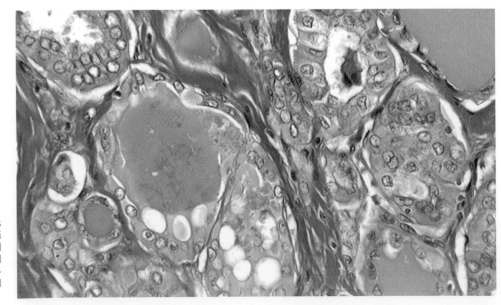

FIGURE 24-20

Follicle formation lined by irregular cells with optically clear nuclei. The nuclei are irregular in shape and size and misplaced around the follicle. Giant cell formation is seen within the hypereosinophilic colloid with scalloping. Tumoral fibrosis separates the follicles.

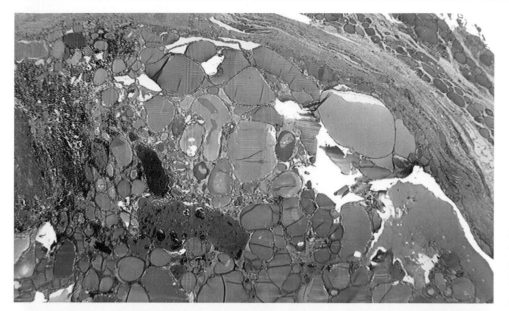

FIGURE 24-21

This macrofollicular variant of papillary carcinoma is surrounded by a capsule, compressing the peripheral parenchyma. The low power resemblance to an adenomatoid nodule is deceiving.

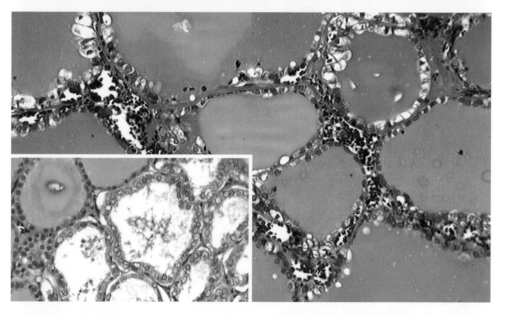

FIGURE 24-22

Large follicles are lined by flattened to atypical follicular cells with scalloped colloid in this macrofollicular variant of papillary carcinoma. Inset demonstrates an area of increased cellularity and the cytologic features of papillary carcinoma.

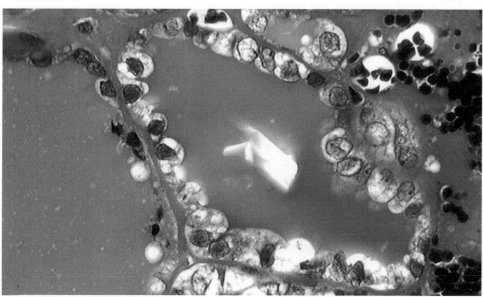

FIGURE 24-23

The nuclear features are well demonstrated in this macrofollicular variant of papillary carcinoma. A crystalloid is seen in the center. Nuclear grooves, nuclear contour irregularities, and nuclear chromatin clearing are accentuated.

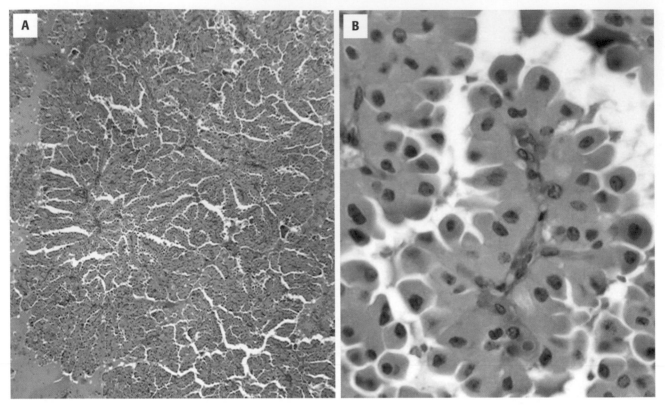

FIGURE 24-24

A, Complex, arborizing papillary structures are composed of oncocytic cells in this oncocytic papillary carcinoma variant. Hemorrhage and degeneration are noted.
B, Tumor nuclei show apical polarization on the papillary fronds, surrounded by deeply eosinophilic cytoplasm in this oncocytic variant of papillary carcinoma.

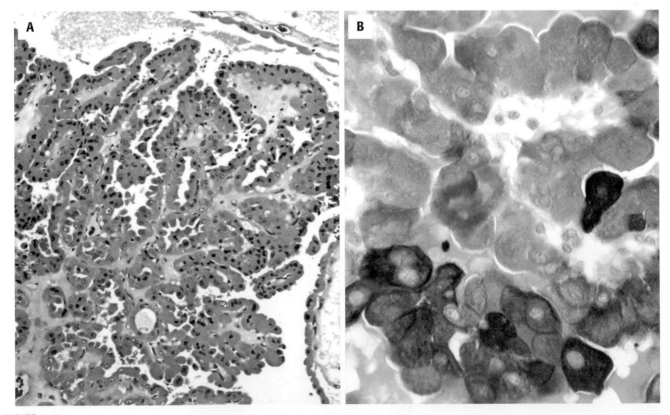

FIGURE 24-25

A, Oncocytic cells within a papillary architecture. Note that the nuclei are luminal. **B**, CK19 is known to be positive in the oncocytic variant of papillary carcinoma, but is not specific or sensitive.

mixture of oncocytic and clear cells may be seen, as clearing results from degeneration of the oncocytic cells. Separation from metastatic renal cell carcinoma or medullary carcinoma can be made by the presence of colloid, but may require the use of TTF-1, thyroglobulin, and calcitonin. The treatment and prognosis are identical to classic papillary carcinoma.

DIFFUSE SCLEROSING VARIANT

Usually developing in young patients (mean, 18 years), the tumor is characterized by diffuse involvement of one or both lobes with nearly 100% of patients demonstrating cervical lymph node metastasis at the time of presentation. The gland is firm, with white streaks and a gritty cut consistency, and an ill-defined border, if a dominant mass is noted. The histology shows an exaggeration of features of papillary carcinoma, with extensive fibrosis, innumerable psammoma bodies, extensive intravascular and extrathyroidal extension, florid squamous metaplasia, and a background of dense lymphocytic thyroiditis (Figures 24-26 and 24-27). Nuclear features of papillary carcinoma are present, often identified in papillary or solid groups of cells within vascular spaces (Figure 24-28). Total thyroidectomy, lymph node dissection, and radioablative therapy will yield an excellent long-term prognosis despite the "biologically" aggressive clinical presentation. Lung metastases occur in up to 25% of patients, necessitating close and careful patient follow-up.

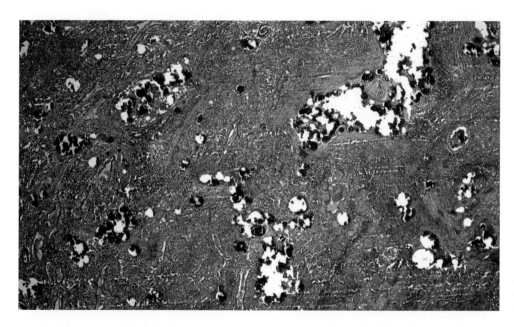

FIGURE 24-26

A low-magnification view demonstrating innumerable psammoma bodies in clusters with lymphocytic thyroiditis. Many of the psammoma bodies are in lymphovascular spaces.

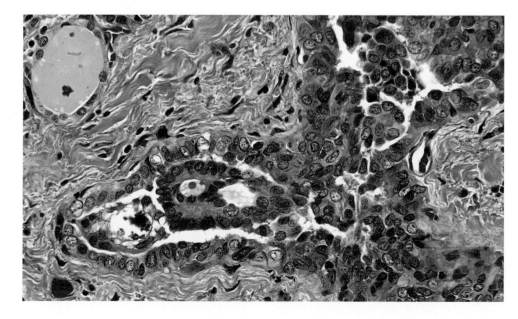

FIGURE 24-27

Dense fibrosis separates the tumor into nodules. Lymphovascular invasion is noted with tumor cells within a vascular space, associated with squamous metaplasia.

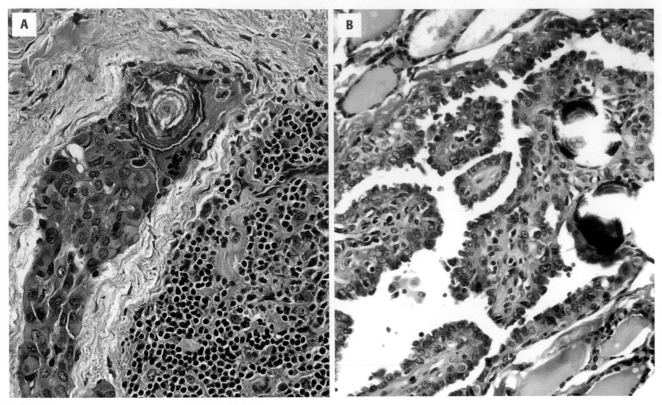

FIGURE 24-28

A, Papillary carcinoma with squamous metaplasia associated with a psammoma body. There is lymphocytic thyroiditis. **B**, Psammoma bodies and papillary carcinoma are noted within a lymphovascular channel.

TALL CELL VARIANT

There is controversy as to whether the "tall cell" is a variant or just a pattern of growth within papillary carcinoma (I believe this is a true variant). When this cell type is the dominant finding in the neoplasm (>70% of the tumor area), the patients tend to be older (>60 years) with an increased proportion of men, and the tumor tends to be large (>5 cm), showing extrathyroidal extension. However, microscopic tumors can occur. Papillary structures and elongated parallel follicles with scant or no colloid are common, along with intratumoral fibrosis. By definition, a tall cell is at least three times as high as it is wide (plane of section must be taken into consideration). There is usually abundant, granular cytoplasm, resulting in an increased number of intranuclear cytoplasmic inclusions and nuclear grooves (Figure 24-29). Intercellular borders are sharply demarcated (Figure 24-30). Necrosis and mitotic activity are present. The nuclei are enlarged with a central position of the nucleus rather than at the luminal aspect as seen in the oncocytic variant. The tall cell variant stains uniquely with Napsin A, while *BRAF* point mutations are common. Since most of these tumors occur in older patients who have large tumors with extrathyroidal extension, perhaps the histologic variant has only a minor influence on the patient's outcome. There does tend to be an increased incidence of lymph node metastasis and hematogenous spread to bone and lung, with a tendency for local recurrence and invasion into adjacent structures. Surgery and adjuvant therapy are necessary, with a worse prognosis than classic papillary carcinoma.

COLUMNAR CELL VARIANT

Men and women are equally affected by this rare variant. Tumors are usually large (>5 cm) and encapsulated but have intrathyroidal and extrathyroidal spread. There is prominent papillary growth with markedly elongated, parallel follicles ("railroad tracks"), which are separated by scant colloid (Figure 24-31). The cells are tall with a syncytial arrangement. There is prominent nuclear stratification of elongated nuclei with coarse and heavy chromatin deposition, distinctly different from classic papillary carcinoma. Subnuclear or supranuclear vacuolization of the cytoplasm is common (Figure 24-32). Squamous metaplasia in the form of "morules" is common ("endometrioid pattern"; Figure 24-33). Mitotic figures may be present, along with necrosis in a few cases. Uniquely, this variant commonly expresses CDX2. If the patient is older with a large tumor that has extrathyroidal extension, more aggressive surgery and radioablative therapy may be necessary. The prognosis is worse than for classic papillary carcinoma.

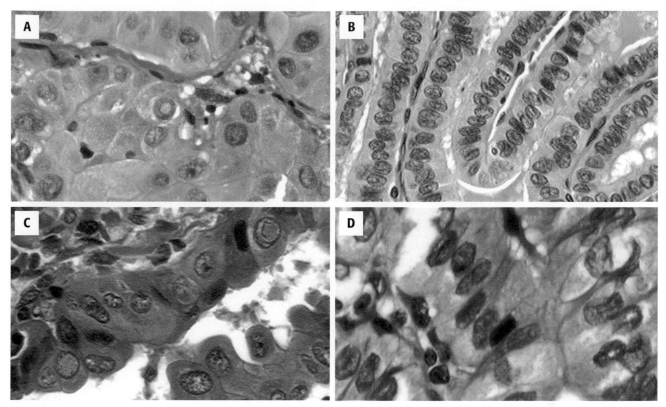

FIGURE 24-29

A-D, Various patterns seen in tall cell variant of papillary carcinoma. The cells are each at least three times taller than they are wide with prominent cellular borders. The cytoplasm ranges from oncocytic, amphophilic, basophilic, and clear. Intranuclear cytoplasmic inclusions are common.

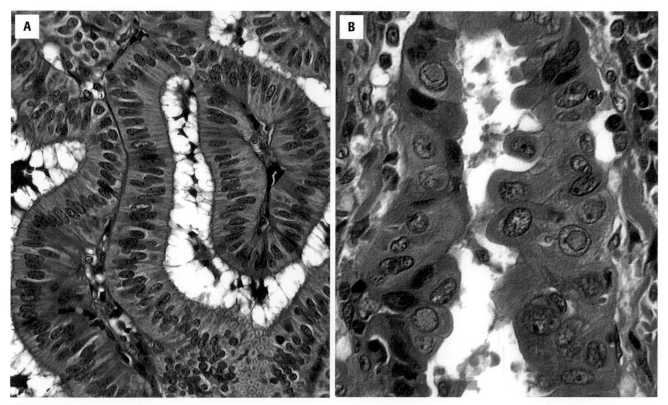

FIGURE 24-30

A, Columnar variant with pseudostratification of nuclei with no colloid present. **B**, Tall cell variant with oncocytic cells, intranuclear cytoplasmic inclusions, and cells three times as tall as they are wide.

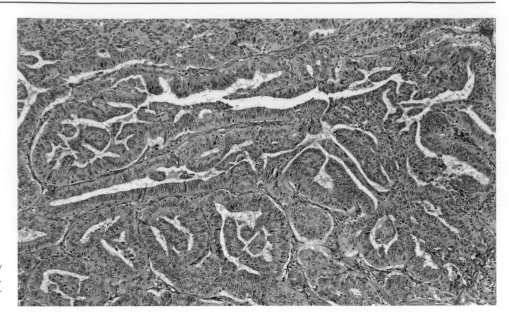

FIGURE 24-31

Papillary structures arranged in markedly elongated, parallel follicles ("railroad tracks"). There is no colloid, but there is well-developed nuclear stratification.

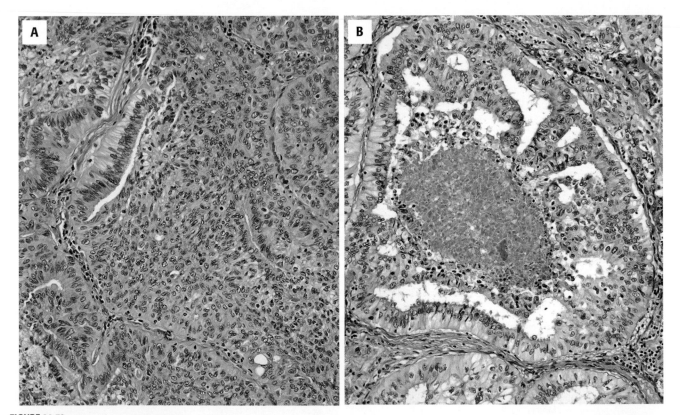

FIGURE 24-32

A, A syncytial architecture predominates in this tumor. Nuclear stratification with subnuclear vacuoles is noted. **B**, The tumor cell nuclei have an elongated shape and demonstrate pronounced pseudostratification. Prominent subnuclear vacuoles are seen in cells arranged in a cribriform architecture. Central comedonecrosis is present.

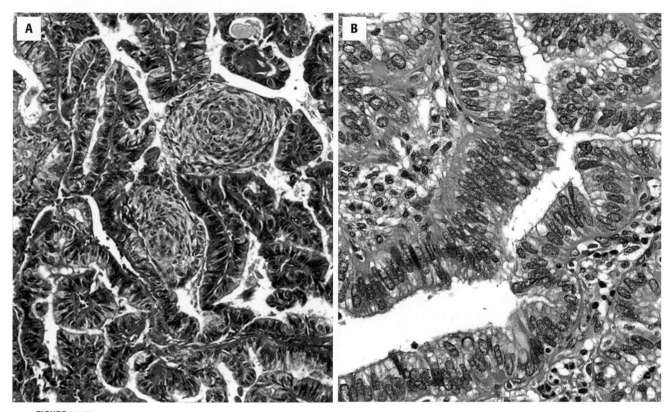

FIGURE 24-33
A, Squamous morules are a unique feature in this papillary carcinoma type. **B**, The elongated nuclei may have coarser, pseudostratified nuclei.

INSULAR/SOLID

Papillary carcinoma may have a solid or insular pattern, with oval nests or islands with scant colloid, and cells with a high nuclear:cytoplasmic ratio (Figure 24-34). Sometimes the pattern is classified as poorly differentiated, but if the nuclear features of papillary carcinoma are present, then this pattern does not influence the management or the outcome.

CRIBRIFORM-MORULA

Usually seen in patients with FAP, a diagnosis of this variant should prompt colonic examination and possibly genetic testing for germline *APC* mutation. There are often multiple encapsulated tumor nodules, showing a mixed pattern of growth: cribriform, trabecular, solid, papillary, and follicular. There are often whorls or morules composed of spindle cells without keratinization. The nuclear features of papillary carcinoma are rare.

PAPILLARY CARCINOMA: SIZE VARIATION

Any of the papillary carcinoma variants may be <1 cm, which is referred to as microscopic papillary carcinoma, or occult, incidental, or microcarcinoma (Figure 24-35). This qualification should only be applied when the tumor is found incidentally in a thyroid gland removed for other reasons. The tumor has a proclivity to develop in the subcapsular region and is frequently sclerotic with a radiating "scar-like" infiltration into the surrounding parenchyma. The term "microcarcinoma" should be used for adult patients, since children with small tumors may still have biologically aggressive neoplasms. Separation from intraglandular metastasis may be difficult, although the intravascular location, lack of capsule and sclerosis, and lack of "stellate" growth support intraglandular metastasis. Most of these tumors are <2 mm and are of limited clinical consequence, with an outcome indistinguishable from the general population. Therefore, no additional therapy is necessary for tumors of this size.

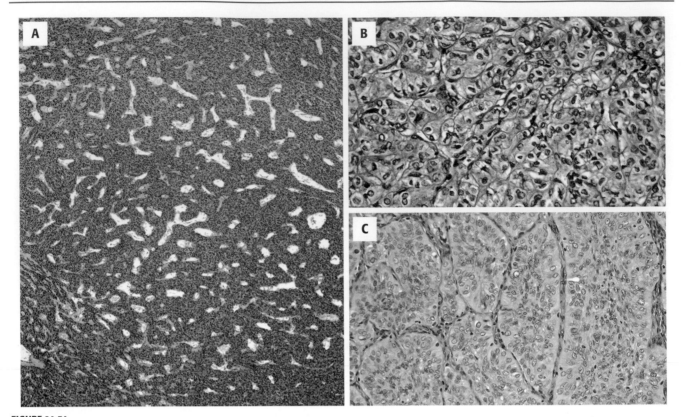

FIGURE 24-34

An insular architecture can be the predominant pattern in any thyroid tumor. **A**, Classic papillary carcinoma with an insular architecture. **B**, Small, tight trabeculae that create an insular appearance. **C**, Columnar variant with an insular pattern.

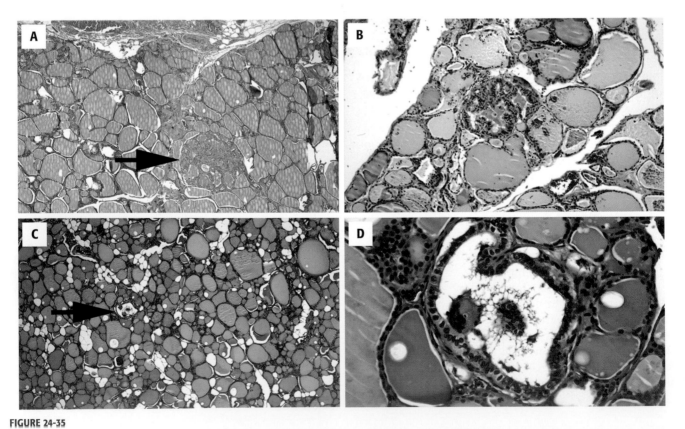

FIGURE 24-35

A and **B**, Microscopic papillary carcinoma is distinct from the surrounding tissue (*arrow*) and has both papillary architecture and shows typical nuclear features. The tumors are frequently only a few follicles large. **C** is a low-power magnification (*tumor at arrow point*), while **D** is a high-power view of the same tumor.

■ FOLLICULAR CARCINOMA

Follicular carcinoma (FC) is the second most common malignant neoplasm of the thyroid gland, defined by invasive growth of a follicular epithelial derived cell that lacks the nuclear features of papillary carcinoma. There is a familial association in up to 4% of FC in the United States, with Cowden disease, Werner syndrome, and Carney complex the most common. Iodine deficiency, radiation exposure (5.2 times relative risk), and preexisting thyroid disease are known risk factors. Specifically, follicular adenoma may be a direct precursor (similar genetic mutations can be seen, although lower frequency) since the histology is identical except for invasion, and patients with FC are about a decade older than patients with adenoma.

CLINICAL FEATURES

About 10% to 15% of thyroid carcinomas are FCs (0.8/100,000 persons/yr), reflecting a downward trend as the recognition of the follicular variant of papillary carcinoma has improved. FC is more common in women than men (~2:1), with a peak incidence in the 5th and 6th decades, although recently the gender difference is not as distinct. The oncocytic type tends to occur in patients about a decade older. Patients usually present with an asymptomatic solitary, painless thyroid mass, which is usually solid on radiographic imaging. Hoarseness, dysphagia, dyspnea, and stridor are rare. FCs tend to be larger than papillary carcinoma. Thyroid function tests are almost always normal. Lymph node metastasis is uncommon although slightly more common in the oncocytic variant, as hematogenous spread is more common than lymphatic spread. Distant metastasis is seen in up to 20% of patients (lung and bone). Imaging cannot reliably distinguish between benign and malignant lesions. Iodinated contrast is to be avoided as it delays ^{131}I therapy. Ultrasound may demonstrate a solid versus cystic lesion and show a nonechogenic halo (capsule). Turbulent intratumoral blood flow is seen more often in carcinoma.

PATHOLOGIC FEATURES

FOLLICULAR CARCINOMA—DISEASE FACT SHEET

Definition
- A malignant epithelial neoplasm with follicular cell differentiation and lacking the nuclear features of papillary carcinoma

Incidence and Location
- ~10% to 15% of thyroid malignancies
- Increased in iodine-deficient areas and in patients with preexisting thyroid disease or syndrome association (Cowden, Werner, Carney)

Morbidity and Mortality
- Recurrent laryngeal nerve damage and hypoparathyroidism

Gender and Age Distribution
- Female > male (2:1)
- Usually in the 5th to 6th decades
- Oncocytic tumors occur in patients about a decade older

Clinical Features
- Usually an asymptomatic, palpable mass
- Rarely dysphagia or hoarseness

Radiologic Features
- Ultrasound shows a solid or cystic mass, a capsule, used to guide fine needle aspiration
- Computed tomography is useful to determine extent of the mass and lymph node disease
- Nuclear scintigraphy infrequently used

Prognosis and Therapy
- Excellent long-term prognosis (~97% 20-year survival)
- Surgery (lobectomy or thyroidectomy) with radioactive iodine

FOLLICULAR CARCINOMA—PATHOLOGIC FEATURES

Gross Findings
- Solitary, encapsulated mass
- Invasion usually difficult to see on gross examination
- Usually <5 cm

Microscopic Findings
- Capsule varies from thin to thick with vessels in the wall
- Capsular invasion: into and through the capsule
- Vascular invasion: within or beyond capsule, showing direct extension, tumor thrombus, or endothelial lining
- Cellular tumors with follicular, solid and trabecular growth
- Slightly enlarged cells with round to oval nuclei and coarse nuclear chromatin
- Oncocytic cells often have large, centrally placed macronucleoli within the nuclei
- Variant patterns and cytologic features

Immunohistochemical Results
- Thyroglobulin, TTF-1, PAX8, CK7 positive

Molecular Results
- *PAX8-PPARγ* commonly identified
- *RAS* in up to 45% of tumors

Fine Needle Aspiration
- Cellular aspirates with dispersed microfollicular arrangements of cells forming small "ring-like" structures; colloid is scant
- Cannot be reliably separated from follicular adenoma and adenomatoid nodules

Pathologic Differential Diagnosis
- Follicular adenoma, papillary carcinoma, medullary carcinoma and adenomatoid nodules

Gross Findings

The tumors are usually solitary, well-circumscribed masses surrounded by a variably thick capsule separating them from the uninvolved parenchyma. The capsule is usually thicker than an adenoma. The cut surface is often bulging and has a light tan to brown appearance (Figure 24-36), although widely invasive tumors often have hemorrhage and necrosis (Figure 24-37). Most tumors are <5 cm in size (generally 2 to 4 cm), although oncocytic tumors are slightly larger. The tumors are rarely multifocal. Oncocytic tumors may be mahogany-brown. In general, usually a minimum of 10 blocks (two or three sections per block) from the capsule-tumor interface are submitted for histologic evaluation.

Microscopic Findings

The tumors are surrounded by a variable fibrous connective tissue capsule, which ranges from thick (0.1 to 0.4 cm) and well-formed to thin, irregular, uneven, and poorly formed. The capsule has parallel layers of collagen containing smooth muscle–walled vessels. The

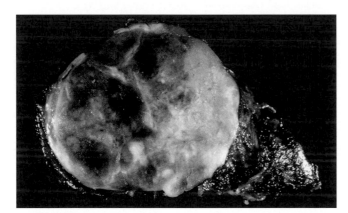

FIGURE 24-36
A solitary mass surrounded by a capsule has a distinctly different appearance from the surrounding uninvolved thyroid parenchyma.

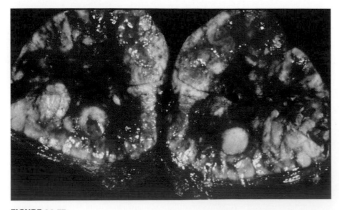

FIGURE 24-37
A widely invasive tumor with central hemorrhage, necrosis, and degeneration.

diagnostic feature of FC is invasion: capsular and/or vascular penetration (either is sufficient for diagnosis). Capsular invasion is classified as single or multiple foci of tumor cells identified penetrating *into* (partial capsule; Figure 24-38) and *through* (entire thickness; Figures 24-39 and 24-40) the capsule. In general, penetration beyond half the capsular thickness or beyond the tumor nodule in an area unassociated with a previous FNA site qualifies as capsular invasion. Parenchymal extension is defined by neoplastic cells surrounded by uninvolved thyroid parenchyma on either side of the protrusion. Deeper sections may be necessary to "connect" satellite nodules. Vascular invasion can involve single or multiple foci within small, medium-sized, or large vessels (Figure 24-41). Small vessels, usually within the capsule, have a limited caliber, while medium-sized vessels with or without smooth muscle walls are noted within or immediately adjacent to the capsule. Vascular invasion is defined by direct extension of tumor cells into the vessel lumen, tumor thrombi adherent to the vessel wall (often associated with blood clot), and/or tumor nests covered by endothelium (Figure 24-42). Tumor plugs in vascular spaces *within* the tumor mass do not qualify as vascular invasion; nor do detached or artifactually dislodged tumor fragments free floating in vascular spaces. An intravascular organizing thrombus (Masson disease) does not qualify as invasion. Also, "penetrating" vessels should not be misinterpreted to represent invasion. There is a movement toward quantifying the number of vessels involved, specifically listing if more than four vessels are involved.

Many different patterns of growth can be seen in follicular carcinoma (microfollicular, trabecular, insular, solid, cystic; Figure 24-43), but usually only one pattern predominates. The tumors are usually cellular with colloid easily identified. Oncocytic cells (oxyphilic, Ashkenazi, or Hürthle cell) have fine to slightly coarse, granular, abundant eosinophilic cytoplasm surrounding round to regular nuclei with coarse nuclear chromatin and eosinophilic, centrally placed nucleoli (Figure 24-43). Colloid is usually less in oncocytic tumors. While the majority of cases will have tumor cells that are round and regular, occasionally, focal tumor cell spindling, tumor cell clearing, signet ring formation, and even pleomorphism may be present (Figure 24-44). Mitotic figures and necrosis can be seen, but degenerative changes are more common, especially in the central regions of the tumor or post FNA. Direct soft tissue and tracheal extension is rare. Extrathyroidal extension should be reported along with involvement of the surgical margin.

A number of variants or qualifiers are used in describing FCs, identified as follows:

• *Minimally invasive:* Limited capsular and/or vascular invasion, although exact number of foci is undefined. Invasion is limited to small or medium-sized capsular or pericapsular vascular spaces.

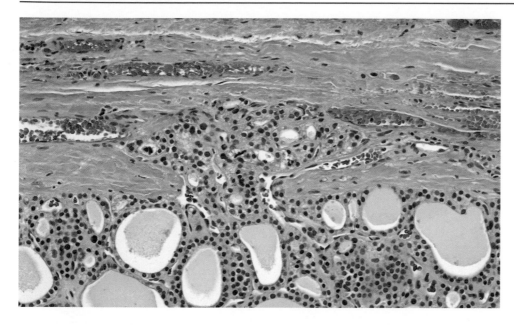

FIGURE 24-38

The tumor capsule is broken by the neoplastic cells penetrating through the capsule, showing a small "mushroom" shape.

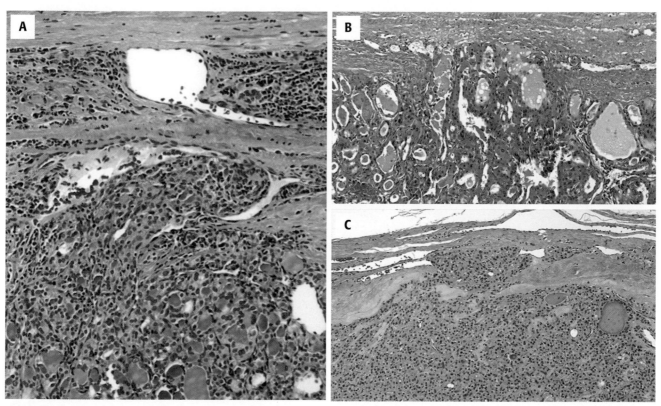

FIGURE 24-39

A, Capsular penetration by the neoplastic cells in association with a vascular space. **B**, Oncocytic tumor cells are invading into the capsule. **C**, Capsular transgression noted on frozen section specimen.

- *Widely invasive:* Uncommon type with extensive infiltration beyond the tumor capsule ("mushroom" invasion), into large vessels, and shows nodules of tumor within the parenchyma. Many times the capsule is attenuated or hard to identify. As the degree of invasion increases, the biologic behavior becomes more aggressive (Figures 24-40 and 24-42).

- *Oncocytic variant (Hürthle, Ashkenazi, oxyphilic):* Greater than 75% of the tumor is composed of large, polygonal, oncocytic cells (Figures 24-39 and 24-43), the cytoplasm of which is filled with abnormal mitochondria (abnormal dense bodies). The cytoplasm is coarse to deeply eosinophilic or "opacified." Due to increased mitochondria, the

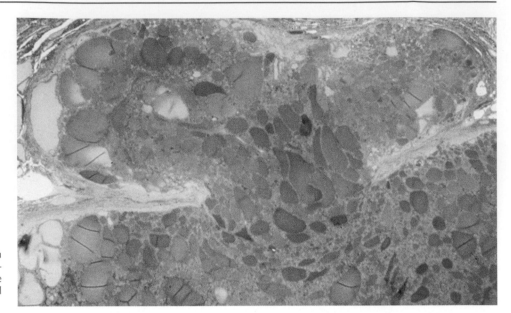

FIGURE 24-40

A large, "mushroom-shaped" projection of neoplastic cells out into the surrounding parenchyma. Note that the capsule has "traveled" with the tumor and is still present at the advancing edge.

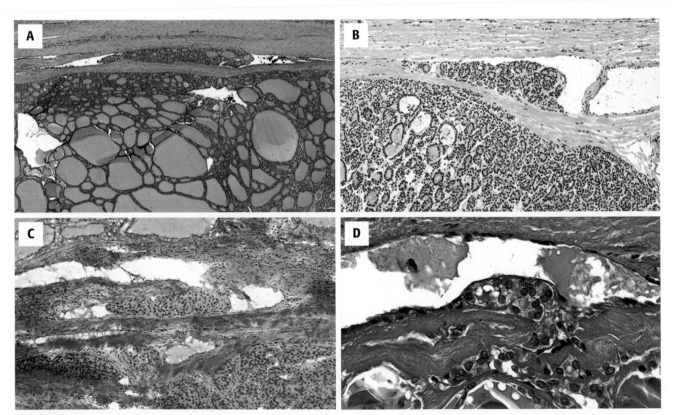

FIGURE 24-41

Vascular invasion in follicular carcinoma. **A**, Tumor thrombus filling a vascular space. **B**, A tumor fragment attached to a vessel wall within the tumor capsule. **C**, A frozen section showing tumor attached to the wall of an intermediate vessel. **D**, The point of vascular invasion is noted, with an endothelial lining covering the tumor nest.

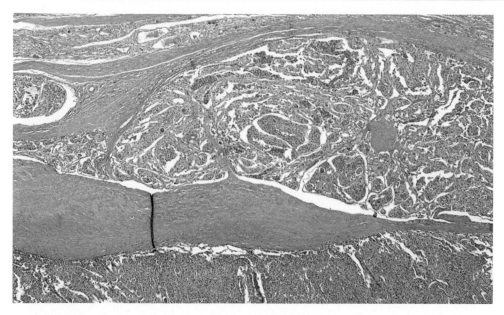

FIGURE 24-42

Large projections of tumor beyond the contour of the lesion with vascular invasion is diagnostic of a widely invasive follicular carcinoma.

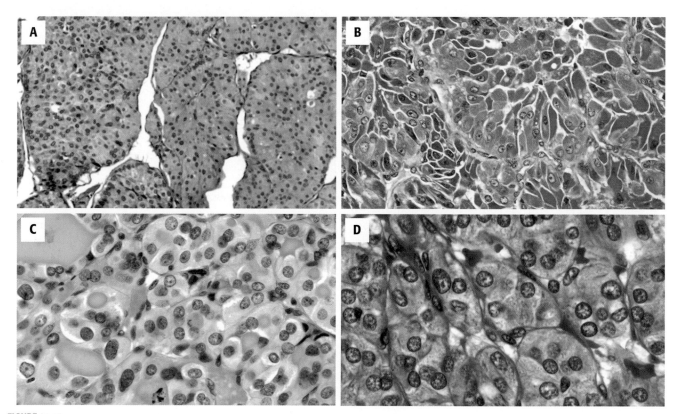

FIGURE 24-43

Patterns of growth and cytoplasmic appearance of follicular carcinoma. **A**, Trabecular pattern with granular cytoplasm. **B**, Solid pattern with oncocytic cytoplasm. **C**, Slight nuclear variability in a follicular pattern. **D**, Insular growth with focal colloid.

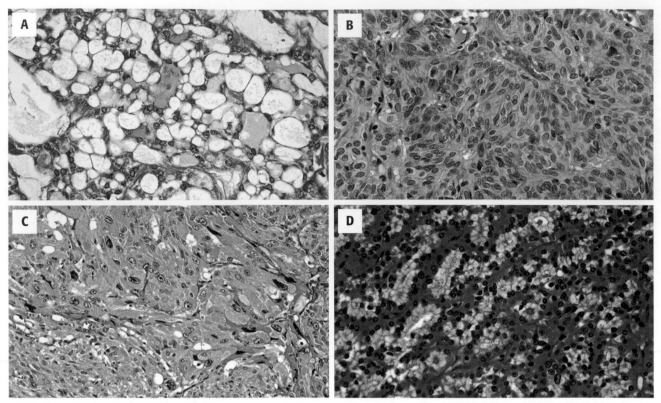

FIGURE 24-44

Uncommon features include: **A**, Signet ring pattern. **B**, Tumor cell spindling without colloid production. **C**, Profound, focal nuclear pleomorphism. **D**, A focal tumor cell clearing in an oncocytic tumor (colloid is seen).

tumors are more prone to infarction or degeneration. The tumors tend to be larger than conventional FC. The tumors have scant to absent colloid. Thyroglobulin or TTF-1 may be required to confirm follicular derivation. There may occasionally be calcifications, which can resemble psammoma bodies. The nuclei often contain large, centrally placed, brightly eosinophilic nucleoli. Pleomorphism tends to be more easily identified. There is no difference in outcome or management, although follicular carcinomas with oncocytic cells tend to occur in older patients, have larger tumors, and more commonly have lymph node metastasis (up to 30%). FNA will frequently result in infarction with associated hemorrhage, cyst formation, and eventual fibrosis.

- *Clear cell variant:* Any tumor may have clear cell change, especially prominent in oncocytic neoplasms (Figure 24-44). It should be the dominant finding (>75%) for this variant to be diagnosed.
- *Spindle cell variant:* Tumor spindling should be the dominant finding (Figure 24-44).
- *Signet-ring cell variant:* The nuclei are compressed and displaced by clear to amphophilic cytoplasm. The material is irregular thyroglobulin (Figure 24-44).

ANCILLARY STUDIES

IMMUNOHISTOCHEMICAL RESULTS

Immunohistochemistry may be of value in confirming that the neoplasm is of follicular derivation, but it is seldom necessary for diagnostic purposes. The cells would be thyroglobulin, TTF-1, PAX8, and CK7 immunoreactive, while chromogranin, calcitonin, and polyclonal carcinoembryonic antigen (pCEA) are negative. Oncocytic tumors can show high background or nonspecific staining, however, so interpreting results should be done with caution. Stains for endothelial markers (CD34, CD31, factor VIII–related antigen [FVIII-RAg]) to accentuate vessels are of only limited value, as the endothelial cells are frequently discontinuous or lost in deeper sections, making interpretation difficult.

FINE NEEDLE ASPIRATION

Separation between adenomatoid nodule, FA, and FC relies on the demonstration of capsular or vascular invasion, making FNA of no value in making such a distinction. However, FNA is an excellent screening tool with a sensitivity of 78%, specificity of 98%, and positive predictive value of 99% for these lesions. The aspirates are hypercellular with a dispersed microfollicular architecture or small, spherical three-dimensional clusters. There are often 6 to 12 nuclei forming a ring-like structure. The cytoplasmic borders are often indistinct. The cells are enlarged with uniform, round nuclei with coarse nuclear chromatin. Nuclear size and shape variability may be present (Figure 24-45). Oncocytic cells may be the dominant finding (Figure 24-45). The cells tend to be larger, with an eccentric nucleus, binucleated or multinucleated, and often with a prominent nucleolus. There is usually scant or absent colloid. These findings are best reported as "follicular neoplasm or suspicious for a follicular neoplasm," which translates into a tumor requiring surgical excision (Bethesda System for Reporting Thyroid Cytopathology: Group IV).

FROZEN SECTION

If an FNA has been performed, then frozen section should be declined. It is nearly completely useless unless you "happen" upon an area of invasion. If a frozen section is demanded, two to three sections of the capsule should be sampled, and then "defer to permanent" can be invoked.

MOLECULAR ANALYSIS

Many FCs (up to 50%) will demonstrate rearrangements of the peroxisome proliferator-activated receptor gamma (*PPARγ*) gene, which produces a number of fusion proteins of which *PAX8-PPARγ* is the most common. This is a fusion between *PAX8* gene on 2q13 and *PPARγ* gene on 3p25 and can be detected with fluorescence in situ hybridization (FISH). Almost never identified concurrently, *RAS* mutations are identified in ~45% of FCs. *GRIM-19* gene mutations can be seen in oncocytic tumors. However, the detection techniques are not universally accepted, and there is some overlap with FAs, papillary carcinoma, and anaplastic carcinoma. This suggests additional studies are necessary before these molecular techniques are incorporated into daily use.

DIFFERENTIAL DIAGNOSIS

FA and *cellular adenomatoid nodules*, especially those with degenerative fibrosis, are sometimes difficult to separate from minimally invasive or low-grade FC. Neoplasms usually have muscle-walled vessels in the fibrous capsule, while an adenomatoid nodule usually does not. Tangential sectioning, irregular tumor contour, FNA, and frozen section artifacts all hamper interpretation. Adequate sampling of the *tumor-to-capsule-to-parenchymal* interface (at least one section per centimeter of tumor) is imperative before resorting to "atypical FA" or "follicular neoplasm

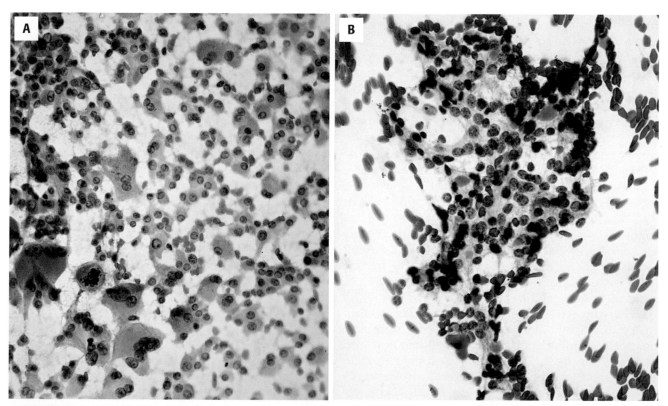

FIGURE 24-45

A, Small follicles and sheets of oncocytic cells showing mitoses and multinucleation in a "favor neoplasm" fine needle aspiration (FNA) (alcohol-fixed, Papanicolaou stain). **B**, An FNA smear showing a microfollicular pattern with nuclear size and shape variability and green droplets of colloid (alcohol-fixed, Papanicolaou stain).

of uncertain malignant potential." Adenomatoid nodules are usually multiple, tend to be less cellular with more colloid than neoplasms, and do not have a true capsule.

Follicular variant of papillary carcinoma may occasionally be a problem, although the nuclear features should assist in the distinction. *Medullary carcinoma* can occasionally be oncocytic, but the nuclei tend to be finely stippled (neuroendocrine) and the cells are chromogranin, calcitonin, and CEA immunoreactive. Tumor cells are frequently ovoid to spindled. Amyloid is often present. C-cell hyperplasia in the background may suggest the diagnosis, especially in inherited tumors. In the clear cell variant, *parathyroid tumors* and *metastatic renal cell carcinoma* may need to be separated from follicular carcinoma by using immunohistochemical studies along with the clinical history. A poorly differentiated carcinoma tends to have a more solid, trabecular or insular growth pattern, shows necrosis and increased mitoses and shows limited to absent colloid production.

PROGNOSIS AND THERAPY

There has been a change in patient outcome over the past decades, especially with more neoplasms being found earlier in their development and with correct classification as minimally invasive. Overall, minimally invasive follicular carcinoma has an ~97% 20-year survival, with survival curves approaching those of normal age- and gender-matched controls. Hypoparathyroidism and recurrent laryngeal nerve damage are seen in up to 3% of patients. Widely invasive tumors, on the other hand, portend a more aggressive biologic behavior with an approximately 50% 20-year survival. In any tumor type or grade, if metastasis develops, it occurs most commonly in lungs and bone, although the oncocytic type may have a higher frequency of lymph node metastases. When follicular carcinomas are stratified by gender, age, size and extent of invasion, there is no difference in recurrence or patient outcome when controlling for variant type, specifically the oncocytic variant. Therefore, "oncocytic" FCs should be managed in a fashion identical to FC. Adverse prognostic factors include age >45 years, extrathyroidal extension, tumor >4 cm, distant metastases, and *RAS* mutations.

Conservative resection (lobectomy) versus radical surgery (total thyroidectomy) does not seem to yield statistically significant differences in patient outcome. Therefore, the most conservative treatment to completely remove the tumor is advocated. However, as radioablative iodine therapy is only effective after total thyroidectomy, there is a tendency toward this management. ^{131}I is not taken up by 25% of conventional FCs and up to 75% of oncocytic FCs, so is ineffective. External beam radiation may be used in some patients.

■ UNDIFFERENTIATED CARCINOMA

Accounting for approximately 2% to 3% of all thyroid gland neoplasms (1 to 2/1 million population), undifferentiated carcinoma (also known as *anaplastic carcinoma* and *pleomorphic carcinoma*), is a highly aggressive malignant neoplasm composed of undifferentiated cells which require immunohistochemical or ultrastructural support to determine their epithelial origin. All are primary thyroid tumors by definition (not metastatic or direct extension). Risk factors include radiation exposure risk, low socioeconomic status, and old age, along with iodine deficiency and a long history of thyroid disease.

CLINICAL FEATURES

The vast majority of patients are >60 years, but the sharp female predilection for other thyroid gland neoplasms is not sustained in this neoplasm: the female to male ratio is 1.5:1. Nearly all of the patients present with a rapidly (1 to 2 weeks) enlarging fixed and hard neck mass (Figure 24-46), often associated with a long history of thyroid disease (goiter, follicular carcinoma, papillary carcinoma). Furthermore, the hoarseness, dysphagia, vocal cord paralysis, and pain often associated with the mass are indications of the widely invasive nature of the neoplasm. Extension into the soft tissues and surrounding organs (esophagus, trachea) is common. Hyperthyroidism may result due to rapid destruction of follicles and hormone release. Metastases to cervical lymph nodes and/or lungs are noted at clinical presentation in ~50% of patients. Leukocytosis can be seen due to the secretion of macrophage colony-stimulating factor. Radiographic studies show the extent of the disease and degree of infiltration (including vessels), along with necrosis and calcifications.

PATHOLOGIC FEATURES

GROSS FINDINGS

The tumors are usually a large (mean: 6 cm), fleshy, pale-tan solitary mass (60%), often fixed and firm. Multifocal (40%) or bilateral (25%) tumors are not as common. Typically completely replacing the thyroid parenchyma, tumors show extensive invasion beyond the thyroid gland into the perithyroidal tissues. Necrosis and hemorrhage are almost ubiquitous (Figure 24-46).

UNDIFFERENTIATED CARCINOMA—DISEASE FACT SHEET

Definition
- Highly aggressive malignant neoplasm composed of undifferentiated cells that exhibit immunohistochemical or ultrastructural epithelial differentiation

Incidence and Location
- 2% to 3% of all thyroid malignancies
- Higher in endemic goiter regions and in Europe
- Radiation exposure risk

Morbidity and Mortality
- Rapidly fatal in nearly all patients

Gender and Age Distribution
- Female > male (1.5:1)
- Most patients are older than 60 years

Clinical Features
- Rapidly expanding neck mass
- Usually have underlying long history of thyroid disease
- Hoarseness, dysphagia, and pain are common
- Frequent metastases identified at presentation

Prognosis and Therapy
- Poor prognosis, >95% die of disease usually in <6 months (accounts for >50% of all thyroid cancer deaths)
- Surgery and combination multimodality therapy

UNDIFFERENTIATED CARCINOMA—PATHOLOGIC FEATURES

Gross Findings
- Large (mean: 6 cm), fleshy masses with necrosis and hemorrhage
- Infiltrating, often into adjacent soft tissues and organs

Microscopic Findings
- Widely invasive with extensive lymphovascular invasion
- Many different patterns of growth
- Poorly differentiated cells: polygonal, spindle, and epithelioid
- Profound pleomorphism
- Tumor giant cells, osteoclast-like giant cells, and squamous differentiation may be seen
- Increased mitotic figures, including atypical forms
- Necrosis, hemorrhage and degeneration

Immunohistochemical Results
- Keratin and EMA, in up to 80% of cases (focal and limited)
- p63 may be positive, but thyroglobulin and TTF-1 are rarely positive
- Vimentin and p53 positive in nearly all cases

Fine Needle Aspiration
- Biphasic population: tumor and uninvolved thyroid
- Highly cellular with single cells and focal clusters composed of remarkable atypical cells; mitotic figures are prominent; background necrosis can be seen

Pathologic Differential Diagnosis
- Exclude metastatic disease to thyroid; primary thyroid sarcomas and anaplastic lymphoma

Adequate sampling to show preexisting or coexisting carcinoma is suggested.

MICROSCOPIC FINDINGS

The remarkably infiltrative tumor is composed of a combination of pleomorphic, spindle, and epithelioid cells arranged in solid sheets to fascicular bundles that nearly completely efface the thyroid parenchyma (Figures 24-47 to 24-49). Extrathyroidal extension, with soft tissue and local organ extension, is common. Extensive lymphovascular invasion is present, along with significant coagulative-type necrosis, hemorrhage, and degeneration. A desmoplastic stroma may be present. It is not

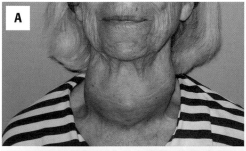
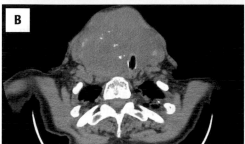
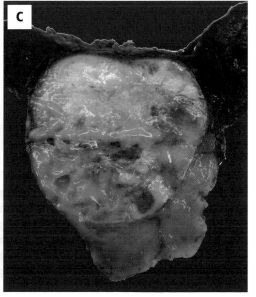

FIGURE 24-46

A, A clinical photograph demonstrates a large thyroid mass with engorged veins. **B**, A large mass nearly entirely replacing the thyroid gland and expanding into the soft tissue with tracheal deviation is seen on computed tomography. **C**, The cut surface shows the thyroid parenchyma invaded by a yellow to tan fleshy tumor, focally showing degeneration. (**A**, *Courtesy of Dr. G. Calzada.*)

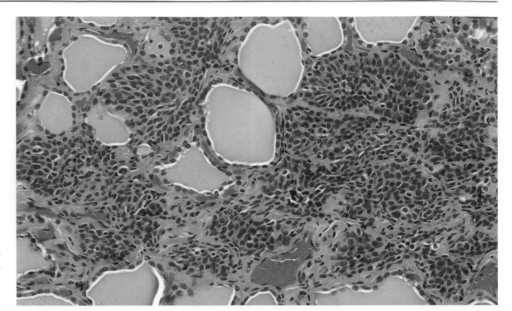

FIGURE 24-53

The ultimobranchial body remnants are called solid cell nests. These structures are seen around normal follicles with oval nuclei, coarse nuclear chromatin, and a lack of intercellular borders.

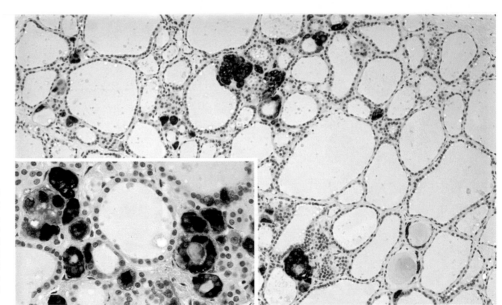

FIGURE 24-54

The small aggregates of C cells are part of a physiologic response to chronic disease, aging, or other abnormalities. No nest contains more than 50 cells, the nodules do not coalesce, and there is no associated fibrosis or amyloid. Inset demonstrates small groups of cells but usually still in a parafollicular distribution without destruction of the parenchyma (calcitonin immunohistochemistry).

noted adjacent to medullary carcinoma. These groups may be focal, diffuse or nodular. Furthermore, if the tumor is <1 cm, the term "microcarcinoma" may be employed (Figure 24-56). In contrast, physiologic C-cell hyperplasia, usually *not* identified by standard hematoxylin and eosin (H&E), is composed of discrete small (<50 cells) aggregates of normal-appearing C cells without associated fibrosis or amyloid. With increased experience, physiologic C cells can be recognized by H&E, with calcitonin used as confirmation. This type of response is seen widely in aging, chronic disease, renal disorders, hyperparathyroidism, and lymphocytic thyroiditis, among others.

- *Medullary carcinoma*: The borders are irregular, circumscribed to encapsulated, with tumor cells extending out into the thyroid parenchyma, entrapping benign, uninvolved follicular epithelium (Figure 24-57). These entrapped areas can be seen quite deep within large tumors (Figure 24-58). In very large tumors, extension into adjacent soft tissues and neck organs may be present. Lymphovascular invasion is usually prominent, often associated with a high incidence of lymph node metastases. A host of different patterns of growth and cell types are observed in medullary carcinoma, including solid sheets, organoid, lobular, trabecular, insular, glandular, tubular, and papillary patterns,

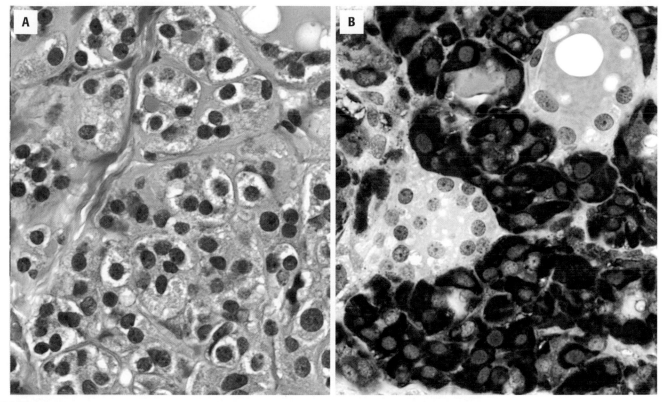

FIGURE 24-55

A, Neoplastic C-cell hyperplasia shows aggregates of >50 C cells with associated fibrosis. A small uninvolved thyroid follicle is present (*upper right*). **B**, Calcitonin immunohistochemistry accentuates the cells around the thyroid follicles.

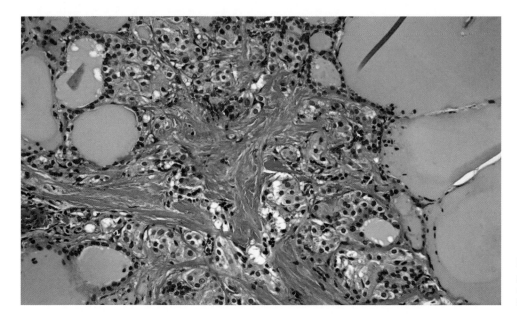

FIGURE 24-56

A microscopic medullary carcinoma shows destructive growth of >50 cells, fibrosis, and focal nuclear pleomorphism.

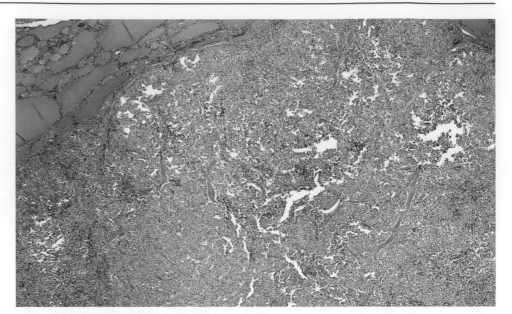

FIGURE 24-57

A predominantly solid growth pattern is noted in this medullary carcinoma. The interface between the tumor and the adjacent thyroid is irregular. Small wisps of pink amyloid are noted.

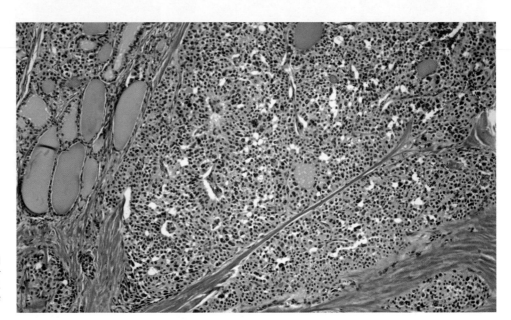

FIGURE 24-58

The medullary carcinoma has entrapped a number of benign thyroid follicular epithelial cells with associated colloid. There are more follicles on the left side of the image.

variably comprising spindle, oncocytic, clear, and amphicrine cell types (Figures 24-59 and 24-60). The various patterns of growth are separated by a fibrovascular stroma. The cells are round to oval, spindled to plasmacytoid with ill-defined eosinophilic or amphophilic, granular cytoplasm. Pigmentation is uncommon. The nuclei are usually round to oval and chromatin is coarse to stippled and "salt-and-pepper" in distribution (Figure 24-61). Nucleoli are not prominent, except in the oncocytic variant. Intranuclear cytoplasmic inclusions can be identified. Bi- and multinucleation are common, with moderate nuclear pleomorphism present. An increased mitotic index and necrosis are usually identified only in large tumors. Amyloid, a

homogeneous, acellular, eosinophilic, extracellular matrix material is seen in most cases (up to 80%; Figure 24-62). It is thought to be calcitonin derived and may be associated with calcifications. Tumors without amyloid tend to have a worse prognosis. Mucin production is occasionally noted, but is of limited amount.

Numerous variants are recognized but are of no specific clinical or management significance: oncocytic cell, papillary/pseudopapillary, glandular or follicular, giant cell, small cell, paraganglioma-like, spindle cell, clear cell, squamous cell, melanin-producing, angiosarcoma-like, and amphicrine. Immunohistochemical confirmation is usually required.

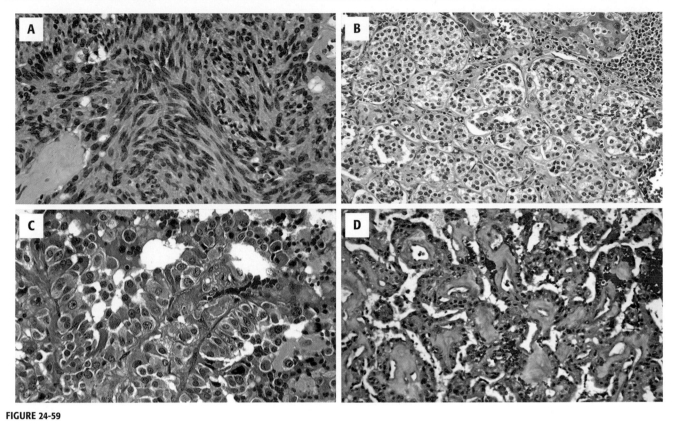

FIGURE 24-59

Patterns of growth in medullary carcinoma: **A**, Spindled to fascicular. **B**, Organoid. **C**, Papillary architecture with basophilic granular cytoplasm. **D**, Angiomatoid, simulating an angiosarcoma.

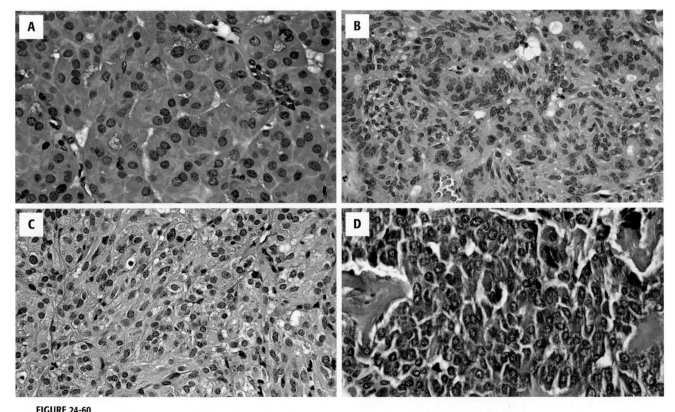

FIGURE 24-60

Cell types in medullary carcinoma: **A**, Oncocytic. **B**, Fusiform to columnar cells with basophilic, granular cytoplasm. **C**, Spindled. **D**, Plasmacytoid.

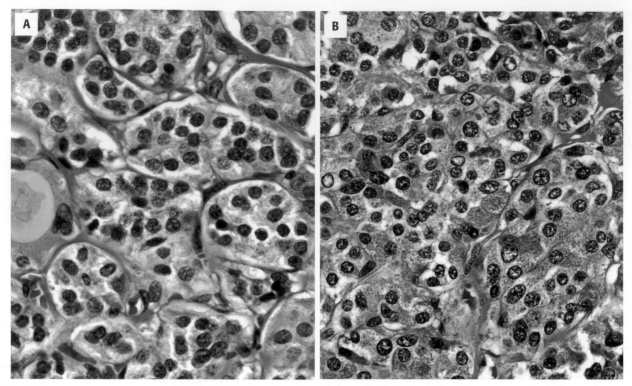

FIGURE 24-61

A, Organoid pattern of growth with basophilic granular cytoplasm noted around nuclei with coarse, salt-and-pepper nuclear chromatin distribution. There is a single follicle on far left. **B**, Follicular growth may mimic a follicular epithelial neoplasm. However, the nuclear chromatin is different.

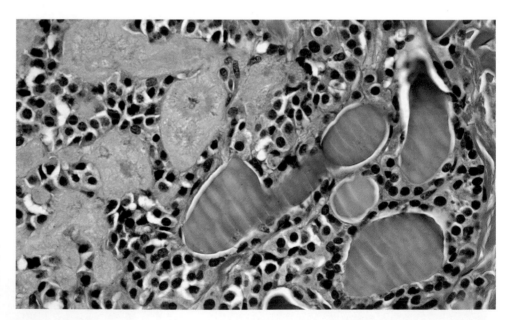

FIGURE 24-62

Amyloid is common. Left side shows eosinophilic, amorphous, extracellular amyloid blending with surrounding tumor cells. Note the difference from the colloid (*right side*), which is more brightly eosinophilic. These are entrapped thyroid follicles.

ANCILLARY STUDIES

HISTOCHEMICAL AND IMMUNOHISTOCHEMICAL RESULTS

C cells are easily accentuated by calcitonin (Figure 24-63), calcitonin-gene-related peptide (CGRP), chromogranin, CD56, and synaptophysin, while keratin and pCEA are also reactive. It is important to know that medullary carcinoma is also TTF-1 reactive although negative with thyroglobulin.

Argyrophilic stains (Grimelius stain) can be employed, while the Fontana-Masson stain is negative. When amyloid is present, polarization of a Congo red stain will give the characteristic apple-green birefringence. Alternatively, crystal violet yields purple metachromatic staining. Occasionally, amyloid immunohistochemistry may be performed, but it is a difficult stain to interpret due to significant diffusion artifact.

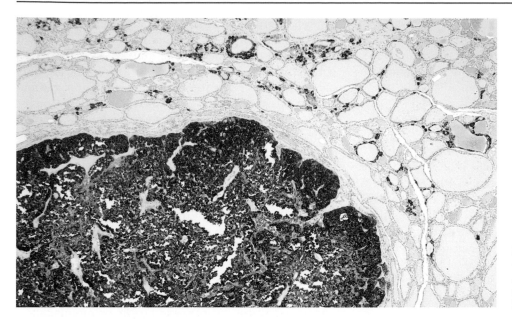

FIGURE 24-63

The medullary carcinoma is strongly and diffusely immunoreactive for calcitonin. Groups of C cells are highlighted around the medullary carcinoma.

FINE NEEDLE ASPIRATION

There is significant cytologic variability from case to case. Most aspirates are cellular with single cells or small, loosely cohesive clusters of cells (Figure 24-64). Colloid is notably absent; however, the extracellular, homogeneous, amorphous eosinophilic clumps or spheres of amyloid (seen in ~60% of aspirates) may sometimes be misinterpreted as colloid (Figure 24-64). The tumor cells vary from round to oval, spindle-shaped, and polygonal. Binucleation and multinucleation can be seen, along with moderate pleomorphism. The nuclear chromatin is stippled or coarsely granular ("salt-and-pepper") with abundant, eosinophilic cytoplasm often

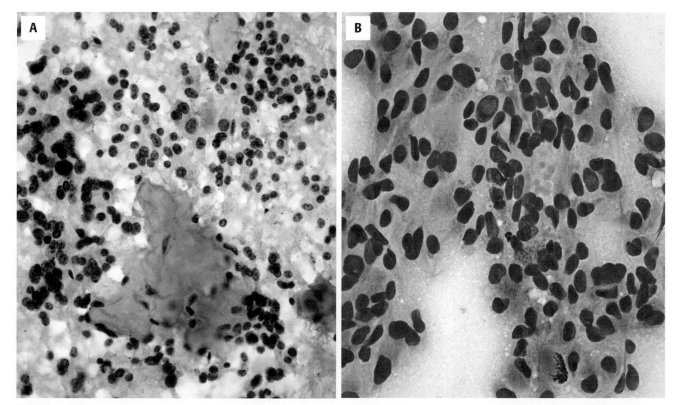

FIGURE 24-64

A, A cellular aspirate with loosely cohesive tumor cells. Plasmacytoid architecture is prominent. There is nuclear pleomorphism as well as amorphous amyloid in the center (alcohol-fixed, Papanicolaou stain). **B**, There are clusters of cells with plasmacytoid and spindled cells. Note the intranuclear cytoplasmic inclusion and mitotic figure (air-dried, Diff-Quik stain).

608

HEAD AND NECK PATHOLOGY

eccentrically surrounding the nucleus. This plasmacy-toid appearance is quite characteristic. Intranuclear cytoplasmic inclusions may be seen (Figure 24-64). Air-dried preparations often highlight the distinctive metachromatic red cytoplasmic granules.

MOLECULAR ANALYSIS

Somatic *RET* mutations, most commonly the M918T mutation, have been shown to occur in 20% to 80% of sporadic medullary thyroid carcinoma (the wide range is due to different detection techniques). Germline *RET* oncogene mutations are identified in all hereditary forms, although the mutations occur in different codons and with different degrees of penetrance. Germline mutations can be detected in peripheral blood samples rather than using tumor cells.

DIFFERENTIAL DIAGNOSIS

Neoplastic C-cell hyperplasia (clusters of >50 cells) may be mistaken for intraglandular spread of medullary carcinoma, since fibrosis may be seen. However, the cells tend to have a more intense calcitonin immunoreactivity. Solid cell nests and palpation thyroiditis can usually be separated by histology alone.

The differential diagnosis of medullary carcinoma includes most of the primary tumors of the thyroid gland. Hyalinizing trabecular tumor, follicular carcinoma, paraganglioma, amyloid goiter, undifferentiated carcinoma, and lymphoma may mimic medullary carcinoma. Metastatic carcinomas are uncommon, although renal cell is the most frequent. Direct extension into the thyroid by laryngeal neuroendocrine carcinomas may occasionally cause diagnostic difficulty. Metastatic foci of medullary carcinoma may be difficult to separate from other carcinomas, although immunohistochemical analysis for calcitonin, CEA, and chromogranin aids in this distinction.

PROGNOSIS AND THERAPY

Clinical stage and inheritance pattern are most important in determining the patient's prognosis. If there is no metastatic disease, patients can enjoy nearly 100% cure rates following surgery. This is especially true in tumors found incidentally (usually small and without metastasis) during screening for familial disease. Metastatic disease to cervical lymph nodes is common, while metastases to liver, lungs, and bone are less commonly identified. However, if there is metastatic disease or elevated calcitonin and/or CEA levels, the prognosis is more guarded and difficult to predict.

Overall, there is between a 70% and 80% 10-year survival. Survival is best for familial non–MEN-related disease, followed by sporadic and MEN2A, which is better than MEN2B. Women and patients <40 years old tend to have a better prognosis. Similarly, tumors rich in calcitonin (>75% of cells) and with abundant amyloid behave less aggressively, lacking in lymph node metastases. In somatic *RET* mutations, those with codon 918 mutations tend to have a more aggressive clinical course.

Total thyroidectomy is the treatment of choice, with central lymph node dissection as clinically or radiographically indicated. Prophylactic thyroidectomy is used in patients with germline mutations. Specific *RET* mutations will dictate the specific age for the thyroidectomy: Mutations in codon 611, 618, 620, and 634 receive thyroidectomy before 5 years of age. Lymph node dissection is performed in tumors >1 cm. Chemotherapy, somatostatin analogs, and targeted molecular therapy (tyrosine kinase inhibitors targeting *RET*) are being used with variable effectiveness.

Parathyroid gland disease may also be present, especially if the medullary carcinoma is familial, necessitating parathyroidectomy. There is no effective chemotherapy and radiation is used only as a palliative measure. [131]I radioablative therapy is useless since there is no thyroid hormone production. Follow-up of the patient's serum calcitonin and CEA levels, especially if elevated, is required to monitor for recurrence. Whenever medullary carcinoma is found, the incidence of discovering a genetic form when evaluating relatives of the proband is ~10% to 15%; thus, genetic testing is a valuable screening tool, irrespective of the specific technique employed (biochemical or molecular).

■ PRIMARY THYROID LYMPHOMA

This is defined as a primary lymphoma arising within the confines of the thyroid gland and usually associated with chronic lymphocytic thyroiditis. These are uncommon neoplasms. The understanding of the "mucosa-associated lymphoid tissue" (MALT) concept suggests that previous plasmacytomas may be within the spectrum of extranodal marginal zone B-cell lymphoma (EMZBCL). Acquired MALT from autoimmune, immune deficiency, or inflammatory processes results in a nodular or diffuse infiltrate of lymphoid cells, frequently with follicles and germinal centers, and associated oncocytic metaplasia of thyroid epithelium. There is a chronicity to the process. The MALT lymphoma cell of origin is a post germinal center (activated), marginal zone B cell. Although there is usually a lack of systemic involvement, regional lymph nodes may be affected. Follicular lymphoma (FL) and Hodgkin lymphoma (HL) are exceptional.

CLINICAL FEATURES

Primary thyroid lymphomas account for ~2-5% of all thyroid gland neoplasms and ~5% of all extranodal lymphomas, and are basically divided into two types: EMZBCL and diffuse large B-cell lymphoma (DLBCL). Primarily a disease of older individuals (mean, 65 years), there is a strong female to male predilection (3 to 7:1). Patients nearly always have a history of chronic lymphocytic thyroiditis (Hashimoto thyroiditis), the MALT setting considered essential for the development of this lymphoma. In fact, there is an 80-fold increased risk of lymphoma in patients who have chronic lymphocytic thyroiditis. By definition, lymph node lymphomas directly extending into the thyroid are not considered primary thyroid lymphomas. Patients' symptoms are generally nonspecific, with the most common complaint being a mass in the thyroid gland, with pain and obstructive symptoms, including dysphagia and/or hoarseness (seen in 30% of patients) related to compression. Hypothyroidism is usually due to underlying Hashimoto thyroiditis rather than the lymphoma. In DLBCL, the "end point" of many other types of B-cell lymphoma, patients often report a rapidly enlarging mass (Figure 24-65). The duration of symptoms is usually short (mean, 4 months). Staging is the same as that used for lymphomas in general, with "E" added for extranodal. The perithyroidal lymph nodes may be involved, resulting in stage IE or IIE, followed by other lymph nodes or bone marrow. Patients usually lack constitutional or "B" symptoms (fever, profound night sweats, weight loss, anorexia).

PATHOLOGIC FEATURES

GROSS FINDINGS

The lymphomas are often large (mean, 7 cm), firm to soft, lobulated and may be either a solid or cystic mass involving one or both thyroid lobes. The cut surface is

---

PRIMARY THYROID LYMPHOMA—DISEASE FACT SHEET

Definition
- Primary lymphoma arising within the thyroid gland and nearly always associated with lymphocytic thyroiditis

Incidence and Location
- ~2% to 5% of thyroid neoplasms
- ~5% of extranodal lymphomas

Morbidity and Mortality
- Most arise within the setting of lymphocytic thyroiditis and/or Hashimoto disease
- Mortality is grade and stage dependent

Gender, Race, and Age Distribution
- Female >> male (3 to 7:1)
- Mean age: 7th decade

Clinical Features
- Mass (often rapidly enlarging) with associated pain, dysphagia, and hoarseness
- Hypothyroidism may develop
- Associated cervical adenopathy in some cases

Prognosis and Therapy
- Overall, ~60% 5-year survival, although type (grade) and stage dependent
- Poor prognosis: >65 years, males, vocal cord paralysis, diffuse large B-cell lymphoma, high stage, diffuse architecture, vascular invasion, high mitoses
- Chemotherapy and radiation employed, dependent on grade and stage

---

PRIMARY THYROID LYMPHOMA—PATHOLOGIC FEATURES

Gross Findings
- Usually large (mean: 7 cm)
- Soft to firm, lobular and multinodular
- Effacement of the normal thyroid
- Cut surface is bulging, tan, and "fish-flesh"
- Usually homogeneous or mottled
- Extension into perithyroidal soft tissues

Microscopic Findings
- Extranodal marginal zone B-cell lymphoma and diffuse large B-cell lymphoma with transitions between the two
- Constant background of lymphocytic thyroiditis
- Extension into fat and skeletal muscle
- Atypical small lymphocytes, centrocytes, monocytoid B cells, and plasma cells
- Dutcher bodies and Russell bodies
- Lymphoepithelial lesions (atypical lymphoid cells within the follicular epithelium) are diagnostic
- Diffuse architecture; large, atypical cells; and increased mitoses suggests transformation into a diffuse large B-cell lymphoma

Immunohistochemical Results
- CD20 (coexpressed with CD43 occasionally)
- CD79a, PAX-5, and CD138
- Bcl-2 in the colonizing B cells within germinal centers
- κ or λ light chain restriction
- Keratin highlights the lymphoepithelial lesions

Fine Needle Aspiration
- Marginal zone B-cell lymphomas are a dispersed, noncohesive admixture of lymphocytes, centrocytes, monocytoid B cells, immunoblasts, plasma cells and histiocytes—perhaps indistinguishable from a lymphocytic thyroiditis
- Diffuse large B-cell lymphoma aspirates are hypercellular with dyscohesive, large, atypical neoplastic cells

Pathologic Differential Diagnosis
- Lymphocytic thyroiditis; undifferentiated carcinoma, myeloid sarcoma and melanoma

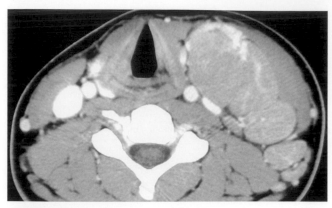

FIGURE 24-65

A computed tomography scan showing a large left thyroid gland mass, with associated lymphadenopathy. This is nonspecific but was part of a thyroid diffuse large B-cell lymphoma.

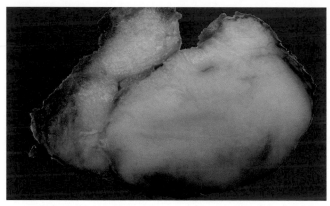

FIGURE 24-66

Malignant lymphoma with a characteristic "fish-flesh" appearance. Note the lack of any significant thyroid gland parenchyma.

FIGURE 24-67

While lymphocytic thyroiditis can be seen in a few areas, there is a pseudofollicular to nodular effacement of the thyroid parenchyma by this mucosa-associated lymphoid tissue lymphoma.

often bulging, pale, with a "fish-flesh," uniform, homogeneous to mottled appearance (Figure 24-66). Foci of hemorrhage and necrosis are frequently noted. Extension into the surrounding soft tissues is common.

MICROSCOPIC FINDINGS

Lymphomas of the thyroid gland virtually always arise in the setting of chronic lymphocytic thyroiditis. There is a vaguely nodular to diffuse heterogeneous effacement of the thyroid gland (Figure 24-67). Perithyroidal extension into fat and skeletal muscle (Figure 24-68) is common, while lymphovascular invasion is more common in higher grade tumors. Atrophy and fibrosis are frequently present. Thyroid lymphoma is divided into two main groups: EMZBCL (30% to 40% of cases) and DLBCL (60% to 70% of cases). In cases of EMZBCL, the B-cell infiltrate is composed of a heterogenous population of atypical small lymphocytes, marginal zone (centrocyte-like) small cleaved cells, monocytoid B cells, scattered large immunoblasts and centroblast-like cells, and plasma cells (Figures 24-69 and 24-70). Monocytoid B cells are monotonous populations of atypical lymphoid cells with abundant, pale cytoplasm with lobulated or kidney-shaped nuclei. Reactive germinal centers, which may often demonstrate colonization or follicle lysis by the neoplastic cells, are invariably present. These cells yield a darker zone within follicles on low-power examination. However, the follicular architecture may recapitulate a follicle center lymphoma. Lymphoepithelial lesions, which represent infiltration of epithelial follicular structures by atypical neoplastic B cells, are a consistent feature and present in two forms: (1) rounded balls or masses, filling and distending the lumen of the thyroid follicles ("MALT balls"; Figure 24-71), or (2) single or

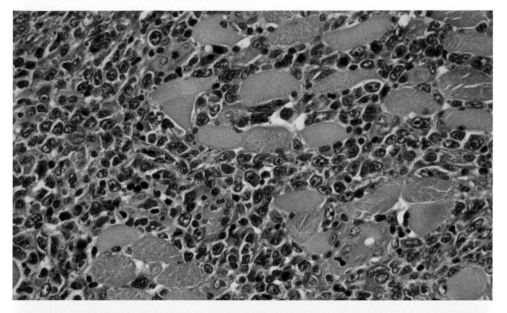

FIGURE 24-68

There are many plasmacytoid to centrocyte-like lymphoid cells infiltrating between skeletal muscle bundles.

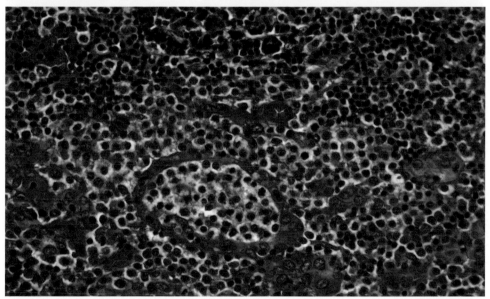

FIGURE 24-69

Atypical small lymphocytes, centrocyte-like cells, and monocytoid B cells are arranged in sheets and small clusters, growing into the follicular epithelium of the thyroid gland (*lower*).

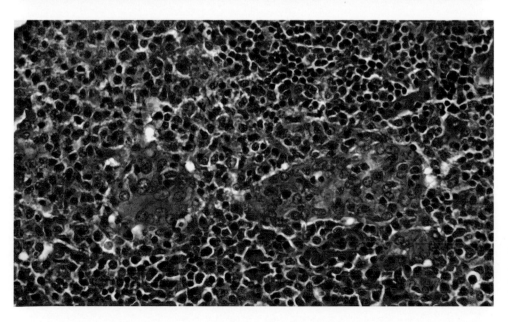

FIGURE 24-70

Monocytoid B cells have an "epithelioid" appearance. Note the thyroid cells in the center, surrounded by plasmacytoid cells (*lower*) and monocytoid cells (*upper*).

aggregated lymphocytes within or between follicular epithelial cells (Figure 24-72). Plasma cells (Figure 24-73) and plasmacytoid cells with Dutcher bodies or cytoplasmic immunoglobulin (Mott cells; Figure 24-74) are also seen, occasionally simulating a plasmacytoma. Concurrent disease within the gastrointestinal tract, salivary gland, lung, or breast may be present.

There may be single or multifocal areas of large cell transformation adjacent to the low-grade component, suggesting a transformation, transition, or "dedifferentiation." Alternatively, DLBCL may occur in the absence of any recognizable, preexistent low-grade areas (Figure 24-75). There are usually sheets of large cells that show a spectrum of cytologic features that resemble centroblasts, immunoblasts, monocytoid B cells and plasmacytoid cells (Figure 24-76). Focal Reed-Sternberg–like

(Figure 24-77) or Burkitt-like cells may be noted that are associated with brisk mitotic activity, apoptosis, and a "starry-sky" pattern (Figure 24-78). Vascular invasion is seen more commonly in higher grade tumors. The uninvolved thyroid parenchyma may have adenomatoid nodules, adenomas, or carcinoma (papillary much more often than follicular carcinoma).

Extramedullary plasmacytoma is rare, lacks evidence of bone marrow involvement, and shows only sheets or nodules of plasma cells, which may be atypical and show light chain restriction (monoclonality).

Classic Hodgkin lymphoma, nodular sclerosis subtype is the only one identified in the thyroid gland, but it is exceedingly rare. Classic Hodgkin-Reed-Sternberg (HRS) cells are identified in a variably cellular background diathesis of plasma cells, eosinophils, and

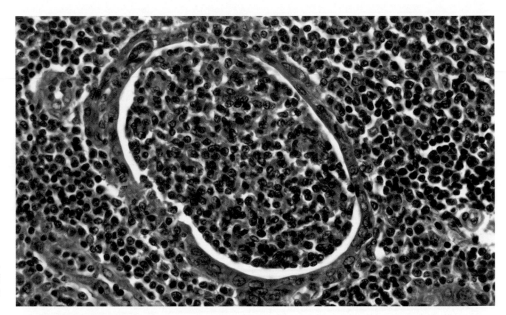

FIGURE 24-71

Masses of lymphoid cells are noted distending a thyroid follicle. This type of lymphoepithelial lesion is referred to as a "MALT ball."

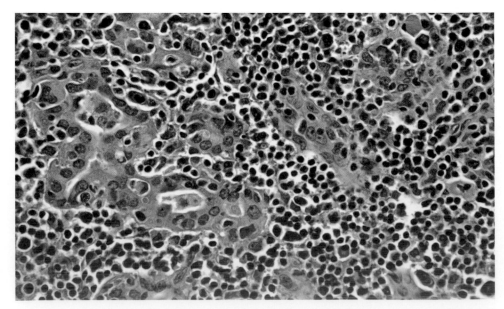

FIGURE 24-72

This lymphoepithelial lesion shows destruction of the follicular epithelium by the atypical lymphoid elements, which are seen effacing the background tissue.

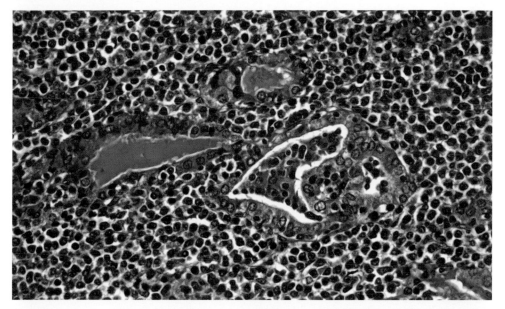

FIGURE 24-73

A prominent plasmacytoid differentiation is noted with Dutcher bodies (intranuclear cytoplasmic inclusions) in this mucosa-associated lymphoid tissue lymphoma. There is also a prominent lymphoepithelial lesion.

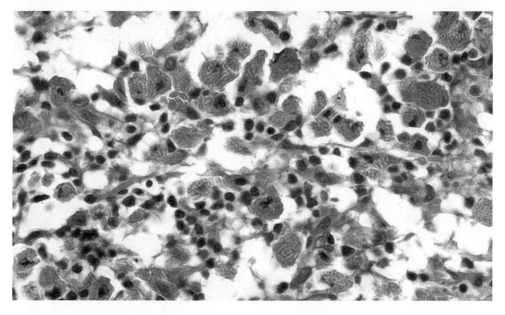

FIGURE 24-74

Crystalline type immunoglobulins are seen filling the cytoplasm of the neoplastic plasmacytoid cells of this mucosa-associated lymphoid tissue lymphoma.

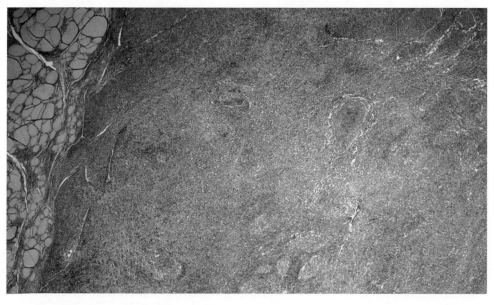

FIGURE 24-75

The thyroid tissue (*left*) has been replaced by a diffuse, large cell population of centroblastic-like B cells in this diffuse large B-cell lymphoma.

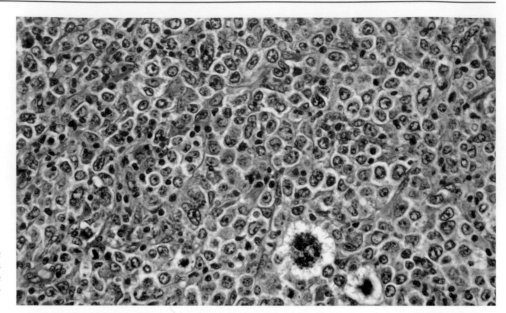

FIGURE 24-76

A sheet-like growth of centroblast-like immunoblasts and monocytoid cells with significant atypia in this diffuse large B-cell lymphoma. Note the pleomorphism and mitoses.

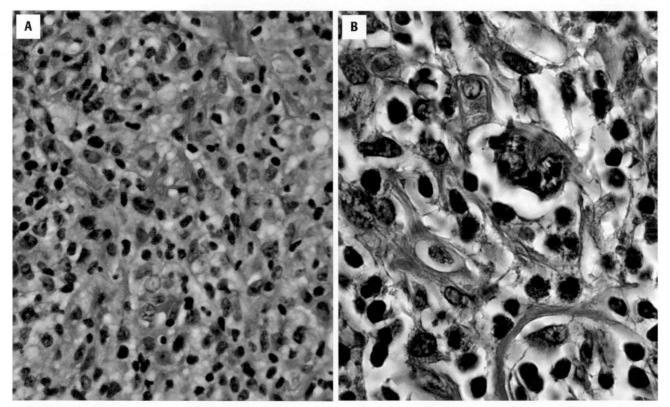

FIGURE 24-77

A, Large, cleaved cells are admixed with small cleaved lymphocytes in this diffuse large B-cell lymphoma (DLBCL). **B**, Eosinophils and Reed-Sternberg–like cells are focally identified in this DLBCL.

neutrophils. There is heavy birefringent collagen fibrosis, with appropriate lacunar and mummified variant HRS cells.

Follicular lymphoma is very uncommon and requires careful immunohistochemistry and molecular studies to prove the diagnosis. Lacking a mantle zone, there is a monotonous population of centrocytes and/or centroblasts without tingible body macrophages.

ANCILLARY STUDIES

IMMUNOHISTOCHEMICAL RESULTS

The B-cell immunophenotypes of EMZBCL and DLBCL are confirmed by immunoreactivity for CD20 (Figure 24-79), CD79a (Figure 24-80), PAX-5, and/or CD138. Bcl-2 reactivity in the neoplastic, colonizing

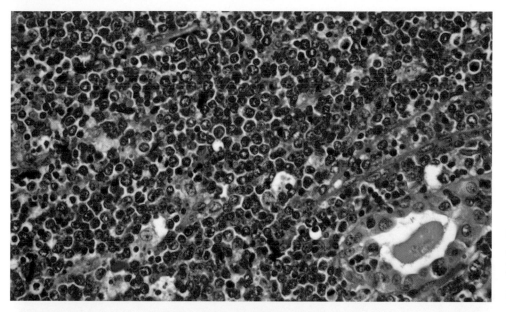

FIGURE 24-78

A Burkitt-like pattern shows brisk mitotic activity, apoptosis, and a "starry-sky" pattern with numerous tingible body macrophages in this diffuse large B-cell lymphoma. There is a thyroid follicle (*lower right*).

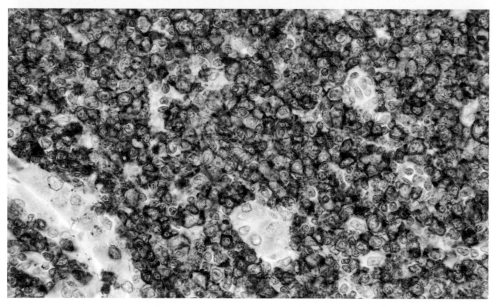

FIGURE 24-79

A CD20 strongly and diffusely highlights the large, cleaved cells in this lymphoma. Note the unstained thyroid follicular epithelium.

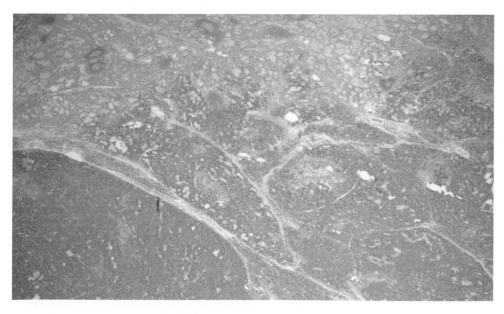

FIGURE 24-80

The chronic lymphocytic thyroiditis (*top*) shows focal CD79a staining, while the mucosa-associated lymphoid tissue lymphoma shows strong and diffuse staining of most of the cells.

B cells (but not in the residual, reactive germinal center cells) is also characteristic. Immunoglobulin light chain restriction for either κ or λ may be demonstrated (Figure 24-81), especially in the plasma cell or plasmacytoid component. Coexpression of CD43 with CD20 may be seen in a small percentage of EMZBCL. An antibody to cytokeratin will highlight the epithelial remnants in the lymphoepithelial lesions (Figure 24-82). Additional

molecular and cytogenetic studies can be performed to confirm the nature of the tumor.

FINE NEEDLE ASPIRATION

The full spectrum of dispersed, noncohesive admixture of lymphoid elements will often be present within the cellular aspirates from an EMZBCL (Figure 24-83),

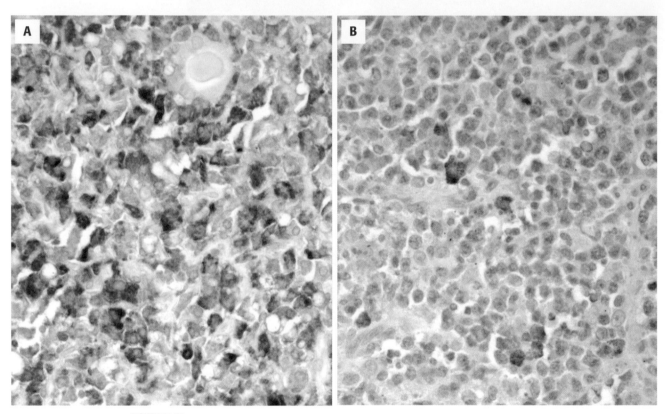

FIGURE 24-81

A, Kappa-restricted population of atypical lymphoid cells. **B**, Lambda highlights only a rare plasma cell.

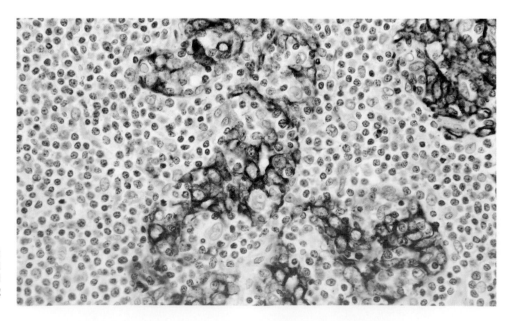

FIGURE 24-82

A malignant lymphoma immunostained for keratin highlights the residual thyroid follicles, which are extensively infiltrated by neoplastic lymphoid cells, creating lymphoepithelial lesions.

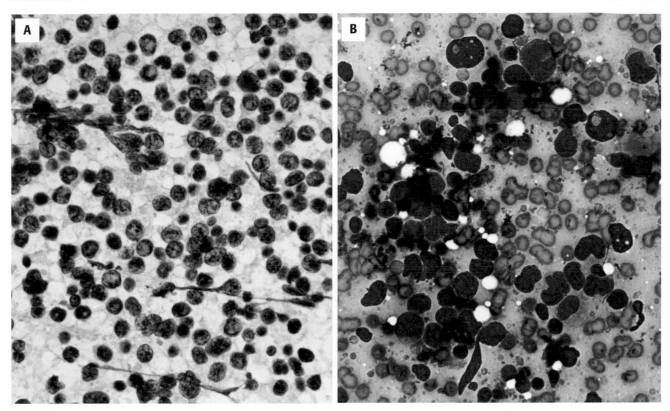

FIGURE 24-83
Fine needle aspiration smears are usually cellular without thyroid epithelial cells. **A**, Enlarged lymphoid cells with lymphoglandular bodies in the background (alcohol-fixed, Papanicolaou stain). **B**, Greatly enlarged atypical lymphoid cells with background lymphoglandular bodies (air-dried, Diff-Quik stain).

making separation from chronic lymphocytic thyroiditis nearly impossible. There may be a better yield if there is a single or dominant mass lesion rather than diffuse enlargement. However, there is usually an absence of tingible body macrophages in lymphoma. Similarly, thyroid follicular epithelium is usually absent. Moreover, the dyscohesive, monotonous population of large atypical cells (2 to 3 times the size of mature lymphocytes) with scant cytoplasm and large nuclei with vesicular nuclear chromatin and background lymphoglandular bodies suggest a diagnosis of DLBCL. Immunohistochemistry, flow cytometry, and/or Ig heavy chain gene rearrangements can be performed on aspiration material.

DIFFERENTIAL DIAGNOSIS

The distinction between EMZBCL and *chronic lymphocytic thyroiditis* may be difficult at times. In EMZBCL, the diffuse pattern, colonization of the benign germinal center, Dutcher bodies, and lymphoepithelial cells should help make the diagnosis. Usually there is no cytologic atypia and there may be oncocytic change in the thyroid follicular epithelial cells. In a few cases, however, immunohistochemical, flow cytometric or molecular genetic

analyses may be required. DLBCL may be indistinguishable from *undifferentiated carcinoma*, *melanoma* or *myeloid sarcoma* by histology alone and may require a more thorough antibody panel, including CD45RB, CD20, cytokeratin, S100 protein, Melan-A and HMB-45, and myelomonocytic markers (CD11B, CD14) to make the correct diagnosis. Rarely, an *ectopic thymoma* has both epithelial and lymphoid elements, but lacks lymphoepithelial lesions, a nondestructive pattern of growth and would be positive with CD5.

PROGNOSIS AND THERAPY

The prognosis of thyroid MALT-type lymphomas is very favorable in general, although the prognosis is stage and histology dependent. In general, localized (stage IE or IIE) tumors with a low grade histology have an excellent prognosis (>95% disease-specific 5-year survival) whereas those with either a large cell component or diffuse large B-cell type, have a worse overall survival (approximately 30% to 70% disease-specific 5-year survival for stage IVE versus IE, respectively) and are much more likely to die of disease. Poor prognostic features include age >65 years, males, vocal cord paralysis, DLBCL, high stage, extrathyroidal extension, vascular invasion, diffuse architecture, and a high mitotic rate. Nearly all patients with stage IVE die with disease. While surgery is used to "debulk" or decompress and obtain tissue for the diagnosis, chemotherapy and radiation (including hyperfractionation) are standard, with the regimen determined by the histologic grade and stage.

UNCOMMON THYROID NEOPLASMS

Mucoepidermoid Carcinoma

UNCOMMON THYROID GLAND EPITHELIAL MALIGNANCIES

Mucoepidermoid Carcinoma

- Low-grade malignant thyroid tumor with histology identical to salivary gland tumor
- Painless neck mass, managed by surgery, with an excellent prognosis
- Unencapsulated tumor with squamous/epidermoid cells and mucous cells

Squamous Cell Carcinoma

- Primary thyroid squamous cell carcinoma without mucocytes or direct extension from adjacent organs
- Older female patients who present with a rapidly enlarging neck mass
- Radical surgery and radiotherapy still have a poor prognosis
- Widely invasive tumor composed of cohesive sheets, ribbons and nests of cells with polygonal to spindle shape
- Keratinization, keratin pearl formation, high mitotic index

SETTLE

- A highly cellular biphasic tumor showing spindle-shaped epithelial cells that blend with glandular structures, showing primitive thymic differentiation
- Occurs in young patients with an asymptomatic thyroid mass
- Prolonged, indolent course after surgery
- Firm to hard, white-tan and fleshy, occasionally with cysts, up to 6 cm
- Spindle-shaped cells arranged in short, reticulated, intersecting and streaming, tight to loose fascicles or bundles which merge with epithelial cells separated into lobules by dense fibrosis
- Epithelial cells are arranged in glands, tubules, papillae or sheets
- Abrupt keratinization can be seen
- Delicate nuclear chromatin in both cell types
- Spindle and epithelial cells are keratin positive

CASTLE

- Primary thyroid gland malignancy that is architecturally and cytologically similar to thymic epithelial tumors
- Slightly more common in women, usually in the 5th decade
- Asymptomatic thyroid mass, often of the lower thyroid lobes
- Metastatic disease at presentation in ~30% of patients
- Prolonged, indolent course after surgery and radiation
- Firm to hard, white-tan and fleshy, up to 6 cm, often infiltrative tumor
- Solid, nests and lobules, with an infiltrative growth
- Epithelioid, syncytial cells with large vesicular-appearing nuclei, pleomorphism and prominent nucleoli
- Squamous differentiation is noted, often abrupt
- Dense fibrosis frequently associated with lymphocytes and plasma cells
- Positive with keratin and CD5

This rare, low-grade malignant thyroid tumor has a histologic appearance similar to the low-grade salivary gland counterpart. There are two histologic variants: mucoepidermoid carcinoma and sclerosing mucoepidermoid carcinoma with eosinophilia. While distinctive histologically, they have a similar indolent clinical behavior. Nearly all cases develop in the setting of chronic lymphocytic thyroiditis (LT), within which there is squamous metaplasia. Females are affected more often than males, with a mean age at presentation in the 5th to 7th decades of life. Patients present nonspecifically with a neck mass. Surgery is the treatment of choice, yielding a good long-term prognosis, although metastatic disease to lymph nodes can be seen.

Tumors are circumscribed but unencapsulated and predominantly composed of a solid mass. However, prominent cystic foci may be seen. The tumor is composed of intertwined cords and nests of cells within a fibrous stroma (Figure 24-84). As its name implies, the proliferation includes squamous cells admixed with mucocytes. The squamous cells have mild pleomorphism, increased nuclear:cytoplasmic ratio, round nuclei with prominent nucleoli, and eosinophilic cytoplasm. Horny pearl formation, individual cell keratinization, and intercellular bridges are present. Mucous cells have abundant clear- to foamy-appearing cytoplasm and peripherally located hyperchromatic nuclei. Ciliated cells may be seen. Hyaline bodies resembling colloid may be seen in the cytoplasm of mucocytes. Eosinophils may predominate. Intratumoral sclerosis composed of thick, acellular hyalinized bands of tissue can be seen. Psammoma bodies are occasionally present. Concurrent thyroid papillary carcinoma is seen in up to 50% of cases, and may show areas of blending-transition, even though it is considered a distinct tumor type. Mucicarmine will highlight intracytoplasmic and intraluminal mucin. The epidermoid cells will be positive with keratins (high and low molecular weight), p63 and CK5/6, while the mucocytes are mCEA positive. Thyroglobulin and TTF-1 may be focally positive. *BRAF* (V600E) mutation is not detected, but *MECT1/TORC1/CRTC1-MAML2* fusion transcript may be identified by RT-PCR. The differential diagnosis includes squamous metaplasia, epithelial cysts in lymphocytic thyroiditis, medullary carcinoma, primary squamous cell carcinoma, undifferentiated carcinoma, and carcinoma showing thymus-like differentiation (CASTLE).

Squamous Cell Carcinoma

A thyroid primary squamous cell carcinoma is composed entirely of squamous cells without mucocytes and without direct invasion from adjacent organs (larynx, esophagus). A history of radiation exposure is occasionally present. This tumor is thought to be derived from

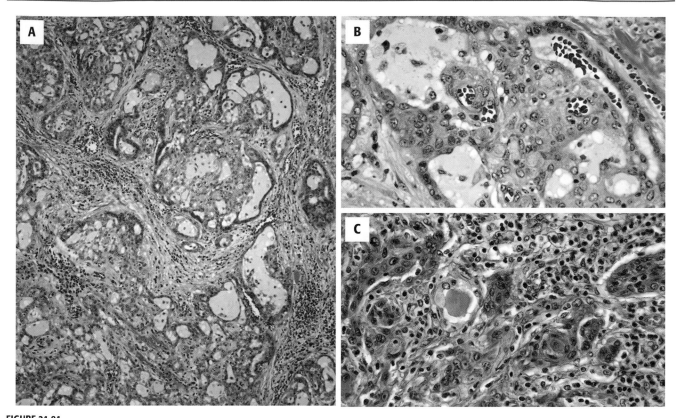

FIGURE 24-84
Mucoepidermoid carcinoma. **A**, Cysts and small glands with intervening fibrosis. **B**, Transitional and epidermoid cells and mucocytes are easily identified. **C**, There are a large number of eosinophils, along with areas of squamous and mucinous differentiation.

thyroid follicular epithelium, via squamous metaplasia compounded by additional genetic alterations resulting in malignant transformation. A rare tumor, females are affected more often than males (3:1), with a mean age at presentation in the 6th and 7th decades. Patients usually present with a rapidly enlarging neck mass after a long history of preexisting thyroid disease. Cervical lymph node enlargement is common.

Early radical resection yields the best outcome by debulking the tumor. Radical dose radiotherapy can be used, as radioiodine therapy does not work. Tumors follow a rapidly declining clinical course, with a very poor prognosis (mean survival: <1 year).

By definition, direct extension or metastasis must be excluded. The tumors are widely invasive and destructive, with extrathyroidal extension, soft tissue invasion, and both vascular and perineural invasion. Tumors are arranged in cohesive sheets, ribbons, or nests, with variable pleomorphism (Figure 24-85). The cells are polygonal, polyhedral and spindled, with keratinization and keratin pearl formation. There is usually a high mitotic index, including atypical forms. An inflammatory infiltrate (Hashimoto thyroiditis) and stromal desmoplasia are common. Other tumors may be present (papillary carcinoma is most common), and in these cases, a diagnosis of "with squamous differentiation" is usually used. Tumors are usually positive with cytokeratin,

CK5/6, CK19, and p63, while negative with thyroglobulin, CEA, calcitonin, and CD5. *Metastatic squamous cell carcinoma* can usually be excluded on clinical or radiographic grounds. Extensive *squamous metaplasia* lacks atypia, does not form a mass, is not infiltrative, and lacks necrosis. *CASTLE* shows a greater degree of tumor cell spindling, has more keloid-like collagen deposition and inflammatory cells, and is positive with CD5 and S100-A9.

THYMIC AND RELATED BRANCHIAL POUCH NEOPLASMS

This is a rare group of tumors that have spindle cells and thymic-like areas of differentiation. They are thought to arise from thymic rests adjacent to or within the thyroid gland or from branchial pouch remnants. Spindle cell tumor with thymus-like differentiation (SETTLE) occurs in young patients (mean, 15 to 20 years), with males affected more often than females (2:1). Patients usually have an asymptomatic neck mass. CASTLE is slightly more common in women than men (1.3:1) and tends to develop in adults in the 5th decade. An asymptomatic neck or thyroid mass, which may or may not be invasive at the time of presentation, is the most common clinical presentation. Metastatic disease can be seen in ~30% of patients.

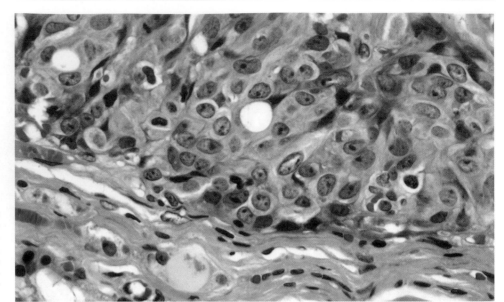

FIGURE 24-88

The thyroid epithelium is noted at the bottom of the image, separated from the neoplastic cells by fibrosis. Note the mitotic figure in the upper left quadrant in this carcinoma showing thymus-like differentiation, composed of large, polygonal, epithelioid cells with vesicular nuclear chromatin distribution.

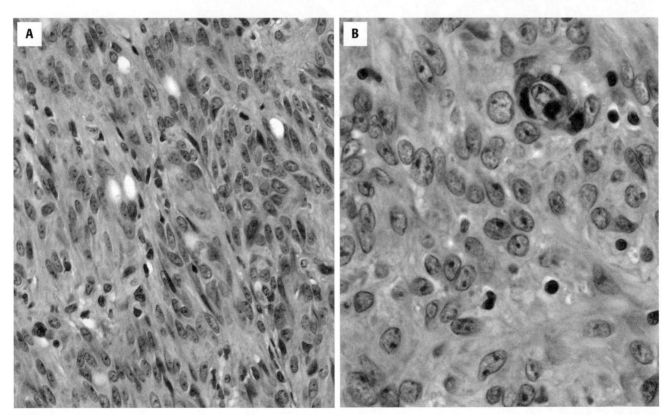

FIGURE 24-89

A, This carcinoma showing thymus-like differentiation (CASTLE) shows a syncytial arrangement of spindled cells. The nuclei are pale with small, but distinct nucleoli. **B**, This CASTLE shows the syncytial arrangement of epithelial cells with open, pale to vesicular nuclear chromatin distribution. There is a hint of "squamous pearl" formation. Nucleoli are easily identified, but are not prominent.

ANCILLARY STUDIES

In SETTLE, both the spindle cells and epithelial cells are cytokeratin, CAM5.2, CK7, CD117, and INI1 positive (Figure 24-90), while in CASTLE the tumor cells are keratin, p63, and CD5 positive (Figure 24-91). In both tumors, the cells are negative for thyroglobulin, TTF-1, calcitonin, carcinoembryonic antigen (CEA), EBER, S100 protein, synaptophysin, and CK20.

DIFFERENTIAL DIAGNOSIS

Thymic carcinoma, ectopic thymoma, synovial sarcoma, solitary fibrous tumor, teratoma, follicular den-

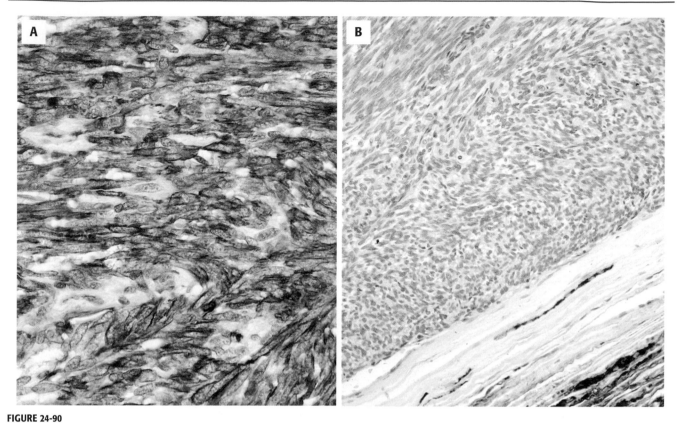

FIGURE 24-90

Keratin is strongly and diffusely immunoreactive in the neoplastic cells of a spindle cell tumor with thymus-like differentiation (**A**), while thyroglobulin is nonreactive (**B**).

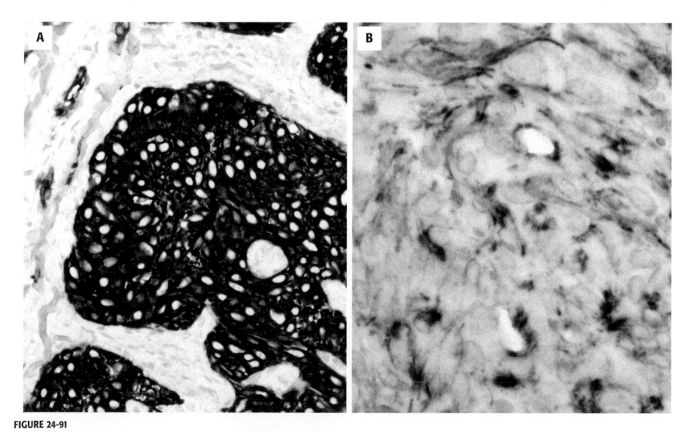

FIGURE 24-91

A carcinoma showing thymus-like differentiation shows strong keratin immunoreactivity (**A**), with a delicate immunoreaction with CD5 (**B**), confirming the thymic-like differentiation.

dritic cell sarcoma, spindle cell carcinoma, squamous cell carcinoma, medullary carcinoma, metastatic lymphoepithelial carcinoma, and undifferentiated carcinoma are all considered in the differential diagnosis of these thymic-like tumors. However, the distinct histologies of these tumors and their respective immunohistochemical profiles help with separation.

PROGNOSIS AND THERAPY

Due to the rare nature of these tumors, a definitive prognosis is difficult to predict, although most pursue a prolonged indolent course (~80% 10-year survival). Local recurrence and regional metastases have been reported more often in CASTLE (30%) than in SETTLE, with delayed metastases seen more often in SETTLE (up to 70% of cases). Surgical excision is the treatment of choice (including selected lymph node dissection and resection of all delayed metastases), with neoadjuvant chemotherapy and radiation occasionally used.

MESENCHYMAL TUMORS

Many different benign and malignant mesenchymal tumors can be seen in the thyroid gland with limited frequency.

Leiomyoma is a benign primary thyroid neoplasm composed of cells with distinct smooth muscle differentiation histologically. They develop from smooth muscle–walled vessels at the thyroid gland periphery. Usually, patients are young with an equal gender distribution. Tumors are small (mean, 2 cm), well-circumscribed, and unencapsulated with a smooth periphery. The cells are arranged in bundles or fascicles of bland smooth muscle fibers that intersect in an orderly fashion (Figure 24-92). Cells are spindled and blunt-ended or cigar-shaped, with centrally placed nuclei. Paranuclear cytoplasmic vacuoles are sometimes prominent. The tumor cells are positive with vimentin, SMA, MSA, and desmin.

Schwannoma is a benign neoplasm composed of cells with evidence of distinct peripheral nerve sheath differentiation histologically. They develop from the sympathetic and parasympathetic or possibly sensory nerves adjacent to the thyroid gland. All ages are affected with an equal gender distribution. Tumors are well circumscribed or encapsulated. The tumor cells show densely packed spindle cell areas (Antoni A) adjacent to loosely arranged, hypocellular degenerated areas (Antoni B; Figure 24-93). The slender spindle cells are arranged in interlacing fascicles with fibrillar cytoplasmic extensions. Nuclear palisading (Verocay bodies) may be seen. The nuclei are wavy and spindled, lacking atypia. There are usually small to medium-sized blood vessels with heavily hyalinized walls. The tumor cells

UNCOMMON THYROID GLAND MESENCHYMAL NEOPLASMS

Leiomyoma
- Primary thyroid gland benign smooth muscle tumor
- Young patients, who present with small tumors
- Bundles or fascicles of bland smooth muscle, intersecting with blunt-ended, cigar-shaped nuclei and paranuclear vacuoles

Schwannoma
- Primary thyroid gland benign peripheral nerve sheath tumor
- Densely packed spindle cell areas adjacent to loosely arranged hypocellular areas
- Slender spindle cells with fibrillar cytoplasm and wavy-spindled nuclei
- Medium-sized vessels with hyalinized walls

Solitary Fibrous Tumor
- Collagen-producing spindle cells arranged in characteristic vascular pattern
- Usually middle-aged female patients
- Large tumors with solid, white-gray-tan cut appearance
- Cellular mesenchymal tumor with syncytial arrangement of bland, spindled and monotonous cells with elongated slender nuclei
- Separated by bundles of collagen and delicate open-patulous vascular spaces

Angiosarcoma
- Primary thyroid gland malignant neoplasm of endothelial cell differentiation
- Increased in areas with iodine deficiency and in occupational exposure to polymeric materials usually in older patients, with females >> males (4:1)
- Poor prognosis with high metastatic rate
- Variegated cut surface with extensive hemorrhage and necrosis, showing invasion
- Freely anastomosing vascular channels with irregular, cleft-like to patulous vascular spaces lined by large, epithelioid polygonal cells
- Neolumen formation with erythrocytes, vesicular nuclear chromatin, prominent macronucleoli
- High mitoses and hemosiderin-laden macrophages

Leiomyosarcoma
- Primary malignant thyroid gland neoplasm with smooth muscle differentiation
- Thought to arise from large vessel walls at the gland periphery
- Older patients who have a poor prognosis
- Large, nodular to bosselated tumor with significant invasion
- Entrapped follicles within the highly cellular, bundles or fascicles of pleomorphic spindled cells, blunt-ended, hyperchromatic nuclei, with perinuclear vacuoles
- Positive with vimentin, actin and desmin, with a high Ki-67 index

Malignant Peripheral Nerve Sheath Tumor
- Primary malignant thyroid gland neoplasm showing peripheral nerve sheath differentiation
- Older patients, who usually have a poor outcome
- Arising from peripheral nerves, they invade, entrap, and destroy the thyroid parenchyma, with significant vascular invasion and necrosis
- Highly cellular, tightly packed fascicles giving a herringbone appearance
- Highly pleomorphic spindled cells with fibrillary cytoplasmic extensions

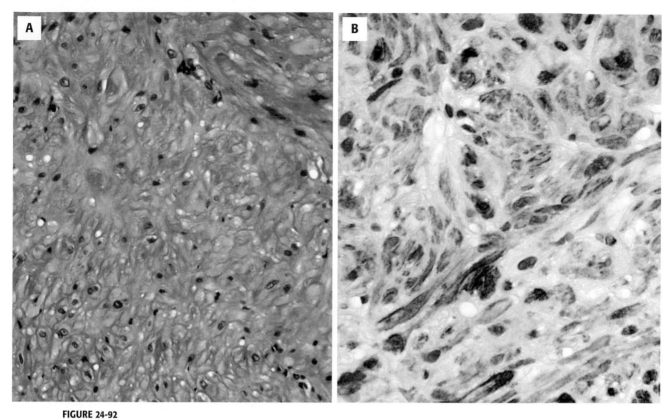

FIGURE 24-92

A, A leiomyoma composed of cytologically bland spindled tumor cells with vacuoles. **B**, Strong and diffuse actin immunoreactivity.

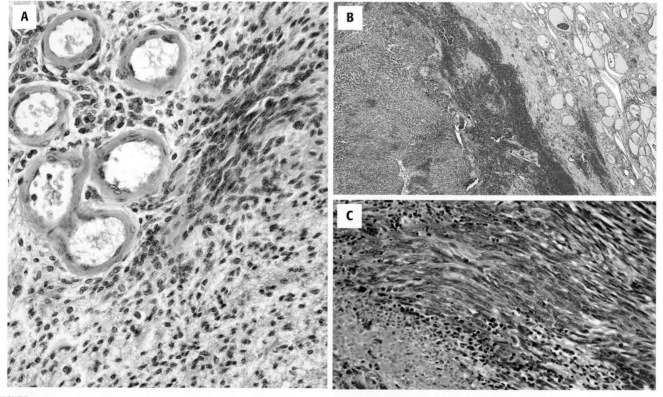

FIGURE 24-93

A, A schwannoma with spindled cells associated with loosely arranged hypocellular areas and heavily hyalinized vessels. **B**, A highly cellular spindled cell malignant peripheral nerve sheath tumor (MPNST) within the thyroid gland. **C**, The fascicles of this MPNST are associated with necrosis and mitoses.

show strong and diffuse S100 protein and vimentin immunoreactivity.

Solitary fibrous tumor is a mesenchymal tumor composed of collagen-producing spindle cells arranged in a characteristic vascular pattern. Females are affected more often than males, usually as middle-aged patients. Tumors are relatively large (mean, 4.5 cm), well circumscribed and frequently encapsulated, with a firm, solid, white-gray-tan cut appearance. Histologically, they are variegated, cellular, mesenchymal tumors, showing hypocellular areas alternating with hypercellular areas. The tumor cells are spindled, bland, and monotonous with elongated, slender nuclei arranged in a syncytial, nonspecific growth pattern (Figure 24-94). The cells are separated by bundles of keloid-like collagen, and delicate, open to patulous vascular spaces. Extravasated erythrocytes, inflammatory cells, and mast cells are common. The neoplastic cells are immunoreactive with vimentin, CD34 (Figure 24-94), CD99, and bcl-2, with weak, variable reactions to actin. Pertinent negatives include S100 protein, CD117, keratin, ALK1, desmin, and other muscle markers.

Angiosarcoma is a primary thyroid gland malignant tumor of endothelial cell differentiation. There is an increased incidence in regions with dietary iodine deficiency, especially in alpine areas of central Europe, and in patients with significant occupational exposure to industrial vinyl chloride and other polymeric materials. The tumors are thought to arise from endothelium and not follicular epithelial cells. Tumors usually present in the 7th decade of life, with women affected more often than men (4:1). Most patients have a long history of goiter, with a painless mass. Rarely, there may be a rapidly growing mass with pressure symptoms. It is important to realize that there may be severe bleeding at primary or metastatic sites which may complicate surgery. Total thyroidectomy is the treatment of choice, with palliative chemotherapy. Adjuvant radiotherapy, frequently administered as brachytherapy with a radiation sensitizer may be used. The overall prognosis is poor, with the majority of patients dying from disease in <6 months. Distant metastases develop to lung, gastrointestinal tract, and bone.

The cut surface is variegated with extensive hemorrhage and necrosis within tumors that tend to be large (up to 12 cm). The periphery is irregular, with blending and invasion of the thyroid parenchyma. Freely anastomosing vascular channels are arranged in solid, spindled, papillary, and pseudoglandular patterns. Tumor necrosis and hemorrhage are usually seen throughout the tumor. There are increased mitoses, including atypical forms. Hemosiderin-laden macrophages are common. There are irregular, cleft-like to patulous vascular channels lined by large, epithelioid polygonal cells (Figure 24-95). There is abundant eosinophilic to vacuolated cytoplasm surrounding round nuclei with vesicular chromatin and prominent macronucleoli. Neolumen formation with erythrocytes within the lumen may be seen. The lesional cells are positive with vascular endothelial markers, including CD31, FVIII-RAg, CD34, and ULEX-1. In a number of cases, keratin may be positive also. It is important to not overinterpret diffusion artifacts. The differential diagnosis includes undifferentiated carcinoma, degenerative adenomatoid nodules, post-FNA artifacts, and even metastatic angiosarcoma.

Leiomyosarcoma (LMS) is a malignant primary thyroid neoplasm composed of cells with distinct smooth muscle differentiation histologically. This is the malignant counterpart of leiomyoma. Patients tend to be older, presenting with a mass at the thyroid gland periphery. Patients usually have a poor prognosis. The tumors are large (up to 12 cm), showing a nodular to bosselated outer surface, and significant soft tissue invasion.

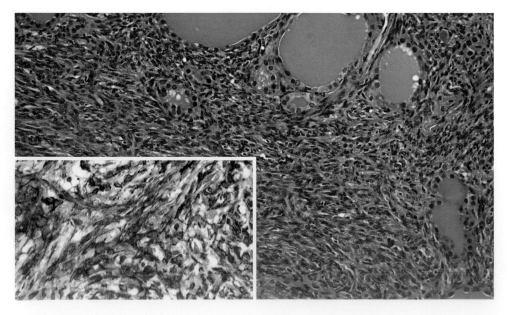

FIGURE 24-94

A solitary fibrous tumor infiltrates around the uninvolved thyroid follicles (*lower right*). The spindle cell population is separated by bands of collagen. Inset demonstrates positivity with CD34.

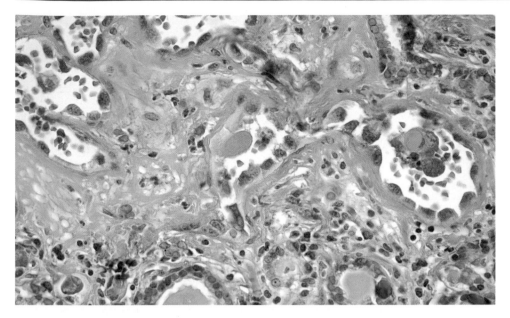

FIGURE 24-95

Pleomorphic endothelial cells lining irregular vascular spaces are the hallmark of angiosarcoma. Note the entrapped thyroid follicular epithelial cells (*bottom*).

There is often entrapment and destruction of thyroid follicles. Perineural and vascular invasion are frequently present, along with tumor necrosis. The tumors are highly cellular, arranged in bundles or disordered fascicles of spindled cells with centrally placed, hyperchromatic, blunt-ended, cigar-shaped nuclei. Perinuclear cytoplasmic vacuoles are quite characteristic (Figure 24-96). Nuclear pleomorphism is usually present, along with increased mitoses. The neoplastic cells are positive with vimentin, SMA, MSA, and desmin, showing a high Ki-67 index. The differential includes medullary carcinoma, undifferentiated carcinoma, and direct extension or metastatic leiomyosarcoma.

Malignant peripheral nerve sheath tumor (MPNST) of the thyroid gland is a malignant neoplasm composed of cells with evidence of distinct peripheral nerve sheath differentiation histologically. This is the malignant counterpart of schwannoma. Most patients have a poor outcome and die from disease. All ages are affected, although patients are usually older at initial presentation. Syndrome-associated tumors tend to develop in patients of younger age. There is an equal gender distribution. Tumors are tan to white and glistening with a "neural" appearance, sometimes showing thyroid gland effacement, cystic change, and necrosis. They may be seen arising from the perithyroidal nerves. The tumors arise within the thyroid gland, invading, entrapping, and destroying the parenchyma. Vascular invasion may be present. The tumors are highly cellular, arranged in tightly packed fascicles that are woven into a vague herringbone pattern, with only isolated Antoni B areas. The cells are spindled, with fibrillar cytoplasmic extensions arranged in a loose background. Pleomorphism, necrosis, increased

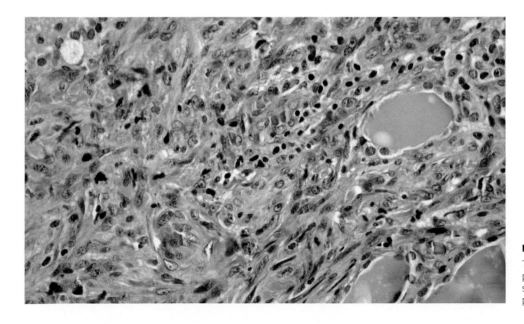

FIGURE 24-96

The thyroid follicles are destroyed by this pleomorphic spindled cell population, showing numerous mitotic figures in this primary leiomyosarcoma.

mitoses (Figure 24-93), and atypical mitoses are all easily identified. The cells are strongly positive with vimentin and p53, showing variable S100 protein reaction (strong, to focal and weak). Other markers are negative. The differential diagnosis includes Riedel thyroiditis, undifferentiated carcinoma, medullary carcinoma, metastatic melanoma, and other sarcomas (both primary and metastatic). Other melanoma markers (HMB-45, Melan-A) should be positive in melanoma.

■ METASTATIC NEOPLASMS

Tumors that occur in the thyroid as a result of lymphovascular spread from distant sites are considered as metastatic disease. While not covered in this section, it should be noted that direct extension into the thyroid from adjacent organs (larynx [squamous cell carcinoma], trachea, esophagus, lymph nodes [lymphoma], soft tissues) may sometimes need to be included in the differential diagnosis of thyroid masses. The thyroid gland is richly vascularized, predisposing to relatively high frequency of metastases.

Seen in up to 7.5 % of surgically removed glands, up to 25 % of autopsied patients with disseminated malignancies will have thyroid gland metastases. This may be due to advances in radiographic techniques, increased use of FNA, or improved treatments resulting in longer survival. In clinical series, metastatic deposits are identified at a higher frequency in abnormal glands: those with adenomatoid nodules, thyroiditis, and follicular neoplasms. Furthermore, the metastatic deposits may be found within primary thyroid tumors (i.e., metastatic renal cell carcinoma to a thyroid papillary carcinoma). All ages are affected, but metastases are more common in older patients (mean, 62 years), and in females more often than in males (1.2:1). A rapidly enlarging thyroid mass may be the presenting sign, although more often the underlying thyroid disease may result in the clinical presentation. In a number of patients (up to 40 %), the thyroid gland metastatic deposit is the initial presentation of the occult primary tumor. The most common primary sites in order of frequency are kidney (Figure 24-97), lung (Figure 24-98), breast (Figure 24-99), stomach, prostate, and skin (melanoma). Kidney tumors are the most likely to present with an occult primary, while also having the longest latency period. Ultrasound can be used to show multifocal disease and bilateral metastases, and to guide biopsy.

CLINICAL FEATURES

METASTATIC NEOPLASMS—DISEASE FACT SHEET

Definition
- Lymphovascular spread from distant sites to the thyroid gland, which is richly vascularized, predisposing to metastatic deposits

Incidence and Location
- Up to 25% in autopsied patients and 7.5% in clinical series
- Increased in peripheral vascular spaces or in other tumors

Morbidity and Mortality
- Usually poor clinical outcome, although exceptions occur

Gender, Race, and Age Distribution
- Female > male, although tumor type specific
- Usually older patients

Clinical Features
- Rapidly enlarging thyroid mass, although sometimes a thyroid disorder may be the clinical presentation
- In up to 40% of patients, the thyroid presentation is the initial manifestation of an occult primary

Prognosis and Therapy
- Usually poor and determined by the underlying primary
- When limited to the thyroid gland, surgery may yield a prolonged survival

PATHOLOGIC FEATURES

METASTATIC NEOPLASMS—PATHOLOGIC FEATURES

Gross Findings
- Usually multifocal and bilateral
- Can metastasize to preexisting thyroid lesions

Microscopic Findings
- Usually resemble the primary tumor, although dedifferentiation can occur
- Kidney > lung > breast > stomach, prostate > skin
- Lymphovascular channels at thyroid gland periphery show tumor most frequently
- Distinctly different architecture and histology from primary thyroid neoplasms (although clear cell metastatic renal cell carcinoma and metastatic neuroendocrine carcinomas may cause difficulty)

Immunohistochemical Results
- Metastatic tumors have unique immunohistochemical profiles, distinctly different from thyroid primaries (caution with TTF-1 results)

Pathologic Differential Diagnosis
- Clear cell adenoma/carcinoma, medullary carcinoma, lymphoma, direct extension

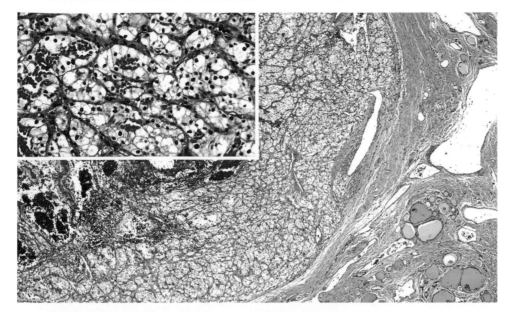

FIGURE 24-97

An encapsulated metastatic clear cell renal cell carcinoma to the thyroid gland may mimic a primary thyroid neoplasm with clear cells. Inset shows erythrocytes in the center of pseudoglands. Prominent cell borders and small hyperchromatic nuclei are present.

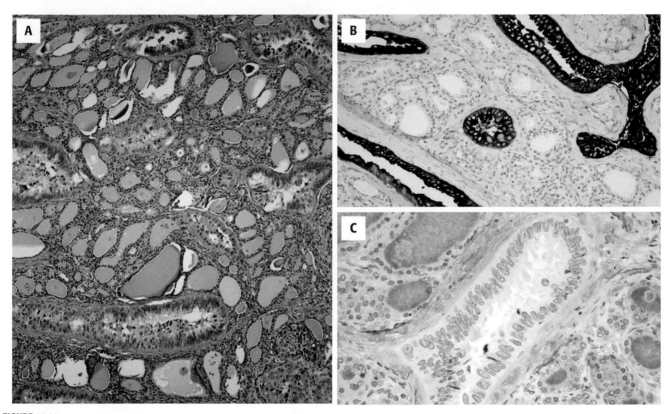

FIGURE 24-98

A, Metastatic lung adenocarcinoma to the thyroid gland within multiple intravascular channels. **B**, Strong and diffuse monoclonal carcinoembryonic antigen in the metastatic tumor. **C**, Thyroglobulin is negative in the tumor but positive in the adjacent follicles.

GROSS FINDINGS

Multifocal and bilateral disease is more common, but in clinically significant metastatic deposits, a unilateral solitary mass is more likely to result in clinical evaluation. There is a predilection for larger vessels at the thyroid gland periphery. Metastatic deposits can be large, up to 15 cm in maximum dimension.

MICROSCOPIC FINDINGS

The thyroid gland is a richly vascularized endocrine organ, hence susceptible to metastatic deposits. For the most part, the metastatic deposits morphologically resemble the primary site, with rare examples of more poorly differentiated tumor in the thyroid. Close examination of the periphery of the thyroid gland, immediately adjacent to the capsule where the vasculature is the most dense, will help to identify intravascular metastatic deposits. Fibrous septa within the gland are widened by tumor within lymphatic channels (Figures 24-98 and 24-99). When the tumor deposits form a mass lesion, they usually have an architecture and cytomorphology distinct from thyroid primaries. Metastatic clear cell renal cell carcinoma is an exception (Figure 24-97). Carcinomas are most common (~80%), while leiomyosarcoma and melanoma are the most common noncarcinomas. Metastatic neuroendocrine (small cell) carcinomas may also pose some difficulty, as they may resemble a medullary thyroid carcinoma; or they may also be TTF-1 immunoreactive if they are from the lung.

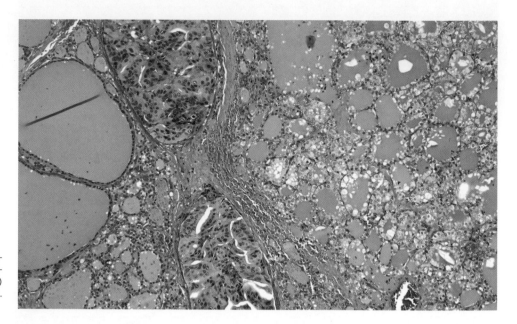

FIGURE 24-99

The vascular spaces are filled with neoplastic cells that have a different appearance from the adenomatoid nodules (*left*) and the papillary thyroid carcinoma (*right*). This is a metastatic breast carcinoma.

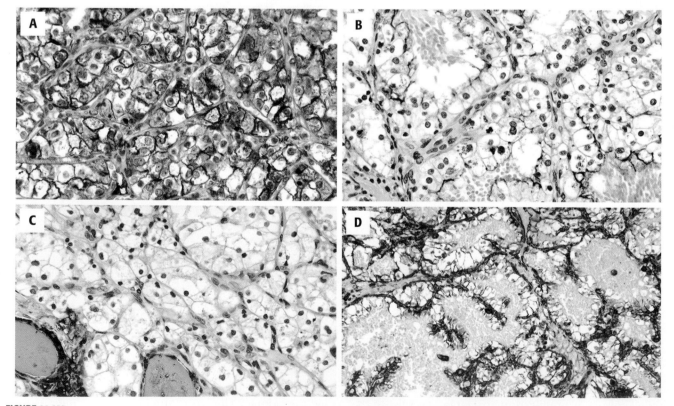

FIGURE 24-100

An immunohistochemical panel can help to separate metastatic from primary neoplasms. This renal cell carcinoma is reactive with CD10 (**A**), negative for thyroglobulin (**C**), and positive with EMA (**B**) and vimentin (**D**).

ANCILLARY STUDIES

Primary thyroid follicular tumors will usually be thyroglobulin, CK7 and TTF-1 immunoreactive, while C-cell–derived tumors will be calcitonin and chromogranin reactive. While there are exceptions, metastatic tumors will not be thyroglobulin reactive (Figures 24-100 and 24-101), and only rare examples of calcitonin immunoreactivity in metastatic neuroendocrine neoplasms are known. Diffusion or entrapment of follicular epithelium within metastatic tumors must be excluded. FNA may help to confirm malignancy but it is frequently misinterpreted as to type. In general, the smears are cellular with two distinct cell populations (Figure 24-102). Molecular studies can be helpful (*RET/PTC*, *PAX8/PPAR*γ, *BRAF*, *RAS*), although there are overlapping results with several tumors.

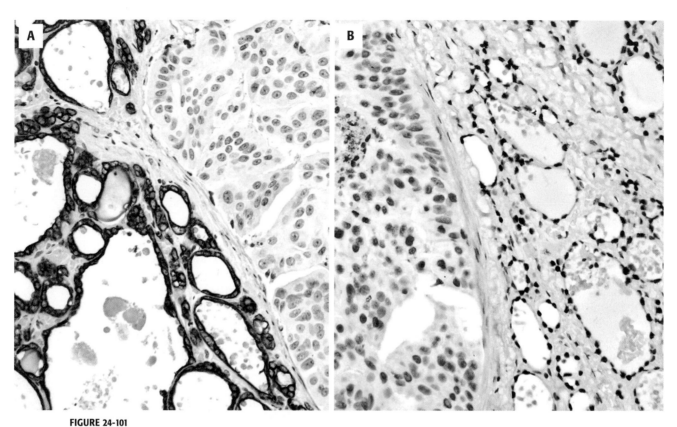

FIGURE 24-101

A metastatic breast carcinoma is nonreactive with thyroglobulin (**A**) and TTF-1 (**B**). The tumor cells are within a vascular space.

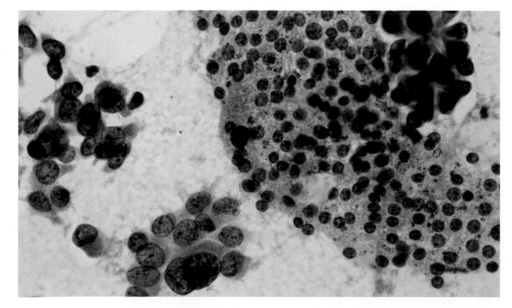

FIGURE 24-102

Two distinct populations are present: the thyroid follicular epithelium and the greatly enlarged, pleomorphic adenocarcinoma population (from a lung primary) (alcohol-fixed, Papanicolaou stain).

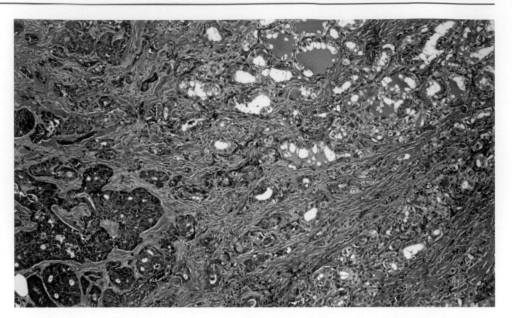

FIGURE 24-103

The adenoid cystic carcinoma is directly invading from a larynx primary, colliding with a primary thyroid papillary carcinoma.

DIFFERENTIAL DIAGNOSIS

A solitary metastatic renal cell carcinoma may be difficult to separate from the clear cell change seen in follicular adenomas or carcinomas, and more rarely in papillary and medullary carcinoma. The prominent vascularity, glandular lumina filled with erythrocytes, lack of colloid, sharp intercellular borders, and small, hyperchromatic nuclei favor a renal cell carcinoma. The neoplastic cells are renal cell carcinoma, CD10, and EMA immunoreactive, while nonreactive for TTF-1 or thyroglobulin. The latter can have diffusion artifacts from the surrounding thyroid parenchyma, requiring careful interpretation. Direct extension from adjacent organs is usually radiographically and clinically distinctive (Figure 24-103).

PROGNOSIS AND THERAPY

For the most part, the outcome is determined by the underlying primary and, almost by dint of metastases, correlates with a poor prognosis. However, if metastatic disease is limited to the thyroid, surgery can result in prolonged survival, especially for renal cell carcinoma, a primary tumor known for capricious behavior. Therefore, surgery is advocated if the tumor is slow growing or it is an isolated metastasis.

SUGGESTED READINGS

The complete suggested readings list is available online at www.expertconsult.com.

25

Non-Neoplastic Lesions of the Parathyroid Gland

■ **Lester D. R. Thompson**

■ GENERAL CONSIDERATIONS

There are a variable number of glands (2 to 10), but usually four are present, symmetrically arranged within the upper and lower poles of the bilateral thyroid gland. About 5% of people have more than four glands. The glands are usually soft and pliable and measure <0.5 cm (5 mm) with a combined weight of ~120 to 140 mg. It is agreed that no single gland should be >60 mg, although the lower glands are often slightly larger than the upper glands. Embryologically, the upper pair arise from the 4th branchial pouch, while the lower pair arise from the 3rd branchial pouch. Notably, glands can be found anywhere along the normal route of migration, resulting in glands embedded within the thymus, pericardium, esophagus, and mediastinum.

The parathyroid gland is composed of four cell types:

- The *chief cell* (6 to 8 microns), a small polygonal cell with central round nuclei and abundant cytoplasmic secretory granules, is the basic functional cell involved in parathyroid hormone (parathormone [PTH]) secretion.
- The *oxyphilic* or *oncocytic cell* (12 microns), is slightly larger than chief cells with abundant granular cytoplasm, ultrastructurally shown to be packed with mitochondria. These cells increase in number as the patient ages and tend to occur in nodules; its function is not entirely known.
- The *water-clear cell* (which is quite rare) has well-defined cell borders and abundant clear cytoplasm due to excessive glycogen.
- *Adipocytes,* which also increase with age, compose up to 80% of the cellular mass.

These cells can be arranged in cords, sheets, and pseudoglandular or pseudoacinar patterns.

In short, the principal function of the parathyroid glands is calcium homeostasis, briefly discussed here (spatial constraints limit this discussion). Calcium homeostasis is maintained within narrow limits (~8 to 10 mg/dL) by the balance between variables increasing serum calcium (dietary intake, intestinal absorption, and bone resorption) and those decreasing serum calcium (bone accretion and urinary/fluid excretion). Nearly 99% of calcium is stored in the skeletal system, and osteoclastic resorption is most important. The three most important hormones are PTH, calcitonin (secreted by thyroid C cells), and vitamin D.

PTH is a polypeptide hormone (84–amino acid residues; the N-terminal is active, while the C-terminal is assayed) that increases blood calcium levels by stimulating osteoclastic resorption of bone and decreasing urinary excretion of calcium, while increasing renal phosphate excretion. This results in hypophosphatemia and can cause metabolic acidosis due to inhibition of bicarbonate (HCO_3^-). The half-life of PTH is 20 to 30 minutes. Abnormal or decreased function of the parathyroid glands results in disorders of calcium metabolism, characterized by too little (e.g., osteomalacia, pseudohypoparathyroidism) or too much (e.g., milk-alkali syndrome, calcinosis) calcium. PTH also stimulates production of 1,25-dihydroxy-cholecalciferol (calcitriol), the hormonally active form of vitamin D, which increases the uptake of calcium from the gut, decreases urinary excretion of calcium, and increases the release of calcium from bone.

Parathyroid non-neoplastic disorders also include aplasia, cysts, parathyroiditis, and hyperplasia. This discussion will be limited to hyperplasia.

Hyperparathyroidism is a state of elevated serum PTH as a result of excessive secretion. It is separated into primary, secondary, and tertiary, with primary hyperparathyroidism caused, most commonly, by adenoma (80%), followed by hyperplasia (15%), and carcinoma (5%). The inappropriately increased PTH is due to an intrinsic abnormality in the gland(s) rather than a known stimulus for PTH secretion. In contrast, most hyperplasia results from secondary hyperparathyroidism, in which there is an increase in parathyroid parenchymal cell mass within multiple glands in response to a known clinical stimulus for increased secretion of PTH, such as chronic renal failure, malabsorption, and abnormalities of vitamin D metabolism. It is usually characterized by hypocalcemia and hyperphosphatemia. Similarly, tertiary hyperparathyroidism is generally characterized by four-gland hyperplasia in a state of autonomous hypersecretion.

■ PRIMARY CHIEF CELL HYPERPLASIA

Primary chief cell hyperplasia is a non-neoplastic increase in the parenchymal cell mass within multiple parathyroid glands without a known clinical stimulus for increased PTH secretion. There is an annual incidence of approximately 0.04/1,000 persons/year in the United States.

CLINICAL FEATURES

About 15% of all primary hyperparathyroidism is caused by primary chief cell hyperplasia. Women are affected much more commonly than men (3:1), with the overall incidence increasing with age (especially in

PRIMARY CHIEF CELL HYPERPLASIA—DISEASE FACT SHEET

Definition
- Non-neoplastic increase in parathyroid parenchymal cell mass within all parathyroid tissue without a known stimulus

Incidence and Location
- Approximately 40/1 million population per year

Morbidity and Mortality
- Calcium metabolism abnormality
- Cardiovascular disease may cause death

Gender, Race, and Age Distribution
- Female > male (3:1)
- Adults, 50 to 70 years

Clinical Features
- 20% may be familial
- Asymptomatic, discovered during multichannel analyzer studies
- If symptomatic: fatigue, lethargy, anorexia, weakness, vomiting, depression, polyuria, polydipsia, hypertension
- "Bones, stones, abdominal moans" not seen often
- Nephrolithiasis, nephrocalcinosis
- Biochemical findings include elevated calcium, decreased inorganic phosphorus, and increased parathyroid hormone levels

Prognosis and Therapy
- Excellent, although recurrences occur (~15%)
- Surgery with autotransplantation

postmenopausal women). The mean age at presentation is the 6th decade. Most patients present with sporadic disease (80%), although ~20% of patients have familial disease (most commonly, multiple endocrine neoplasia [MEN] syndromes). MEN1 (Wermer syndrome) is the most common syndrome, with nearly 90% of patients having parathyroid hyperplasia. The MEN1 gene is localized on chromosome 11q13. Up to ~40% of patients with MEN2A (Sipple syndrome) have parathyroid proliferative disease, but it is rare in MEN2B. Patients may also present as part of autosomal dominant familial hyperparathyroidism without other endocrine abnormalities.

A fair number of patients are asymptomatic, the disorder discovered incidentally during routine multiphasic screening for other reasons. The presentation is often varied but vague, including fatigue, lethargy, anorexia, weakness, nausea, vomiting, constipation, polyuria, polydipsia, hypertension, arthralgias, and psychiatric symptoms. The classic triad of "bones, stones, and abdominal moans" is not commonly seen in modern care but refers to osteitis fibrosa cystica (brown tumor of bone), kidney stones, and peptic ulcer disease, respectively. Workup often reveals nephrocalcinosis, nephrolithiasis, and metastatic calcifications. Psychiatric or mental changes are frequent and include emotional instability, depression, psychosis, and confusion. Symptoms relate specifically to the degree (serum level) and duration of calcium elevation. Rarely, patients will present with a neck mass.

Biochemical findings include an elevation of serum ionized calcium levels, with corresponding decrease in serum inorganic phosphorus concentrations and associated high serum alkaline phosphatase. Serum PTH levels, using the intact hormone assay, will usually be increased above the normal range of 210 to 310 pg/mL. Additionally, there will be a high urine calcium, cyclic adenosine monophosphate, hydroxyproline, and phosphate.

RADIOLOGIC FEATURES

Technetium-99m sestamibi (^{99m}Tc sestamibi) imaging has gained significant favor as the preferred technique for detecting the topographic location of parathyroid tissue (Figure 25-1). However, the technique is limited in detecting hyperplasia, with greater clinical utility for detecting adenoma or carcinoma. In general, radiographic studies are primarily used in the setting of recurrent disease after failed surgery. Single-photon emission computed tomography with the use of ^{99m}Tc sestamibi as the radiotracer, especially when combined with computed tomography, can help with preoperative localization. Unusual locations of (ectopic) parathyroid tissue may be identified with magnetic resonance imaging using gadolinium and fat suppression techniques. Hyperplasia, however, does not enhance as much with gadolinium as

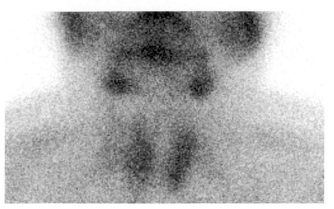

FIGURE 25-1

A delayed ⁹⁹ᵐTc sestamibi image demonstrates uneven, increased uptake in all glands, consistent with hyperplasia. *(Courtesy of Dr W. Chen.)*

does an adenoma. Ultrasound (US), when used by an experienced investigator, can be a good alternative if scintigraphic studies are inconclusive. Furthermore, US may be used to guide fine needle aspiration (FNA) or guide venous sampling to determine PTH levels.

PATHOLOGIC FEATURES

GROSS FINDINGS

In hyperplasia, all four glands will be affected, although sometimes not to the same degree, creating uneven or nodular hyperplasia or asymmetric enlargement. At least two glands *should* be sampled, including a "normal" gland to accurately separate adenoma and hyperplasia. However, with significant improvements in radiographic studies and intraoperative rapid PTH assessments, reliable and accurate separation may be

---

PRIMARY CHIEF CELL HYPERPLASIA—PATHOLOGIC FEATURES

Gross Findings

- All glands affected, although not equally (at least two glands are sampled for accurate diagnosis)
- Diffuse or nodular enlargement
- Soft, tan-brown glands

Microscopic Findings

- Variance between glands is common, but all are affected
- Parenchyma increased with decreased fat content
- Cellularity increased
- Chief and oncocytic cells are increased
- Solid, follicular, and cord-like patterns can be seen
- Secondary changes are common

Pathologic Differential Diagnosis

- Parathyroid adenoma, parathyroid carcinoma, metastatic renal cell carcinoma

---

achieved. Diffuse or nodular enlargement is noted, with cystic change occasionally identified. The glands are usually (~50% of cases) <1 g in total weight, although ~30% are 1 to 5 g, and the remaining 20% are >5 g. The glands are soft and tan-brown.

MICROSCOPIC FINDINGS

Primary Chief Cell Hyperplasia

The histology of all the glands is similarly affected, although variance is not uncommon. The parenchymal component shows increased cellularity with a commensurate decrease in stromal fat (Figures 25-2 and 25-3). The process can appear nodular, multinodular, or diffuse

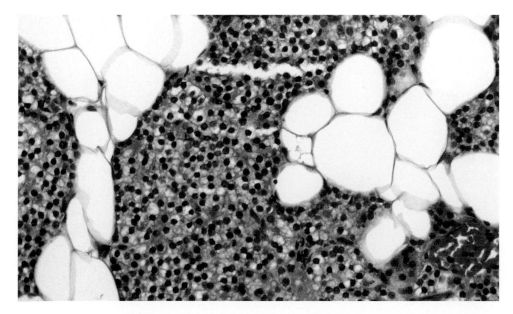

FIGURE 25-2

Normal parathyroid gland tissue showing an appropriate distribution of parathyroid parenchyma and stromal fat. There are chief cells and oncocytic cells within the parenchyma. The cellularity is ~50% and appropriate for a 50-year-old patient without health problems.

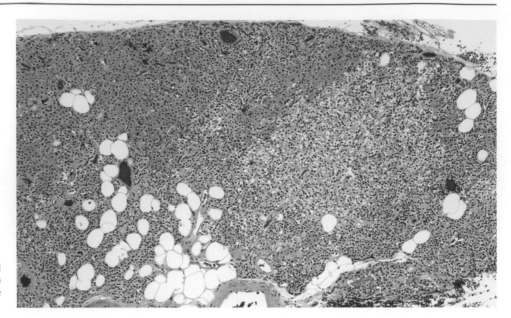

FIGURE 25-3

The entire gland reveals an increased parenchymal cellularity with a decrease in the amount of stromal adipose tissue in this hyperplastic parathyroid gland.

depending on the increasing proportion of the gland involved (Figures 25-4 and 25-5). Notably, the process may extend into the soft tissue surrounding the parathyroid gland and should not be overinterpreted as "invasive." Overall, the cellularity is increased, even if it varies between glands. In general, both chief and oncocytic cell components will be increased with varying degrees of cellularity (Figure 25-6). A variety of different architectural patterns, including solid, follicular (Figure 25-7), and cord-like patterns (Figure 25-8) are noted, in addition to a vaguely nodular appearance (Figure 25-9). Chief cells are polyhedral, with round, centrally located nuclei. The cytoplasm can be amphophilic, clear, or vacuolated. Oncocytic cells are much larger, with abundant eosinophilic, granular cytoplasm surrounding slightly larger nuclei. Cellular atypia can be seen (Figure 25-10),

but it is usually not widespread or profound. Mitoses can be seen but are usually <5/10 high-power fields, without atypical forms. Secondary changes including fibrosis, hemorrhage, and hemosiderin-laden macrophages are common findings (Figure 25-11). Intracellular glycogen is often increased in hyperplastic glands above what is seen in atrophy or adenoma.

Water-Clear Cell Hyperplasia

This is a very uncommon type of hyperplasia seen slightly more commonly in men, most commonly in the 5th decade of life. The upper glands tend to be preferentially involved, and all reported cases have a combined gland weight of >1 g. The large cells have cytoplasm that is completely clear on hematoxylin and eosin staining (Figure 25-12). The feature is usually present on

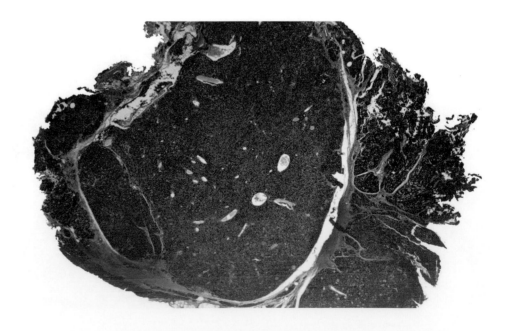

FIGURE 25-4

Multiple nodules are noted within this cellular parathyroid gland. There is fibrosis, but not capsule formation. Note the presence of chief and oncocytic cells, arranged in variably sized nodules.

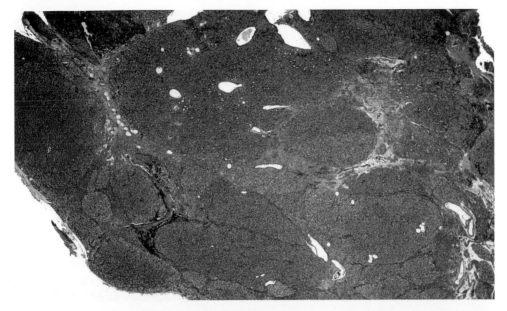

FIGURE 25-5

A hyperplastic gland shows a multinodular appearance, with variably sized nodules of both chief and oncocytic cells. There is virtually no stromal adipose tissue in this gland.

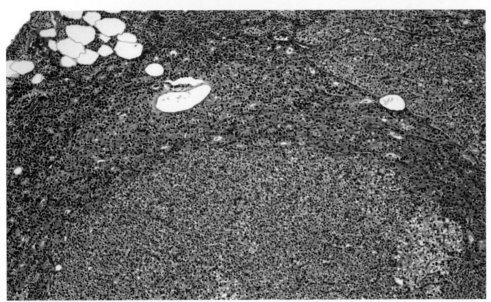

FIGURE 25-6

Increased parenchymal cellularity and decreased fat in this example of hyperplasia. Both chief and oncocytic cell increase is noted, forming cords and nodules.

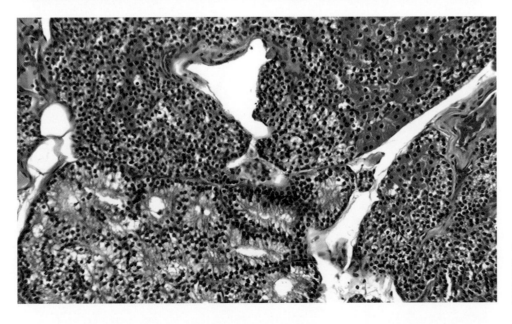

FIGURE 25-7

Solid and follicular patterns of growth are identified. A few oncocytic cells are also identified in the predominantly chief cell hyperplasia.

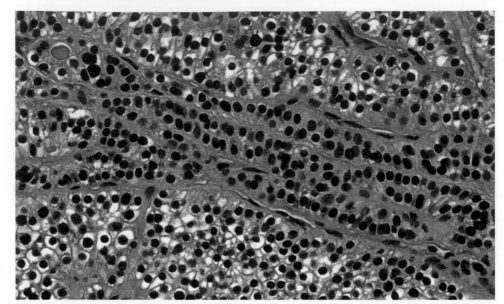

FIGURE 25-8

Cord and "follicular" growth are present within areas of sheet-like growth in this example of parathyroid hyperplasia.

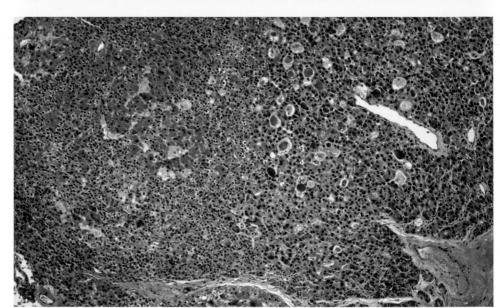

FIGURE 25-9

A nodule of oncocytic cells is noted in this sample of hyperplasia. However, immediately adjacent (right-sided) is a follicular architecture, composed of cells that are a different oncocytic appearance from the nodule.

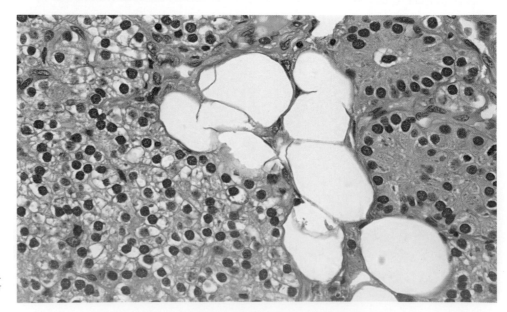

FIGURE 25-10

Fat can be seen within hyperplastic tissue. Slight nuclear atypia is present in the far right of the field.

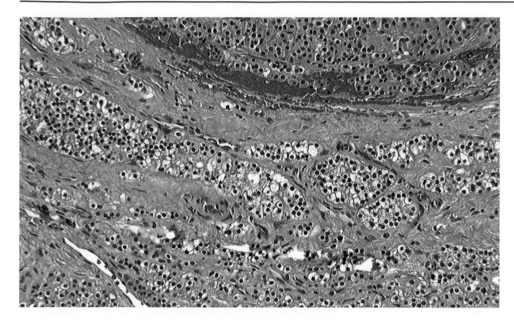

FIGURE 25-11
Fibrosis and hemorrhage are seen within this example of parathyroid hyperplasia.

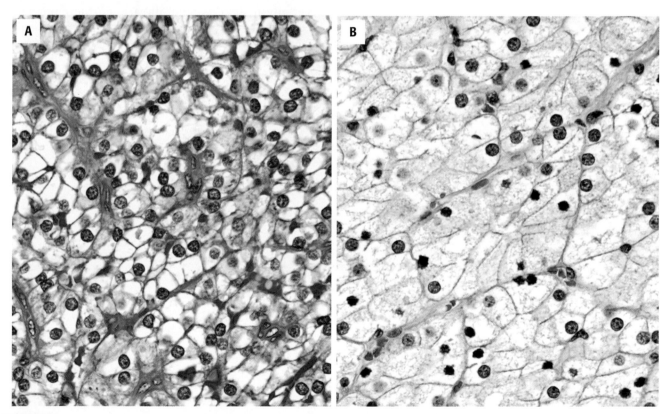

FIGURE 25-12
Water-clear cell hyperplasia presents with optically clear cytoplasm on frozen section material (**A**), but standard processing yields a finely reticulated cytoplasm on routine processing (**B**). The cell borders are prominent and the nuclei tend to be basally oriented.

frozen section material, while usual processing may cause the artifact to be lost, resulting in a finely reticulated cytoplasm composed of numerous small vacuoles. Cell borders are prominent. The nuclei tend to be basally oriented. There is no adipose tissue present. Neutral fat stains are negative, but glycogen is present in the cytoplasm.

ANCILLARY STUDIES

FNA does not reliably separate between adenoma and hyperplasia, and so is not of value. Ultrastructural examination usually shows abundant mitochondria and endoplasmic reticulum with interdigitating cell membranes but is not useful in diagnosis. The chief cells will be positive for keratin, chromogranin, synaptophysin, CD56, and PTH (Figure 25-13), but immunohistochemical studies do not help with the principal differential diagnostic consideration: adenoma. CD4 may be positive on the cell surface (membranous pattern), usually of only chief cells. Fat staining of cryostat sections may help to discriminate between normal and slightly hyperplastic glands (less *intracytoplasmic* fat than normal cells) but is not always helpful. Cyclin D1 overexpression is seen in up to 30 % of hyperplastic glands.

The use of intraoperative PTH assays has profoundly altered the management of parathyroid disease. An intraoperative decline of PTH to normal levels at 10 minutes and >50 % of the initial baseline value suggests surgical cure. Furthermore, the use of chemical evaluation is resulting in a decrease of intraoperative frozen section consultation in parathyroid surgery.

DIFFERENTIAL DIAGNOSIS

The principal differential is with parathyroid adenoma, although sometimes in recurrent disease, separation from parathyroid carcinoma may be more difficult. Tiny glandular biopsy samples from normal associated glands are difficult to interpret since the distribution of parenchymal and fat cells is often irregular. Identification of a capsule, a single cell population, pseudoacinar growth, secretions, and cellular monotony are features seen more commonly in adenoma. While not diagnostic, pleomorphism when seen in multiple foci suggests an adenoma. Reactive fibrosis is seen in recurrent hyperplasia, while dense, acellular, perivascular fibrosis is seen in carcinoma. Other considerations include parathyromatosis or nests of hyperplastic epithelium usually within the soft tissues of the neck, lacking any fibroblastic reaction or an infiltrative pattern. These collections may be iatrogenic remnants from surgery for previous hyperparathyroidism, or may be embryonic rests of parathyroid tissue that are stimulated by the underlying primary hyperparathyroidism. There is no pleomorphism, no intravascular location, and no other histologic features to suggest malignancy. Clear cell hyperplasia may be confused with metastatic renal cell carcinoma, especially if there is renal disease. Furthermore, bony metastasis, in general, may result in hypercalcemia due to the osteolytic effect, but these patients do not have hyperparathyroidism per se. Last, lithium has been known to produce hyperparathyroidism, but it resolves with drug discontinuance.

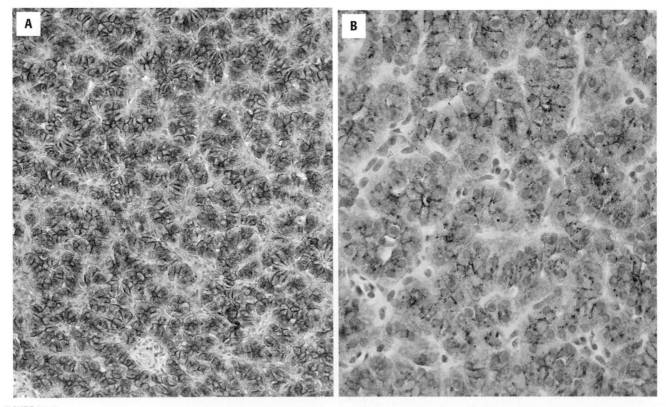

FIGURE 25-13
This example of parathyroid hyperplasia shows the normal staining of the cells with chromogranin (**A**) and parathyroid hormone (**B**). Staining may be useful in separating between primary parathyroid diseases and metastases.

PROGNOSIS AND THERAPY

The serum calcium level can be lowered by hydration and by a variety of pharmacologic agents, including bisphosphonates (inhibition of bone resorption), hormone replacement (inhibition of PTH-related bone resorption), and calcimimetics (negative feedback inhibition). However, no long-term correction is achieved without surgery. Minimally invasive radio-guided parathyroidectomy is generally used for adenoma rather than hyperplasia (usually coupled with specialized radiographic studies, such as single photon emission computed tomography). Complete removal of three glands, while leaving a remnant of the fourth gland, is the most widely used surgery (subtotal parathyroidectomy). Autotransplantation into the forearm may also be performed to avoid neck dissection if recurrence develops. Recurrence may develop in ~15% of patients but may take years to develop. If there is asymmetric involvement and previous history is unknown, the diagnosis of an "adenoma" may be rendered. It is important to consider the presence of supernumerary glands, ectopic glands, or parathyromatosis whenever considering the recurrence or persistence of hyperplasia. Hypoparathyroidism may rarely result if all glands are removed. Subtotal parathyroidectomy is preferred for water-clear cell hyperplasia.

■ SECONDARY AND TERTIARY PARATHYROID HYPERPLASIA

Secondary hyperparathyroidism is a non-neoplastic increase in the parenchymal cell mass within all of the parathyroid tissue in response to a known clinical stimulus for increased PTH secretion. Tertiary hyperparathyroidism is characterized by increased parathyroid parenchymal cell mass associated with autonomous hyperfunction in patients with a history of chronic secondary hyperparathyroidism who are on dialysis or have undergone renal transplantation (the hypertrophied parathyroid glands fail to return to normal after therapy).

CLINICAL FEATURES

The most common cause of secondary hyperparathyroidism is chronic renal failure, which results in abnormally low serum calcium levels—the clinical stimulus that results in the adaptive (compensatory) increase in production of PTH. Alternatively, other causes

SECONDARY AND TERTIARY PARATHYROID HYPERPLASIA—DISEASE FACT SHEET

Definition
- Non-neoplastic increase in parathyroid parenchymal cell mass within all parathyroid tissue with a known stimulus

Incidence and Location
- Especially common in patients with renal failure and/or on dialysis

Morbidity and Mortality
- Control of calcium level may be difficult, leading to skeletal deformities and vessel calcification

Gender, Race, and Age Distribution
- Female > male (3:1)
- Older patients in general, but renal disease occurs in all ages

Clinical Features
- Chronic renal failure, malabsorption, vitamin D metabolism abnormalities, and pseudohypoparathyroidism can all cause disease
- Serum calcium level is decreased
- Symptoms reflect underlying disease

Prognosis and Therapy
- Depends on underlying renal disease
- Subtotal parathyroidectomy performed early to avoid skeletal deformities and vessel calcification

resulting in hyperparathyroidism include abnormalities of vitamin D metabolism, calcium deficiency, malabsorption, and low serum magnesium. Lithium therapy may result in reversible hyperparathyroidism. A broad age spectrum is affected, reflecting the underlying renal disease. Patients present with symptoms of increased PTH, which often results in osteomalacia and periarticular abnormal calcium deposition. The serum calcium level is usually decreased. In renal failure, parathyroid glands seem to expand diffusely and polyclonally, while later developing areas of nodular hyperplasia with diminished expression of both the vitamin D receptor and calcium-sensing receptor. When more than one parathyroid gland progresses to nodular hyperplasia, the hyperparathyroidism is often refractory to medical treatment.

Tertiary hyperparathyroidism usually occurs after years of renal failure and is purported to be an autonomous parathyroid hyperfunction occurring in a setting of known secondary hyperparathyroidism. Most cases result from diffuse or nodular chief cell hyperplasia affecting multiple glands. The hypercalcemia that can result often threatens the kidney transplant graft function, requiring prompt treatment.

PATHOLOGIC FEATURES

SECONDARY AND TERTIARY PARATHYROID HYPERPLASIA—PATHOLOGIC FEATURES

Gross Findings
- Identical to primary hyperplasia although gland enlargement may be huge

Microscopic Findings
- Increased parenchyma with decreased adipocytes
- Nodular or diffuse growth
- Oncocytic cell increase may be more noticeable than chief cell
- Secondary changes are common

Pathologic Differential Diagnosis
- Primary chief cell hyperplasia, parathyroid adenoma, parathyroid carcinoma

---

GROSS FINDINGS

The findings are no different from primary hyperplasia, with all of the glands affected, whether it is uniform, nodular, or asymmetric. The glands are yellow to tan-brown. In tertiary disease, asymmetry can be quite startling, with glands often reaching up to 40 times the size of normal glands.

MICROSCOPIC FINDINGS

There is an overall increase of parenchymal cells, including chief, oxyphilic, and transitional (intermediate between chief and oxyphilic cells) types

(Figure 25-14), while there is a decrease in the amount of stromal adipocytes. The adipocyte decrease seems more pronounced if the disease has been present for a long duration (Figure 25-15). Nodular or diffuse growth is present, with sheets, cords, and acinar structures noted. The cells are quite enlarged in comparison to normal cells. Oxyphilic cells tend to be increased more than chief cells. However, in tertiary hyperparathyroidism, the chief cells are more frequently affected. Fibrosis, calcification, and hemorrhage are seen in many cases.

DIFFERENTIAL DIAGNOSIS

Primary chief cell hyperplasia is the main differential diagnostic consideration, although this is a clinical separation in most cases. Parathyroid adenoma and carcinoma are also considered in the differential diagnosis but are usually eliminated with clinical information. With recurrence of hyperparathyroidism, small islands of residual parenchyma within the fat may take on an atypical and "invasive" appearance, which should not be overinterpreted as carcinoma.

PROGNOSIS AND THERAPY

Prevention and treatment of secondary hyperparathyroidism is a continual management predicament for the nephrologist and endocrinologist. Subtotal parathyroidectomy is the treatment of choice, with a small remnant of tissue left or autotransplanted. However, it

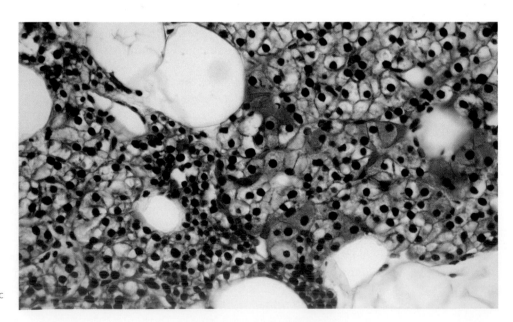

FIGURE 25-14
Hyperplasia shows chief cells, oncocytic cells, and transitional cells.

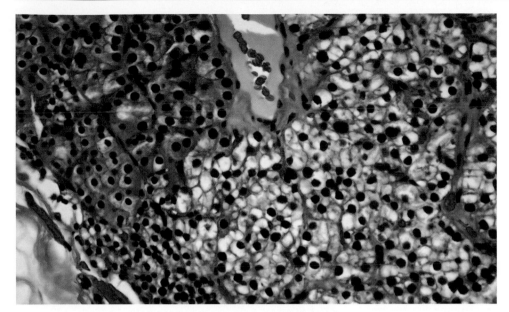

FIGURE 25-15
There are nodules of both oncocytic and chief cells, although no fat is present in this high-power view in a patient with long-standing disease.

is important to perform surgery early to avoid skeletal deformities and vessel calcifications, since these changes will not involute after surgery. Recurrence of hyperparathyroidism is an ongoing management problem with renal failure patients. Likewise, the autonomous hyperfunction of the parathyroid glands results in an alteration of the "set-point" of serum calcium levels, which causes stimulation of the parathyroid tissue despite "normal" calcium levels.

SUGGESTED READINGS

The complete suggested readings list is available online at www.expertconsult.com.

26

Benign Neoplasms of the Parathyroid Gland

■ Lester D. R. Thompson

■ PARATHYROID ADENOMA

A parathyroid adenoma is an encapsulated benign neoplasm of the parathyroid parenchymal cells (either chief or oncocytic cells). Parathyroid disease is separated into primary, secondary, or tertiary, based on whether the parathyroid gland is primarily the source of the disease or if the gland is reacting to exogenous stimulation, such as renal disease (see Chapter 25). This distinction is sometimes quite difficult on histology alone, and even more so if only a single gland is sampled. Intraoperative selective venous parathyroid hormone (PTH) assay is a clinical parameter that may assist with the distinction. Isolated cases of adenoma are associated with exposure to ionizing radiation, but the majority have no specific etiology. A few cases present as part of the hyperparathyroidism-jaw tumor (HPT-JT) syndrome, an autosomal dominant disorder characterized by parathyroid adenoma or carcinoma, various fibro-osseous lesions of jaw (ossifying fibroma), and renal cysts or tumors. Up to 80% of the patients will have HPT. The gene (*HRPT2*) is found on 1q25-q31.

CLINICAL FEATURES

Early detection of parathyroid disease has improved dramatically with increased use of multichannel autoanalyzers, with calcium levels determined as part of routine blood chemistries. Therefore, a true incidence is difficult to determine, although 1/1,000 patients per year is considered an approximate incidence. Parathyroid adenomas are the most common cause of HPT, accounting for ~80% to 85% of primary HPT. Women are affected more frequently than men (~3 to 4:1), with a peak incidence in the 4th to 6th decades. There is a rare association with inherited syndromes (multiple endocrine neoplasia [MEN1], MEN2, and HPT-JT syndrome). The existence of two simultaneous adenomas is quite uncommon and difficult to prove by histology alone. About 90% of tumors develop in normally situated

parathyroid glands, with the lower glands affected more commonly; however, mediastinal, esophageal, and other anatomic site tumors are recognized along with intrathyroidal neoplasms. Symptoms of excess calcium and/or PTH may yield a nonspecific clinical presentation that includes fatigue, malaise, weakness, abdominal pain, depression, constipation, peptic ulcer disease, kidney stones, and/or pancreatitis. Nephrolithiasis is about twice as common in men as in women. However, calculi are not seen as frequently since biochemical screening frequently results in early identification of the tumor before symptoms are well developed. A palpable mass is an uncommon finding.

By laboratory investigation, patients tend to have *higher* serum calcium levels than detected in patients with primary chief cell hyperplasia. Patients will also have elevated serum PTH levels, hypophosphatemia, and hyperphosphaturia.

RADIOGRAPHIC FEATURES

A variety of techniques can be used to detect and localize abnormal parathyroid glands, including ultrasonography, computed tomography, magnetic resonance imaging, thallium subtraction scanning, and nuclear scintigraphy, specifically with ^{99m}Tc sestamibi. Technetium seems to be the most useful in practical application, and it is concentrated by parathyroid tissue (Figure 26-1), effectively identifying adenomas in up to 90% of cases. Still, this suggests it cannot be used in isolation. Specifically, with a greater tendency to use minimally invasive parathyroid surgery, it is much more important to use scintigraphic studies, combined with ultrasound and intraoperative PTH measurement or gamma probe testing. Ultrasound-guided fine needle aspiration or venous sampling can also be of value in evaluating parathyroid disease.

PATHOLOGIC FEATURES

GROSS FINDINGS

Almost always solitary, the gland is typically enlarged, and often ovoid, with a mean weight of ~1 g.

PARATHYROID ADENOMA—PATHOLOGIC FEATURES

Gross Findings
- A single enlarged parathyroid gland (rarely, two adenomas may occur)
- Smooth, encapsulated mass
- Reddish brown, with rim of uninvolved parenchyma adjacent to proliferation
- Usually up to ~1 g

Microscopic Findings
- Single mass
- Encapsulated (although often a thin, irregular capsule)
- Fatless nodule
- Distinct histology within the neoplasm different from remaining gland
- Atrophy or compression of parathyroid parenchyma
- Usually a single histologic population of enlarged cells
- Glandular architecture with "secretions" more common in adenoma than hyperplasia
- Oncocytic adenoma is all oncocytes

Immunohistochemical Results
- Parathyroid hormone, chromogranin, and synaptophysin positive
- Parafibromin strong nuclear reaction
- CD4 surface membrane of chief cells only
- Ki-67: low proliferation index
- TTF-1 and calcitonin negative

Fine Needle Aspiration
- Similar to thyroid follicular lesions
- Clear cytoplasm and distinct cell borders are helpful

Molecular Findings
- CCND1 overexpression (20% to 40%) or translocation (~8%)
- Somatic mutations of MEN1 in up to 40%
- RET mutational activation in MEN2A patients

Pathologic Differential Diagnosis
- Parathyroid hyperplasia, thyroid adenoma, medullary thyroid carcinoma, metastatic renal cell carcinoma

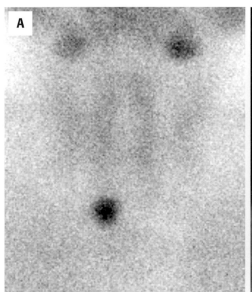
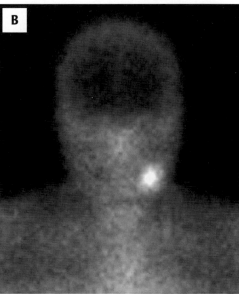

FIGURE 26-1

A ^{99m}Tc sestamibi scan shows increased uptake disproportionate to the other parathyroid glands, a finding consistent with adenoma. **A** was obtained at 20 minutes, while **B** was obtained at 4 hours (different patients).

The surface is smooth and surrounded by a thin capsule (Figure 26-2), although multinodularity and multilobularity may develop. The cut surface is smooth, soft, and reddish-brown, often distinct from the yellowish-brown surrounding periphery of parathyroid parenchyma. If the adenoma is large, degenerative or cystic changes are noted (Figure 26-2), sometimes masking the true nature of the process.

MICROSCOPIC FINDINGS

A single gland is usually affected by a well-circumscribed and usually encapsulated mass with a fatless population of cells within the tumor, distinct from the uninvolved, compressed or atrophic parathyroid parenchyma

(Figures 26-3 and 26-4). The capsule is sometimes extremely thin and attenuated (Figures 26-5 to 26-6). The tumor is usually composed of a single-cell proliferation of enlarged oncocytic (Figure 26-7) or chief cells (Figure 26-8), with the latter the most common, although occasionally a mixture of both can be seen. The cells are often arranged in a solid or acinarglandular (follicular) distribution, a finding uncommon in hyperplasia (Figures 26-9 through 26-11). Peritheliomatous palisading (tumor growth centered around vessels) is occasionally identified. The neoplastic cells tend to be larger than the non-neoplastic cells in the adjacent parathyroid parenchyma. The chief cells have ample clear to slightly eosinophilic cytoplasm surrounding nuclei that are round to oval

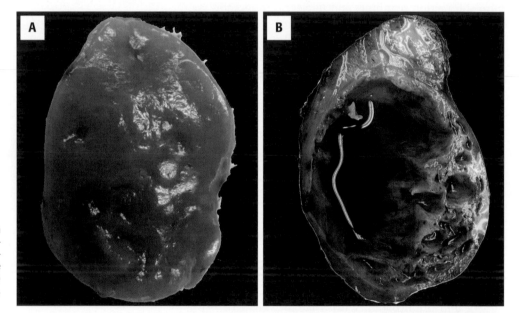

FIGURE 26-2

A, This parathyroid gland adenoma weighed 4.5 g, showing a homogeneous cut surface. No areas of atrophic or compressed parenchyma are seen. **B**, This large adenoma (4.5 cm) has undergone cystic degeneration, showing multiple, variable sized cysts.

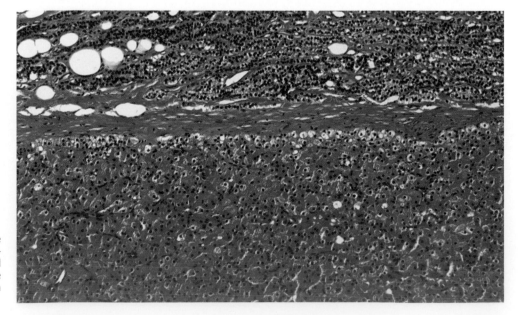

FIGURE 26-3

A well-formed capsule separates the oncocytic neoplasm from the surrounding, compressed uninvolved parathyroid parenchyma which contains fat. The cells of the neoplasm are oncocytic with a monotonous appearance.

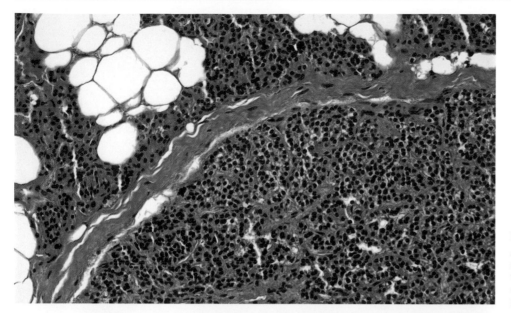

FIGURE 26-4

A thin but well-formed fibrous capsule separates this chief cell adenoma from the surrounding nonatrophic parenchyma. Fat is seen in the uninvolved parenchyma.

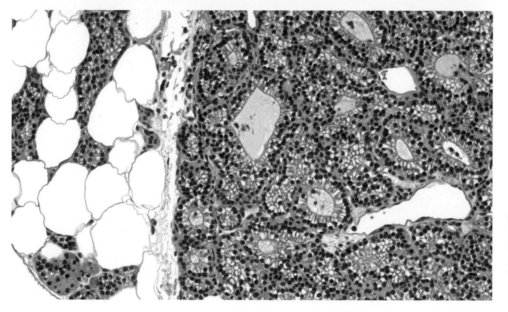

FIGURE 26-5

A nearly nonexistent capsule separates the adenoma from the surrounding parenchyma. The parenchyma contains cells that are smaller than the neoplasm and has fat. The neoplastic cells are arranged in a pseudoglandular distribution.

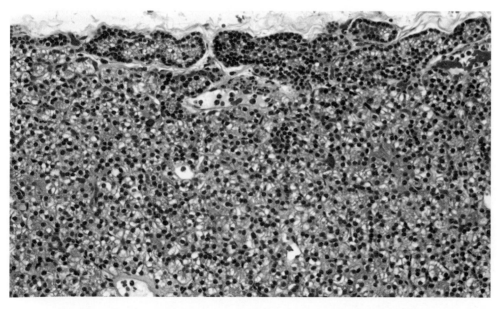

FIGURE 26-6

Compressed parenchyma is noted at the superior portion of the field. A true capsule is not present in this example of an adenoma.

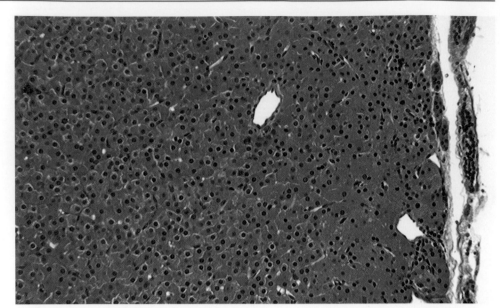

FIGURE 26-7

Sometimes the compressed parenchyma looks like lymphocytes at the periphery (*right side*). However, a delicate capsule separates this adenoma from the surrounding atrophic parenchyma. This is an oncocytic type of adenoma.

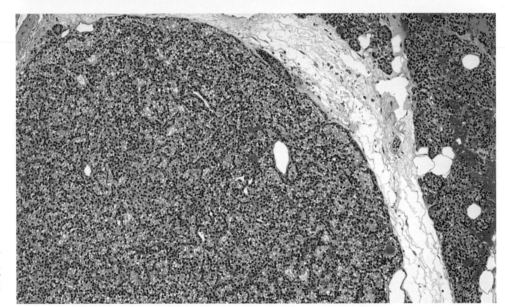

FIGURE 26-8

Chief cells compose this adenoma without any fat cells present. There is a thin, edematous capsule separating the tumor from uninvolved parenchyma that still contains adipocytes.

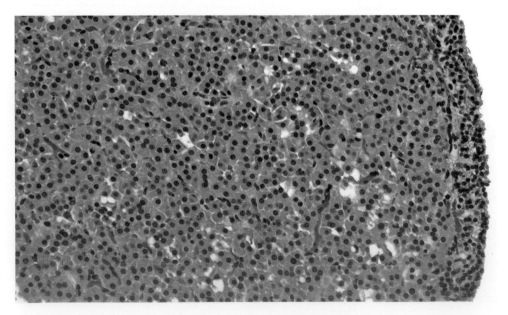

FIGURE 26-9

This oncocytic adenoma shows a rim of atrophic parenchyma at the periphery (*right side*), with only a hint of an attenuated capsule noted.

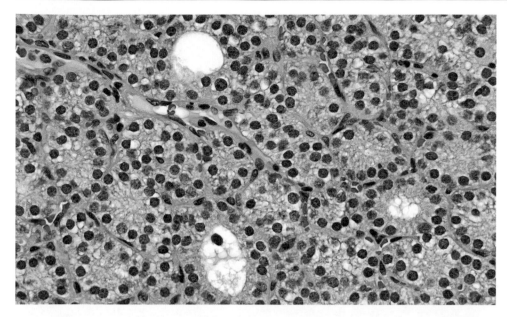

FIGURE 26-10

A glandular pattern is commonly seen in adenomas, with cells arranged around a lumen.

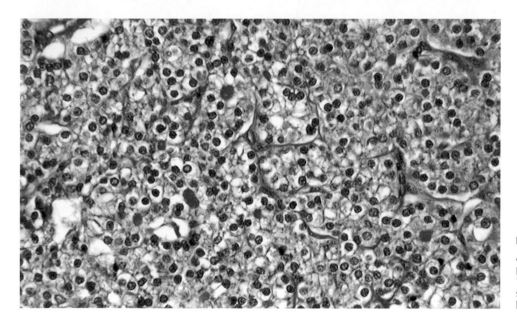

FIGURE 26-11

A pseudofollicular pattern of growth is present in this adenoma. Inspissated "colloid-like" material is noted. In a case such as this, immunohistochemistry may be of value.

with heavy nuclear chromatin distribution (Figure 26-12). Nucleoli are small to inconspicuous. Intracellular lipid (fat) within the cytoplasm is limited if present at all.

Nuclear pleomorphism can be seen, although it is usually focal or arranged in clusters. Multinucleated giant cells are also seen in isolation. Mitotic figures are inconspicuous, with usually ≤1 mitotic figures/10 high-power fields. Eosinophilic "secretions" may be mistaken for colloid (Figure 26-13) and may occasionally calcify, simulating a psammoma body. Amyloid may occasionally be identified between the neoplastic cells. Stroma is scant, but delicate fibrovascular bands separate the neoplastic cells. Hemosiderin-laden macrophages, inflammation, and fibrosis may be part of degenerative changes, especially in large tumors (Figure 26-14).

Oncocytic (oxyphilic) cell adenomas are arranged in sheets, cords, nests, or glandular structures, composed of cells with abundant eosinophilic, granular cytoplasm and may have prominent, centrally placed eosinophilic nucleoli (Figure 26-13); otherwise, there is no difference from chief cell adenomas. There may be adenomas with a mixture of chief and oncocytic cells, but this is a feature much more frequently seen in hyperplasia. Clear cell adenoma and lipoadenoma are recognized but are exceedingly uncommon. Lipoadenoma (hamartoma) is a proliferation of parenchymal and stromal adipose cells in an encapsulated tumor, separate from the rest of the gland. The diagnosis is exceedingly difficult in small biopsy samples, as it may appear to be normal tissue. Sometimes the presence of myxoid stroma or degeneration may be helpful.

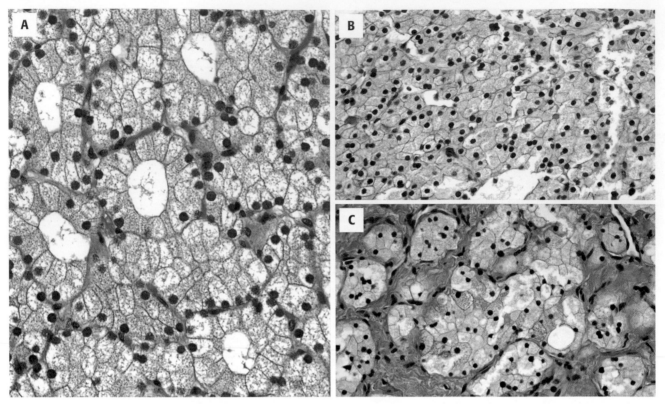

FIGURE 26-12

A and **B**, Cytoplasmic clearing can be seen in parathyroid adenoma, although a slightly granular or vacuolated appearance may remain. Note the increased intralesional fibrosis (**C**).

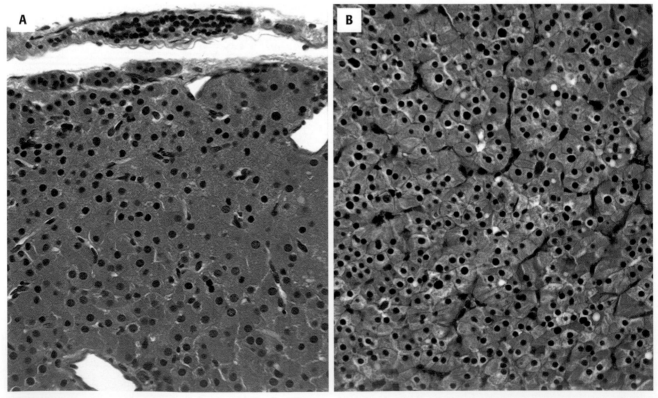

FIGURE 26-13

Granular, oncocytic, or oxyphilic cytoplasm may be seen in adenoma (compressed uninvolved parathyroid is present at the upper region of **A**). Note the "inspissated" material in **B**.

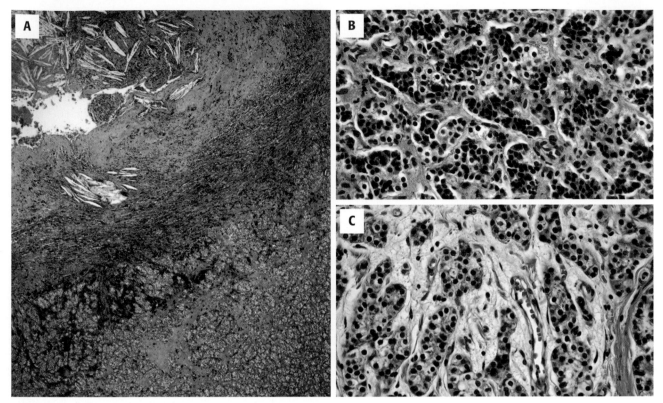

FIGURE 26-14

Degenerative changes are not uncommon in adenoma. **A**, Large area of degeneration with fibrosis, hemosiderin-laden macrophages, and cholesterol clefts. **B**, This "pseudoalveolar" pattern is associated with numerous hemosiderin-laden macrophages. **C**, A myxoid-mucinous degeneration of the stroma is noted in this adenoma.

ANCILLARY STUDIES

ULTRASTRUCTURAL FEATURES

The cells tend to have more abundant rough endoplasmic reticulum and Golgi apparatus than in non-neoplastic cells, while also showing a large number of microvilli. Annulated lamellae, structures resembling cell membranes, singly or in groups, may be seen infrequently.

IMMUNOHISTOCHEMICAL RESULTS

The parenchymal cells will be chromogranin, synaptophysin, and PTH immunoreactive, although the interpretation of the PTH reaction is fraught with diffusion artifacts and serum reactions. Parafibromin will show a strong nuclear reaction in adenoma. TTF-1 and thyroglobulin are nonreactive, while specific keratins may be positive. Interestingly, CD4 will give a surface membrane reaction in chief cells. Ki-67 yields a low proliferation index.

HISTOCHEMISTRY

Fat stains (oil red O, Sudan black) have been used historically to show decreased intracellular fat in hyperfunctioning tumor cells but are of limited practical value.

FINE NEEDLE ASPIRATION

Ultrasound-guided parathyroid sampling is used in some settings. Separation of a thyroid follicular neoplasm from a parathyroid proliferation is difficult. There are usually naked nuclei set within a few small sheets of cells, sometimes forming acinar or follicular structures. The nuclei are usually small and hyperchromatic, with isolated atypical cells. Secretions and "colloid-like" substances may suggest a thyroid lesion. Cleared cytoplasm may be noted, but separation from a metastatic renal cell tumor or a thyroid gland neoplasm may be difficult. Fluid PTH levels may help, but only if fluid is obtained from a cystic lesion. If cell block material is obtained, immunohistochemistry can be used. Furthermore, molecular techniques can be used to confirm a parathyroid or thyroid neoplasm in certain settings.

MOLECULAR FINDINGS

A number of molecular findings are seen in adenoma, which is considered a monoclonal proliferation. There are alterations involving cyclin D1 (*CCND1*), including translocations (8%) or overexpression (20% to 40%). Adenomas tend to show adenomatous polyposis coli (*APC*) expression, while it is lost in carcinoma. Tumor suppressor gene *MEN1* (11q13) frequently shows somatic (rather than germline) mutations in the second wild-type allele in ~25% to 40% of patients with adenoma, with an additional inactivating mutation of the remaining allele. The gene codes for menin, a nuclear protein that has been shown to inhibit transcriptional activity. *RET* will show mutational activation in adenomas of patients with MEN2A.

DIFFERENTIAL DIAGNOSIS

Parathyroid hyperplasia and carcinoma are occasionally difficult to separate from an adenoma, while thyroid neoplasms and metastatic renal cell carcinoma may also occasionally enter the differential diagnosis. Uneven, nodular hyperplasia will mimic an adenoma, especially if only a single gland is sampled. A "remnant" can be seen in both lesions. The easiest way to separate hyperplasia and adenoma is to sample more than one gland. Hyperplasia should be considered (1) if more than one gland is enlarged or abnormal, (2) if there is an increase in the parenchyma:stromal fat ratio (age variability considered), and (3) if there is nodular distribution of both chief and oncocytic cells. Clinical information about renal status, serum calcium, and/or PTH levels and condition of the remaining "in situ" glands will help to make the separation. Intraoperative changes in the serum PTH levels may also serve to confirm the diagnosis of adenoma (levels decrease after removal) versus hyperplasia (elevated level persists).

Carcinoma usually has a trabecular architecture and demonstrates thick, acellular bands of fibrosis; a thick capsule; capsular, vascular, or perineural invasion; profound nuclear pleomorphism; increased mitotic figures, including atypical forms; and the presence of necrosis. Adherence to the thyroid gland, difficulty in removing the tumor, and extremely elevated serum calcium levels should elevate the suspicion of parathyroid carcinoma. In sites of previous surgery, however, the reactive changes in the stroma may also simulate invasive growth or result in attachment to the surrounding tissues, factors that should be weighed carefully in determining the final diagnosis. Ancillary studies show a reduced to absent nuclear expression of parafibromin and a loss of APC in carcinoma. Occasionally, in cases that cannot be definitively separated, the term "atypical adenoma" can be used, while detailing the histologic features of concern. It is interesting to note that when these tumors are followed, there is usually a benign clinical outcome.

Thyroid lesions, which can cause diagnostic difficulty, do not have a rim of uninvolved parathyroid tissue, may have birefringent oxalate crystals, and will be TTF-1 or thyroglobulin immunoreactive.

PROGNOSIS AND THERAPY

Surgery is the treatment of choice if there is significant calcium elevation or other complications of HPT or if the patient is younger than 50 years. In the past, removal of the adenoma and sampling of a second gland were advocated. With the use of minimally invasive radio-guided parathyroidectomy, removal of a single gland can now be done with success. However, preoperative definitive anatomic and functional localization must be achieved, accompanied by intraoperative gamma probe readings and rapid intact PTH determination. Surgery ameliorates the calcium effects of HPT, specifically those affecting the cardiovascular system. Recurrent HPT may be due to incomplete removal, parathyromatosis (ruptured, implanted, or remnant parathyroid adenoma tissue), or hyperfunction of the autografted parathyroid tissue.

SUGGESTED READINGS

The complete suggested readings list is available online at www.expertconsult.com.

27

Malignant Neoplasms of the Parathyroid Gland

■ Lester D. R. Thompson

■ PARATHYROID CARCINOMA

Parathyroid carcinoma comprises <2% of all primary hyperparathyroidism (HPT) cases and is a rare tumor. This is a malignant neoplasm of parathyroid parenchymal cells (no malignant adipose tumors are recognized in the parathyroid). Secondary parathyroid hyperplasia and neck irradiation are suggested as etiologic factors. There is also an increased incidence of carcinoma in patients with hereditary HPT-jaw tumor (HPT-JT) syndrome. There are no well-accepted histologic features that are used alone to diagnose carcinoma, but a constellation of features can help to secure the diagnosis.

CLINICAL FEATURES

Parathyroid carcinoma occurs in all ages, although more frequently in older adults, and up to a decade earlier than adenoma. There is no gender bias, distinctly different from the marked female predominance in patients with parathyroid adenoma. Japanese patients show a higher incidence of carcinoma than other races. The clinical features are due primarily to the effects of excessive parathyroid hormone (PTH) secretion and hypercalcemia. Laboratory values of >1,000 ng/L for PTH and >16 mg/dL for serum calcium are very concerning for parathyroid carcinoma. The nonspecific symptoms (weakness, fatigue, anorexia, weight loss, nausea, polyuria, polydipsia) overlap with adenoma, but excessively high serum calcium levels (>16 mg/dL) are associated with nephrolithiasis, renal insufficiency, and bone "brown tumors." Concurrent bone and kidney stone disease are more common in patients with carcinoma than adenoma. A palpable neck mass, often difficult to remove at surgery due to adherence to the soft tissues, nerves (recurrent laryngeal nerve involvement gives hoarseness), and/or thyroid gland, suggests carcinoma. Carcinoma can develop in any parathyroid gland, but

PARATHYROID CARCINOMA—DISEASE FACT SHEET

Definition
- A malignant neoplasm derived from parathyroid parenchymal cells

Incidence and Location
- Accounts for <2% of primary hyperparathyroidism
- Slightly higher frequency in lower parathyroid glands

Morbidity and Mortality
- Adverse effects of hypercalcemia on the cardiovascular system
- Indolent tumor with recurrences and metastases, up to 15% mortality at 5 years

Gender, Race, and Age Distribution
- Equal gender distribution
- Wide age range, although predominantly older patients; still ~10 years younger than patients with adenoma
- Japanese patients have a higher incidence

Clinical Features
- Symptoms referable to excess calcium and parathyroid hormone
- Nephrolithiasis and bone "brown tumors"
- Palpable neck mass, often difficult to remove surgically
- Hoarseness is common with recurrent laryngeal nerve involvement
- May be part of hereditary hyperparathyroidism-jaw tumor syndrome
- High serum calcium and parathyroid hormone levels

Prognosis and Therapy
- Indolent with recurrences common (up to 60% of patients, usually within 3 years)
- About 50% 10-year survival
- Surgery

it is slightly more common in the *lower* parathyroid glands. Interestingly, there are recurrent losses of chromosome 13q, the same region known to contain the retinoblastoma (*RB1*) and *BRCA2* tumor suppressor genes. A genomic region frequently lost in parathyroid adenomas is 11q, the location of *MEN1*, but it is almost never identified in carcinoma, supporting the contention that parathyroid carcinomas arise de novo rather than from preexisting adenomas. Carcinoma is a component of HPT-JT syndrome. Radiographic studies are usually unreliable in separating adenoma from carcinoma, but can aid in planning surgery.

PATHOLOGIC FEATURES

GROSS FINDINGS

Carcinoma is usually large and adherent to the surrounding soft tissues, nerves, and thyroid gland. If there has been previous surgery, scarring and hemorrhage may simulate "invasion." The cut surface is firm and white-tan and may have areas of necrosis. Tumors range from 1.5 to 6 cm (mean, 3 cm).

MICROSCOPIC FINDINGS

No one histologic feature, other than metastatic disease, is considered diagnostic for parathyroid carcinoma. However, a constellation of features can usually be used to support the diagnosis. Reliable features of malignancy include (1) definitive vascular invasion (endothelial lined space with attachment to the wall by the neoplastic cells; Figure 27-1), (2) capsular invasion (Figure 27-2), (3) extension into the uninvolved periparathyroidal adipose tissue (Figure 27-3), (4) invasion-attachment to the thyroid parenchyma (Figures 27-4 and 27-5), and (5) perineural invasion, which is almost diagnostic of carcinoma (Figure 27-6), although this feature is not commonly identified (~5%). Epithelial

---

PARATHYROID CARCINOMA—PATHOLOGIC FEATURES

Gross Findings

- Large tumors (mean, 3 cm)
- Adherent to soft tissues and thyroid gland
- Firm, gray-white cut surface
- Central necrosis may be present

Microscopic Findings

- Adherence to the thyroid gland
- Capsular, vascular or perineural invasion
- Soft tissue extension
- Tumor cell necrosis (comedonecrosis)
- Trabecular growth with thick, acellular bands of fibrosis
- Tumor cell monotony, although profound pleomorphism can be seen
- High nuclear:cytoplasmic ratio
- Spindling of tumor cells
- Prominent, eosinophilic, irregular macronucleoli
- Increased mitotic figures, including atypical forms

Immunohistochemical Results

- Chromogranin and parathyroid hormone, along with keratins
- *Loss* of parafibromin
- Increased Ki-67 labeling index
- Cyclin D1 overexpression
- Negative TTF-1 and thyroglobulin

Molecular Findings

- Recurrent losses in chromosome 13q (region of *RB1* and *BRCA2*)
- *HRPT2* shows germline inactivating mutations
- *CCND1* is overexpressed

Pathologic Differential Diagnosis

- Parathyroid adenoma, medullary carcinoma, thyroid follicular neoplasms, metastatic renal cell carcinoma

---

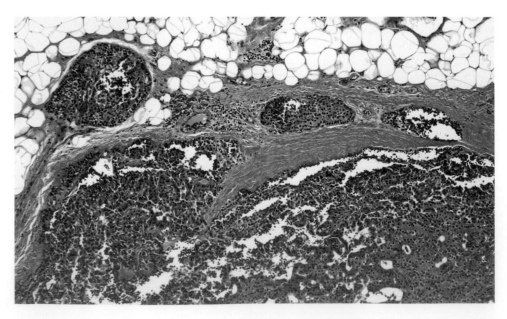

FIGURE 27-1

Neoplastic cells are identified within vascular spaces of the fibrous connective tissue capsule of this parathyroid carcinoma.

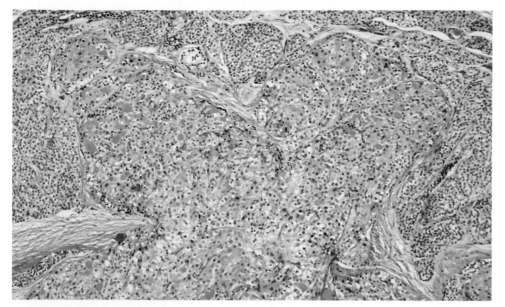

FIGURE 27-2

A "mushroom" projection of neoplastic cells through the capsule into the surrounding parathyroid parenchyma is seen in this parathyroid carcinoma.

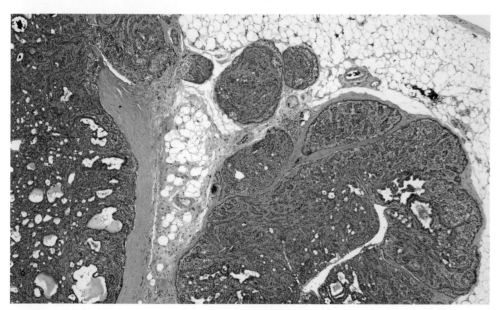

FIGURE 27-3

A thick capsule surrounding the neoplasm, with areas of invasion and direct extension into the surrounding periparathyroidal adipose tissue.

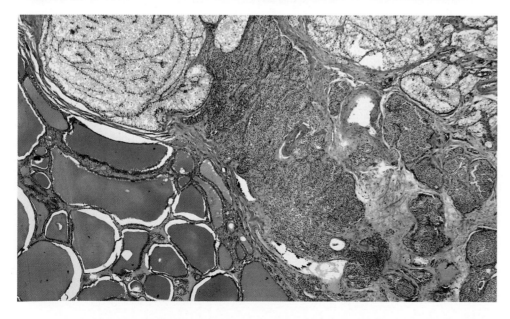

FIGURE 27-4

Different morphologic patterns of parathyroid carcinoma are identified immediately adjacent to thyroid parenchyma (*lower left quadrant*).

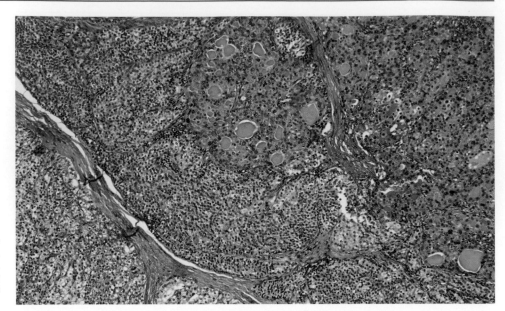

FIGURE 27-5

The neoplastic parathyroid cells are intimately associated with thyroid tissue. Thyroid tissue is in the upper right. Bands of fibrosis are dissecting between the parathyroid neoplasm and within the thyroid parenchyma.

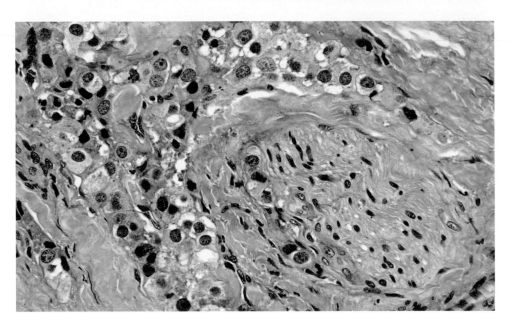

FIGURE 27-6

Perineural invasion, including intraneural invasion, is diagnostic of a parathyroid carcinoma in this example.

entrapment in fibrosis (usually secondary to degenerative changes) can mimic invasion and may be nigh unto impossible to separate from true invasion in some cases. A thick capsule is frequently associated with band-like acellular, dense fibrosis, with occasional hemosiderin-laden macrophages or hemorrhage (Figure 27-7). The fibrosis often shows a perivascular distribution, with collagen expanding into the tumor. Small compartments are often formed by the fibrosis (Figure 27-8). True tumor necrosis, often in a central, comedo necrosis pattern, also suggests malignancy (Figure 27-9). The tumor cells are arranged in solid, diffuse (Figure 27-10) or organoid groups, with a trabecular pattern noted in a number of cases (Figure 27-11). Many different patterns of growth can be seen in parathyroid carcinoma, including glandular, pseudoacinar, spindle cell, peritheliomatous (perivascular palisade), and papillary

(Figure 27-12). Chief cell neoplasms are more common than oncocytic neoplasms, although the cytoplasmic quality does not influence patient outcome (Figure 27-13). Tumor cell spindling, "watermelon seeds," and pyknosis are seen more frequently in carcinoma, but not exclusively (Figure 27-14). A monotonous cellular population (in which the cells may be atypical or not) suggests malignancy. There is an increased nuclear:cytoplasmic ratio, cellular enlargement, profound pleomorphism, and prominent, irregular, eosinophilic macronucleoli (Figure 27-15). Remarkably increased mitotic activity, including atypical forms, is more likely in carcinoma (Figure 27-16), but mitotic figures alone cannot separate between adenoma and carcinoma. Frozen section is discouraged, especially if it is an incisional biopsy, as it results in tumor cell seeding, with recurrent HPT, whether the original disease was benign or malignant.

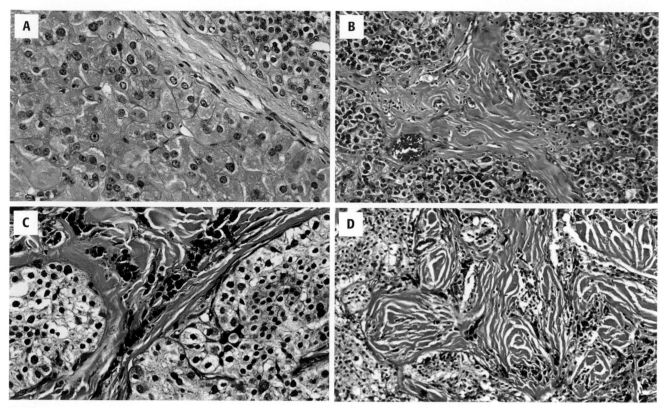

FIGURE 27-7

Fibrosis is common in parathyroid carcinoma. Scant fibrosis (**A**) to dense, acellular, eosinophilic perivascular fibrosis (**C**) is seen in parathyroid carcinoma. Hemosiderin may be deposited within the fibrosis to a variable degree (**B** and **D**).

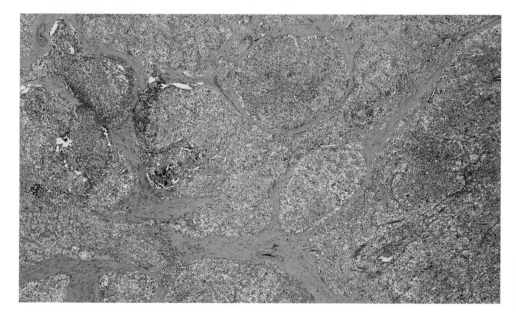

FIGURE 27-8

Multiple nodules of monotonous cells are separated by dense fibrosis in this parathyroid carcinoma.

ANCILLARY STUDIES

IMMUNOHISTOCHEMISTRY

The neoplastic cells are chromogranin and PTH immunoreactive (Figure 27-17), while nonreactive with TTF-1 and thyroglobulin. There is a loss of parafibromin immunoreactivity in carcinoma, although it is not universal, and may show decreased expression instead. Increased Ki-67 (Figure 27-18) and cyclin D1 overexpression are seen more commonly in parathyroid carcinoma. A variety of other markers may occasionally be

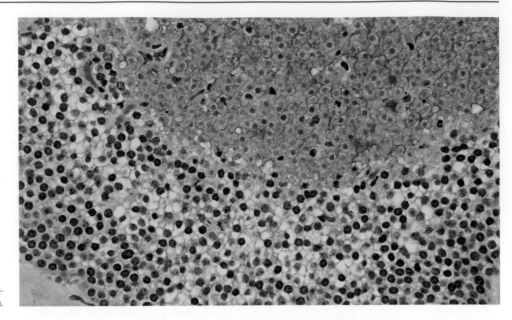

FIGURE 27-9

Comedonecrosis showing "ghost-cell" outlines is not a feature of a benign condition.

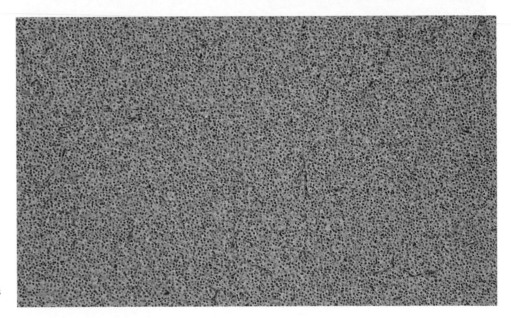

FIGURE 27-10

A monotonous, diffuse pattern suggests a neoplasm rather than hyperplasia.

expressed in parathyroid carcinoma, and include CK7, CK18, muc-1, epithelial membrane antigen, p16, and renal cell marker, among others (Figures 27-19 and 27-20). The clinical utility of these markers is limited at present.

Molecular Findings

A variety of different genes are involved to a variable degree in parathyroid tumorigenesis (Table 27-1), along with related syndromes. Menin protein (encoded by *MEN1*) is required for the transforming growth factor (TGF)-beta to effectively inhibit parathyroid cell proliferation and PTH production. The high rate of somatic mutations in menin within tumors supports this contention. Approximately 15% of patients with

the HPT-JT syndrome develop parathyroid carcinoma. The tumor suppressor gene *HRPT2* (1q25) shows a germline inactivating mutation in many cases of HPT-JT, but ~20% of patients with seemingly sporadic parathyroid carcinoma also have germline mutations. Somatic mutations are also known. *HRPT2* encodes the protein parafibromin, a nuclear protein, that is lost with mutation. Therefore, nuclear parafibromin reaction is lost in many, but not all carcinomas, while remaining expressed in adenoma. Cyclin D1 (*CCND1*, formerly known as *PRAD1*: parathyroid adenomatosis 1) is overexpressed in both adenomas (20% to 40%) and carcinomas (up to 70%), but somatic rearrangements or germline translocations or rearrangements have not been detected in carcinoma.

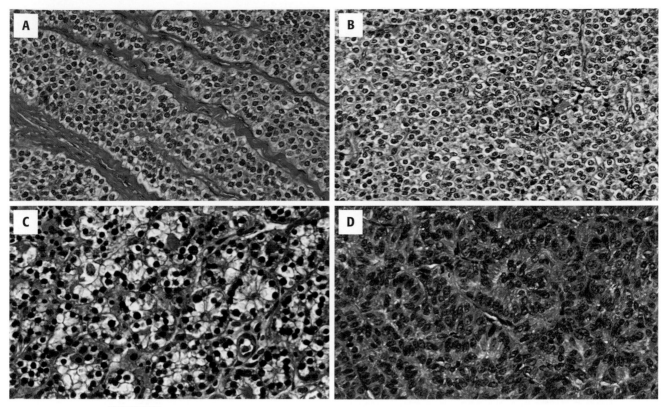

FIGURE 27-11
Many patterns can be seen in carcinoma, including trabecular (**A**), solid (**B**), follicular (**C**), and festoons (**D**).

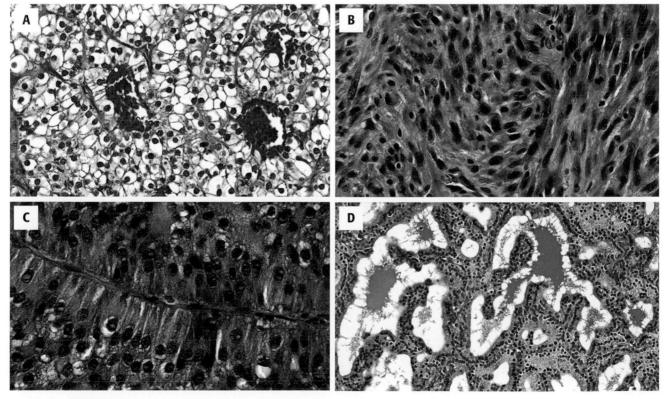

FIGURE 27-12
Many patterns can be seen in carcinoma, including pseudoglandular (**A**), spindled (**B**), peritheliomatous (**C**), and papillary (**D**).

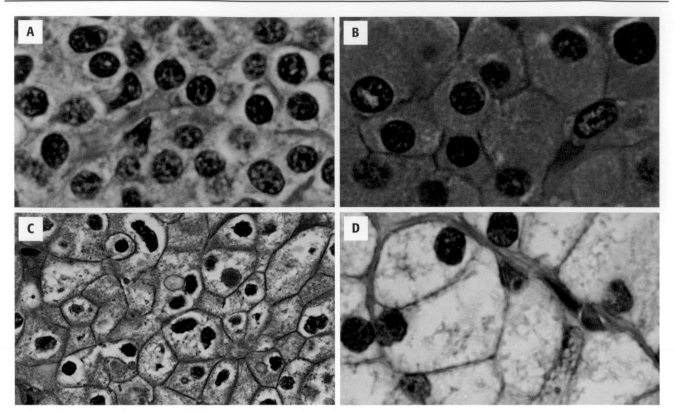

FIGURE 27-13
The cytoplasmic quality can range from amphophilic (**A**), oxyphilic (**B**), partially cleared (**C**), to completely clear (**D**). Note how the cell membranes are prominent in all types of cytoplasm.

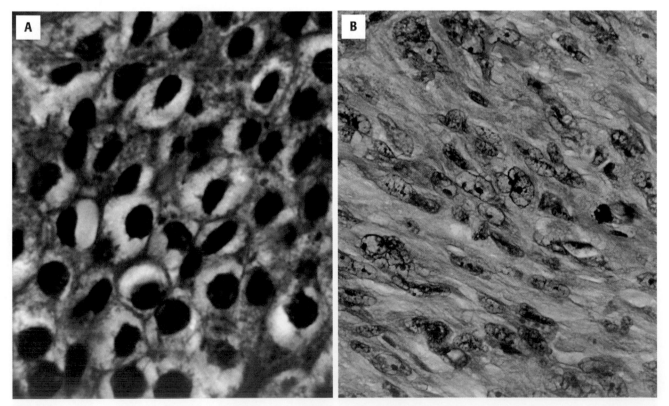

FIGURE 27-14
A, Pyknotic, "watermelon seed" appearance to the nuclei is common in carcinoma. **B**, Tumor cell spindling and remarkable anaplasia are seen in this parathyroid carcinoma.

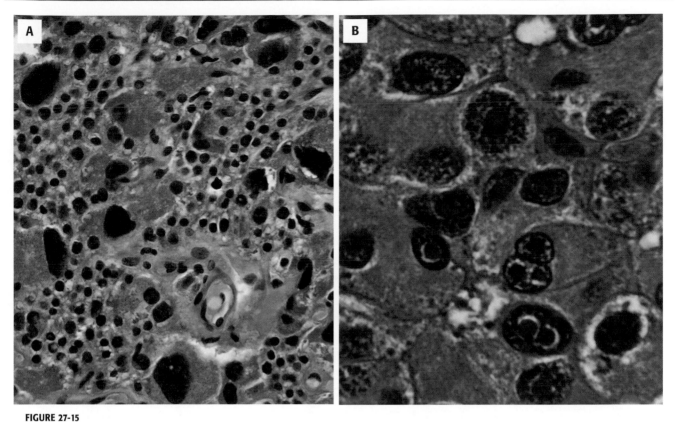

FIGURE 27-15
A, Profound nuclear pleomorphism. **B**, Prominent, irregular, macro, eosinophilic nucleoli with perinucleolar halos are almost diagnostic of carcinoma.

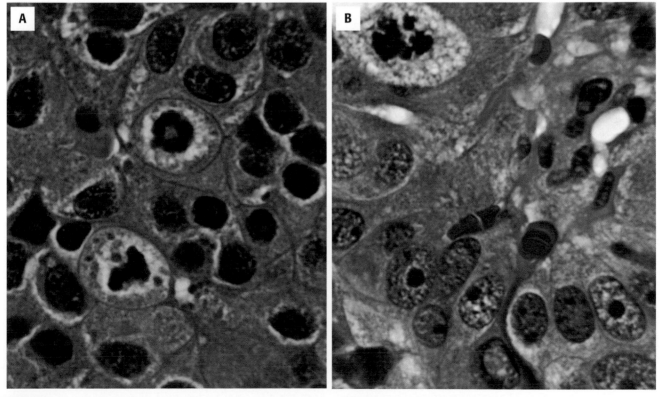

FIGURE 27-16
A, Mitotic figures, including atypical forms, are seen in carcinoma. **B**, Prominent nucleoli and intranuclear cytoplasmic inclusions (*lower field*) are common in carcinoma.

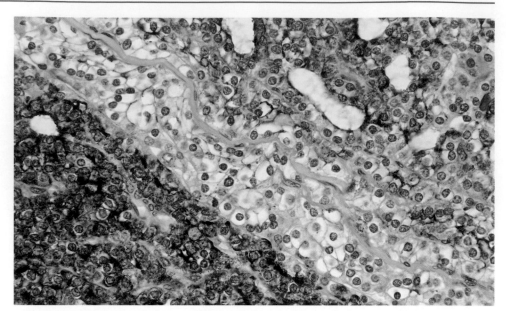

FIGURE 27-17
Variable expression of chromogranin is seen in this carcinoma, with heavy reaction in the lower left, focal reaction in the middle, and intermediate staining in the upper right.

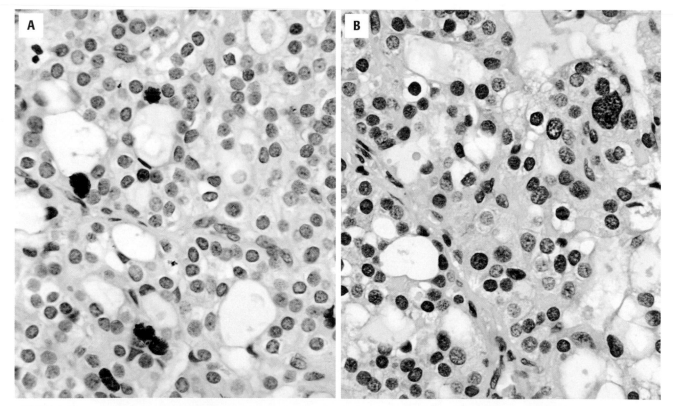

FIGURE 27-18
A, Ki-67 is strongly reactive within the nuclei of a number of cells. **B**, p16 is strongly and diffusely immunoreactive in nearly all of the neoplastic nuclei.

DIFFERENTIAL DIAGNOSIS

The difficulty with the diagnosis of parathyroid carcinoma is the separation of parathyroid adenoma from carcinoma, especially in the setting of previous surgery or with "neck manipulation." Parathyroid carcinoma must be separated from parathyroid adenoma, thyroid conditions, and metastatic neoplasms. The most difficult separation is from parathyroid adenoma. Adenomas are usually smaller, but with increased use of screening laboratory studies, this feature is not as useful in present medical practice. Unfortunately, large adenomas

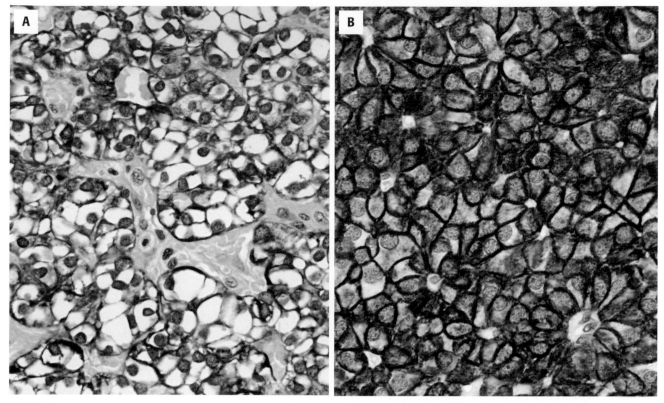

FIGURE 27-19

A, CK7 shows a predominantly membrane reactivity in this clear cell parathyroid carcinoma. **B**, CK18 has both membrane and cytoplasmic reactivity, with accentuation of the cell membranes.

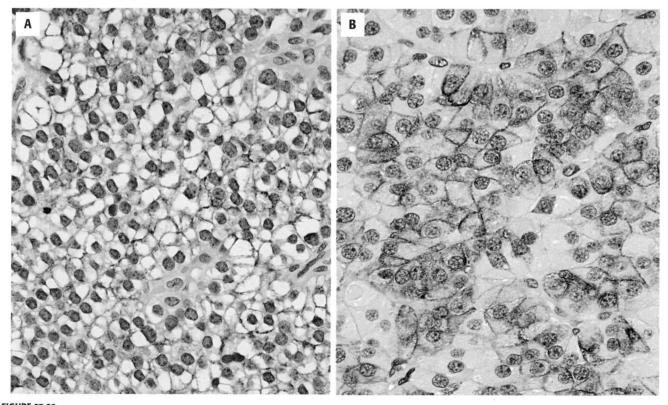

FIGURE 27-20

Renal cell marker reacts along the membranes of parathyroid carcinoma cells in some cases (**A**), while also yielding a positive reaction in the cytoplasm of other cases (**B**).

TABLE 27-1

Genes Associated With Syndromic and Sporadic Parathyroid Neoplasms

Gene	Location	Protein Encoded	Syndrome-Associated Parathyroid Disease	Sporadic Parathyroid Disease
MEN1	11q13	Menin	MEN1, typical adenomas	Inactivating mutation in up to 35% of adenomas
HRPT2	1q25-q31	Parafibromin	Hyperparathyroidism-jaw tumor syndrome	Inactivation in ~70% of carcinomas
			Parathyroid carcinoma in up to 15% of patients	
RET	10q11.2	c-Ret	MEN2a	Very rare
			Parathyroid adenoma in >99%	
CCND1	11q13	Cyclin D1	N/A	Overexpression in adenoma and carcinoma

will frequently display fibrosis, hemosiderin deposits, and cystic degeneration, thereby mimicking carcinoma. Moreover, although a rim of uninvolved parathyroid parenchyma is rarely seen in parathyroid carcinoma, in large adenomas it may be more difficult to detect. When adenoma cells are arranged in acinar or glandular-type structures, eosinophilic material can be seen, a feature uncommon in carcinoma. The cells of an adenoma are enlarged, but do not usually have the increased nuclear:cytoplasmic ratio of a carcinoma; nucleoli are usually small and inconspicuous. Mitotic activity is usually low in adenomas, but mitotic figures alone cannot be used to separate benign from malignant tumors. Adenomas will be positive with parafibromin, p27, bcl-2, and MDM2.

A thyroid follicular neoplasm may be simulated by the "follicular" pattern of growth and by inspissated material within the lumen in parathyroid carcinoma (Figure 27-21). Parathyroid tissue usually has clear cytoplasm and will display very prominent and easy-to-detect cell borders. Intrathyroidal parathyroid tissue often lacks a well-defined capsule and may show pseudoinvasive growth patterns. Immunohistochemistry will also help with separation. Medullary carcinoma

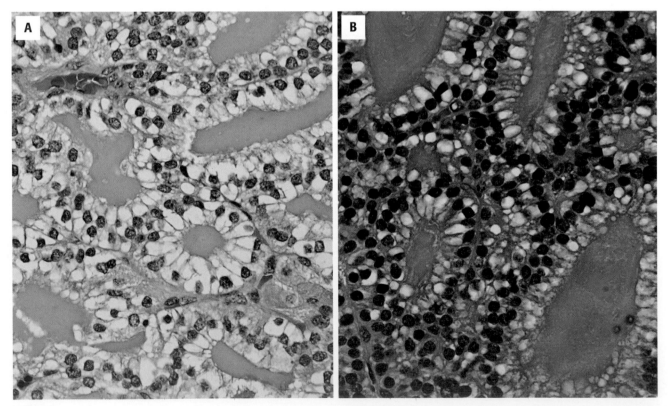

FIGURE 27-21

Parathyroid carcinoma can have inspissated secretions that can mimic a thyroid neoplasm (**A**). The prominent cell borders and clear cytoplasm (**B**) will help with the separation from a thyroid neoplasm.

665

may metastasize or directly invade into parathyroid tissue and will be chromogranin immunoreactive, but will be calcitonin and carcinoembryonic antigen–positive. Metastatic renal cell carcinoma may present as a "clear cell neoplasm" in the parathyroid gland (Figure 27-21). However, the vascular pattern, sinusoidal growth, and immunoreactivity with vimentin, CD10, PAX8, and epithelial membrane antigen without other markers will probably help to make this distinction in the correct clinical context.

As nice as it would be to have a definitive diagnosis in each case, the concept of an intermediate category must be addressed. The term "atypical adenoma" is suggested for a parathyroid neoplasm lacking unequivocal evidence of invasiveness, even though it may be adherent to surrounding tissues, but showing some other feature(s) suspicious for malignancy. These tumors are considered of uncertain malignant potential, requiring close clinical follow-up. The use of parafibromin for these difficult tumors may help limit the use of this noncommittal term. Curiously, these cases, where follow-up is available, show a benign clinical outcome.

PROGNOSIS AND THERAPY

Overall, there is a 5-year survival up to 85% with a 10-year survival of ~50%. Local recurrence can occur in up to 60% of patients, usually within 3 years. Recurrences should be documented by localization studies in a patient with recurrent hypercalcemia, but a prolonged survival can still be expected after palliative surgery. Disruption of the capsule during surgery may cause seeding of parathyroid tissue and give rise to persistent or recurrent HPT, referred to as parathyromatosis. There are possible factors associated with a worse prognosis, including male gender, vascular invasion, and lymph node metastasis. The best outcome for parathyroid carcinoma occurs when there is complete resection at the first surgery. Adjuvant therapy does not play much of a role in management, since it is the management of the metabolic effects of PTH and hypercalcemia which are important. When metastatic disease develops, lung and mediastinum are affected more often than bone and liver. While axiomatic, benign "brown tumors" caused by profound HPT may mimic bone metastases.

■ METASTATIC TUMORS

By definition, tumors that metastasize to or directly invade the parathyroid parenchyma or gland are considered metastatic tumors. Although the glands are vascular, lymphatic spread is uncommon. Abnormal glands

(hyperplasia, adenoma, carcinoma) are more likely to contain metastatic deposits than normal tissue, suggesting there is perhaps an alteration in vascularity, vessel permeability, or blood flow in the abnormal tissue. Lymphomas and leukemias are excluded by definition.

CLINICAL FEATURES

Metastases are uncommon, present in <0.1% of surgically removed parathyroids. The vast majority of patients are asymptomatic, although occasionally a mass in the neck, hoarseness, and pain may be the presenting finding. Multiple glands may be involved. Hypoparathyroidism is exceptionally rare. Women are affected slightly more frequently. Patients tend to be older (7th decade). The most common metastatic primary sites include breast (lobular > ductal carcinoma), melanoma, lung, kidney, and soft tissue primaries. Direct extension from a laryngeal or esophageal squamous cell carcinoma or lymphoma may also be identified.

PATHOLOGIC FEATURES

GROSS FINDINGS

The gland may be slightly enlarged, but metastases are usually not identified at macroscopic examination. Direct extension may result in "attachment" to thyroid, larynx, or esophagus.

METASTATIC TUMORS—DISEASE FACT SHEET

Definition
- Tumors that metastasize to, or directly invade, the parathyroid gland

Incidence and Location
- Unknown due to asymptomatic presentation

Morbidity and Mortality
- Usually poor clinical outcome, although exceptions occur

Gender, Race, and Age Distribution
- Women slightly more commonly
- Tend to be older age at initial presentation

Clinical Features
- Vast majority of patients are asymptomatic

Prognosis and Therapy
- Usually poor and determined by the underlying primary

METASTATIC TUMORS—PATHOLOGIC FEATURES

Gross Findings

- Direct extension may have "attached" thyroid, larynx, or esophagus
- Metastases may be multinodular

Microscopic Findings

- Features of primary tumor are usually maintained
- Lymphomas and squamous cell carcinomas are easy to distinguish from primary lesions

Pathologic Differential Diagnosis

- Clear cell neoplasms including follicular or medullary thyroid tumors and metastatic renal cell carcinoma

MICROSCOPIC FINDINGS

The lymphatic or vascular location of tumor emboli will help to separate a primary lesion from metastatic disease. The histologic features of the primary site are usually maintained in the metastatic focus (Figures 27-22 and 27-23). When there is direct extension (Figure 27-24), the tumor is usually large, and the parathyroid gland involvement is incidental. Separation from thyroid gland (follicular or medullary) primary clear cell tumors and metastatic renal cell carcinoma may occasionally warrant the use of immunohistochemical studies to achieve the correct diagnosis.

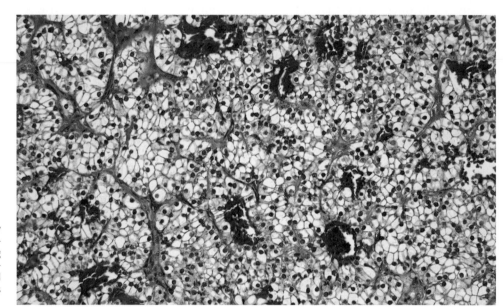

FIGURE 27-22

Parathyroid carcinoma may occasionally have a sinusoidal pattern of growth, including prominent cell borders, making separation from metastatic renal cell carcinoma a challenge. This metastatic renal cell carcinoma has prominent cell borders and a pseudoglandular pattern.

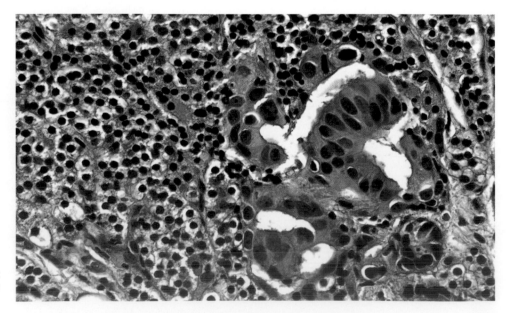

FIGURE 27-23

A neoplastic gland from a metastatic breast carcinoma is noted within the background parathyroid parenchyma.

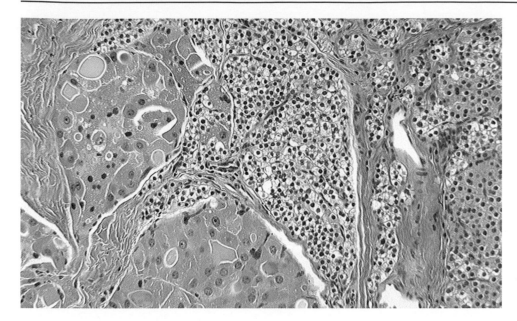

FIGURE 27-24
Metastatic thyroid follicular carcinoma creates nodules of oncocytic epithelium within a cellular parathyroid gland. Immunohistochemistry may be required to confirm the diagnosis.

PROGNOSIS AND THERAPY

The prognosis is usually guarded, with the nature of the underlying primary determining the overall outcome. In light of the metastatic nature of the disorder at time of presentation, the management is symptomatic or palliative, with surgery usually employed to remove the tumor and obtain a histologic diagnosis.

SUGGESTED READINGS

The complete suggested readings list is available online at www.expertconsult.com.

28

Diseases of the Paraganglia System

■ Jennifer L. Hunt

■ PARAGANGLIOMA

Extra-adrenal paragangliomas arise from paraganglia distributed along the paravertebral sympathetic and parasympathetic chains and include tumors arising in the carotid body, jugulotympanic body, orbit, nasopharynx, larynx, vagal body, paraspinal chain (aortico-sympathetic and visceral-autonomic), urinary bladder, and the organ of Zuckerkandl. While the most common site of paraganglioma is within the adrenal gland (referred to as pheochromocytoma), this discussion will be limited to head and neck sites.

The pathogenesis of paraganglioma is not entirely understood. The best-studied tumor is the carotid body tumor, which is derived from the oxygen-sensing chemoreceptive organ at the bifurcation of the carotid artery. In people who live at high altitudes, this organ can become hyperplastic, presumably secondary to chronic hypoxia. The oxygen-sensing activity in the carotid body led investigators to identify germline mutations associated with hereditary paragangliomatosis. These mutations are located in genes (*PLG1* to *PLG4*) encoding the various subunits of the succinate-ubiquinone oxidoreductase gene (*SDH*), which is an enzyme in the mitochondrial respiratory chain complex II. These genes include *SDHD* (on 11q23), *SDHC* (on 1q21), *SDHB* (on 1p36), and several newly identified rare mutations. Interestingly, point mutations and/or deletion mutations in these genes can also be identified in up to 20 % of patients with presumed spontaneous paragangliomas. Newly identified immunohistochemical markers for several of the SDH subunits have been used to identify hereditary tumors. There are also known associations with *VHL*, *NF1*, and *RET* genes.

PARAGANGLIOMA—DISEASE FACT SHEET

Definition
- Tumors arising from the paraganglia along the parasympathetic or sympathetic nerves

Incidence and Location
- Rare (incidence estimate of 0.2 to 1/100,000 population)
- Carotid body, vagal body, middle ear (jugulotympanic), organ of Zuckerkandl, aorticopulmonary, larynx

Morbidity and Mortality
- Infiltrative growth and local recurrence can lead to death
- <10% are malignant

Gender and Age Distribution
- Females >> males (especially at high altitude for carotid body tumors)
- 5th to 6th decades

Clinical Features
- Slowly growing, painless mass
- Ear lesions may produce tinnitus, hearing loss, and nerve dysfunction
- Occasionally may be a pulsatile lesion
- Abdominal cavity lesions may produce headache, perspiration, palpitation, pallor, and hypertension secondary to hypersecretion
- About 10% are bilateral, multiple, familial, pediatric, and malignant

Radiographic Findings
- Computed tomography shows enhancing mass in characteristic location
- Hyperintense T2-weighted magnetic resonance imaging
- Angiography shows splaying of the internal and external carotid arteries with a tumor blush
- 123I-MIBG localizes tumor(s)

Prognosis and Treatment
- Good prognosis if completely resected, although may be indolent and recur/metastasize years later
- Surgery with preoperative adrenergic blockage and/or embolization

CLINICAL FEATURES

Because normal paraganglia are located throughout the body, paragangliomas have been described in nearly every anatomic location. The head and neck are the most common locations for extra-adrenal paragangliomas, accounting for up to 70 % of tumors. The most common subsites are the carotid body, the middle ear (glomus tympanicum or glomus jugulare), and around the vagus nerve (glomus vagale). In the head and neck, normal paraganglia are associated with the parasympathetic nervous system and are adjacent to cranial nerves or the arterial vasculature. It must be stressed that cervical or thoracic sympathetic paragangliomas are separated from parasympathetic paragangliomas arising in nearby locations. Cervical sympathetic paragangliomas are separate from the carotid body and other structures and are vanishingly rare.

Most patients with head and neck paragangliomas are in the 5th to 6th decades with females affected more often than males (5:1), although males are affected more often with inherited or familial tumors. Patients present with a slowly growing, painless mass and may have related symptoms, most commonly tinnitus, hearing loss, or cranial nerve dysfunction depending on the location of the tumor. Only rare head and neck paragangliomas are biochemically active (up to 4%). In superficial locations, paragangliomas are often described clinically as a pulsatile mass. In the middle ear, for instance, otic examination may demonstrate a pulsatile, reddish-purple mass behind the tympanic membrane. About 10% of tumors are bilateral, multiple, familial, pediatric, and malignant, respectively.

In the abdomen (nonadrenal), the neoplasms are most often associated with the sympathetic nervous system. Tumors in the abdomen are more often functional and the secretion of catecholamines can produce clinical symptoms, such as headache, perspiration, palpitations, pallor, and hypertension. The majority of abdominal, extra-adrenal, sympathetic paragangliomas arise from the organ of Zuckerkandl (at the aortic bifurcation or origin of inferior mesenteric artery). These may be discovered incidentally when radiologic surveys are performed for other reasons. Abdominal paragangliomas can also be associated with hereditary paragangliomatosis. Tumors arising in patients with a genetic

syndrome are more likely to be multiple and bilateral (Table 28-1). Pheochromocytomas, a term reserved for paragangliomas of the adrenal gland proper, are more commonly syndrome associated.

RADIOLOGIC FEATURES

The most common studies used to assess paragangliomas are angiography, computed tomography (CT), magnetic resonance imaging (MRI), and ^{131}I-meta-iodobenzylguanidine (MIBG) scans. These studies usually accurately define location, size, and extent of the tumor. Contrast-enhanced CT scans will demonstrate an enhancing mass in characteristic locations and are better for detailing fine osseous changes (Figure 28-1). Contrast-enhanced MRI is also characteristic, showing a hyperintense T2-weighted image. Due to their vascularity, paragangliomas have a characteristic "salt-and-pepper" pattern on MR caused by high-velocity flow voids (black dots) and foci of hemorrhage or slow flow (white dots).

Angiography is often used for patients who are undergoing operative resection and this type of imaging will demonstrate the characteristic pronounced tumor vascularity. In carotid body paragangliomas, the tumor will splay the internal and external carotid arteries, which is a diagnostic feature of paraganglioma (Figure 28-1). In some cases, ultrasound may be helpful in localizing superficial paragangliomas. ^{123}I-MIBG scans have been reported to aid in localization of paragangliomas, especially in occult or familial settings. ^{111}In octreotide (a somatostatin analog) may also be sensitive for tumors >1.5 cm. Positron emission tomography (PET) using

TABLE 28-1

Genetic Syndromes Associated with Paraganglioma and Pheochromocytoma

Syndrome	Gene Locus	Gene	Paraganglia Tumor	Other Abnormalities
von Hippel-Lindau	3p26	VHL	Pheochromocytoma in 10%-20%	Renal cysts and renal cell carcinoma Visceral organ cysts Hemangioblastomas
Hereditary paragangliomatosis	11q23 11q13 1q21 1p36	PGL1 PGL2 PGL3 PGL4	Multiple paragangliomas (100%)	
Neurofibromatosis type I (von Recklinghausen disease)	17q11.2	Neurofibromin	Pheochromocytoma in 1%-5%	Neurofibromas Schwannomas Central nervous system gliomas
MEN2A	10q11.2	RET	Pheochromocytoma in 50%-70%	Parathyroid hyperplasia Medullary thyroid carcinoma
MEN2B	10q11.2	RET	Pheochromocytoma in 50%-70%	Medullary thyroid carcinoma Mucosal neuromas Skeletal abnormalities

Hemorrhage may be present in these tumors, but frank necrosis is not a common feature. In embolized tumors, there may also be an infarct, as well as foreign material within the vascular channels (Figure 28-4).

The cytomorphology of paraganglioma tumor cells varies. The main cell type is the chief cell (type I cells, chemoreceptive cells). These cells are neuroectodermal in origin (Figure 28-5). The cytoplasm can vary from a finely granular eosinophilic to deeply basophilic appearance; occasionally, clear cytoplasm may be seen (Figure 28-6). Similarly, the nuclei vary from small, round, and inconspicuous to large and vesicular with random, bizarre pleomorphism. Mitoses are sparse and they should not be atypical.

A characteristic feature in paragangliomas is the supporting network of stromal cells and vessels that surround

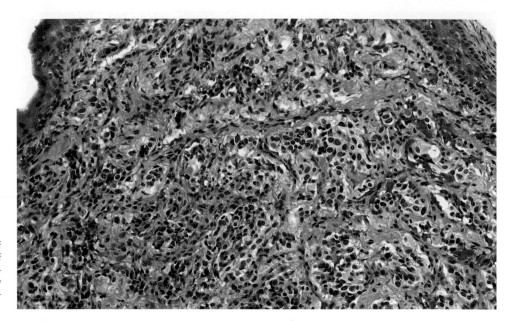

FIGURE 28-5

A squamous epithelium overlies nests of paraganglia cells in this paraganglioma of the middle ear. The zellballen and neuroendocrine nature of the tumor is easily identified in this example. There is a fibrovascular stroma.

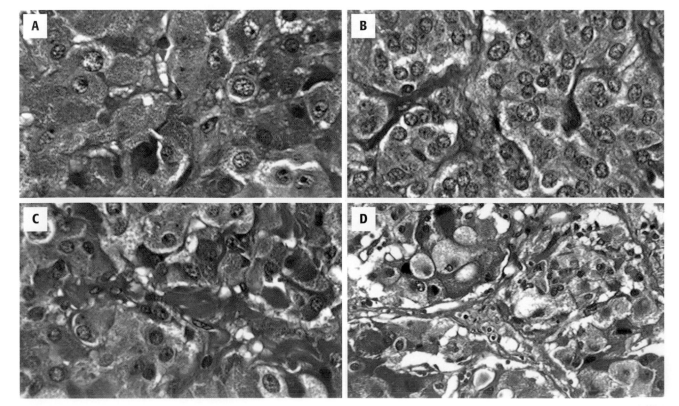

FIGURE 28-6

The various cytomorphologic features include basophilic cytoplasm (**A**), a syncytial architecture (**B**), granular cytoplasm with fibrosis (**C**), and focal clearing in cells that are moderately pleomorphic (**D**).

the nests of neoplastic cells. These surrounding cells are called "sustentacular" (supporting) cells, also referred to as type II cells. They are histologically and ultrastructurally nondistinct but are highlighted with S100 protein immunohistochemistry, while also highlighted with glial fibrillary acidic protein (GFAP) in some cases.

Middle ear and laryngeal paragangliomas deserve special mention, as the histologic features can be difficult to identify in these locations. Because of the fragmentation of jugulotympanic paragangliomas and the fact that they tend to have smaller nests and higher vascularity (Figure 28-7), they can be mistaken for other middle ear tumors (neuroendocrine adenoma of the middle ear/middle ear adenoma). Laryngeal paragangliomas are extremely rare and must be differentiated from other neuroendocrine tumors of the larynx (atypical carcinoid and neuroendocrine carcinoma). Occasionally, paragangliomas can have pigment, which is thought to be neuromelanin, or they

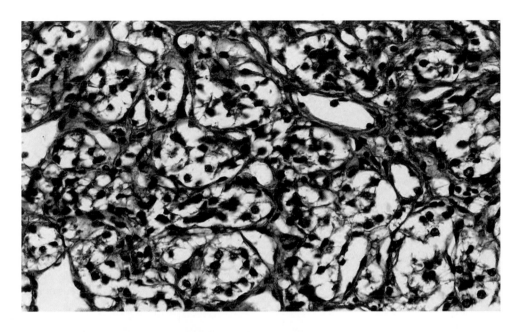

FIGURE 28-7
A jugulotympanic paraganglioma showing small nests and high vascularity.

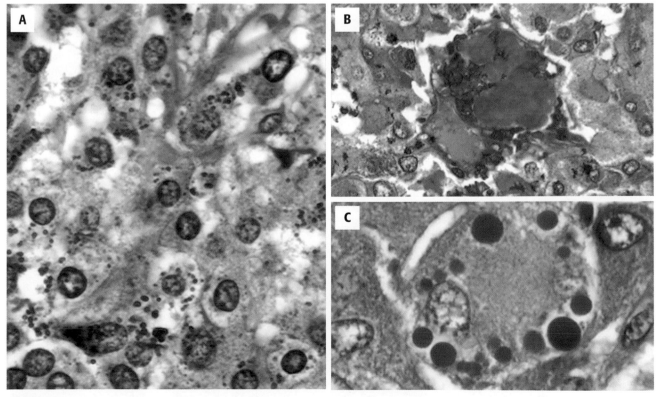

FIGURE 28-8
A, Melanin pigment may be found in paraganglioma. **B**, Amyloid deposition in a paraganglioma. **C**, Eosinophilic cytoplasmic globules in a paraganglioma.

can contain amyloid (Figure 28-8). While these features do not alter the prognosis, they may be a pitfall for correct diagnosis.

ANCILLARY STUDIES

ULTRASTRUCTURAL FEATURES

Electron microscopy is not used often but shows the characteristic dense-core neurosecretory granules of neuroendocrine cells. The granules can vary in number and size, often correlating with the secretory characteristics.

IMMUNOHISTOCHEMICAL FEATURES

The "nonchromaffin" cells of paragangliomas will invariably stain for neuroendocrine immunohistochemical markers, including chromogranin, synaptophysin, neuron-specific enolase (NSE), CD56, leu-7, S100 protein, and a variety of specialized neuropeptides in a smaller subset of tumors (i.e., somatostatin, substance P, adrenocorticotropic hormone, and calcitonin). The supporting sustentacular cells have a unique staining pattern in that they are uniformly S100 protein positive, highlighting the periphery of the tumor (Figure 28-9). GFAP also highlights the sustentacular cells in a number of cases.

FINE NEEDLE ASPIRATION

Fine needle aspiration (FNA) of paraganglioma is generally not recommended as it may result in significant hemorrhage or potentially a vasovagal reaction. Furthermore, manipulation of a functional tumor can induce a hypertensive crisis. Nonetheless, aspiration specimens in unsuspected cases show moderate cellularity, composed of single cells or small groups arranged in a "pseudorosette" pattern (Figure 28-10). The cells are small to medium-sized and polygonal with wispy, pale cytoplasm and variably sized and shaped nuclei. Binucleated, multinucleated, or giant cells may be seen.

DIFFERENTIAL DIAGNOSIS

The differential diagnosis for paraganglioma depends on the location of the tumor.

JUGULOTYMPANIC PARAGANGLIOMA

Paraganglioma may be difficult to separate from other tumors when biopsy samples are small and possibly crushed. The differential diagnosis includes neuroendocrine adenoma of the middle ear, ceruminous adenoma,

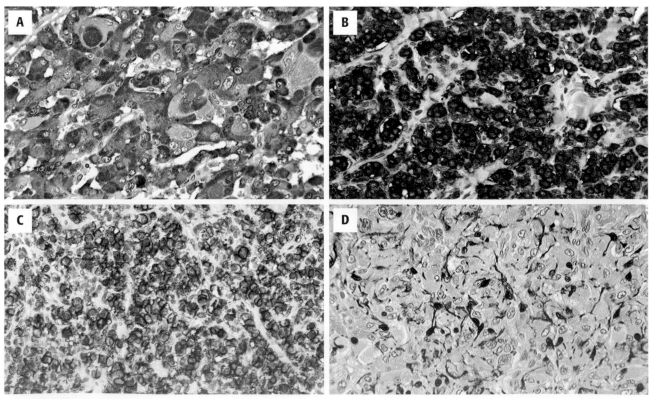

FIGURE 28-9

The paraganglia cells will be positive with chromogranin (**A**), synaptophysin (**B**), and CD56 (**C**); S100 protein highlights the sustentacular cells (**D**).

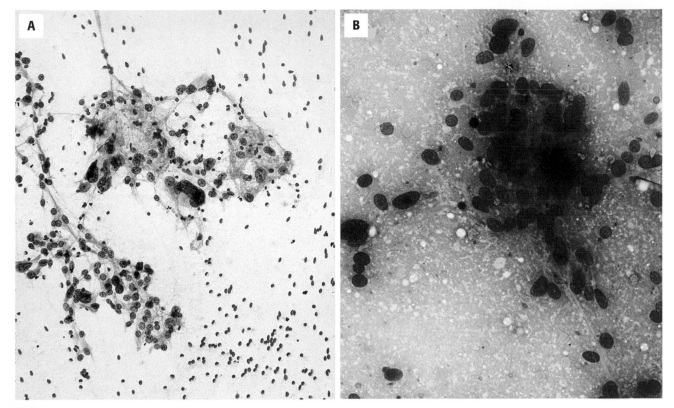

FIGURE 28-10

A, A Papanicolaou-stained, alcohol-fixed smear of a paraganglioma showing a small "rosette" of cells with variable, hyperchromatic nuclei. Focal spindling is noted. **B,** An air-dried, Diff-Quik–stained smear shows a pseudorosette with cells having moderate pleomorphism and wispy cytoplasm.

meningioma, schwannoma, or metastasis, such as metastatic renal cell carcinoma. Morphologic overlap can usually be resolved through use of a pertinent panel of immunohistochemistry studies (Table 28-2). Paraganglioma is negative for keratin and epithelial membrane antigen, which can help separate a number of these tumors.

small cell neuroendocrine carcinomas, as well as other neuroendocrine tumors that can secondarily involve the larynx, such as medullary thyroid carcinoma, or metastases. However, different patterns of growth, increased nuclear pleomorphism, necrosis, increased mitoses, and a carefully selected immunohistochemical panel will help in this differential.

LARYNGEAL PARAGANGLIOMA

Laryngeal paraganglioma is very uncommon. The differential includes carcinoid, atypical carcinoid, and

VAGAL AND CAROTID BODY TUMORS

In this location, paraganglioma must be differentiated from other neuroendocrine tumors, including medullary

TABLE 28-2

Immunohistochemical Separation of Ear Tumors

Stain	Paraganglioma	Neuroendocrine Adenoma of the Middle Ear	Meningioma	Metastatic Renal Cell Carcinoma
Chromogranin	+	+	−	−
Synaptophysin	+	+	−	−
S100 protein	+ (sustentacular)	−	−/+ (rare)	−
Cytokeratin	−	+	−/+ (rare)	+
EMA	−	+	+	+
CD10	Unknown	Unknown	Unknown	+

thyroid carcinoma, hyalinizing trabecular tumor of the thyroid, and neuroendocrine carcinoma. Medullary thyroid carcinoma will be positive for calcitonin, TTF-1, and carcinoembryonic antigen. Hyalinizing trabecular tumor of the thyroid shows distinctive Ki-67 membrane staining. Furthermore, these entities, as well as neuroendocrine carcinomas, will be positive for cytokeratin (Table 28-3), unlike paraganglioma. Clinical and radiographic correlation will also be of use in separating these tumors.

PROGNOSIS AND THERAPY

Paragangliomas are indolent tumors (estimated to have a 7-year doubling time) and generally have a good clinical outcome, particularly in the sporadic setting. However, there are not very well-established histologic criteria for malignancy. Thus, even with histologically benign tumors, lifelong clinical follow-up (including biochemical and/or radiographic studies) is probably essential to monitor for potential recurrence or metastasis. If recurrence or metastasis develops, the overall >90 % 5-year survival will decrease substantially to approximately 60 % 5-year survival.

Surgery is the treatment of choice but must be individualized by taking into consideration the patient's age, medical status, tumor site and size, history of recurrences, and evidence of any cranial nerve deficits. Patients frequently experience stroke or cranial nerve injury as a complication of the surgery (35 %), which has a recurrence rate of ~5 %. Generally, there is preoperative treatment (2 to 3 weeks prior) with alpha and beta blockers to suppress malignant hypertension and/or embolization to avoid excess bleeding. Gamma knife radiation has been used with mixed results, but radiation can be used effectively for poor surgical candidates and older adults.

■ MALIGNANT PARAGANGLIOMA

Malignant paragangliomas are relatively uncommon, although in some studies of extra-adrenal paragangliomas, malignancy rates are as high as 50 %. The pathologist is rarely able to make the diagnosis of malignancy in the primary tumor based on histology alone, as there are no reproducible, reliable, and well-accepted criteria for malignancy. Furthermore, the occurrence of multifocal,

MALIGNANT PARAGANGLIOMA—DISEASE FACT SHEET

Definition
- Malignant tumor arising from the paraganglia along the parasympathetic or sympathetic nerves

Incidence and Location
- Very rare
- Most malignant paragangliomas are abdominal

Morbidity and Mortality
- Protracted clinical course with late recurrences
- Functional tumors have symptomatic recurrences

Gender, Race, and Age Distribution
- Equal gender distribution
- 4th to 5th decades

Clinical Features
- May be larger than benign tumors
- More likely to be functional (catecholamine secretion)

Prognosis and Treatment
- <60% 10-yr survival
- Regional lymph nodes are usual location of metastases
- Recurrences and metastases in up to 50%, often late
- Surgery (debulking), radiation, and radiolabeled analogs showing promise

TABLE 28-3

Immunohistochemical Separation of Neck Neuroendocrine Tumors

Stain	Paraganglioma	Medullary Thyroid Carcinoma	Larynx Neuroendocrine Carcinoma	Metastatic Neuroendocrine Carcinoma
Chromogranin	+	+	+	+
Synaptophysin	+	+	+	+
S100 protein	+ (sustentacular)	−	−	−
Cytokeratin	−	+	+	+
CEA	−	+	+	+
Calcitonin	−	+	+/−	+/−
TTF-1	−	+	−	+/−

multiple, and bilateral tumors, in as many as 10% of cases, can make the determination of metastatic disease a greater challenge. Therefore, malignancy is narrowly defined as the presence of metastatic disease in sites *not normally known* to have chromaffin tissue. The most common sites for diagnosis of true metastatic disease are regional lymph nodes, bone, and lungs. However, despite known metastatic disease, the clinical course is indolent and prolonged in many patients. Functional tumors allow for biochemical monitoring (urine or plasma levels) to identify recurrence.

CLINICAL FEATURES

The clinical parameters of malignant tumors may be indistinguishable from benign tumors, although patients may be slightly younger (mean, 44 years) and without the same gender bias of benign tumors. However, patients are more likely to be symptomatic than patients with benign tumors. Interestingly, patients with inherited syndromes have malignancies *less often* than patients with sporadic disease.

RADIOLOGIC FEATURES

The principle role of radiographic studies is to define the extent of disease and presence of multifocal or metastatic deposits preoperatively to allow for appropriate intervention (Figure 28-11). Metastatic deposits can be FDG-avid, suggesting PET scanning may be useful. ^{123}I-MIBG studies or a labeled dopamine analog tracer may be useful for imaging as well as therapy.

PATHOLOGIC FEATURES

GROSS FINDINGS

Malignant paragangliomas tend to be large, demonstrating areas of confluent necrosis and hemorrhage. Extensive and significant gross capsular and/or vascular invasion may be noted.

MICROSCOPIC FINDINGS

While no features are absolute, a few histologic features correlate with metastatic potential: extensive capsular or

---

MALIGNANT PARAGANGLIOMA—PATHOLOGIC FEATURES

Gross Findings
- Usually larger tumors with hemorrhage and necrosis

Microscopic Findings
- Widely invasive lesions (capsule, vessels, into surrounding parenchyma/soft tissue)
- Confluent necrosis
- Large nests or diffuse growth
- Profound pleomorphism
- Increased mitotic figures and atypical forms

Immunohistochemical Features
- *Decreased* S100 protein–positive sustentacular cells suggests malignancy
- *Increased* Ki-67 labeling index suggests malignancy

Pathologic Differential Diagnosis
- Benign paraganglioma, atypical carcinoid, neuroendocrine carcinoma, medullary thyroid carcinoma

---

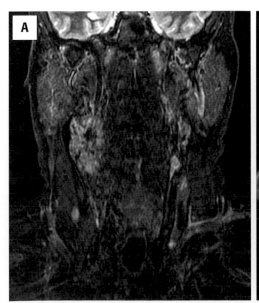
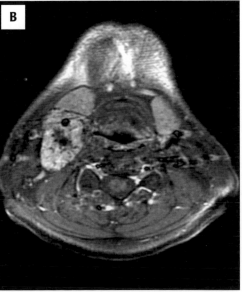

FIGURE 28-11

A malignant paraganglioma with known metastases to the lymph nodes. Note the bright signal on magnetic resonance imaging without contrast (**A**). The T1-WI post contrast image shows a much brighter signal, with flow voids (**B**).

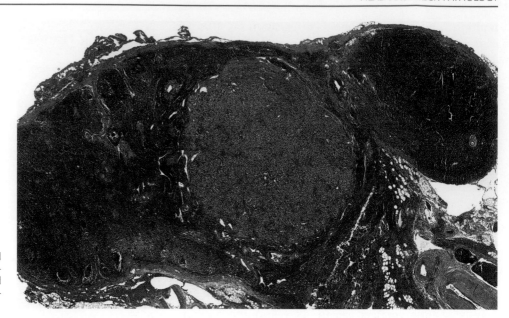

FIGURE 28-12

There is a tumor deposit within a cervical lymph node. Note the well-defined zellballen architecture and relatively bland cytology, underscoring that definitive features of malignancy are usually absent.

vascular invasion, confluent necrosis, increased cellularity, large nests or diffuse growth, profound pleomorphism, increased mitoses (>3/10 high-power fields), and atypical mitotic figures. Otherwise, the histologic features are identical to those of a benign paraganglioma. Metastases are generally to the regional lymph nodes (70 %), a figure that is even higher in carotid body tumors (>92 %) (Figure 28-12).

ANCILLARY STUDIES

There are no currently available histochemical, immunohistochemical, ploidy, or molecular/genetic markers that accurately predict a malignant paraganglioma. However, malignancy is suggested when there is a *loss* of S100 protein–positive sustentacular cells, correlating with a diffuse growth or large nest pattern, and if there is an increased proliferation index (Ki-67). While the level is not absolute, a mitotic index >5 % to 8 % suggests malignancy.

DIFFERENTIAL DIAGNOSIS

Separation between benign and malignant paraganglioma causes the most difficulty and may be impossible to accurately diagnose. Paragangliomatosis may sometimes be mistaken for metastatic tumor. Malignant paraganglioma may mimic other neuroendocrine tumors, such as medullary thyroid carcinoma, but these are easily resolved using immunohistochemistry, as previously discussed (also see Table 28-3).

PROGNOSIS AND THERAPY

Malignant paragangliomas are indolent, but progressive, resulting in <50 % 10-year overall survival. When metastasis develops, the most common sites are lymph node, bone, liver, and lung. Surgery, especially debulking procedures, is the treatment of choice for metastatic disease, with symptomatic management of the excess catecholamines (alpha and beta blockade). Radiation may slow disease progression. Radiolabeled analogs (including tyrosine kinase inhibitors) may be used in functional tumors, but chemotherapy and radiation do not seem to impact survival. Ultimately, without accepted histologic criteria for malignancy in the primary tumors, all patients with paraganglioma need lifelong clinical follow-up to monitor for evidence of metastatic or recurrent disease.

SUGGESTED READINGS

The complete suggested readings list is available online at www.expertconsult.com.

Index

Note: Page numbers followed by f indicate figures; t, tables; b, boxes.